SPEECH MOTOR CONTROL IN NORMAL AND DISORDERED SPEECH

SPEECH MOTOR CONTROL IN NORMAL AND DISORDERED SPEECH

Edited by

Ben Maassen

Radboud University Nijmegen Medical Center, The Netherlands

Ray D. Kent

Waisman Center, University of Winsconsin-Madison, USA

Herman F. M. Peters

Radboud University Nijmegen Medical Center, The Netherlands

Pascal H. H. M. van Lieshout

Oral Dynamics Lab, Graduate Department of Speech-Language Pathology, University of Toronto, Canada

Wouter Hulstijn

Nijmegen Institute for Cognition and Information, Radboud University Nijmegen, The Netherlands

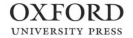

OXFORD

UNIVERSITY PRESS

OXFORD
UNIVERSITY PRESS

Great Clarendon Street, Oxford OX2 6DP

Oxford University Press is a department of the University of Oxford.
It furthers the University's objective of excellence in research, scholarship,
and education by publishing worldwide in

Oxford   New York
Auckland   Bangkok   Buenos Aires   Cape Town   Chennai
Dar es Salaam   Delhi   Hong Kong   Istanbul   Karachi   Kolkata
Kuala Lumpur   Madrid   Melbourne   Mexico City   Mumbai   Nairobi
São Paulo   Shanghai   Taipei   Tokyo   Toronto

Oxford is a registered trade mark of Oxford University Press
in the UK and in certain other countries

Published in the United States
by Oxford University Press Inc., New York

A catalogue record for this title is available from the British Library

ISBN 0 19 8526261 (Hbk)

10 9 8 7 6 5 4 3 2 1

Typeset by EXPO Holdings, Malaysia
Printed in Great Britain
on acid-free paper by
Biddles Ltd, King's Lynn

PREFACE

The purpose of this volume is to present recent theoretical developments in the area of speech motor control and to offer a state of the art review of research devoted to the understanding of the nature of speech disorders. Progress in studies on speech motor control in normal and disordered speech was boosted in the late 1970s and early 1980s by models on motor planning that were inspired by hierarchical computational designs, implemented in the emerging computer technology of those days. This can perhaps best be illustrated in the field of stuttering research. In those early days, the psychosomatic (psychology and learning theory) approach to explain stuttering was reaching an impasse. Influenced by the theoretical and practical developments of studies in motor control, the focus then shifted to speech motor processes in stuttering, especially with respect to the execution stages. In the past two decades, time has witnessed three important developments. First, it became apparent that speech motor execution alone could not explain the complex symptoms as found in stuttering. Higher order psycholinguistic and motor planning processes proved to be relevant as well. Second, historical boundaries between the fields of stuttering and other motor speech disorders no longer appeared valid and were crossed from both sides. To date, we witness a situation in which theories about underlying deficits in stuttering and other motor speech disorders show overlap in all aspects: motor planning, motor execution, and in the role of feedback. Third, a rapid growth of experimental approaches and techniques has taken place, due to developments in information technology, tools for acoustic and kinematic measurements, brain imaging techniques, and methods for psycholinguistic experimentation and developmental modelling.

The basis for this volume was laid at the International Conference on Speech Motor Control, which was held in Nijmegen, June 13-16, 2001. This conference was the fourth in a series that started in 1985; a series of international speech motor conferences that clearly reflected the course of research sketched above. In 1985, the focus was on initial applications of the just expanding field of motor control in stuttering. The second conference (1990) highlighted the development of more general motor control models and the inclusion of higher order psychomotor and psycholinguistic functions, and broadened the scope to normal speech motor control and to other motor speech disorders than stuttering. At the third conference (1996), emphasis was put on the upcoming field of brain imaging, and on fine-tuning existing models of speech production. In addition, the development of speech motor control became a prominent topic. At the last conference (2001), we witnessed the introduction of neurophysiological and neurobehavioral concepts, and a strong growing interest in higher order cognitive and psycholinguistic processes, including the 'interface' between motor and linguistic stages of speech production. Still, the core orientation of this conference remained a speech motor one, if only because our observations and measurements very much depend on the end products of the production process: speech movements and the resulting acoustic consequences.

At the moment time seems ripe to publish a book that summarizes the tremendous progress that has been made in modelling the facilitation and control of speech movements and understanding the underlying processes, neurological correlates, and pathological conditions. Presenters of the highlights of the last conference were invited to write a chapter for this book. The result is the present volume, that exposes recent progress in the field of speech motor control, discusses the major methodological concerns, and looks into the future at the challenges lying ahead of us. The volume is divided into five sections: models of speech motor control; neural processes; speech motor development; the interface between motor, linguistic, and cognitive processes; and disorders of speech motor control. Following is a brief characterization of the individual chapters in each section.

The intriguing common denominator of Part 1, on models of speech production, is the focus on neurobehavioral modelling. It is clear that motor control models based on behavioral studies on the one hand and neural network models on the other are moving towards each other, in correspondence with the natural link that exists between behavior and neural processes.

In the first Chapter on the implications from recent developments in neurophysiological and neurobehavioral science, Kent argues against a peripheral notion of motor control. Motor behavior is invested with cognitive influences. Further, these influences offer important insights into motor performance and learning, neural mechanisms of motor control, treatment of motor impairments in neurological patients, and the development of motor abilities in children. The author applies the same line of thinking to speech, including its disorders and development. Accordingly, theories of the neural (motor) control of speech should take cognitive factors into account. Kent reviews several studies to support this claim. For instance, it has been shown in monkeys that neurons in motor cortex, the now famous mirror neurons, discharge *either* when the monkey *performs* an action or when it *observes* the experimenter performing the action, suggesting that the motor system is responsible not only for executing actions but also for their internal representation.

In the second Chapter, Guenther and Perkell present a detailed neural network model of speech production. Auditory feedback plays an important role in their model, and studies of its role in the planning of speech movements are reviewed. The model consists of three kinds of information transformations or mappings. The first mapping provides for each phoneme the auditory (and orosensory) targets. It is phoneme (or language) specific. The other two mappings are systemic (or speaker-specific). The second one transforms auditory and orosensory targets in articulator movements. The third mapping, or 'forward model', is necessary for the control of fast speech movements when the processing of auditory feedback would take too much time. These mappings are acquired with the use of auditory feedback and rely on auditory feedback for their maintenance over the course of a lifetime. The authors provide a description of the model and its neural correlates, and further present experimental evidence in support of their model which suggests that, once learned, the neural mappings are stable, even in the absence of hearing.

In the third Chapter, van Lieshout presents a condensed review of the Dynamical Systems Theory (DST) as applied to speech. The chapter provides an introduction to the main concepts of DST. It briefly sketches the history of DST, its current status, and its relation with the well-known Task Dynamics model. In DST, the central tenet is to relate the existence and maintenance of complex patterns in living systems to principles of self-organization, similar to what is found in non-living systems. The author also discusses 'Chaos in speech' and he ends with setting out lines for the future of DST's application to speech and speech disorders. He concludes that DST has powerful concepts and tools to offer research in speech motor control, and that it provides a refreshing new view on notions of stability, flexibility, and variability in motor control, and their relationship between brain and behavior. Some examples of his own research are provided to illustrate these notions.

Part 2, on brain imaging and neurological diseases, focuses more directly on the neural aspects of speech. In Chapter 4, Ackermann, Riecker, and Wildgruber present a review of imaging techniques, and a series of PET and fMRI studies from their own lab looking at functional aspects of speech motor control at the central nervous system level. The findings suggest that automated overt speech yields bilateral activation of the sensory motor cortex (SMC) and cerebellar hemispheres in association with the left anterior insula. By contrast, silent production of the same test materials (auditory verbal imagery, inner speech) results in a more limited response pattern encompassing left SMC and right cerebellum, but excluding intrasylvian cortex. Series of studies are presented contrasting activation patterns not only for overt speech as compared to silent speech, but also for speech and singing, and for dysartric as compared to normal speech. These and other findings are discussed in a larger framework of neural control of speech production.

Chapter 5, by De Nil, is a review of neuro-imaging studies in the field of stuttering. The overall picture suggests that differences in activation levels in brain regions of interest between stuttering and nonstuttering speakers not only involve areas associated with motor planning and execution, but also include regions important for the processing of sensory feedback. The author suggests that the observation of increased recruitment of both cortical and sub-cortical areas during non-manipulated speech in stuttering adults may suggest a less automatized form of motor control compared to nonstuttering individuals. The author concludes that the availability of functional imaging tools has provided new opportunities to study the neural processes underlying stuttering, which despite current limitations of the technique have already indicated potential relationships between brain processes and speech disfluencies.

In Chapter 6, Murdoch presents a review on what is known about the role of subcortical structures in speech motor control. The author discusses potential reasons for discrepancies in the treatment success of limb and speech control problems in diseases with subcortical involvement. For example, the often reported observation that speech motor function benefits less from surgical or medical treatment (e.g. in Parkinson's disease) may relate to the fact that it is not under predominant dopaminergic control. To provide more insight into the complex functions of subcortical structures in speech motor control, the author argues in favor of a combined approach of stereotactic neurosurgical procedures and deep brain stimulation with functional neuroimaging techniques.

Part 3 approaches speech motor development from various perspectives. In Chapter 7, Locke takes us back in phylogenetic history, looking for the "antecedent activities of the vocal tract", in order better to comprehend the processes by which infants first appropriate these systems for the new purpose of linguistic sound making. Core concepts are displacement and emancipation, processes by which pre-existing movements, that is, actions that are linked in evolution and development to an "original" function, become available for other uses. It is argued that the means of shifting from prelexical sound making to speech was worked out evolutionarily, leaving the human infant with an endowment adequate to the task. In the Chapter the nature of this endowment and its mode of activation are further explored in relation to work on phonological universals.

In Chapter 8, Moore takes a dynamic systems perspective to the study of early physiologic development of respiratory, phonatory, and articulatory systems, the motor infrastructure upon which developing speech is built. The dynamic systems perspective is primarily interested in the search for developmental periods of marked stability demarcated by intervals of marked instability. By means of time series analyses on physiologic signals, instabilities are demonstrated while comparing, among others, mastication and babbling, rest breathing and speech breathing, and the increasing contribution of lip activity relative to jaw activity during lip closure gestures. Moore concludes that the hypothesis that infants capitalize on an existing coordinative organization to generate new behaviors (e.g. adapting the motor organization of chewing and sucking to babbling) is not supported by these physiologic findings.

Chapter 9, by Barlow, Finan and So-Young Park, delves even deeper into the biological mechanisms underlying motor patterns, taking the perspective that motor behavior evolves from so-called central pattern generating circuits (CPGs). CPGs are involved in locomotion, respiration, swallowing, mastication, sucking, vocalization; for speech motor development, it is likely that different central pattern generating networks are coordinated with one another with respect to phase and frequency. Barlow *et al.* report on a series of experiments with neonates showing adaptive *entrainment*: the synchronization of an endogenous oscillator to external periodic events. A rudimentary understanding of such pattern-generating circuitry provokes some intriguing options for the dynamic assembly of CPGs from relatively early appearing motor behaviors into the ontogeny of speech production.

Part 4 provides the reader with recent insights into the possible relevance and influence of linguistic processes on speech motor control. In Chapter 10, Smith and Goffman focus on language/motor interactions in an attempt to provide a theoretical account of how various levels of linguistic processing and their units are related to speech motor processes. The central argument proposed by the authors is that there is a much closer link between speech motor processes and linguistic processes than suggested in earlier models of speech. Specifically, based on experimental findings from their lab on movement pattern stability, they argue that there are multiple, parallel units operating in the preparation of command signals for speech production. During development, these mappings between linguistic units and motor output change, suggesting that the late maturation of articulatory motor processes is driven by the interplay between speech motor control and co-developing cognitive/linguistic systems.

Chapter 11, by the authors Conture, Zackheim, Anderson, and Pellowski, provides a theoretical base for a programmatic study of linguistic processes in children who stutter. In this Chapter, the authors take the basic assumption that any theoretical account of stuttering must begin by accounting for the behavior or symptoms of the disorder itself. While the authors acknowledge that stuttering involves changes in speech motor behaviors, they believe that the most common instances of childhood stuttering (e.g. sound/syllable repetitions, sound prolongations, and single-syllable whole-word repetitions) reflect relatively slow and inefficient (when compared to normal) linguistic processing preceding the preparations and execution of speech motor actions. Conture and his colleagues review previous studies and preliminary findings from their own lab to support their claim, and argue that the link between symptoms of childhood stuttering and the linguistic system warrants serious consideration and further empirical study.

Whereas speech motor disorders are addressed by way of example in the previous four sections, Part 5 concentrates on gaining a deeper understanding of speech disorders through insight into underlying speech motor control deficits. The whole spectrum of speech motor disorders is discussed: stuttering, dysarthria, and apraxia of speech. The section starts with a methodological Chapter by Kent and Rosen (Chapter 12) for the assessment of speech motor disorders in general. The authors aim to relate auditory perceptual features with the underlying pathophysiology, such that perceptual assessment is a reliable guide to physiologic abnormality and, perhaps, vice versa. If successful, it would be possible to "hear" the manifestations of hypotonus, weakness, slow movement, and dyscoordination. The emphasis is on disorders of rate, strength and endurance, and coordination. For each of these, the authors argue, there is a clear lack in understanding the relationships between perceptual measures of speech deficiency and physiologic measures of speech motor function. The discussion also addresses other challenging issues like the compensations used by the speaker to overcome the neurologic disorder, and the difficulty to distinguish pathophysiology from changes that typically occur with aging.

In Chapter 13, van Lieshout, Hulstijn, and Peters argue that stuttering can be linked to the speech motor system, but not necessarily in terms of a "speech motor disorder". Rather, the central theme is that for people who stutter, the speech motor control system is the weak link in the chain of events that leads to the production of speech. This link is weak in terms of limited skill or ability to prepare and perform the motor actions that are required for speech. Evidence is provided that the motor system of stutterers tends to be less effective, more variable, and more basic, perhaps even "immature", in handling the complex coordination between individual articulators. The authors introduce the term "speech clumsi-ness", thereby indicating that speech motor skill is not a dichotomy but a contin-uum. Individuals can be traced along the entire continuum, and some stuttering individuals could be fairly close to "normals" in their performance and responses to demands.

In Chapter 14, Max suggests the possibility that the onset and maintenance of stuttering is essentially related to the use of feedback, namely difficulties with the formation or updating of internal models that correspond to neural mappings between central motor commands and the sensory consequences resulting from movements. Speech disfluencies, the core characteristics of stuttering, are consid-ered maladaptive attempts to correct for discrepancies between the anticipated and the actual sensory consequences of the unfolding movements. From this per-spective, speech and nonspeech experiments are reviewed which suggest that stuttering and nonstuttering speakers differ with regard to how much detail about the movement consequences is taken into account during motor planning.

In Chapter 15, McNeil, Pratt, and Fossett raise the provocative point that it is not a lack of theory nor the inability to select the correct theory from the known alter-natives that limits understanding of apraxia of speech (AOS). Neither is it the inability to select the appropriate level of description or contrast with the appro-priate comparison group that limits understanding of AOS. According to the authors, the most important impediment to theoretical and clinical advancement in AOS is the lack of a comprehensive and clear definition of AOS that leads to an agreed-upon set of criteria for subject selection. Based on a review of models of phonological encoding and speech production, the authors argue for the develop-ment of criteria that can distinguish phonemic dysfunctions from those of motor processing, thereby allowing for easier distinction between behaviors attributable to AOS from those characteristic of phonemic paraphasia.

In Chapter 16, Ziegler and Maassen do not take a particular speech disorder as starting point, but discuss the role of the syllable as an organizing structure in spoken language production and understanding, as well as its disorders. Evidence for this comes from different sources: from phonological theory, phonetics, theories of language development, and psycholinguistic studies of speaking and of language comprehension in adults. The chapter reviews results from studies of aphasic patients with phonological encoding problems, patients with apraxia of speech, or with other motor speech problems, and children with developmental speech motor disorders. It is shown that the patterns of breakdown provide additional evidence for the assumption that speaking is heavily based on the rhythmical structure of syllabified language.

As editors of this book, we are very pleased and grateful that we were able to get the commitment of all the authors in this book to provide us not only with a state-of-the-art review on speech motor control in normal and disordered speech, but also to give a glimpse of their views on future developments in these areas. We think that anyone who has a scientific or clinical interest in speech motor control issues will find something of his or her liking in the Chapters that are presented in the various sections. It is our hope that this volume will provide direction in handling complex clinical problems, but modesty urges us to emphasize that our main expectation is to bring forward intriguing research questions and challenges. We further hope that at the next Nijmegen conference on speech motor control, we will witness how the ideas, suggestions, and questions have found solid ground in the various exciting and innovative new studies that will be initiated in the very near future and beyond.

Acknowledgements

The editors of this book would like to acknowledge the generous financial and/or administrative support from the Dutch Royal Academy of Science (KNAW), the National Institute on Deafness and Other Communication Disorders (National Institutes of Health), the Departments of ENT, Medical Psychology, and Paediatric Neurology of the Radboud University Nijmegen Medical Center, and the Nijmegen Institute for Cognition and Information (NICI) in the planning and implementation of the 4th International Conference on Speech Motor Control including the editorial support to publish this book.

Ben Maassen
Pascal van Lieshout
Ray Kent
Herman Peters
Wouter hulstijn   Nijmegen/Toronto/Madison,
                                                      September 2003

CONTENTS

CONTRIBUTORS

Hermann Ackermann
Department of Neurology,
University of Tuebingen,
Hoppe-Seyler-Str. 3,
D-72076 Tuebingen,
Germany

Julie D. Anderson
Department of Speech and Hearing
Sciences,
Indiana University,
200 South Jordan Avenue,
Bloomington, Indiana 47405-7002,
USA

Steven M. Barlow
Department of Speech-Language-
Hearing: Sciences and Disorders
Communication Neuroscience
Laboratories,
University of Kansas,
1000 Sunnyside Avenue,
Lawrence, Kansas 66045-7555,
USA

Edward G. Conture
Department of Speech and Hearing
Sciences,
Vanderbilt University,
1114 19th Avenue South,
Nashville, Tennessee 37212,
USA

Luc F. De Nil
Graduate Department of Speech-
Language Pathology,
Rehabilitation Sciences Building,
Centre for Function and Well-Being,
University of Toronto,
500 University Avenue, 10th Floor,
Toronto, ON M5G 1V7,
Canada

Donald S. Finan
Department of Speech, Language, and
Hearing Sciences,
The Center for Neurosciences,
University of Colorado,
2501 Kittredge Loop Road,
Campus Box 409,
Boulder, Colorado 80309-0409,
USA

Tepanta R. D. Fossett
Department of Communication Science
and Disorders,
4033 Forbes Tower,
University of Pittsburgh,
Pittsburgh, PA 15260,
USA

Lisa Goffman
Audiology & Speech Sciences,
Purdue University Heavilon Hall,
500 Oval Drive, West Lafayette,
Indianapolis 47907-1353,
USA

Frank H. Guenther
Department of Cognitive and Neural
Systems,
Boston University,
677 Beacon Street,
Boston, Massachusetts 02215,
USA

Wouter Hulstijn
Nijmegen Institute for Cognition and
Information,
Radbound University Nijmegen,
P.O. Box 9104,
6500 HE Nijmegen,
The Netherlands

Ray D. Kent
Waisman Center,
University of Wisconsin-Madison,
1500 Highland Avenue,
Madison, Wisconsin 53705–2280,
USA

Pascal H. H. M. van Lieshout
Oral Dynamics Lab
Graduate Dept. of Speech-Language
Pathology, Rehabilitation Sciences
Building,
Centre for Function and Well-Being,
University of Toronto,
500 University Avenue, 10th Floor,
Toronto, ON M5G 1V7
Canada

John Locke
Department of Speech-Language-
Hearing Sciences,
Lehman College,
City University of New York,
250 Bedford Park Blvd. West,
Bronx, New York 10468,
USA

Ben Maassen
Child Neurology Center/ ENT/ Medical
Psychology,
Radboud University Nijmegen Medical
Center,
P.O. Box 9101,
6500 HB Nijmegen,
The Netherlands

Ludo Max
Laboratory for Speech Physiology and
Motor Control, Department of
Communication Sciences,
University of Connecticut,
850 Bolton Road Unit 1085,
Storrs, Connecticut 06269-1085,
USA

Malcolm R. McNeil
Department of Communication Science
and Disorders,
University of Pittsburgh,
4033 Forbes Tower,
Pittsburgh, Pennsylvania 15260,
USA

Christopher A. Moore
Department of Speech and Hearing
Sciences,
University of Washington,
1417 NE 42nd Street,
Seattle, Washington 98105,
USA

Bruce E. Murdoch
Motor Speech Research Unit,
Department of Speech Pathology and
Audiology,
The University of Queensland,
Brisbane, Queensland 4072,
Australia

So-Young Park
Voice-Speech-Swallowing Center,
Otolaryngology/Head & Neck Surgery,
2521 Stockton Blvd.,
Sacramento, California 95817,
USA

Mark W. Pellowski
Department of Communication
Sciences and Disorders,
109E Van Bokkelen Hall,
Towson University,
Towson, Maryland 21252-0001,
USA

Joseph S. Perkell
Speech Communication Group,
Research Laboratory of Electronics,
Massachussetts Institute of Technology,
50 Vassar St.,
Cambridge, Massachussetts 02139-
4307,
USA

Herman F. M. Peters
ENT/Medical Psychology,
Radboud University Nijmegen Medical
Center,
P.O. Box 9101,
6500 HB Nijmegen,
The Netherlands

Sheila R. Pratt
Department of Communication Science
and Disorders,
4033 Forbes Tower,
University of Pittsburgh,
Pittsburgh, Pennsylvania 15260,
USA

Axel Riecker
Department of Neurology and Section
Experimental Magnetic Resonance of
the CNS,
Department of Neuroradiology,
University of Tuebingen,
Hoppe-Seyler-Str. 3,
D-72076 Tuebingen,
Germany

Kristin Rosen
Waisman Center,
University of Wisconsin-Madison,
1500 Highland Avenue,
Madison, Wisconsin 53705-2280,
USA

Anne Smith
Audiology & Speech Sciences,
Purdue University Heavilon Hall,
500 Oval Drive,
West Lafayette, Indianapolis 47907-
1353,
USA

Dirk Wildgruber
Department of Neurology and Section
Experimental Magnetic Resonance of
the CNS,
Department of Neuroradiology,
University of Tuebingen,
Hoppe-Seyler-Str. 3,
D-72076 Tuebingen,
Germany

Courtney T. Zackheim
Department of Hearing and Speech
Sciences,
Vanderbilt University,
1114 19th Avenue South,
Nashville, Tennessee 37212,
USA

Wolfram Ziegler
Clinical Neuropsychology Research
Group,
Department of Neuropsychology,
City Hospital Bogenhausen,
Dachauer Str. 164,
D-80992 München,
Germany

ABBREVIATIONS

ADHD	attention deficit hyperactivity disorder
ALS	amyotrophic lateral sclerosis
AMR	alternating motion rate
AOS	apraxia of speech
AVS	average vowel spacing
BC	bilabial closure
CD	coordination dynamics
CI	cochlear implant
CN	caudate nucleus
CNS	central nervous system
COP	constriction order parameter
CPGs	central pattern generators
CRH	covert repair hypothesis
CWS	children who stutter
DAF	delayed auditory feedback
DAS	developmental apraxia of speech
DCD	developmental coordination disorder
DI	devoicing interval
DST	dynamical systems theory
EEG	electroencephalograph(y)
EGG	electroglottography
EMG	electromyogram
EMMA	electro-magnetic midsagittal articulograph
EPG	electro-palatographic
EPI	echoplanar imaging
ERP	evoked response potential
FAF	frequency altered feedback
FDG	fluorodeoxyglucose
fMRI	functional magnetic resonance imaging
GMP	generalized motor programs
GP	globus pallidus
GPe	external segment of the globus pallidus
GPi	internal segment of the GP
HKB	Haken–Kelso–Bunz model
IEMG	integrated electromyogram
IS	interfering stimulus
lCMRGlc	local cerebral metabolic rates for glucose
LSVT	Lee Silverman Voice Treatment

MEG	magnetoencephalograph(y)
MPTP	1-methyl-4-phenyl-1,2,3,6 tetra-hydropyridine
mRGs	medullary respiratory pattern generators
NIRS	near-infrared spectroscopy
NS	neostriatum
PET	positron emission tomography
PNS	people who do not stutter
PP	phonemic paraphasias
PRC	phrase repetition cycle
PWS	people who stutter
rCBF	regional cerebral blood flow
ROI	region of interest
SAAD	simple active affirmative declarative (structure)
SD	speech delay
SLI	specific language impairment
SMA	supplementary motor area
SMC	sensorimotor cortex
SNPC	substantia nigra pars compacta
SNPR	substantia nigra pars reticulata
SOA	stimulus–onset asynchrony
SPE	sound pattern of English
SPL	sound pressure level
SPM	statistical parametric mapping
STF	slow tonic muscle fibers
STI	spatiotemporal index
STN	subthalamic nucleus
TB	tongue body
TBI	traumatic brain injury
TD	task dynamics
VIM	ventral intermedius
VOT	voice onset time

PART 1

MODELLING OF SPEECH PRODUCTION

CHAPTER 1

MODELS OF SPEECH MOTOR CONTROL: IMPLICATIONS FROM RECENT DEVELOPMENTS IN NEUROPHYSIOLOGICAL AND NEUROBEHAVIORAL SCIENCE

RAY D. KENT

1.1 Introduction

The study of motor control is entering a new phase of integration that carries important implications for the study of communication and its disorders. An intriguing part of this integration is the synthesis of motor control and cognition. Historically, the theoretical understanding of motor control, including the motor control of speech, was dominated by generalized motor programs (GMP), or the idea that movement is guided by a mental representation of some kind (Kent *et al.* 1996). But within the past 25 years, the hegemony of GMP was seriously challenged by the theory of coordination dynamics (or dynamic systems), which, in the minds of many, displaced GMP as the predominant view of motor control. Coordination dynamics offered many advantages, including a formal mathematical structure, an appealing parsimony, and a widespread scientific and clinical application. The proponents of coordination dynamics generally rejected a role of cognition (mental representation) in motor control. Indeed, many of them argued strongly against cognitive participation, which was seen as unnecessary and cumbersome. Recently, coordination dynamics itself has been challenged because of mounting evidence of cognitive influences on motor control. These influences can be seen in behavioral, neurophysiological, clinical, and developmental studies, and a primary goal of this chapter is to review this evidence and to consider implications for the study of speech and its disorders. The crux of the present argument is that cognition exerts strong influences on motor control, and speech, or any motor behavior, is best viewed as a cognitive–motor accomplishment. This perspective holds important implications for the understanding of speech development and speech disorders.

1.2 Behavioral studies of motor control in healthy subjects

In behavioral studies, the evidence for motor–cognitive interactions includes the effects of nonmovement practice (such as observational practice), reversal effects (through feedback and contextual interference), and intention (cognitive mediating strategies such as goal setting, attentional focus, self-control, and instructions). See Wulf et al. (1999) for a cogent review of this evidence, including references to relevant studies. For a discussion of the application of these ideas to one field (sport and exercise), see Holmes and Collins (2001). Only a very brief summary is given here.

Data on these aforementioned phenomena are difficult to reconcile with the standard view of coordination dynamics, which often predicts contradictory outcomes. For example, coordination dynamics does not predict that merely observing a motor act would be beneficial in the subsequent performance of that act, especially because observation does not supply critical information on muscle synergies related to the biodynamics of the effector system in performing a particular task. If evidence is presented that observing a motor act performed by another individual facilitates performance of that act by the observer, this evidence is a challenge to coordination dynamics. In fact, a growing number of studies have established that observing a motor act often is advantageous to the subsequent performance of that act (Wulf et al. 1999; Blandin and Proteau 2000; Heyes and Foster 2002). Similarly, coordination dynamics does not predict that limited or delayed feedback would be more beneficial in motor learning than unrestricted or immediate feedback. For most versions of coordination dynamics, feedback should be readily available to insure both rapid learning and successful retention. But several studies have shown that reduced frequency of feedback or delayed feedback leads to better retention of a new motor skill than does frequent and immediate feedback (Wulf et al. 1999; Anderson et al. 2001). Further, most accounts of coordination dynamics are not compatible with evidence that motor performance is influenced by the cognitive acts of instructions, goal setting, or attentional focus. Coordination dynamics has given little consideration to such cognitive factors. But, again, recent studies have demonstrated that cognitive acts such as goal setting and attentional focus can have important effects on motor performance (Wulf et al. 1999, 2001). In view of empirical results pointing to cognitive influences, some advocates of coordination dynamics have allowed that the theory must accommodate cognition. Recently, Pressing (1999) introduced a new theory, referential dynamics, that embraces aspects of information processing while retaining properties of coordination dynamics.

Is there evidence that the same kinds of effects apply to speech? Adams and Page (2000) reported on a task in which subjects learned a phrase with a specified target duration under different conditions of feedback and practice. The subjects showed better retention: (1) when summary feedback was given after every five trials as opposed to after every trial; (2) for random as opposed to blocked practice; and (3) for multiple as opposed to single tasks. Steinhauer and Grayhack (2000) studied the effects of different rates of feedback (100%, 50%, or no knowledge of results) on a task of novel vowel nasalization. They observed a decrease in motor performance and learning as the relative frequency of feedback was increased, with the worst condition being 100% knowledge of results. A similar study with 18 subjects with Parkinson's disease showed that 2-day retention scores were better for subjects who received summary feedback after five trials than for subjects who received summary feedback after every trial (Adams *et al.* 2002). In a study of severe apraxia of speech, Knock *et al.* (2000) reported that two patients receiving speech treatment showed better retention under random practice compared with blocked practice. Admittedly, there are relatively few relevant studies published at this time, but those that have been reported conform with the conclusions from more general studies of motor control.

1.3 Neurophysiological studies in healthy subjects

The behavioral evidence does not stand alone. Recent investigations of the neurophysiology of movement control point in the same direction of cognitive–motor interactions. Hauert's (1986) assertion that 'motor function is a cognitive function' is gaining support from a variety of neurophysiological studies on both animals and humans. The interaction of cognition and motor control is evident in recent research on neural processes of motor skill acquisition and performance.

1.3.1 Motor cortex functions

It is now recognized that the motor cortex serves both motor and cognitive functions. This cortical area, often considered to be the exclusive province of motor control, is involved in many functions that have a distinctively cognitive flavor, including spatial transformations, serial order coding, stimulus–response incompatibility, motor learning, and motor imagery (Georgopoulos 2000). Moreover, it appears that the motor cortex is highly plastic, with modifications resulting from motor skill learning and cognitive motor actions (Sanes and Donoghue 2000). In short, it appears that the motor cortex should be more appropriately labeled the cognitive–motor cortex.

1.3.2 Basal ganglia and cerebellar functions

Like the motor cortex, the basal ganglia and cerebellum traditionally have been viewed as dedicated largely to motor control. But a newer view is emerging, especially because of research showing that there are cognitive contributions from these structures, and because of research showing connections between these structures and the cerebral cortex (Hikosaka *et al.* 2002). With respect to the basal ganglia, it has been shown that: (1) these structures participate in multiple circuits with cognitive areas of the cerebral cortex; (2) neuronal activity in selected regions of the basal ganglia is related more to cognitive and sensory operations than to motor functions; and (3) certain lesions to the basal ganglia result in cognitive or sensory dysfunctions without gross motor disturbances (Middleton and Strick, 2000). Similarly, many recent articles conclude that the cerebellum participates in cognitive functions (Decety *et al.* 1990; Leiner *et al.* 1991; Bloedel and Bracha 1997; Schmahmann 1997; Rapoport *et al.* 2000). Bloedel and Bracha make the point clearly in stating that a cerebellar role in cognition is not only expected but necessary.

1.3.3 Mirror neurons

It has been known for some time that neurons in the rostral part of monkey inferior area 6 (area F5) discharge during active movements of the hand, mouth, or both (Kurata and Tanji 1986; Rizzolatti *et al.* 1988). Interestingly, neurons in the same area discharge *either* when the monkey *performs* an action or when it *observes* the experimenter performing the action (Rizzolatti *et al.* 1996a; Fadiga *et al.* 2000). Rizzolatti and Arbib (1998) concluded, 'These neurons (mirror neurons) appear to represent a system that matches observed events to similar, internally generated actions, and in this way forms a link between the observer and the actor' (p. 152).

A similar neural system appears to exist in humans. A mirror system for gesture recognition has been identified using transcranial magnetic stimulation (Fadiga *et al.* 1995), positron emission tomography (Grafton *et al.* 1996; Rizzolatti *et al.* 1996a, b), functional magnetic resonance imaging (Binkofski *et al.* 2000), and neuromagnetic recordings (Nishitani and Hari 2000; Jarvelainen *et al.* 2001). Importantly, Broca's area is part of this system and perhaps even central to it. Nishitani and Hari (2000) referred to Broca's area as the 'orchestrator of the human mirror neuron system' (p. 913) and noted that it is strongly activated in imitation of actions. In addition, electroencephalography (EEG) associated with finger movements indicates that observation and execution of movement share the same cortical network (Cochin *et al.* 1999). Wohlschlager and Bekkering (2002) concluded that 'imitation emerged from C, the mirror-neurone system of the common ancestor of monkeys and humans' (p. 335). These studies show that humans, like monkeys, activate the same cortical region when observing a movement or in performing that movement. One way of explaining the coexistence of motor and sensory properties in the same neurons is that the motor system is responsible not only for executing actions but also for the internal representation (Fadiga *et al.* 2000). The specificity of this representation is becoming clear. Jarvelainen *et al.* (2001) reported that the mirror neuron system in humans differentiates natural (live) as opposed to artificially presented (videotaped) movements. In addition, the frontal mirror-neuron system has the capability to modulate somatosensory inputs that are directed to precentral areas (Rossi *et al.* 2002), and a phase-specific modulation of cortical motor output accompanies movement observation (Gangitano *et al.* 2001).

Motor imagery and motor performance also have similar neural substrates (Grafton *et al.* 1996; Lotze *et al.* 1999; Binkofski *et al.* 2000; Kosslyn *et al.* 2001). The shared neural resources for these different tasks lend unity and efficiency to motor behavior. Observing, imaging, and performing a movement are represented in a common neural circuit that reflects the cognitive–motoric integrity of learned movements.

The central point is that several lines of evidence point to a neural system in both humans and monkeys that is activated by *observing, imagining,* or *performing* a movement. The hypothesis for speech is that one or more neural areas are activated both by hearing a speech pattern and by producing or imagining a similar pattern. This neural system underlies the auditory–motor integrity of speech. Skoyles (1998) wrote of this possibility in his assertion that speech is a 'replication code'. Imitation is a means to establishing such a code. The auditory–motor linkage for speech is supported by the observation that listening to speech specifically modulates the excitability of tongue muscles (Fadiga *et al.* 2002). A visual–motor linkage is indicated by research demonstrating that Brodmann areas 44 and 45 are bilaterally activated when subjects observe silent speech (Ryding *et al.* 1996; Campbell 1998; Campbell *et al.* 2001).

1.3.4 Broca's area (Brodmann areas 44 and 45)

The hypothesized location of mirror neurons in Broca's area prompts a reconsideration of the functional importance of this cortical region. Classically, Broca's area was thought to be a center for the motor control of speech. However, research has shown that Broca's area is not necessarily active in all speech behavior. It is not active in the production of single words for nouns (Raichle 1996; Wise *et al.* 1999), but it is more likely to be activated in verb generation (Raichle 1996), sentence reading (Muller *et al.* 1997), and verbal fluency tasks (Phelps *et al.* 1997; Schlosser *et al.* 1998). Jurgens (2002) concluded that the planning of longer purposeful utterances depends on the ventral premotor and prefrontal cortex, including Broca's area. Perhaps this region is activated in tasks that require analysis of hierarchical structure (e.g. sentences) or complex sequences (e.g. extracting and manipulating phonetic segments; Zatorre *et al.* 1996). Single words may not require activation of Broca's area because they can be produced through automatized motor plans. More complex hierarchical or sequential patterns require Broca's area, most likely working in cooperation with other regions, especially the insula and premotor cortex (Wise *et al.* 1999). The attribution of mirror neurons to Broca's area means that it plays a role in perceptual–motor linkage, and therefore in the acquisition of motor skills, especially those involving the hands or mouth. Rizzolatti and Arbib (1998) proposed that Broca's area derives phylogenetically from premotor areas controlling arm and hand movements. Studies of double grasp preparation with hand and mouth demonstrate that humans, like monkeys, have premotor neurons that participate in grasp preparation (Gentilucci *et al.* 2001). This result prompted the authors to suggest that 'circuits involved in double grasp preparation might have been the neural substrate where hand motor patterns used as primitive communication signs were transferred to mouth articulation system' (p. 1685).

1.3.5 Cortical connections of Broca's and Wernicke's areas

Recently, some authors have questioned the classic proposition that the two major language areas, Broca's and Wernicke's, are connected primarily via the arcuate fasciculus. Aboitiz and Garcia (1997*a, b*) noted that there may be few direct connections between Broca's and Wernicke's areas, and that the functional link between them may well be inferior parietal areas. They hypothesized a connectional pattern for language that strongly resembles the network of parieto-temporal–prefrontal connections thought to serve working memory. This type of memory, applied to immediate cognitive processing, may well be called upon to support early imitative behaviors, which would then foster the development of neural connections for language learning. The imitation of modeled actions may help in establishing networks for representation of meaning, because it may contribute to understanding the actions of others and to learning the semantic categorization of objects (Fadiga *et al.* 2000). Interestingly, some cortical regions traditionally associated with speech and language functions are activated with the performance of nonverbal motor tasks. These include Broca's area, as already discussed, but also the angular gyrus (Grezes *et al.* 1999).

1.3.6 Mirror neurons and imitation across species

The identification of mirror neurons in monkeys prompts the idea that monkeys should imitate readily and successfully ('monkey see, monkey do'), but, in fact, the role of imitation in nonhuman species is controversial. Perhaps the most remarkable thing about imitation in animals is the debate over whether it occurs (Hauser 1996; Byrne and Russon 1998; Miklosi 1999). Imitation has not been abundantly observed, and much of the commentary pertains to why this should be so. Although the present chapter does not presume to point to evolutionary precedents of imitation in humans, it is interesting to note that a recent proposal to explain learning by imitation in nonhuman primates asserts that imitation can occur at various levels, two of which are an *action level* (a detailed, linear specification of sequential acts) and a *program level* (a more general description of subroutine structure and the hierarchical pattern of a behavioral program) (Byrne and Russon 1998). Some elements of imitation may be common between humans and other species, but it is also possible that imitation in humans is part of the unique biological adaptation for culture in *Homo sapiens*. Tomasello (1999) pointed to a key adaptation as that enabling individuals to comprehend other individuals as intentional agents like the self. This adaptation is a form of social cognition that appears in human infants at about 1 year of age, 'as infants begin to engage with other persons in various kinds of joint attentional activities involving gaze following, social referencing, and gestural communication' (p. 509). One role of imitation in this social cognition is the recognition of self as distinct, yet similar to others, and capable of intentional action. (For further discussion of philosophical conceptions of self, see Gallagher 2000; for a re-examination of the issue of cultural variation in nonhuman primates, see Whiten *et al.* 1999.)

1.3.7 Corticospinal excitabilty

Motor imagery enhances corticospinal excitability, especially in the lower limb muscles for tasks such as knee movements (Tremblay *et al.* 2001), arm and hand movements (Fadiga *et al.* 1999), and wrist flexion and extension movements (Hashimoto and Rothwell 1999). The general conclusion is that motor imagery can influence the excitability of the motor cortex in much the same way as actual motor performance.

1.4 Clinical studies

Support for cognitive penetration of motor behavior is also seen in clinical studies on paralysis due to stroke, Parkinson's disease, developmental coordination disorder, apraxia of speech and adaptations to altered structures (as in surgical ablation). The following review is necessarily selective; for general perspectives on potentials for clinical intervention, see Hummelsheim (1999) and Jackson *et al.* (2001).

1.4.1 Stroke

Many adults with left or right upper-limb paralysis have a preserved ability to represent accurate prehensile movements of the impaired limb (Johnson 2000). A clinical implication is that patients with stroke can use motor imagery to activate partially damaged motor networks, which may be a useful step in functional recovery. In a study of recovery of motor function in stroke, Yoo *et al.* (2001) examined the effect of mental practice on line tracing by three persons with right hemiparesis. The task was to trace a line 5.9 inches long with and without cognitive rehearsal. Line length errors were reduced for all three individuals after cognitive rehearsal. A similar benefit was reported for a 56-year-old man who had stable motor deficits 5 months after a parietal infarct (Page *et al.* 2001). A reduction in impairment and improved arm function was observed following physical therapy and audiotape instruction that the patient imagine himself using the affected limb.

The potency of motor imagery has been demonstrated in research on brain-to-computer rehabilitation for paralyzed patients. EEG changes during motor imagery were used to control a hand orthosis in a tetraplegic individual (Pfurtscheller and

Neuper 2001). The authors reported nearly 100% accuracy with this form of EEG-based control. Preserved motor imagery has also been reported for a patient with locked-in syndrome resulting from a large pontine infarction (Cincotta *et al.* 1999).

Studies of patients with different lesions are beginning to define the neural network that mediates motor imagery. Li (2000) studied patients with putaminal or cortical lesions who were asked to imagine themselves (first-person task) or another person (third-person task) performing a sequence of three movements, and then to select, from four photos, the end posture of the movement to be imagined. Impairments of limb-specific imagery were observed in both putaminal and cortical lesions in the first-person task, but not the third-person task. Interestingly, the majority of errors committed by the patients with cortical lesions involved the first movement, which was taken as evidence that the motor cortex participates in memory processes.

Finally, motor learning following unilateral stroke appears to follow the same principles described earlier in this chapter. Specifically, patients with chronic hemiparesis secondary to a single unilateral cerebral stroke demonstrated better retention of a functional movement sequence with random practice as opposed to blocked practice (Hanlon 1996).

1.4.2 Parkinson's disease

Studies of Parkinson's disease lend further support to a role of motor representation in the understanding of motor impairment. Filippi *et al.* (2001) used transcranial magnetic stimulation to map the cortical representations of the abductor digiti minimi during rest, contraction, and motor imagery in individuals with Parkinson's disease and neurologically normal controls. The subjects with Parkinson's disease had a reduced area of representation elicited by motor imagery in the clinically affected hemisphere. A positron emission tomography (PET) study of regional cerebral blood flow showed that individuals with Parkinson's disease had a relative reduction of activation in dorsolateral and mesial frontal cortex during a task of motor imagery (Samuel *et al.* 2001). Similarly, Cunnington *et al.* (2001) reported that subjects with Parkinson's disease in the clinically 'off' phase of dopaminergic stimulation had reduced activation of several regions, including the dorsolateral prefrontal cortex ipsilateral with the imagined movement. It was concluded that subjects with Parkinson's disease have: (1) deficits in pre-supplementary motor area (pre-SMA) function (especially dorsolateral prefrontal cortex and anterior cingulate) but preserved function of the SMA proper; and (2) compensatory over-activity in ipsilateral premotor and inferior parietal cortex. Another PET study revealed that subjects with asymmetrical Parkinson's disease had abnormal patterns of brain activation for motor imagery involving both the akinetic and non-akinetic hand (Thobois *et al.* 2000). Motor imagery with the akinetic hand was associated with absence of activation in the contralateral primary sensorimotor cortex and the cerebellum, persistent activation of the SMA, and bilateral activation of the superior parietal cortex. Motor imagery with the non-akinetic hand was associated with a lack of activation of the SMA. These studies indicate that abnormalities associated with Parkinson's disease can be detected in tasks of motor imagery.

As noted earlier, a study by Adams *et al.* (2002) demonstrated that individuals with Parkinson's disease had better retention scores in a speech motor learning task when they were provided with summary feedback after every five trials as opposed to summary feedback after every trial. Although few studies of this kind have been reported, the results are encouraging and suggest that clinical intervention may be guided by the same principles that have emerged in the study of motor learning in neurologically healthy individuals.

1.4.3 Developmental coordination disorder

Evidence of impaired internal representations in developmental coordination disorder (DCD) was reported by Wilson *et al.* (2001). Subjects with DCD and normal controls performed a visually guided pointing task with and without a weight attached to a pen. The controls conformed to Fitts' law for both real and imagined performances, but the subjects with DCD conformed to Fitts' law only for real movements.

1.4.4 Ideomotor apraxia

Because apraxia is typically thought to involve an impaired motor representation or motor programming for movement, the question arises if motor imagery is affected in apraxia. In a study of one patient with severe ideomotor apraxia but intact language, Ochipa *et al.* (1997) determined that the patient was impaired both in her ability to make transitive movements to demonstrate tool usage, and in her ability to answer imagery questions about joint movement or hand position during the action. Yet her visual object imagery was unaffected. The authors concluded that the same representations that guide gesture execution are activated during imagery of the movements.

1.4.5 Stuttering

Overt and imagined stuttering were investigated in a PET study by Ingham *et al.* (2000). In subjects who stutter, patterns of activation and deactivation were quite similar for overt stuttering and imagined stuttering. Furthermore, the regional activations generally changed in the same direction when overt stuttering diminished during a task of chorus reading, and when subjects imagined that they were not stuttering (also during chorus reading). The authors concluded that overt stuttering is not prerequisite to the regional activations and deactivations associated with stuttering. But this study also shows that speech disorders may be evident even during the imagined production of speech.

1.5 Developmental studies (humans and robotics)

Research shows that cognitive and motor development are fundamentally interrelated. Diamond (2000) concluded that both have protracted developmental timetables and that disturbances of cognitive development frequently affect motor development. The neurophysiological correlate of these developmental interactions is thought to be the 'close activation of the neocerebellum and dorsolateral prefrontal cortex' (Diamond 2000, p. 44). This section explores cognitive–motoric interactions in early development of speech and speech-related behaviors, beginning with imitation and observational learning. It also considers the role of observational learning and imitation in the design of robotics.

1.5.1 Imitation and observational learning in early speech development

Cognitive–motoric interaction can be seen in early infancy. It is well established that newborns imitate the lip and tongue movements that they see others perform (Meltzoff 1999). The same proclivity is observed in infants with Down syndrome, up to the age of about 4 months (Heimann *et al.* 1998). This seemingly precocious imitative ability demands a reconsideration of classic views of cognitive development (Meltzoff and Moore 1993; Meltzoff 1999). Because infants often spontaneously imitate speech sounds produced by adults, it is sometimes supposed that vocal imitation is a route to the learning of speech. Infants as young as 12 weeks imitate vowels produced by adults (Kuhl and Meltzoff 1996), and infants who are 18 weeks old spontaneously mimic vocal expressions if the accompanying voice matches the expression (Kuhl and Meltzoff 1982; Patterson and Werker 1999). This latter ability must reflect a capacity to judge auditory–motor correspondence (i.e. judging the match between facial expression and concurrent vocalization). Visual information on speech production is, in fact, quite rich, as studies show that approximately 80% of the variance in vocal tract activity can be estimated from facial movements (Yehia *et al.* 1998). In typical development, infants are exposed to the human face and human speech, often simultaneously, so that facial expression is paired with the hearing of speech. Slater and Kirby (1998) proposed that the human face is 'special' to newborns, who respond to the face holistically and not as a collection of stimulus elements (eyes, nose, etc.). Furthermore, the authors present evidence that newborns form auditory–visual associations after a brief exposure to a stimulus. These observations were viewed as evidence of innate capacities (modules) that 'facilitate and direct early learning' (p. 90). Attention to the face also provides cues for determining the speaker's emotional state, and there may be a general human tendency to mimic emotional facial expressions (Blairy *et al.* 1999).

Meltzoff (1999) remarked that, vocal imitation 'is a principal vehicle for infants' learning of the phonetic inventory and prosodic structure of their native language'. Curiously, vocal imitation by infants has not been systematically or widely studied.

The neglect of imitation in some accounts of language development is therefore not surprising, even though common wisdom ascribes a role of imitation in infants' progress toward the skills of speech.

Children demonstrate a preference for motor actions that match their own capabilities. For example, both deaf infants and hearing infants who *have never been exposed to sign* show greater attentional and affective responsiveness to infant-directed ('motherese') signing than to adult-directed signing (Masataka 1998). Remarkably, even infants who have no experience in the sign modality seem to recognize and prefer signing that is directed to infants. Perhaps this preference involves the mirror neurons that connect observed action with performed action. That is, assuming that infant-directed signing is more compatible with the infant's motor capabilities than is adult-directed signing, the infant would naturally prefer the former.

Imitation may take different forms as a child's skill and knowledge increase. Speidel and Nelson (1989) remarked that, 'If we study how different forms of imitation change over time, how they are a function of the developing neural substrate, and how they interweave with other cognitive functions, with memory, with psychological and social needs and motivations, our understanding of language phenomena will become fuller' (p. 18). Imitation is perhaps best viewed as a complex behavior, parts of which can be exercised independently (such as observational learning without demonstrable imitation), and which is adapted to the child's repertoire of skills and knowledge (e.g. beginning with individual sounds or gestures and proceeding to complex sound or gesture sequences). The facial and vocal imitations evident in the first few months of infancy lay down basic capacities for the registration of other-produced and self-produced behaviors. These capacities evolve to support observational learning of other components of language. Imitation does not need to be exact in order that it can be useful. Hauser (1996) pointed out that, 'Imitation allows individuals to pick up the meaning of a new signal quickly and also provides a foundation for generating variation' (p. 650).

1.5.2 Cognitive aspects of sensory–motor experience in typically developing children

Rochat (1998) reviews research showing that in the first weeks of life, infants develop an ability to detect intermodal invariants and regularities in their sensori-motor experience. This ability would contribute to the learning of sensory–motor associations and it might also be means to self-recognition. Rochat proposed that 'young infants' propensity to engage in self-perception and systematic exploration of the perceptual consequences of their own action plays an important role in the intermodal calibration of the body and is probably at the origin of an early sense of self: the ecological self' (p. 102). It is likely that imitation of other's actions reinforces this sense of self as infants come to understand themselves as separate agents capable of behaviors homologous to those they observe external to themselves.

Imitation may be a means by which infants: (1) recognize themselves as independent beings; (2) realize that they can replicate the actions of others and therefore see themselves and others as intentional agents; (3) can efficiently learn motor skills; (4) acquire basic aspects of spoken, signed, or tactile language; and (5) develop a theory of minds (theirs and others). A cross-disciplinary view of imitation reveals a number of common features that motivate the principled study of imitation as a behavior that mediates skill acquisition. The general ethological value of imitation was summarized by Hauser (1996), who remarked that imitation has been regarded as a powerful social learning mechanism because it 'enables individuals to accurately reproduce a particular motor action in the absence of a demonstrator, thereby facilitating the rapidity and fidelity with which information can be transmitted ...' (p. 650).

1.5.3 Development of speech and gesture in children who are blind or deaf

If observational learning and imitation play a role in language learning, then children who are blind, deaf, or both, present a unique opportunity to determine what the role of these factors might be. As is readily demonstrated by language acquisition in the blind, individuals do not need to see speech movements in order to learn speech. However, studies have shown that children who are blind or have severe visual impairment develop expressive language later than do sighted children (Landau and Gleitman 1985; McConachie and Moore 1994; Preisler 1995). Apparently, visual information facilitates the development of spoken language, but it is not absolutely necessary to it. The nature of visual facilitation is not entirely clear, but, as noted previously, about 80% of the variance in vocal-tract activity can be estimated from facial movements (Yehia *et al.* 1998). At the very least, visual information would reinforce information derived from the acoustic signal of speech. It is interesting that although blind children do not produce gestures in as many contexts as do sighted children, the gestures they do produce resemble those of sighted children in both form and content (Iverson and Goldin-Meadow 1997).

Curiously, imitation of sign language has not been studied in detail, although it would seem that imitation is a necessary route to learning of sign in children who are deaf. At the minimum, observational learning is needed to acquire sign, but it is highly likely that imitation also plays a role. Bonvillian and Siedlecki (1998) reported on the acquisition of the movement aspect of American Sign Language signs in nine young children of deaf parents. The most frequently produced movement was contacting action. A somewhat similar preference was reported in a study of the imitation of manipulatory actions in chimpanzees, with superior performance occurring for actions in which an object was directed toward an external location, such as another object or one's own body (Myowa-Yamakoshi and Matsuzawa 1999). Weeks *et al.* (1996) studied the effects of various arrange-ments of demonstration and imitation of modeled actions on the learning of the 26 handshapes of the American manual alphabet. It is particularly interesting to compare the group of subjects who imitated the handshapes concurrently as they were demonstrated with the group who delayed imitation until three handshapes had been displayed. The latter had superior performance, presumably because deferred imitation 'required subjects to expend more cognitive effort to retain and produce handshapes' (p. 348). Imitation was a route to the learning of handshapes, but deferred imitation is preferable to skill learning. For children who are deaf–blind, a movement-based approach to language development was outlined by Wheeler and Griffin (1997). The approach is based on four coactive movement phases: resonance, coactive movement, nonrepresentation reference, and deferred imitation.

1.5.4 Imitation and observational learning in robotics and neural network models

Robotics and computer models, too, provide evidence of the value of perceiving and doing as a means to learning, and perhaps even self-recognition. In some respects, the design of robotics is inspired by studies from human performance and skill learning by children. Efforts to design autonomous humanoid robots have focused on imitation learning because it pertains to the three important issues of: (1) efficient motor learning; (2) the connection between action and perception; and (3) modular motor control in the form of movement primitives (Schaal 1999). Kalveram (1999) introduced a modified model of the Hebbian synapse in which motor learning was accomplished with an algorithm called 'auto-imitation' (defined as a non goal-oriented inductive learning algorithm that enables a controller to adopt a general rule from seeing a few examples of that rule). Studies of robots indicate the importance of imitation in 'high-level cognitive abilities linked to self-recognition and to the recognition of others as something similar' (Gaussier *et al.* 1998). It is interesting that ideas emerging in the science of robot-ics have a parallel in the study of human cognition. Whether the agent is machine or human, one means by which the agent can learn a skill is to see that skill performed by a similar, or at least comparable, agent in the environment. This is a kind of perspective taking, in which the imitator takes the perspective of another who is performing an action and also appreciates the intentionality of the act. Another similarity is in the goal-oriented nature of imitation for both robots (Kalveram 1999) and human children (Bekkering *et al.* 2000).

If robots can learn skilled movement from observing ('seeing') movements performed by humans, then is it also possible for computers to learn speech by imitating acoustic patterns in human speech? This appears to be the case. Bailly (1997) developed a computer-based articulatory model that learns to speak using four steps (Fig. 1.1). First, babbling is used to build up a model of forward transforms that will guide articulatory actions. Implicit in this step is the achievement of a sensory–motor calibration that underlies movement selection but also contributes to refinement of internal representations. Secondly, imitation is the means by which sound sequences can be reproduced using audio-visual to articulatory inversion. Imitation is a valuable testing ground because it requires that a child uses internal mechanisms to replicate an externally generated sound pattern. Thirdly, a process referred to as shaping determines the most efficient sensorimotor representation. This can be accomplished by response selection and tuning. And, finally, rhythmic coordination is applied to assemble sequences of motor patterns for linguistic expression. Rhythmic activity is a powerful phenomenon that has been exploited in other neural network models of human behavior. In a model for early sensorimotor development, van Heijst *et al.* (1999) demonstrated that the model's neural circuits accomplish a self-organization based on rhythmic activity generated spontaneously in the model. Gasser *et al.* (1999) used a network of coupled oscillators to perceive and produce patterns of pulses that conform to particular meters relevant to speech and music. Proceeding from an initial state with no biases, the model learns a particular meter to which it has been exposed. The emphasis on rhythm in neural network models has a counterpart in theories that rely on rhythmic processes to facilitate speech development (Kent *et al.* 1991). The various steps illustrated in Fig. 1.1 represent increasing degrees of movement sophistication that prefigure the essential requirements of speech as a precisely coordinated motor behavior that is reliably keyed to internally and externally generated sensory information.

1.5.5 Compatibility with internal models

The foregoing observations are compatible with recent theories of speech motor control that emphasize internal models as a means of representing and controlling speech movements (Perkell *et al.* 1997; Guenther *et al.* 1998; Callan *et al.* 2000). Indeed, much of what has been discussed to this point can be taken as a design for the construction and refinement of internal models.

1.5.6 A model of imitative behavior

As we have seen, imitation is a fundamental motor behavior that integrates different types of information into a capacity for efficient motor learning. Figure 1.2 is a simplified model of the major components of imitation identified in the foregoing discussion. Modeled behavior is the motor action to be reproduced. Initially, this behavior is analyzed by the appropriate sensory system(s), primarily visual or auditory, but also tactile under some conditions. The result of this sensory analysis is an initial representation that contains salient aspects of the observed movement. Perspective taking can contribute to the formation of the initial representation. If no attempt is made to imitate the action, then only this initial representation is

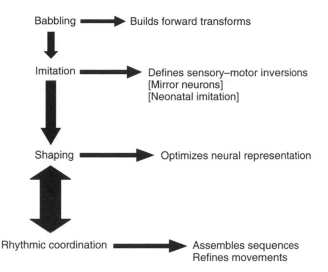

Fig. 1.1 Steps in early speech development in children, based on proposals from Bailly (1997). Babbling, imitation, shaping, and rhythmic coordination all contribute to the establishment of sensorimotor patterns for speech.

formed. But if the observer imitates the modeled action, then a movement sequence is prepared from information in the initial representation, and this sequence gives rise to a motor program with various motor subroutines (SR_i). Execution of the full set of subroutines produces a replica of the modeled action and the generation of multimodal sensory information. Several opportunities arise for feedback to modify the components of the motor representation.

1.6 Conclusion

The evidence is substantial that motor behavior is invested with cognitive influences, and, further, that these influences offer important insights into motor performance and learning, neural mechanisms of motor control, treatment of motor impairments in neurological patients, and the development of motor abilities in children. It appears reasonable that the same insights apply to speech, including its disorders and development. Accordingly, theories of the neural control of speech should take into account a role of cognitive factors in motor processes.

But there is much more to the cognitive story. Studies of brain function in other domains also reflect a growing appreciation of cognitive influence. Current theories of perceptual learning emphasize cue informativeness, modulation of contextual influences, plasticity of neuronal populations in sensory cortex, and the interaction among multiple cortical areas (Sathian 1998; Treisman 1999; Gilbert

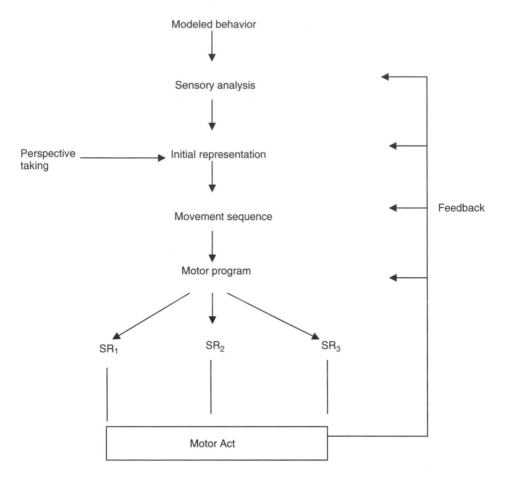

Fig. 1.2 A simplified model of imitation, including stages that account for observational learning in addition to actual imitation of a motor act (see the text for a description).

et al. 2001). For both perceptual and motor learning, the underlying sensory and motor maps are dynamic and plastic, and the course of learning is affected by the emotional and cognitive context in which the new behavior is acquired (Das *et al.* 2001). The current understanding of pain is another example. The gate control theory of pain (which itself emphasized that the brain actively filters, selects, and modulates sensory inputs) has been replaced by the body-self neuromatrix theory, which was formulated especially to account for the integration of multiple inputs related to an ultimate pain perception (Melzack 1999; Melzack *et al.* 1999). As suggested by Vandervert (1999), this corticalized neuromatrix may contribute to a number of other faculties, including consciousness, linguistic representation, and mathematical cognition. Speech and language may be pinnacle functions that derive information from several components of the hypothesized neuromatrix.

Parallel progress in neuroscience has identified brain regions that are activated by functionally equivalent or overlapping behaviors, especially observing, imagining, performing, or verbalizing actions. The accumulated evidence points to specific regions that are activated across a variety of tasks (Grezes and Decety 2001). Broca's area has received particular attention because of its fairly consistent activation in motor tasks of observing, imaging, and performing movement. This research motivates a new understanding of Broca's area and its role in learning of several kinds. At the very least, these ideas suggest a new leverage for the study of brain function. But beyond that, they promise an integrated view that may encompass issues in development, plasticity in the mature brain, and compensations for brain damage.

Observation and imagery of motor actions have received growing attention in both behavioral and brain imaging studies, with the result that these cognitive behaviors are becoming among the best understood within the domain of cognitive science. Furthermore, these behaviors have consequences for the understanding of many different phenomena, including phoneme perception, speech shadowing, imitation in neonates, echoic memory, stimulus–response compatibility, maintenance rehearsal, language learning, social learning, and perspective taking (Skoyles 1998; Wilson *et al.* 2001). Observation and imitation may be the means to diverse cognitive accomplishments, which build on partly isomorphic input–output representations to achieve action–perception linkage, efficient selection of sensory cues and motor responses, and insight into tool and object usage and the motor behaviors in other individuals.

The importance of these discoveries to speech is evident in several respects, including: (1) principles of speech motor learning that parallel those of motor learning in general; (2) the role of cognitive factors in explaining speech motor acquisition, retention, and revision; (3) neural circuits that represent speech movements in both developing and mature individuals; and (4) potentials for treatment of communication disorders.

Acknowledgments

This work was supported in part by research grant No. 5 R01 DC 00319 from the National Institute on Deafness and Other Communicative Disorders (NIDCD-NIH).

Bibliography

Aboitiz, F. and **Garcia, V. R.** (1997a). The evolutionary origin of the language areas of the human brain: a neuroanatomical perspective. *Brain Research—Brain Research Reviews*, 25, 381–396.

Aboitiz, F. and **Garcia, V. R.** (1997b). The anatomy of language revisited. *Biological Research*, 30, 171–183.

Adams, S. G. and **Page, A.** (2000). Effects of selected practice and feedback variables on speech motor learning. *Journal of Medical Speech–Language Pathology*, 8, 215–220.

Adams, S. G., Page, A., and **Jog, M.** (2002). Summary feedback schedules and speech motor learning in Parkinson's disease. *Journal of Medical Speech–Language Pathology*, 10, 215–220.

Anderson, D. I., Magill, R. A., and **Sekiya, H.** (2001). Motor learning as a function of KR schedule and characteristics of task-intrinsic feedback. *Journal of Motor Behavior*, 33, 59–66.

Andry, P., Gaussier, P., Moga, S., Banquet, J. P., and **Nadel, J.** (2001). Learning and communication via imitation: An autonomous robot perspective. *IEEE Transactions on Systems, Man, and Cybernetics Part A: Systems and Humans*, 31, 431–442.

Bailly, G. (1997). Learning to speak—sensori-motor control of speech movements. *Speech Communication*, 22, 251–267.

Bekkering, H., Wohlschlager, A., and **Gattis, M.** (2000). Imitation of gestures in children is goal-directed. *Quarterly Journal of Experimental Psychology Section A— Human Experimental Psychology*, 53, 153–164.

Binkofski, F., Amunts, K., Stephan, K. M., Posse, S., Schormann, T., Freund, H. J., Zilles, K., and **Seitz, R. J.** (2000). Broca's region subserves imagery of motion: A combined cytoarchitectonic and fMRI study. *Human Brain Mapping*, 11, 273–285.

Blairy, S., Herrera, P., and **Hess, U.** (1999). Mimicry and the judgment of emotional facial expressions. *Journal of Nonverbal Behavior*, 23, 5–41.

Blandin, Y. and **Proteau, L.** (2000). On the cognitive basis of observation learning: Development of mechanisms for the detection and correction of errors. *Quarterly Journal of Experimental Psychology. A, Human Experimental Psychology*, 53, 846–867.

Bloedel, J. R. and **Bracha, V.** (1997). Duality of cerebellar motor and cognitive functions. *International Review of Neurobiology*, 41, 613–634.

Bonvillian, J. D. and **Siedlecki, T.** (1998). Young children's acquisition of the movement aspect in American Sign Language—parental report findings. *Journal of Speech, Language, and Hearing Research*, 41, 588–602.

Byrne, R. W. and **Russon, A. E.** (1998). Learning by imitation: A hierarchical approach. *Behavioral and Brain Sciences*, 21, 667–684.

Callan, D. E., Kent, R. D., Guenther, F. H., and **Vorperian, H. K.** (2000). An auditory-feedback-based neural network model of speech production that is robust to developmental changes in the size and shape of the articulatory system. *Journal of Speech, Language, and Hearing Research*, 43, 721–736.

Campbell, R. (1998). Speech reading: advances in understanding its cortical bases and implications for deafness and speech rehabilitation. *Scandinavian Audiology*, 27, 80–86.

Campbell, R., MacSweeney, M., Surguladze, S., Calvert, G., McGuire, P., Suckling, J., Brammer, M. J., and **David, A. S.** (2001). Cortical substrates for the perception of face actions: An fMRI study of the specificity of activation for seen speech and for meaningless lower-face acts (gurning). *Cognitive Brain Research*, 12, 233–243.

Cincotta, M., Tozzi, F., Zaccara, G., Borgheresi, A., Lori, S. Cosottini, M., and Cantello, R. (1999). Motor imagery in a locked-in patient: Evidence from transcranial magnetic stimulation. *Italian Journal of Neurological Sciences*, 20, 37–41.

Cochin, S., Barthelmy, C., Roux, S., and Martineau, J. (1999). Observation and execution of movement: similarities demonstrated by quantified electroencephalography. *European Journal of Neuroscience*, 11, 1839–1842.

Cochin, S., Barthelmy, C., Roux, S., and Martineau, J. (2001). Electroencephalographic activity during perception of motion in childhood. *European Journal of Neuroscience*, 13, 1791–1796.

Cunnington, R., Iansek, R., Johnson, K. A., and Bradshaw, J. L. (1997). Movement-related potentials in Parkinson's disease. Motor imagery and movement preparation. *Brain*, 120, 1339–1353.

Cunnington, R., Egan, G. F., O'Sullivan, J. C., Hughes, A. J., Bradshaw, J. L., and Colebatch, J. G. (2001). Motor imagery in Parkinson's disease: A PET study *Movement Disorders*, 16, 849–857.

Curio, G., Neuloh, G., Numminen, J., Jousmaki, V., and Hari, R. (2000). Speaking modifies voice-evoked activity in the human auditory cortex. *Human Brain Mapping*, 9, 183–191.

Das, A., Franca, J. G., Gattas, R., Kaas, J. H., Nicolelis, M. A. L., Timo-Iaria, C., Vargas, C. D., Weinberger, N. M., and Volchan, E. (2001). The brain decade in debate: VI. Sensory and motor maps: dynamics and plasticity. *Brazilian Journal of Medical and Biological Research*, 34, 1497–1508.

Decety, J., Sjoholm, H., Ryding, E., Stenberg, G., and Invar, D. H. (1990). The cerebellum participates in mental activity: Tomographic measurements of regional cerebral blood flow. *Brain Research*, 535, 313–317.

Diamond, A. (2000). Close interaction of motor development and cognitive development and of the cerebellum and prefrontal cortex. *Child Development*, 71, 44–56.

Fadiga, L., Fogassi, L., Pavesi, G., and Rizzolatti, G. (1995). Motor facilitation during action observation: a magnetic stimulation study. *Journal of Neurophysiology*, 73, 2608–2611.

Fadiga, L., Buccino, G., Craighero, L., Fogassi, L., Gallese, V., and Pavesi, G. (1999). Corticospinal excitability is specifically modulated by motor imagery: A magnetic stimulation study. *Neuropsychologia*, 37, 147–158.

Fadiga, L., Fogassi, L., Gallese, V., and Rizzolatti, G. (2000). Visuomotor neurons: ambiguity of the discharge or 'motor' perception? *International Journal of Psychophysiology*, 35, 165–177.

Fadiga, L., Craighero, L., Buccino, G., and Rizzolatti, G. (2002). Speech listening specifically modulates the excitability of tongue muscles: A TMS study. *European Journal of Neuroscience*, 15, 399–402.

Filippi, M.M., Oliveri, M., Pasqualetti, P., Cicinelli, P., Traversa, R., Vernieri, F., Palmieri, M.G., and **Rossini, P.M.** (2001). Effects of motor imagery on motor cortical output topography in Parkinson's disease. *Neurology*, 57, 55–61.

Galef, B. G., Jr (1992). The question of animal culture. *Human Nature*, 3, 157–178.

Gallagher, S. (2000). Philosophical conceptions of the self: implications for cognitive science. *Trends in Cognitive Sciences*, 4, 14–21.

Gangitano, M., Mottoghy, F. M., and **Pascual-Leone, A.** (2001). Phase-specific modulation of cortical motor output during movement observation. *Neuroreport*, 12, 1489–1492.

Gasser, M., Eck, D., and **Port, R.** (1999). Meter as mechanism: a neural network model that learns metrical patterns. *Connection Science: Journal of Neural Computing, Artificial Intelligence and Cognitive Research*, 11, 187–216.

Gaussier, P., Moga, S., Quoy, M., and **Banquet, J. P.** (1998). From perception–action loops to imitation processes—a bottom-up approach of learning by imitation. *Applied Artificial Intelligence*, 12, 701–727.

Gentilucci, M., Benuzzi, F., Gangitano, M., and **Grimaldi, S.** (2001). Grasp with hand and mouth: A kinematic study. *Journal of Neurophysiology*, 86, 1685–1699.

Georgopoulos, A.P. (2000). Neural aspects of cogntive motor control. *Current Opinion in Neurobiology*, 10, 238–241.

Gilbert, C. D., Sigman, M., and **Crist, R. E.** (2001). The neural basis of perceptual learning. *Neuron*, 31, 681–697.

Grafton, S. T., Arbib, M. A., Fadiga, L., and **Rizzolatti, G.** (1996). Localization of grasp representations in humans by positron emission tomography. 2. Observation compared with imagination. *Experimental Brain Research*, 112, 103–111.

Grezes, J. and **Decety, J.** (2001). Functional anatomy of execution, mental stimulation, observation, and verb generation of actions: A meta-analysis. *Human Brain Mapping*, 12, 1–19.

Grezes, J., Costes, N., and **Decety, J.** (1999). The effects of learning and intention on the neural network involved in the perception of meaningless actions. *Brain*, 122, 1875–1887.

Guenther, F. H., Hampson, M., and **Johnson, D.** (1998). A theoretical investigation of reference frames for the planning of speech movements. *Psychological Review*, 105, 611–633.

Hanlon, R. E. (1996). Motor learning following unilateral stroke. *Archives of Physical Medicine and Rehabilitation*, 77, 811–815.

Hashimoto, R. and **Rothwell, J. C.** (1999). Dynamic changes in corticospinal excitability during motor imagery. *Experimental Brain Research*, 125, 75–81.

Hauert, C. A. (1986). The relationship between motor function and cognition in the developmental perspective. *Italian Journal of Neurological Science*, Suppl. 5, 101–107.

Hauser, M. D. (1996). *The evolution of communication*. Cambridge, MA: MIT Press.

Heijst, J. J. van, Touwen, B. C. L., and **Vos, J. E.** (1999). Implications of a neural network model of early sensori-motor development for the field of developmental neurology. *Early Human Development,* 55, 77–95.

Heimann, M., Ullstadius, E., and **Swerlander, A.** (1998). Imitation in eight young infants with Downs-syndrome. *Pediatric Research,* 44, 780–784.

Heyes, C. (2001). Causes and consequences of imitation. *Trends in Cognitive Sciences,* 5, 253–261.

Heyes, C. M. and **Foster, C. L.** (2002). Motor learning by observation: Evidence from a serial reaction time task. *Quarterly Journal of Experimental Psychology. A., Human Experimental Psychology,* 55, 593–607.

Hikosaka, O., Nakamura, K., Sakai, K., and **Nakahara, H.** (2002). Central mechanisms of motor skill learning. *Current Opinion in Neurobiology,* 12, 217–222.

Holmes, P. S. and **Collins, D. J.** (2001). The PETTLEP approach to motor imagery. A functional equivalence model for sport psychologists. *Journal of Applied Sport Psychology,* 13, 60–83.

Hummelsheim, H. (1999). Rationales for improving motor function. *Current Opinion in Neurology,* 12, 697–701.

Ingham, R. J., Fox, P. T., Costello Ingham, J., and **Zamarripa, F.** (2000). Is overt stuttered speech a prerequisite for the neural activations associated with chronic developmental stuttering? *Brain and Language,* 75, 163–194.

Iverson, J. M. and **Goldin-Meadow, S.** (1997). What's communication got to do with it? Gesture in children blind from birth. *Developmental Psychology,* 33, 453–467.

Jackson, P. L., Lafluer, A. F., Malouin, F., Richards, C., and **Doyon, J.** (2001). Potential role of mental practice using motor imagery in neurologic rehabilitation. *Archives of Physical Medicine and Rehabilitation,* 82, 1133–1141.

Jarvelainen, J., Schurmann, M., Avikainen, S., and **Hari, R.** (2001). Stronger reactivity of the human primary motor cortex during observation of live rather than video motor acts. *Neuroreport,* 12, 3493–3495.

Jeannerod, M. (2001). Neural simulation of action: A unifying mechanism for motor cognition. *Neuroimage,* 14, 103–109.

Johnson, S. H. (2000). Imagining the impossible: intact motor representations in hemiplegics. *Neuroreport,* 11, 729–732.

Jurgens, U. (2002). Neural pathways underlying vocal control. *Neuroscience and Biobehavioral Reviews,* 26, 235–258.

Kalveram, K. T. (1999). A modified model of the Hebbian synapse and its role in motor learning. *Human Movement Science,* 18, 185–199.

Kent, R. D., Mitchell, P. R., and **Sancier, M.** (1991). Evidence and role of rhythmic organization in early vocal development in human infants. In J. Fagard and P. Wolff (eds) *The development of timing control and temporal organization in coordinated action* (pp. 135–149). Amsterdam: Elsevier.

Kent, R. D., Adams, S. G., and **Turner, G.** (1996). Models of speech production. In N. J. Lass (ed.) *Principles of experimental phonetics.* St. Louis: Mosby.

Knock, T. R., Ballard, K. J., Robin, D. A., and **Schmidt, R. A.** (2000). Influence of order of stimulus presentation on speech motor learning: A principled approach to treatment for apraxia of speech. *Aphasiology*, 14, 653–668.

Koopmans-van Beinum, F. J., Clement, C. J., and **van den Dikkenberg-Pot, I.** (2001). Babbling and the lack of auditory speech perception: a matter of coordination? *Developmental Science*, 4, 61–70.

Kosslyn, S. M., Ganis, G., and **Thompson, W. L.** (2001). Neural foundations of imagery. *Nature Reviews Neuroscience*, 2, 635–642.

Kuhl, P. K. and **Meltzoff, A. N.** (1982). The bimodal perception of speech in infancy. *Science*, 218, 1138–1141.

Kuhl, P. K. and **Meltzoff, A. N.** (1996). Infant vocalizations in response to speech— vocal imitation and developmental change. *Journal of the Acoustical Society of America*, 100, 2425–2438.

Kurata, K. and **Tanji, J.** (1986). Premotor cortex neurons in macaques: activity before distal and proximal forelimb movements. *Journal of Neuroscience*, 6, 403–411.

Landau, B. and **Gleitman, L. R.** (1985). *Language and experience: Evidence from the blind child*. Cambridge, MA: Harvard University Press.

Leiner, H. C., Leiner, A. L., and **Dow, R. S.** (1991). The human cerebro-cerebellar system: Its computing, cognitive and language skills. *Behavioral and Brain Research*, 44, 113–128.

Li, C. R. (2000). Impairment of motor imagery in putamen lesions in humans. *Neuroscience Letters*, 287, 13–16.

Lotze, M., Montoya, P., Erb, M., Hulsmann, E., Flor, H., Klose, U., Birbaumer, N., and **Grodd, W.** (1999). Activation of cortical and cerebellar motor areas during executed and imagined hand movements: An fMRI study. *Journal of Cognitive Neuroscience*, 11, 491–501.

Masataka, N. (1998). Perception of motherese in Japanese sign language by 6-month-old hearing infants. *Developmental Psychology*, 34, 241–246.

McConachie, H. R. and **Moore, V.** (1994). Early expressive language of severely visually impaired children. *Developmental Medicine and Child Neurology*, 36, 230–240.

McLennan, N. L., Georgiou, N. L., Mattingley, J. L., Bradshaw, J. L., and **Chiu, E.** (2000). Motor imagery in Huntington's disease. *Journal of Clinical and Experimental Neuropsychology*, 22, 379–390.

Meltzoff, A. N. (1999). Origins of theory of mind, cognition and communication. *Journal of Communication Disorders*, 32, 251–269.

Meltzoff, A. N. and **Moore, M. K.** (1993). Why faces are special to infants—on connecting the attraction of faces and infants' ability for imitation and cross-modal processing. In B. de Boysson-Bardies, S. de Schonen, P. Jusczyk, P. McNeilage, and J. Morton (eds) *Developmental neurocognition: Speech and face processing in the first year of life* (pp. 211–225). Dordrecht, The Netherlands: Kluwer Academic Publishers.

Melzack, R. (1999). From the gate to the neuromatrix. *Pain*, Suppl. 6, S121–S126.

Melzack, R., Coderre, T. J., Vaccarino, A. L., and **Katx, J.** (1999). Pain and neuro-plasticity. In J. Grafman and Y. Christen, (eds) *Neuronal plasticity: Building a bridge from the laboratory to the clinic* (pp. 35–52). Springer Verlag: New York.

Middleton, F. A. and **Strick, P. L.** (2000). Basal ganglia output and cognition: evidence from anatomical, behavioral, and clinical studies. *Brain and Cognition*, 42, 183–200.

Miklosi, A. (1999). The ethological analysis of imitation. *Biological Reviews of the Cambridge Philosophical Society*, 74, 347–374.

Muller, R.-A., Rothermel, R. D., Behen, M. E., Muzik, O., Mangner, T. J., and **Chugani, H. T.** (1997). Receptive and expressive activations for sentences: a PET study. *Neuroreport*, 8, 3767–3770.

Myowa-Yamakoshi, M. and **Matsuzawa, T.** (1999). Factors influencing initation of manipulatory actions in chimpanzees (Pan troglodytes). *Journal of Comparative Psychology*, 113, 128–136.

Nishitani, N. and **Hari, R.** (2000). Temporal dynamics of cortical representation for action. *Proceedings of the National Academy of Sciences of the United States of America*, 97, 913–918.

Nudo, R. J., Plautz, E. J., and **Frost, S. B.** (2001). Role of adaptive plasticity in recovery of function after damage to motor cortex. *Muscle and Nerve*, 24, 1000–1019.

Numminen, J., Salmelin, R., and **Hari, R.** (1999). Subject's own speech reduces reactivity of the human auditory cortex. *Neuroscience Letters*, 265, 119–122.

Ochipa, C., Rapcsak, S. Z., Maher, L. M., Rothi, L. J., Bowers, D., and **Heilman, K. M.** (1997). Selective deficit of praxis imagery in ideomotor apraxia. *Neurology*, 49, 474–480.

Page, S. J., Levine, P., Sisto, S. A., and **Johnston, M. V.** (2001). Mental practice combined with physical practice for upper-limb motor deficit in subacute stroke. *Physical Therapy*, 81, 1455–1462.

Patterson, M. L. and **Werker, J. F.** (1999). Matching phonetic information in lips and voice is robust in 4.5-month-old infants. *Infant Behavior and Development*, 22, 237–248.

Paus, T., Perry, D. W., Zatorre, R. J., Worsley, K. J., and **Evans, A. C.** (1996). Modulation of cerebral blood flow in the human auditory cortex during speech: role of motor-to-sensory discharges. *European Journal of Neuroscience*, 8, 2236–2246.

Perkell, J., Matthies, M., Lane, H., Guenther, F., Wilhelms-Tricarico, R., Wozniak, J., and **Guiod, P.** (1997). Speech motor control: Acoustic goals, saturation effects, auditory feedback and internal models. *Speech Communication*, 22, 227–250.

Pfurtscheller, G. and **Neuper, C.** (2001). Motor imagery and direct brain–computer communication. *Proceedings of the IEEE*, 89, 1123–1134.

Phelps, E. A., Hyder, F., Blamire, A. M., and **Shulman, R. G.** (1997). FMRI of the prefrontal cortex during overt verbal fluency. *Neuroreport*, 8, 561–565.

Plummer, T. K. and **Striedter, G. F.** (2000). Auditory responses in the vocal motor system of budgerigars. *Journal of Neurobiology*, 42, 79–94.

Preisler, G. M. (1995). The development of communication in blind and deaf infants—similarities and differences. *Child: Care, Health and Development*, 21, 79–110.

Pressing, J. (1999). The referential dynamics of cognition and action. *Psychological Review*, 106, 714–747.

Raichle, M. E. (1996). What words are telling us about the brain. *Cold Spring Harbor Symposium on Quantitative Biology* (Vol. 61) (pp. 9–14). Cold Spring Harbor Laboratory Press: New York.

Rapoport, M., van Reekum, R., and **Mayberg, H.** (2000). The role of the cerebellum in cognition and behavior: A selective review. *Journal of Neuropsychiatry and Clinical Neurosciences*, 12, 193–198.

Rizzolatti, G. and **Arbib, M. A.** (1998). From grasping to speech: imitation might provide a missing link—Reply. *Trends in Neurosciences*, 22, 152.

Rizzolatti, G., Camarda, R., Fogassi, L., Gentilucci, M., Luppino G., and **Matelli, M.** (1988). Functional organization of inferior area 6 in the macaque monkey. II. Area F5 and the control of distal movements. *Experimental Brain Research*, 71, 491–507.

Rizzolatti, G., Fadiga, L., Gallese, V., and **Fogassi, L.** (1996*a*). Premotor cortex and the recognition of motor actions. *Cognitive Brain Research*, 3, 131–141.

Rizzolatti, G., Fadiga, L., Matelli, M., Bettinardi, V., Paulesu, E., Perani, C., and **Fazio, F.** (1996*b*). Localization of grasp representation in humans by PET: 1. Observation versus execution. *Experimental Brain Research*, 111, 246–252.

Rizzolatti, G., Fogassi, L., and **Gallese, V.** (2002). Motor and cognitive functions of the ventral premotor cortex. *Current Opinion in Neurobiology*, 12, 149–154.

Rochat, P. (1998). Self-perception and action in infancy. *Experimental Brain Research*, 123, 102–109.

Rossi, S., Tecchio, F., Pasqualetti, P., Ulivelli, M., Pizzella, V., Romani, G. L., Passero, S., Battistini, N., and **Rossini, P. M.** (2002). Somatosensory processing during movement observation in humans. *Clinical Neurophysiology*, 113, 16–24.

Ryding, E., Bradvik, B., and **Ingvar, D. H.** (1996). Silent speech activates prefrontal cortical regions asymmetrically, as well as speech-related areas in the dominant hemisphere. *Brain and Language*, 52, 435–451.

Samuel, M., Ceballos-Baumann, A. O., Boecker, H., and **Brooks, D. J.** (2001). Motor imagery in normal subjects and Parkinson's disease patients; an (H_2OPET)-O-15 study. *Neuroreport*, 12, 821–828.

Sanes, J. N. and **Donoghue, J. P.** (2000). Plasticity and primary motor cortex. *Annual Review of Neuroscience*, 23, 393–415.

Sathian, K. (1998). Perceptual learning. *Current Science*, 75, 451–457.

Sathian, K., Greenspan, A. I., and **Wolf, S. L.** (2000). Doing it with mirrors: a case study of a novel approach to neurorehabilitation. *Neurorehabilitation and Neural Repair*, 14, 73–76.

Schaal, S. (1999). Is imitation learning the route to humanoid robots? *Trends in Cognitive Sciences*, 3, 233–242.

Schlosser, R., Hutinchson, M., Joseffer, S., Rusinek, H., Saarimaki, A., Stevenson, J., Dewey, S. L., and Brodie, J. D. (1998). Functional magnetic resonance imaging of human brain activity in a verbal fluency task. *Journal of Neurology, Neurosurgery, and Psychiatry*, 64, 492–498.

Schmahmann, J. D. (1997). Therapeutic and research implications. *International Review of Neurobiology*, 41, 637–647.

Seitz, R. J., Stephan, K. M., and Binkofski, F. (2000). Control of action as mediated by the human frontal lobe. *Experimental Brain Research*, 133, 71–80.

Skoyles, J. R. (1998). Speech phones are a replication code. *Medical Hypotheses*, 50, 167–173.

Slater, A. and Kirby, R. (1998). Innate and learned perceptual abilities in the newborn infant. *Experimental Brain Research*, 123, 90–94.

Speidel, G. E. and Nelson, K. E. (1989). A fresh look at imitation in language learning. In G. E. Speidel and K. E. Nelson (eds) *The many faces of language learning* (pp. 1–21). New York: Springer Verlag.

Steinhauer, K. and Grayhack, J. P. (2000). The role of knowledge of results in performance and learning of a voice motor task. *Journal of Voice*, 14, 137–145.

Thobois, S., Dominey, P. E., Decety, P. J., Pollak, P. P., Gregoire, M. C., Le Bars, P. D., and Broussole, E. (2000). Motor imagery in normal subjects and in asymmetrical Parkinson's disease: A PET study. *Neurology*, 55, 996–1002.

Tomasello, M. (1999). The human adaptation for culture. *Annual Review of Anthropology*, 28, 509–529.

Treisman, M. (1999). There are two types of psychometric function: A theory of cue combination in the processing of complex stimuli with implications for categorical perception. *Journal of Experimental Psychology: General*, 128, 517–546.

Tremblay, F., Tremblay, L. E., and Colcer, D. E. (2001). Modulation of corticospinal excitability during imagined knee movements. *Journal of Rehabilitation Medicine*, 33, 230–234.

Umilta, M. A., Kohler, E., Gallese, V., Fogassi, L., Fadiga, L., Keysers, C. and Rizzolatti, G. (2001). I know what you are doing: A neurophysiological study. *Neuron*, 31, 155–165.

Vandervert, L. R. (1999). A motor theory of how consciousness within language evolution led to mathematical cognition: The origin of mathematics in the brain. *New Ideas in Psychology*, 17, 215–235.

Wilson, M. (2001). Perceiving imitatible stimuli: Consequences of isomorphism between input and output. *Psychological Bulletin*, 127, 543–553.

Wheeler, L. and Griffin, H. C. (1997). A movement-based approach to language development in children who are deaf-blind. *American Annals of the Deaf*, 142, 387–390.

Whiten, A., Goodal, J., McGrew, W. C., Nishida, T., Reynolds, V., Sugiyama, Y., Tutin, C. E. G., Wrangham, R. W., and Boesch, C. (1999). Cultures in chimpanzees. *Nature*, 399, 682–685.

Williams, J. H. G., Whiten, A., Suddendorf, T., and Perrett, D. I. (2001). Imitation, mirror neurons and autism. *Neuroscience and Biobehavioral Reviews*, 25, 287–295.

Weeks, D. L., Hall, A. K., and Anderson, L. P. (1996). A comparison of imitation strategies in observational learning of action patterns. *Journal of Motor Behavior*, 28, 348–358.

Wilson, P. H., Maruff, P., Ives, S., and Currie, J. (2001). Abnormalities of motor and praxis imagery in children with DCD. *Human Movement Science*, 20(11–12), 135–159.

Wise, R. J., Greene, J., Buchel, C., and Scott, S. K. (1999). Brain regions involved in articulation. *Lancet*, 353, 1057–1061.

Wohlschlager, W. and Bekkering, H. (2002). Is human imitation based on a mirror-neurone system? Some behavioural evidence. *Experimental Brain Research*, 143, 335–341.

Wolf, N. S., Gales, M. E., Shane, E., and Shane, M. (2001). The developmental trajectory from amodal perception to empathy and communication: The role of mirror neurons in this process. *Psychoanalytic Inquiry*, 21, 94–112.

Wulf, G., McNevin, N., Shea, C. H., and Wright, D. L. (1999). Learning phenomena: Future challenges for the dynamical systems approach to understanding the learning of complex motor skills. *International Journal of Sport Psychology*, 30, 531–557.

Wulf, G., Shea, C., and Park, J. H. (2001). Attention and motor performance: Preferences for and advantages of an external focus. *Research Quarterly for Exercise and Sport*, 72, 335–344.

Yaguez, L., Canavan, A. G., Lange, H. W., and Homberg, V. (1999). Motor learning by imagery is differentially affected in Parkinson's and Huntington's diseases. *Behavioural Brain Research*, 102, 115–127.

Yehia, H., Rubin P., and Vatikiotis-Bateson, E. (1998). Quantitative association of vocal-tract and facial behavior. *Speech Communication*, 26, 23–43.

Yoo, E., Park, E., and Chung, B. (2001). Mental practice effect on line-tracing accuracy in persons with hemiparetic stroke: A preliminary study. *Archives of Physical Medicine and Rehabilitation*, 82, 1213–1218.

Zatorre, R. J., Meyer, E., Gjedde, A., and Evans, A. C. (1996). PET studies of phonetic processing of speech — Review, replication, and reanalysis. *Cerebral Cortex*, 6, 21–30.

CHAPTER 2

A NEURAL MODEL OF SPEECH PRODUCTION AND ITS APPLICATION TO STUDIES OF THE ROLE OF AUDITORY FEEDBACK IN SPEECH

FRANK H. GUENTHER AND JOSEPH S. PERKELL

2.1 The DIVA model of speech production

The overall objective of our research is to model the brain activity and the motor, biomechanical and sensory processes involved in speech production. Our approach is to use a combination of computational models and to develop and test them with brain imaging, psychophysical, physiological, anatomical and acoustic data. In particular, we have developed a neural network model of speech motor skill acquisition and speech production, called the DIVA model, that explains a wide range of data on contextual variability, motor equivalence, coarticulation and speaking rate effects (Guenther 1994, 1995a, b; Guenther and Micci Barreca 1997; Guenther et al. 1998; Perkell et al. 2000). This model is schematized in Fig. 2.1. In this chapter we provide a description of the model and its neural correlates, and we present results of studies on an important aspect of the model: the role of auditory feedback in the planning of speech movements.

Each block in Fig. 2.1 corresponds to a set of neurons that constitute a neural representation. Model parameters, corresponding to synaptic weights, are tuned during a babbling phase in which random movements of the speech articulators provide tactile, proprioceptive, and auditory feedback signals that are used to train three neural mappings, indicated by filled semicircles in the figure. These mappings are later used for phoneme production.

The synaptic weights of the first mapping, labeled 'convex region targets' in the figure, encode auditory and orosensory targets for each phoneme the model learned during babbling. To explain how infants learn phoneme-specific and language-specific limits on acceptable articulatory and acoustic variability, the learned speech sound targets take the form of multidimensional regions, rather than points, in auditory and orosensory spaces. This 'convex region theory' of

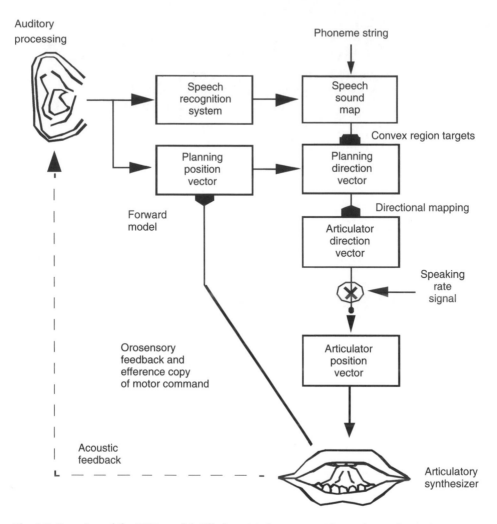

Fig. 2.1 Overview of the DIVA model. Filled semicircles represent learned neural mappings.

phonemic targets as multidimensional regions provides a simple and unified explanation for many long-studied speech phenomena, including aspects of anticipatory and carryover coarticulation, contextual variability, motor equivalence, velocity/distance relationships, and speaking rate effects (Guenther 1995a).

The second neural mapping, labeled 'directional mapping' in the figure, transforms desired movement directions in auditory and orosensory spaces into movement directions in an articulator space closely related to the vocal tract musculature. This mapping is related to the Moore–Penrose (MP) pseudoinverse of the Jacobian matrix relating the auditory and articulatory spaces (in effect, the model learns an approximation of the MP pseudoinverse during babbling); the model is thus closely related to pseudoinverse-style control techniques described in the robotics literature (e.g. Liégeois 1977). The Jacobian matrix defines the transform between changes in articulator positions and the corresponding changes in auditory parameters (e.g. changes in formant frequencies). This relationship is many-to-one; that is, many different articulator movements will lead to the same changes in the auditory parameters. To control speech movements, one needs to invert this relationship; i.e. one needs to compute articulatory changes to carry out desired changes in the auditory parameters. Since this inversion process is one-to-many, a unique inverse to the Jacobian transformation cannot be calculated. Instead, a pseudoinverse must be calculated. The Moore–Penrose pseudoinverse is the pseudoinverse that commands the smallest amount of articulatory movement that can be used to achieve the desired changes in the auditory signal. The model learns an approximation to the MP pseudoinverse and uses this to map desired auditory changes into articulatory movements. The resulting controller is capable of automatically compensating for constraints and/or perturbations applied to the articulators (Guenther 1994, 1995a; Guenther and Micci Barreca 1997), thus accounting for the motor equivalent capabilities observed in humans when speaking with a bite block or lip perturbation.

The third mapping, labeled 'forward model' in Fig. 2.1, transforms orosensory feedback from the vocal tract and an efference copy of the motor outflow commands into a neural representation of the auditory signal that corresponds to the current vocal tract shape. This forward model allows the system to control speech movements without relying on auditory feedback, which may be absent or too slow for use in controlling ongoing articulator movements.

Computer simulations have been used to verify that the model provides a unified explanation for a wide range of data on articulator kinematics and motor skill development (Guenther 1994, 1995a, b; Guenther et al. 1998; Callan et al., 2000) that were previously addressed individually rather than in a single model. The model's explanations for several speech production phenomena are discussed below, with reference to an important issue addressed by the model: the nature of the brain's 'targets' for speech motor control.

2.1.1 The nature of speech sound targets

Most accounts of speech production involve some sort of 'target' that the motor system hopes to achieve in order to produce a particular speech sound. For example, phoneme targets in the task-dynamic model (Saltzman and Munhall 1989) take the form of locations and degrees of key constrictions of the vocal tract. Targets in the DIVA model take the form of regions in a planning space consisting of auditory and orosensory dimensions (e.g. formant ratios and vocal tract constrictions). Each cell in the model's speech sound map (see Fig. 2.1) represents a different sound (phoneme or syllable). The synaptic weights on the pathways projecting from a speech sound map cell to cells in the planning direction vector represent a target for the corresponding speech sound in planning space. When the changing vocal tract configuration is identified by the speech recognition system as producing a speech sound during babbling, the appropriate speech sound map cell's activity is set to 1. This, in turn, causes learning to occur in the synaptic weights of the pathways projecting from that cell, thereby allowing the model to modify the target for the speech sound based on the current configuration of the vocal tract.

To explain how infants learn phoneme-specific and language-specific limits on acceptable articulatory variability, the targets take the form of convex regions in planning space. This 'convex region theory' is a generalization of Keating's (1990) 'window model' of coarticulation to a multidimensional movement planning space, consisting of auditory and constriction dimensions in addition to articulatory dimensions (for further discussion of this topic, see Guenther 1995a). Figure 2.2 schematizes the learning sequence for the vowel /i/ along two dimensions of planning space, corresponding to lip aperture and tongue body height. The first time the phoneme is produced during babbling, synaptic weights that project from the speech sound map cell for /i/ are adjusted to encode the position in planning space that led to proper production of the phoneme on this trial. In other words, the model has learned a target for /i/ that consists of a single point in the planning space, as schematized in Fig. 2.2a. The next time the phoneme is babbled, the speech sound map cell expands its learned target to be a convex region that encompasses the previous point and the new point in planning space, as shown in Fig. 2.2b; this can occur via a simple and biologically plausible learning law (Guenther 1995a). In this way, the model is constantly expanding its convex region target for /i/ to encompass all of the various vocal tract configurations that can be used to produce /i/.

An important aspect of this work concerns how the nervous system extracts the appropriate forms of auditory and orosensory information that define the different speech sounds. For example, how is it that the nervous system 'knows' that it is lip aperture, and not lower lip height or upper lip height, that is the important articulatory variable for stop consonant production? How does the nervous system know that whereas lip aperture must be strictly controlled for bilabial stops, it can be allowed to vary over a large range for many other speech sounds, including not only vowels but also velar, alveolar, and dental stops? How does the nervous system of a Japanese speaker know that tongue tip location during production of Japanese /r/ can often vary widely, while the nervous system of an English speaker knows to control tongue tip location more strictly when producing /r/ so that /l/ is not produced instead?

The manner in which targets are learned in the DIVA model provides a unified answer to these questions. Consider the convex regions that result after many instances of producing the vowel /i/ and the bilabial stop /p/ (Fig. 2.2c). The convex region for /p/ does not vary over the dimension of lip aperture but varies largely over the dimension of tongue body height; this is because all bilabial stops that the model has produced have the same lip aperture (corresponding to full

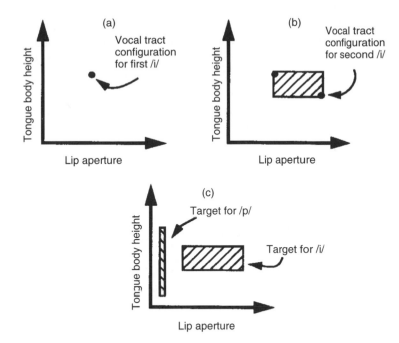

Fig. 2.2 Learning of the convex region target for the vowel /i/ along planning dimensions corresponding to lip aperture and tongue body height. (a) The first time /i/ is produced during babbling, the learned target is simply the configuration of the vocal tract when the sound was produced. (b) The second time /i/ is babbled, the convex region target is expanded to encompass both vocal tract configurations used to produce the sound. (c) Schematized convex regions for /i/ and /p/ after many productions of each sound during babbling. Whereas the target for /i/ allows large variation along the dimension of lip aperture, the target for the bilabial stop /p/ requires strict control of this dimension, indicating that the model has learned that lip aperture is an important aspect of /p/ but not /i/.

closure of the lips), but tongue body height has varied. In other words, the model has learned that lip aperture is the important dimension for producing the bilabial stop /p/. Furthermore, whereas lip aperture is the important dimension for /p/, the model has learned that this dimension is not very important for /i/, as indicated by the wide range of lip aperture in the target for /i/ in Fig. 2.2c. Finally, since convex region learning relies on language-specific recognition of phonemes by the infant, the shapes of the resulting convex regions will vary from language to language.

The convex region theory of the targets of speech provides a unified explanation for a number of long-studied speech production phenomena. A brief summary of some of these data explanations is provided below; see Guenther (1995a) for further details.

2.1.2 Articulatory variability

Convex region targets provide a natural framework for interpreting data on motor variability in speech: the motor system is careful to control movements along dimensions that are important for a sound (i.e. dimensions with small target ranges), but not movements along dimensions that are not important (those with large target ranges). The model accordingly shows more variability for acoustically unimportant dimensions as compared to acoustically important dimensions. Experimental support for this comes from the study of Perkell and Nelson (1985), who found more articulatory variability along acoustically less important dimensions for the vowels /i/ and /a/. Specifically, this study showed more variability in tongue position along a direction parallel to the vocal tract midline than for the acoustically more important tongue position along a direction perpendicular to the vocal tract midline when subjects produced /i/ and /a/ sounds in different phonetic contexts and at different speaking rates.

2.1.3 Carryover coarticulation

The model's explanation for carryover coarticulation is simple and straightforward: when producing a phoneme from different initial configurations of the vocal tract, different positions on the convex region target will be reached, since the model moves to the closest point on the target region. The end effect of this is that the configuration used to produce a sound will depend on which sound precedes it, with the model choosing a configuration that is as close as possible to the preceding configuration. Figure 2.3 schematizes the situation for the target /k/ in the words 'luke' and 'leak'. The initial front–back position of the tongue body for the

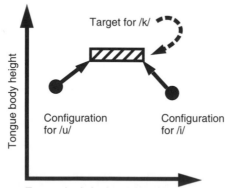

Fig. 2.3 Convex region theory account of carryover coarticulation in /k/ production. Approaching the target for /k/ from the configuration corresponding to the back vowel /u/ in 'luke' leads to a final tongue body configuration that is further back than when approaching from the configuration corresponding to the front vowel /i/ in 'leak'.

preceding vowel determines the configuration of the vocal tract reached for the consonant /k/. When the back vowel /u/ precedes /k/ as in 'luke', the tongue body is further back during /k/ than when the front vowel /i/ precedes /k/ as in 'leak', as seen when English-speaking subjects speak these words (e.g.; Kent and Minifie 1977; Daniloff *et al.* 1980).

2.1.4 Anticipatory coarticulation

The model's explanation of anticipatory coarticulation posits that the target region for a speech sound is reduced in size based on context in order to provide a more efficient sequence of articulator movements. Because the amount of anticipatory coarticulation is limited by the size of the convex region targets in the model, it accounts for experimental results showing decreased coarticulation in cases where smaller targets are necessitated, including speech in languages with more crowded vowel spaces (Manuel 1990), speech hyperarticulated for clarity (Picheney *et al.* 1985, 1986; Lindblom and MacNeilage 1986) and speech hyperarticulated for stress (De Jong *et al.* 1993).

2.2 Hypothesized neural correlates of the DIVA model

One advantage of the neural network approach is that it allows one to analyze the brain regions involved in speech in terms of a well-defined theoretical framework, thus allowing a deeper understanding of the brain mechanisms underlying speech. Figure 2.4 illustrates hypothesized neural correlates for several central components of the DIVA model. These hypotheses are based on a number of neuroanatomical and neurophysiological studies, including lesion/aphasia studies, magnetocn-cephalography (MEG), positron emission tomography (PET), and functional magnetic resonance imaging (fMRI) studies, and single-cell recordings from cortical and subcortical areas in animals.

The pathway labeled 'a' in the figure corresponds to projections from premotor cortex to primary motor cortex, hypothesized to underlie feedforward control of the speech articulators. Pathway b represents hypothesized projections from premotor cortex (lateral BA 6) to higher-order auditory cortical areas in the superior temporal gyrus (BA 22) and orosensory areas in the somatosensory cortex (BA 1,2,3; pathway not shown in figure for clarity) and supramarginal gyrus (BA 40). These 'efference copy' projections are hypothesized to carry target sensations associated with motor plans in premotor cortex. For example, premotor cortex cells representing the syllable /bi/ are hypothesized to project to higher-order auditory cortex cells; these projections represent an expected sound pattern (i.e. the auditory representation of the speaker's own voice while producing /bi/). Similarly, projections from premotor cortex to orosensory areas in the somatosensory cortex and supramarginal gyrus represent the expected pattern of somatosensory

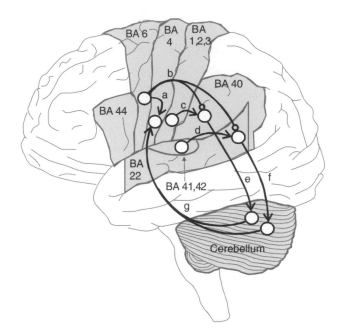

Fig. 2.4 Hypothesized neural correlates of several central components of the DIVA model. BA, Brodmann's Area. See text for details.

stimulation during /bi/ production. Pathway b is hypothesized to encode the convex region targets for speech sounds in the DIVA model, corresponding to the pathway between the 'speech sound map' and 'planning direction vector' in Fig. 2.1.

One interesting aspect of the model in Fig. 2.4 is the role of auditory cortical areas in speech production as well as speech perception. According to the model, auditory 'targets' project from premotor cortical areas to the posterior superior temporal gyrus (pathway b), where they are compared to incoming auditory information from primary auditory cortex (pathway d, corresponding to the pathway between the 'planning position vector' and 'planning direction vector' in Fig. 2.1). The difference between the target and the actual auditory signal represents an 'error' signal that is mapped through the cerebellum (pathway f), which transforms the auditory error into a motor velocity signal that can act to zero this error (pathway g; pathways f and g correspond to the 'directional mapping' in Fig. 2.1). This projection through the cerebellum to motor cortex forms a component of the Directions Into Velocities of Articulators mapping that gives the DIVA model its name. Evidence that auditory cortical areas in the superior temporal gyrus and temporal plane are involved in speech production comes from a number of neuroimaging studies. For example, Hickok *et al.* (2000) report activation in left posterior STG areas (planum temporale, superior temporal sulcus) during a PET visual object naming task in which the subject's auditory feedback of his/her own productions was masked with noise. Bookheimer *et al.* (1995) report activations near primary auditory cortex in a similar task. Paus *et al.* (1996) also reported activation in the area of the left planum temporale during a PET object naming task. These authors attributed this activation to 'motor-to-sensory discharges', compatible with pathway b in Fig. 2.4. This interpretation also receives support from an MEG study by Levelt *et al.* (1998), who showed that the auditory cortical activations during speech production slightly preceded the initiation of articulatory processes. All of these results provide support for the notion of auditory perceptual targets for speech production, in keeping with a central aspect of the DIVA model (e.g. Guenther 1995*b*; Guenther *et al.* 1998; see also Bailly *et al.* 1991; Perkell *et al.* 1995*b*).

The model also proposes a role for the supramarginal gyrus (BA 40) in speech production. This brain region has been implicated in phonological processing for speech perception (e.g. Caplan *et al.* 1995; Celsis *et al.* 1999), as well as speech production (Geschwind 1965; Damasio and Damasio 1980). The current model proposes that, among other things, the supramarginal gyrus represents the difference between target oral sensations (projecting from premotor cortex via pathway b in Fig. 2.4) and the current state of the vocal tract (projecting from somatosensory cortex via pathway c). This difference represents the desired movement direction in orosensory coordinates and is hypothesized to map through the cerebellum to motor cortex, thus constituting a second component of the DIVA mapping.

Not shown in Fig. 2.4, for the sake of clarity, is the insular cortex, buried within the sylvian fissure. The anterior insula has been shown to play an important role in speech articulation (e.g. Dronkers 1996). This region is contiguous with the frontal and central opercula, which include portions of the premotor and motor cortices related to oral movements. We adopt the view that the anterior insula has similar functional properties to the premotor and motor cortices. This view receives support from fMRI studies showing activation of anterior insula during non-speech tongue movements (Corfield *et al.* 1999), PET results showing concurrent primary motor cortex and anterior insula activations during articulation (Fox *et al.* 2001), and PET results showing concurrent lateral premotor cortex and anterior insula activations during articulation (Wise *et al.* 1999).

Also not shown in Fig. 2.4 are the 'forward model' pathways (see Fig. 2.1), which are hypothesized to project from the primary motor cortex (BA 4) to the somatosensory and auditory cortical areas. These pathways are proposed to be used in place of incoming sensory information during rapid speech, when sensory feedback is too slow for the control of ongoing movements.

An important purpose of the model outlined in Fig. 2.4 is to generate predictions that serve as the basis for focused functional imaging studies of brain function during speech. For example, the model of Fig. 2.4 predicts that perturbation of a speech articulator such as the lip during speech should cause an increase in activation in the somatosensory cortex and supramarginal gyrus, since the perturbation will cause a mismatch between orosensory expectations and the actual orosensory feedback signal. The model further predicts that extra activation will be seen in the cerebellum and motor cortex under the perturbed condition, since pathway e in Fig. 2.4 would transmit the extra supramarginal gyrus activation to the cerebellum and on to motor cortex (pathways e, g). We are currently testing these and other predictions of the model using fMRI and MEG.

2.3 Auditory feedback in adult speech production

The model in Fig. 2.1 includes an auditory feedback pathway (left side of figure) that is responsible for the learning and maintenance of three mappings between information in different reference frames. First, articulatory commands are mapped into their expected auditory consequences (the mapping labeled 'forward model' in Fig. 2.1). Secondly, desired movement directions in auditory space are mapped into articulator movements (the 'directional mapping' of Fig. 2.1). These two mappings in the model are 'systemic' mappings, in that they are used for the production of all speech sounds. Auditory feedback is also used to learn a third, 'phoneme-specific' mapping between cells representing speech sounds and corresponding regions in auditory perceptual space (the 'convex region targets' in Fig. 2.1). The components of this mapping are specific to a particular phoneme or syllable. For example, a cell representing the phoneme /i/ in the model's speech sound map will be mapped into a target region of auditory space that corresponds to the sound /i/.

It is well known that people born deaf usually have a very difficult time learning how to speak intelligibly. On the other hand, if someone is born with hearing, learns how to speak, and then becomes deaf, that person is often able to continue speaking intelligibly for decades without being able to hear. These basic observations support the idea that learning how to speak involves establishing neural mappings such as those shown in Fig. 2.1 under conditions of auditory feedback, and that if deafness occurs after establishment of these mappings, they can remain fairly accurate for years as long as the relationship between articulatory and auditory parameters remains constant. Thus, a full-grown adult who becomes deaf would be expected to maintain fairly accurate mappings, while a child that becomes deaf would be expected to show degradation of the mappings relating articulatory and auditory parameters, due to growth-induced changes in the geometry of the vocal tract (which change the auditory–articulatory relationship).

In order to better characterize these mappings, we have been investigating the role of auditory feedback in adult speech production by observing changes in speech that occur in response to changes in hearing status, such as the loss of hearing due to disease or the acquisition of some hearing from a cochlear implant (CI). Six of these studies are described briefly below, along with observations about how their results are related to the model.

2.3.1 Learned neural mappings are generally stable after onset of deafness

The long-term stability of learned neural mappings is exemplified by the predominantly normal vowel formant patterns seen for two female CI users, FA and FB, in Fig. 2.5. The figure shows sets of average F1 and F2 values (upper and lower panels) arranged by vowel for the two speakers (left and right panels). The small squares connected by dotted lines show normative values from Peterson and Barney (1952). The values indicated by unfilled circles are pre-implant, and those indicated by filled circles are 1–2 years post-implant. The error bars indicate one standard error about the mean.

For the most part, overall vowel formant patterns (relations of formant values to one another among the vowels) appear to be relatively congruent with the normative patterns, even years after the onset of profound hearing loss (Perkell *et al.* 1992). The most prominent exception to this observation is for FA. Eighteen years after the onset of her profound hearing loss, pre-implant F2 values among her front vowels /i/, /I/, /ɛ/ and /æ/ were somewhat disordered with respect to the Peterson and Barney data, primarily due to relatively high values for /ɛ/ and especially /æ/. As indicated by the filled circles, after about a year with prosthetic

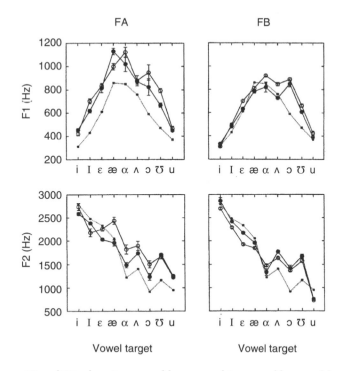

Fig. 2.5 Average F1 and F2 values (upper and lower panels) arranged by vowel for two female CI users (left and right panels).

hearing, these F2 values are more in line with the Peterson and Barney pattern. Thus, FA's abnormal pre-implant F2 pattern was 'corrected' toward the normative pattern after some months of implant use. We hypothesize that this correction was due to a retuning of neural mappings using auditory feedback available from the cochlear implant.

2.3.2 Goals for the fricative consonants /s/ and /ʃ/ are also generally stable

Figure 2.6 shows values of spectral median and symmetry for /s/ and /ʃ/ produced in carrier phrases by three of five cochlear implant users studied by Matthies *et al.* (1994). The measurements, which reflect acoustically and perceptually salient differences between /s/ and /ʃ/, were made pre-implant, within a few months after implant and 6 months post-implant. Pre-implant, as exemplified by FA and MB, four of the five subjects had higher values of spectral median for /s/ than for /ʃ/, higher values of symmetry for /ʃ/ than /s/ and clear separation between the /s/ and /ʃ/ values. These results indicate a good distinction between the two consonants pre-implant—even decades following the onset of profound deafness.

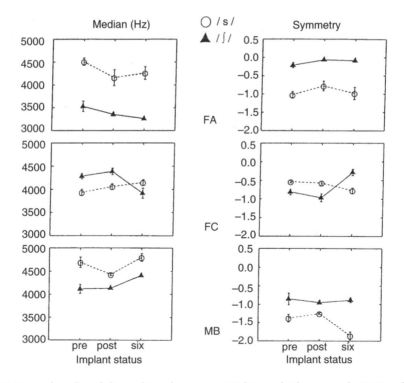

Fig. 2.6 Spectral median (left panels) and symmetry (right panels) for one male (MB) and two female (FA, FC) CI users.

The good pre-implant distinctions between the sibilants in four of the subjects indicate that their systemic and phoneme-specific mappings for the production of /s/ and /ʃ/ were generally quite stable, even in the prolonged absence of auditory feedback. On the other hand, the fifth subject (FC) had reversed values of the two measures pre-implant (consistent with the experimenters' impression that her sibilants were quite distorted), indicating an unusually extreme distortion of her neural mappings. After months of implant use, FC's spectral median and symmetry values were greatly improved. We believe this improvement resulted from a corrective retuning of the neural mappings after she received the cochlear implant.

2.3.3 There are systematic relations among changes in perception, production, and intelligibility

We have hypothesized that if changes are observed in phonemic contrasts after speakers gain hearing with a CI, those changes are in the direction of improved contrast and they are driven by the speaker's motivation to enhance intelligibility. To test this hypothesis in some detail, we gathered speech production, perception, and intelligibility data for the liquids /r/ and /l/ spoken in carrier phrases by eight postlingually deaf adults, pre- and post-implant with a CI. Formant transition analysis for the CI speakers and two speakers with normal hearing indicated that /r/ and /l/ could be differentiated by the extent of the F3 transition from vowel beginning to mid-vowel and the distance in Hz between F2 and F3 at the C–V boundary. Speakers who had a limited contrast between /r/ and /l/ pre-implant and who showed improvement in their perception of these consonants with prosthetic hearing were found to demonstrate greatly improved production of /r/ and /l/ 6 months post-CI. The speech production changes noted in the acoustic analyses were corroborated by intelligibility improvements in the post-CI speech, as measured with a panel of normal-hearing listeners. Figure 2.7 shows an example of enhanced contrast between /r/ and /l/ for a male CI user, from pre- to post-implant (Matthies *et al.* 2003). We have also observed similar results for vowels: significant covariation of perception and production, and of production and intelligibility (Vick *et al.* 2001*a*; see also Gould *et al.* 2001).

Intelligibility is usually quite good in postlingually deafened candidates for cochlear implants; nevertheless, we have observed gains in sentence intelligibility in subjects who had some room for improvement (Vick *et al.* 2001*b*). Such findings indicate that speakers are quite sensitive to intelligibility decrements after implantation and presumably can retune neural mappings even with the relatively crude auditory stimulation supplied by implants.

2.3.4 A change in the vocal tract may invalidate systemic mappings

We have made another observation of the /s–ʃ/ contrast, from a subject, FD, who lost hearing due to bilateral acoustic neuromas (NF-2). The subject had tumor-removal

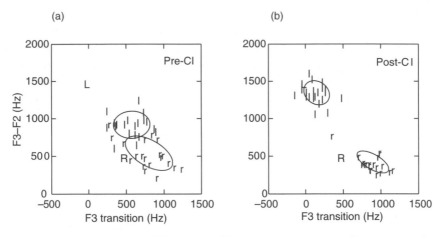

Fig. 2.7 Separation between F3 and F2 at vowel beginning versus extent of F3 transition from vowel beginning to mid-vowel for preceding /r/ and /l/ in a carrier phrase, spoken by a male CI user. (Capital letters indicate normative data.) (a) Pre-implant; (b) data pooled from 6 and 12 months post-implant.

surgery that severed her remaining auditory nerve (Perkell *et al*. 1995a). At the time of surgery, she received an early version of an auditory brainstem implant, which effectively provided her with auditory envelope but not spectral cues. Figure 2.8 shows spectral median versus week from her onset of hearing loss (OHL) for /s/ and /ʃ/. Before OHL, and continuing for over 70 weeks post-OHL, FD maintained a good contrast between the two sounds.

At week 72, FD had another surgery, this time to anastomose her left hypoglossal nerve to the facial nerve, in an attempt to restore some facial function that had also been lost at the time of tumor-removal surgery. The anastomosis surgery denervated some tongue muscles on the left side, producing a slight tongue weakness that effectively altered a functional property of the vocal tract. Without auditory feedback about the sibilant contrast to help the control mechanism develop a compensatory adaptation to the tongue weakness, the contrast gradually collapsed. In terms of the model in Fig. 2.1, the anastomosis surgery invalidated systemic mappings between auditory and articulatory parameters by changing a characteristic of the low-level control of the 'biomechanical plant'. Due to the subject's hearing loss, it was then impossible for her to update the mappings by making auditorily based adjustments. Since people with normal hearing are capable of compensating for significant changes in vocal-tract morphology (e.g. with the initial insertion of dentures), we assume that if this speaker had adequate hearing, she would have been able to compensate for the surgery, even though it resulted in some slight tongue weakness.

The fact that the collapse in contrast was gradual after the tongue surgery may be due to the speaker relying on a combination of auditory and somatosensory

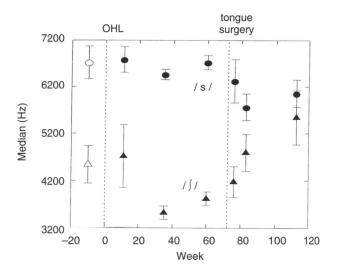

Fig. 2.8 Spectral median for /s/ and /{P1}/ versus time in weeks from a subject who lost hearing (at time OHL) due to removal of an acoustic neuroma.

feedback. Without auditory spectral feedback to reinforce the somatosensory input, the latter gradually became inadequate to maintain the contrast. Although the model as presented in this paper deals primarily with auditory goals and feedback, other versions incorporate the idea that the goals for some sounds, especially consonants, include orosensory components (Guenther 1995a; Perkell 1997).

2.3.5 Language-specific, hearing-related changes in vowel spaces may reflect a trade-off between phonemic contrast and economy of effort

Another important feature of the model summarized in Fig. 2.1 is that movements for a sequence of phonemes are planned to afford an economy of effort (Guenther 1995a; see also Lindblom 1983; Keating 1990). This is accomplished by planning an auditory trajectory that passes through the parts of the auditory goal regions that are closest to those of the neighboring sounds in the sequence. In this study, two hypotheses were tested that are derived from the view that vowel production is influenced by competing demands of intelligibility for the listener and least effort in the speaker:

1. Hearing enables a CI user to produce vowels distinctly from one another; without hearing, the speaker may give more weight to economy of effort, leading to reduced vowel distinctiveness.
2. Speakers may need to produce vowels more distinctly from one another in a language with a relatively 'crowded' vowel space, such as American English, than in a language with relatively few vowels, such as Spanish. Thus, when

switching between hearing and non-hearing states, English speakers may show a trade-off between vowel distinctiveness and least effort, while Spanish speakers may not.

To test these hypotheses, we predicted that there would be a reduction of average vowel spacing (AVS, average inter-vowel distance in the F1–F2 plane) with inter-rupted hearing for English-speaking CI users, but no systematic change in AVS for Spanish CI users. We recorded vowel productions of seven English- and seven Spanish-speaking CI users, who had been using their implants for at least 1 year. When their implant speech processors were turned off and on several times in two sessions, we found that AVS was consistently larger for the English speakers with hearing than without hearing. The presence and direction of AVS change was more variable for the Spanish speakers, both within and between subjects. Thus, vowel distinctiveness was enhanced with the provision of some hearing in the language group with a more crowded vowel space but not in the language group with fewer vowels. This result supports the view that speakers seek to minimize effort while maintaining the distinctiveness of auditory goals.

2.3.6 Changes in phonemic contrasts can be quite rapid

We have observed previously that the kinds of contrast changes cited above can occur quite rapidly, almost as soon as a CI user's speech processor is switched on or off (Svirsky *et al.* 1992). In this study, we investigated such changes in more detail, comparing changes in vowel sound pressure level (SPL) and duration with those in phonemic contrasts between the vowels /ɛ/ and /æ/ and the sibilants /s/ and /ʃ/. An apparatus was built to switch the speech processor of a subject's implant on and off a number of times in a single experimental session while the subject repeated a large number of utterances containing the target sounds. Two normal-hearing subjects performed the same paradigm, except that the 'on' condition consisted of hearing their own speech fed back to them over a set of headphones and the 'off' condition consisted of hearing loud noise that masked their speech. Using the times of on–off or off–on switches as line-up points for averaging, param-eters were compared across the switches.

The speakers' vowel SPL and duration had changed by the first utterance follow-ing the switch. The top half of Fig. 2.9 shows changes in vowel contrast, defined as the Euclidian distance in F1–F2 space between /ɛ/ and /æ/. The bottom half shows change in sibilant contrast, defined as the difference between the spectral median of /s/ and /ʃ/. There are four bars for each subject, corresponding to the change from the off to on condition averaged over 50 s on either side of the switch (1), the change from the tokens immediately before to immediately after the switch (2), and the corresponding on-to-off changes (3 and 4). Shaded bars represent significant changes ($P < 0.05$). All the significant changes but two (vowel contrasts for subject FH, bars 1 and 3) are consistent with the prediction that contrast is

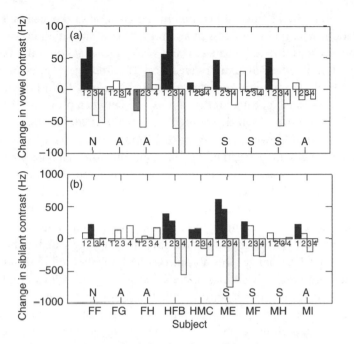

Fig. 2.9 (a) Change in vowel contrast, defined as the Euclidian distance in F1–F2 space between /e/ and /æ/. (b) Change in sibilant contrast, defined as the difference between the spectral median of /s/ and /{P1}/. Subjects HFB and HMC have normal hearing. The darkest gray bars indicate significant off-to-on changes in the predicted direction; the lightest gray bars indicate significant on-to-off changes; the bars with intermediate shading indicate significant changes opposite to the predicted direction.

enhanced in the presence of hearing and diminished without hearing. Further, the changes in phonemic parameters are just as rapid as those for SPL. The model has a mechanism for making phonemic changes as rapid as those described here. This is done using a control parameter that rapidly scales the sizes of all goal regions (Guenther 1995*a*).

2.4 Summary and discussion

Section 2.3 described studies and interpretations that are largely compatible with the model of speech motor control outlined in Sections 2.1 and 2.2. In the model, speech movements are planned to achieve sequences of auditory goals, in a way that provides an economy of effort. The planning utilizes two kinds of mappings, phoneme-specific (language-specific) and systemic (speaker-specific). The mappings are acquired with the use of auditory feedback and rely on auditory feedback for their maintenance over the course of a lifetime. In general, the experimental results support the interpretation that, once learned, the neural mappings are stable, even in the absence of hearing. In the collapse of the sibilant contrast in an NF-2 patient who had lost access to auditory spectral information, we suggested that the collapse was due to a change in the vocal tract that could not be compensated for without the needed auditory feedback. The finding of systematic increases in average vowel spacing with the provision of hearing by a CI in English speakers, but not in Spanish speakers, may reflect a trade-off between phonemic contrast and economy of effort, both of which are predicted by the model to guide articulatory trajectories. Studies of vowels and the /r/–/l/ contrast demonstrated systematic relations among changes in perception, production, and intelligibility, leading to the inference that speakers are quite sensitive to decrements in their intelligibility and can correct them with access to even the relatively crude auditory stimulation provided by a CI. Finally, the rapid changes in phonemic contrasts described in Section 2.3.6 suggest that, although full retuning of systemic mappings may take a long time, some aspects of the phoneme-specific mapping can be changed very rapidly. In the model, changes this abrupt can be implemented by a single neural control signal that effectively shrinks or expands all the goal regions simultaneously.

We are still far from being able to establish quantitative relations between the modeling and experimental work in this area. Nevertheless, when considered collectively, our experimental results provide strong qualitative support for the modeling approach, and as exemplified by the above-cited examples, they can provide insights that may strongly influence model development. In the long run, we believe that this combination of modeling and experimentation will move us closer to understanding neural processes underlying relations between speech perception and production, and to a coherent account of speech processes in people with normal speech and hearing and in clinical populations.

Acknowledgements

This research was supported by the National Institute on Deafness and other Communication Disorders (grants R01 DC02852 to F. Guenther; R01 DC03007 to J. Perkell).

References

Bailly, G., Laboissière, R., and **Schwartz, J.L.** (1991). Formant trajectories as audible gestures: An alternative for speech synthesis. *Journal of Phonetics*, **19**, 9–23.

Bookheimer, S.Y., Zeffiro, T.A., Blaxton, T., Gaillard, W., and **Theodore, W.** (1995). Regional cerebral blood flow during object naming and word reading. *Human Brain Mapping*, **3**, 93–106.

Callan, D., Kent, R., Guenther, F.H., and **Vorperian, H.K.** (2000). An auditory-feedback-based neural network model of speech production that is robust to developmental changes in the size and shape of the articulatory system. *Journal of Speech, Language and Hearing Research,* **43**, 721–736.

Caplan, D., Gow, D., and Makris, N. (1995). Analysis of lesions by MRI in stroke patients with acoustic–phonetic processing deficits. *Neurology,* **45**, 293–298.

Celsis, P., Boulanouar, K., Ranjeva, J.P., Berry, I., Nespoulous, J.L., and Chollet, F. (1999). Differential fMRI responses in the left posterior superior temporal gyrus and left supramarginal gyrus to habituation and change detection in syllables and tones. *NeuroImage,* **9**, 135–144.

Corfield, D.R., Murphy, K., Josephs, O., Fink, G.R., Frackowiak, R.S.J., Guz, A., Adams, L., and Turner, R. (1999). Cortical and subcortical control of tongue movement in humans: A functional neuroimaging study using fMRI. *Journal of Applied Physiology,* **85**, 1468–1477.

Damasio, H. and Damasio, A.R. (1980). The anatomical basis of conduction aphasia. *Brain,* **103**, 337–350.

Daniloff, R., Schuckers, G., and Feth, L. (1980). *The Physiology of Speech and Hearing: An Introduction.* Englewood Cliffs NJ: Prentice-Hall.

De Jong, K., Beckman, M.E., and Edwards, J. (1993). The interplay between prosodic structure and coarticulation. *Language and Speech,* **36**, 197–212.

Dronkers, N.F. (1996). A new brain region for coordinating speech articulation. *Nature,* **384**, 159–161.

Fox, P.T., Huang, A., Parsons, L.M., Xiong, J., Zamarippa, F., Rainey, L., and Lancaster, J.L. (2001). Location-probability profiles for the mouth region of human primary motor-sensory cortex: Model and validation. *NeuroImage,* **13**, 196–209.

Geschwind, N. (1965). Disconnexion syndromes in animals and man. I. *Brain,* **88**, 237–294.

Gould, J., Lane, H., Perkell, J., Vick, J., Matthies, M., and Zandipour, M. (2001). Changes in the intelligibility of postlingually deaf adults after cochlear implantation. *Ear and Hearing,* **22**, 453–460.

Guenther, F.H. (1994). A neural network model of speech acquisition and motor equivalent speech production. *Biological Cybernetics,* **72**, 43–53.

Guenther, F.H. (1995a). Speech sound acquisition, coarticulation, and rate effects in a neural network model of speech production. *Psychological Review,* **102**, 594–621.

Guenther, F.H. (1995b). A modeling framework for speech motor development and kinematic articulator control. *Proceedings of the XIIIth International Conference of Phonetic Sciences* (vol. 2, pp. 92–99). Stockholm, Sweden: KTH and Stockholm University.

Guenther, F.H. and Micci Barreca, D. (1997). Neural models for flexible control of redundant systems. In P. Morasso and V. Sanguineti (eds), *Self-organization, Computational Maps, and Motor Control* (pp. 383–421). Amsterdam: Elsevier-North Holland.

Guenther, F.H., Hampson, M., and **Johnson, D.** (1998). A theoretical investigation of reference frames for the planning of speech movements. *Psychological Review,* **105,** 611–633.

Hickok, G., Erhard, P., Kassubek, J., Helms-Tillery, A.K., Naeve-Velguth, S., Strupp, J.P., Strick, P.L., and **Ugurbil, K.** (2000). A functional magnetic resonance imaging study of the role of left posterior superior temporal gyrus in speech production: Implications for the explanation of conduction aphasia. *Neuroscience Letters,* **287,** 156–160.

Keating, P.A. (1990). The window model of coarticulation: Articulatory evidence. In J. Kingston and M.E. Beckman (eds), *Papers in Laboratory Phonology I: Between the Grammar and Physics of Speech* (pp. 451–470). Cambridge: Cambridge University Press.

Kent, R.D. and **Minifie, F.D.** (1977). Coarticulation in recent speech production models. *Journal of Phonetics,* **5,** 115–133.

Levelt, W.J.M., Praamstra, P., Meyer, A.S., Helenius, P., and **Salmelin, R.** (1998). An MEG study of picture naming. *Journal of Cognitive Neuroscience,* **10,** 553–567.

Liégeois, A. (1977). Automatic supervisory control of the configuration and behavior of multibody mechanisms. *IEEE Transactions on Systems, Man, and Cybernetics,* **7**(12), 869–871.

Lindblom, B. (1983). Economy of speech gestures. In P.F. MacNeilage (ed.), *The production of speech* (pp. 217–245). New York: Springer-Verlag.

Lindblom, B. and **MacNeilage, P.F.** (1986). Action theory: Problems and alternative approaches. *Journal of Phonetics,* **14,** 117–132.

Manuel, S.Y. (1990). The role of contrast in limiting vowel-to-vowel coarticulation in different languages. *Journal of the Acoustical Society of America,* **88,** 1286–1298.

Matthies, M.L., Svirsky, M.A., Lane, H., and **Perkell, J.S.** (1994). A preliminary study of the effects of cochlear implants on the production of sibilants. *Journal of the Acoustical Society of America,* **96,** 1367–1373.

Matthies, M., Vick, J., Perkell, J., Lane, H., Zandipour, M., and **Gould, J.** (2003). Effects of cochlear implants on the speech production, perception, and intelligibility of the liquids /r/ and /l/, in preparation.

Paus, T., Perry, D.W., Zatorre, R.J., Worsley, K.J., and **Evans, A.C.** (1996). Modulation of cerebral blood flow in the human auditory cortex during speech: Role of motor-to-sensory discharges. *European Journal of Neuroscience,* **8,** 2236–2246.

Perkell, J.S. (1997). Articulatory processes. In W. Hardcastle and J. Laver (eds) *The Handbook of Phonetic Sciences,* (pp. 333–370). Oxford, UK: Blackwell.

Perkell, J.S. and **Nelson, W.L.** (1985). Variability in production of the vowels /i/ and /a/. *Journal of the Acoustical Society of America,* **77,** 1889–1895.

Perkell, J., Lane, H., Svirsky, M., and **Webster, J.** (1992). Speech of cochlear implant patients: A longitudinal study of vowel production. *Journal of the Acoustical Society of America,* **91,** 2961–2979.

Perkell, J., Manzella, J., Wozniak, J., Matthies, M., Lane, H., Svirsky, M., Guiod, P., Delhorne, L., Short, P., MacCollin, M., and **Mitchell, C.** (1995a). Changes in speech production following hearing loss due to bilateral acoustic neuromas. *Proceedings of the XIIIth International Congress of Phonetic Sciences,* (vol. 3, pp. 194–197). Stockholm, Sweden: KTH and Stockholm University.

Perkell, J.S., Matthies, M.L., Svirsky, M.A., and **Jordan, M.I.** (1995b). Goal-based speech motor control: A theoretical framework and some preliminary data. *Journal of Phonetics,* **23**, 23–35.

Perkell, J., Guenther, F., Lane, H., Matthies, M., Perrier, P., Vick, J., Wilhelms-Tricarico, R., and **Zandipour, M.** (2000). A theory of speech motor control and supporting data from speakers with normal hearing and with profound hearing loss. *Journal of Phonetics,* **28**, 233–272.

Peterson, G.E. and **Barney, H.L.** (1952). Control methods used in a study of the vowels. *Journal of the Acoustical Society of America,* **24**, 175–184.

Picheny, M.A., Durlach, N.I., and **Braida, L.D.** (1985). Speaking clearly for the hard of hearing I: Intelligibility differences between clear and conversational speech. *Journal of Speech and Hearing Research,* **28**, 96–103.

Picheny, M.A., Durlach, N.I., and **Braida, L.D.** (1986). Speaking clearly for the hard of hearing II: Acoustic characteristics of clear and conversational speech. *Journal of Speech and Hearing Research,* **29**, 434–446.

Saltzman, E.L. and **Munhall, K.G.** (1989). A dynamical approach to gestural patterning in speech production. *Ecological Psychology,* **1**, 333–382.

Svirsky, M., Lane, H., Perkell, J., and **Webster, J.** (1992). Speech of cochlear implant patients: Results of a short-term auditory deprivation study. *Journal of the Acoustical Society of America,* **92**, 1284–1300.

Vick, J., Lane, H., Perkell, J., Matthies, M., Gould, J., and **Zandipour, M.** (2001a). Speech perception, production and intelligibility improvements in vowel-pair contrasts in adults who receive cochlear implants. *Journal of Speech, Language and Hearing Research,* **44**, 1257–1268.

Vick, J., Lane, H., Perkell, J., Zandipour, M. and **Matthies, M.** (2001b). Sentence intelligibility in adults who receive cochlear implants. Poster presented at the 2001 Conference on Implanted Auditory Prostheses, Asilomar, CA.

Wise, R.J., Greene, J., Buchel, C., and **Scott, S.K.** (1999). Brain regions involved in articulation. *Lancet,* **353**, 1057–1061.

CHAPTER 3

DYNAMICAL SYSTEMS THEORY AND ITS APPLICATION IN SPEECH

PASCAL H.H.M. VAN LIESHOUT

3.1 Introduction

In our daily activities, we accomplish a great number of different, often complex tasks without giving them much thought, while we execute them in a seemingly effortless way. We walk, we pick up objects, we write or type, we chew and swallow, and, unlike other animals, we speak. Speech is probably the most complex motor behaviour humans can perform. This complexity alone is a formidable challenge to any theoretical approach to motor control, but in addition, speech lends itself less to the specific type of manipulations that are commonly used to study underlying control mechanisms in other motor tasks. Other complicating issues for speech research are potential influences of cognitive/linguistic processes on motor control in using real words or longer utterances (e.g. van Lieshout *et al.* 1995; Maner *et al.* 2000).

This chapter will review the application of a particular theoretical background to speech production. This theoretical background consists of a group of different views that, for the sake of convenience, are summarized in the term 'dynamical systems theory' (DST). DST has major applications in motor control and other areas of research. This review will highlight those DST studies that have been conducted in the area of speech (Section 3.2) and discuss some potential future developments (Section 3.3). A short historical outline of this approach will be presented first.

3.1.1 The history of DST

A basic way to address the underlying mechanisms of motor actions is in terms of 'control', with the understanding that 'one process (the controller) controlling another (the plant) in the service of some goal or desired end state' (Pressing 1998, p. 362). In the post-Second World War era of the twentieth century, partly due to a tremendous boost from significant developments in computers, the concept of a 'motor program' became immensely popular. The 'motor program' (or as some prefer 'motor plan') has gone through many stages in its history (for recent reviews, see, for example, Summers 1992; Pressing 1998). This approach is characterized by a heavy 'loan' on intelligence, using metaphorical terms like 'executive', 'comparator' and 'observer' to explain organized patterns of behaviour. In other words, there is always something (the so-called 'homunculus') that needs to be in control of the controller. Basically, a motor program approach focuses on discrete features for (a) particular (class of) actions, but it does not provide an account of how these actions actually evolve in time, space, and context. Organized behaviour (pattern formation) is imposed externally by heuristically derived memory-based instructions, ignoring the fact that many patterns in nature may evolve spontaneously in the appropriate context without the need, or even availability, of such instructions (see below).

In response to the issues mentioned above, a radically different view towards motor control and its coupling to perceptual information was formulated in the early 1980s in a, now classic, paper by Kugler *et al.* (1980). These authors and their colleagues (for reviews, see Beek *et al.* 1995; Sternad 2000) promoted the notions of synergy and self-organization in perception–action coupling, or in more general pattern formation. They also referred to the ecological approach as defined by Gibson (Gibson 1966; for a review, see Michaels and Beek 1995), stressing the intimate relationship between an action and the environment in which it takes place.

The concept of a synergy or coordinative structure is originally derived from Bernstein (1967) and can be defined as 'highly evolved task-specific ensembles of neuromuscular and skeletal components constrained to act as a single unit' (Kelso 1998, p. 205). Kugler *et al.* (1982) specifically tied the concept of coordinative structures to the notion of spontaneous pattern formation or self-organization derived from existing theories on non-equilibrium thermodynamics and synergetics in physics (Haken 1983). Self-organization in non-animate, so-called open systems refers to the fact that due to the number and nature of interactions between the individual components of such a system, patterns can form and dissolve spontaneously (cf. Kelso 2000). In such dynamical systems, the pattern that eventually will emerge is defined by current values of so-called *control parameters*, which, depending on the kind of system, can be anything from naturally occurring environmental influences to specific externally imposed manipulations that move the system through certain states. For example, if a person is required to increase pace (= control parameter) during walking, he/she will show transitions to well-defined relatively stable gait patterns (walking → jogging → running; these labels are just used for easy reference) at specific, individually based, velocity thresholds. For certain velocity ranges, a pattern will be maintained until it is no longer efficient (in terms of, for example, energy costs). At that point, the system would tend to move away from the existing pattern towards a more optimal pattern. These behavioural states (walking, jogging, running) reflect the presence of inherently preferred solutions or attractors, induced by physical (e.g.

Diedrich and Warren 1995) and/or functional constraints (Kelso 1995). The latter illustrates that one can opt to maintain the same pattern or elect to establish a different solution (like speed walking), even at a cost (e.g. more effort or physical discomfort). That is, functional constraints are based on intention or purpose, thus defining an attractor in the control space within the range of possibilities as determined by the physically based attractors (referred to as intrinsic) of a given system.

A more formalized illustration of how a dynamical system can generate quite different patterns based on changes in a (in this case) single control parameter is shown in Fig. 3.1. The patterns are generated using the logistic map, a one-dimensional discrete dynamical system expressed by the following difference equation:

$$X_{n+1} = rX_n[1 - X_n] \tag{3.1}$$

This equation describes a lawful relationship between previous and current states of this system or, in other words, the system is deterministic. For example, it can be used to model population dynamics, in which case parameter r is the control parameter for growth rate. A particular value for r influences the nature of changes in number of individuals in biological populations (X) from one time period to the next. What is typical for this model is that for higher values of r, these changes make a very dramatic shift from ordinary quasi-regular behaviour. Compare the output of this system for different values of r, as shown in Fig. 3.1 for $r = 0.5$; 2.0; 3.2; 3.54; and 3.9 (initial value $X_0 = 0.2$) for a small number ($n = 100$) of iterations.

For $r < 0$ (Fig. 3.1AI), the system converges to a zero output (a point attractor effectively); for $0 < r < 3$ the system also converges to a single value or point attractor, but this time it is not zero (Fig. 3.1AII). In fact, it will differ with r. In general, for $r < 3$ all outputs eventually converge to a stable steady-state solution. For $3 < r < 3.5$ the system will alternate between two values, which can be referred to as a two-point attractor (Fig. 3.1B). The period doubling that occurs at this stage, is technically referred to as a *bifurcation*, although the term has been given a somewhat broader interpretation in other literature (Kelso 1995). Increasing r beyond 3.5 will induce a more complicated behaviour, which is evident of the presence of multiple attractors (in this case 4; Fig. 3.1C). With values of $r > 3.99$, the system essentially turns chaotic (Fig. 3.1D), a concept that will be explained in more detail in Section 3.2.4. Being chaotic, the system is highly sensitive to differences in initial conditions, as shown in Fig. 3.2 for near identical values of X_0 (2.0 versus 2.1). Notice how even after a small number of iterations, the two trajectories clearly diverge (for an excellent introduction to these topics, see Liebovitch 1998).

Similar to the way in which water changes from ice to steady-state liquid to a boiling state as we vary water temperature (control parameter), the patterns and changes shown in Fig. 3.1, as they unfold in time, are not prescribed by an external representation or plan; they emerge from the intrinsic properties of the system itself for a specific control parameter value. The logistic map equation is used as a

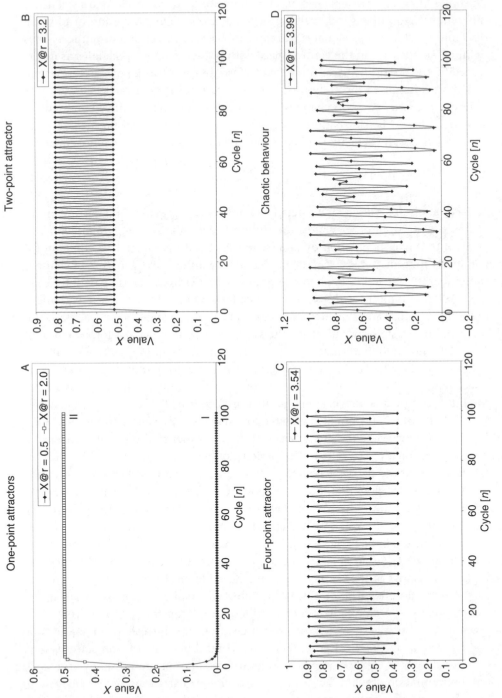

Fig. 3.1 Logistic map output for different control parameter (*r*) values (see text for more details).

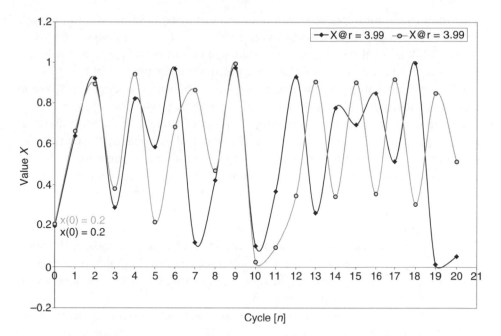

Fig. 3.2 Logistic map output for same r-value (3.99), but with different initial values ($X_0 = 0.21$ or 0.20), showing sensitivity to initial conditions in the way patterns quickly diverge from common trajectories (see the text for more details).

model for changes in rhythmic aspects of speech, as will be discussed in Section 3.2.

Although control parameters influence the nature of behaviours that will emerge from a system, the relationship between behaviours and control parameter settings is not a simple linear one, as the logistic map example clearly shows. For a given range of control parameter values, the system can display similar behaviours, which will only change in a qualitative sense after a critical value is reached. In order to capture these changes in behavioural states within a system, DST uses the concept of an *order parameter* or collective variable (Kelso 2000). For example, returning to the gait example described above, the different gait patterns (walking, jogging, running) can be characterized by specific values for an appropriate order parameter (e.g. relative phase relationships between components of the limbs), which remain relatively stable within certain velocity ranges, but become unstable (more variable) and eventually change at the bifurcation points (e.g. Diedrich and Warren 1995). Whereas control parameters govern change in a system, order parameters reflect, and at the same time prescribe the limits for, the behaviours in a system under the specified values of the control parameter(s). This phenomenon has been dubbed the principle of *circular causality* (Kelso 1995).

As mentioned, there are numerous examples of systems in physics and biology where spontaneous pattern formations can be observed (see, for example, Liebovitch 1998). Think about the weather, the coordinated behaviour of a school of fish or a flock of birds, the orbit of a moon around a planet, the distribution of blood vessels in the lungs, etc. Thus, it seems a small step to extrapolate the same principle and apply it to movement coordination as being the orderly product of 'complex organizations that are composed of a very large number of interacting elements and that may adapt in a flexible manner to changing internal and external conditions by adopting a flexible coordination pattern without any explicit prescription of this pattern' (Beek *et al.* 1995, p. 577). As mentioned before, in a DST perspective actions do not stand on their own, but rather reflect a coupling with the environment in which they occur (Gibson 1966, 1979). If we interact with our environment, information is provided that specifies possibilities for further action ('affordance' in Gibson's terms) in relationship to our own frame of reference (Morasso *et al.* 1998). Action–perception coupling has been studied most extensively in different kinds of non-speech tasks, but speech may provide another fruitful domain for research in this area, as will be discussed in Section 3.2.

This synopsis shows that the DST approach that was promoted originally by Michael Turvey and colleagues (Kugler *et al.* 1982) integrated existing notions from physics and psychology into a coherent new way of thinking on action and perception in complex living systems such as humans. This chapter will not delve into past and existing controversies between opponents of motor programming views and DST, as many reviews have been written on this issue (e.g. Summers 1992; Beek *et al.* 1995; Michaels and Beek 1995; Kelso 1998; Pressing 1998; Sternad 2000; Schöner 2002). Nor will it go into broader applications of DST outside the realm of speech, as this falls outside the scope of this chapter (but see Port and van Gelder 1995; Guastello 2001). Although certain issues remain controversial, in particular with respect to the interpretation of noise in neural systems (Kelso 1998; Newell and Slifkin 1998; Riley and Turvey 2002; see also Section 3.3), there is a tendency for more mutual understanding and convergence, as indicated in a recent special issue of *Brain and Cognition* (**48**, 2002). Some have even argued that there is no controversy between representation and self-organization, and we could allow for both mechanisms in control systems (van Ingen Schenau *et al.* 1995; Pressing 1998) as long as we can agree on the nature of 'representation'. For example, the model proposed by Morasso *et al.* (1998) integrates dynamical systems theory with internal representations as defined by neural activation patterns (referred to as 'population codes') that emerge as attractor states within highly interconnected neural networks.

3.2 Non-linear dynamical systems theory as applied to speech

This section will highlight the role of dynamical systems theory as applied to speech production and perception. Although the number of papers in this area is relatively small, several original contributions have emerged in the past 10–15 years. For space limitations, this review will focus on the notion of a synergy, coupling dynamics and self-organization, and Chaos in speech. The first model that will be discussed is task dynamics (TD), as it is probably the best-known example of a DST perspective on speech.

3.2.1 The task dynamics model

The notion of a synergy entails a form of corporation among muscles and joints that act together as a functional unit to accomplish certain task goals (Bernstein 1967; Kugler *et al.* 1982). A popular way to test the presence of a synergy is to perturb the system, which, in the case of an existing synergy, would be followed by an immediate and task-specific compensation, such as to preserve the intended task goal. This principle was tested and confirmed for speech-related movements in a number of experiments in the early and mid-1980s (e.g. Folkins and Zimmermann 1982; Abbs and Gracco 1984; Kelso *et al.* 1984). More recent work has also demonstrated that such synergies might even extend beyond the components within a specific subsystem in the form of functional couplings between the anatomically and physiologically diverse subsystems of phonation and articulation (Bauer *et al.* 1995; Saltzman *et al.* 1998). The study by Saltzman and colleagues demonstrated that mechanical perturbations to the lower lip elicited an immediate phase shift within and between (but smaller) bilabial and laryngeal gestures, which persisted even after the system returned to its pre-perturbation steady-state rhythm. This was true especially when the perturbation was delivered at the initiation or acceleration of the bilabial closing movement. These data supported the claim that the control of intergestural timing (bilabial and laryngeal) can be influenced by changes in peripheral articulatory events. This indicates a bi-directional coupling between central and peripheral processes (see also Section 3.3), a hallmark characteristic of complex dynamical systems. The data also indicated that phasing relationships within gestures are more stable than those between gestures (where the largest phase shifts were found). These findings in speech, as well as in other motor tasks, led to the formulation and further development of the task-dynamics approach (Fowler *et al.* 1980; Saltzman and Kelso 1987; Saltzman and Munhall 1989; Saltzman and Byrd 2000).

The task-dynamics model has a very specific goal, namely to 'reconcile the linguistic hypothesis that speech involves an underlying sequence of abstract, discrete, context-independent units, with the empirical observation of continuous, context-dependent interleaving of articulatory movements' (Saltzman and Munhall 1989, p. 333; see also Fowler 1995). Instead of the more traditional linguistic units (phonemes or distinctive features), the task-dynamics approach promotes invariant speech-related action units, called gestural primitives or, simply, gestures. The task-dynamic model specifies three levels of coordination (for specific examples see Saltzman and Munhall 1989). The highest level involves the *gestural score*, which details the abstract task-specific activation patterns for different gestures over time. It is at this level that language-specific details can be implemented, and since this is traditionally the domain of phonology, the gestural score level has been developed separately in a linguistic model called the gestural or articulatory phonology model (e.g. Browman and Goldstein 1992). Each gestural activation pattern maps onto a specific *tract variable*, which translates task requirements to changes in a specific vocal tract dimension (location and degree of constriction). The dynamics of these tract variables are modelled in terms of single point attractors as typically found for critically damped mass-spring systems. The parameters of a tract variable map onto individual articulator coordinates, where context-specific influences can be implemented (Saltzman and Munhall 1989). The actual involvement of individual articulators for a specific gesture varies a lot from subject to subject or even within a subject across time (Alfonso and van Lieshout 1997). Potential factors that generate such individual behaviours may include idiosyncrasies at the anatomical and physiological level (e.g. Alfonso and van Lieshout 1997; van Lieshout *et al.* 2002), specific demands at the linguistic task level (e.g. van Lieshout *et al.* 1999), and higher-order aspects as related to, for example, the intention of the speaker.

Although the dynamics of the coordination between individual articulators (e.g. the two lips) are well defined in TD, the dynamics of coordination between gestures at the level of the gestural score are more problematic (see Fowler 1995 for a discussion on this topic). Saltzman and Munhall (1989) tried to address this issue by implementing a connectionist model of serial order as developed by Jordan (1986). In such a network, 'temporal ordering among the output elements of a gestural sequence is an implicit consequence of the network architecture' (Saltzman and Munhall 1989, p. 358). That is, the sequencing of gestures reflects relative phase relationships (the order parameter; Kelso *et al.* 1986) corresponding to preferred stable solutions (attractors) defined by physical and, in this case more likely, intentional constraints. These intentional constraints can be driven by language-specific requirements (e.g. amount of gestural overlap as a function of linguistic boundaries) as well as speaker-specific preferences (e.g. speaking style).

The use of single-point attractors (as in the TD model) entails the concept of a specific vocal tract target (both in terms of location and degree of constriction). However, this is not a necessary concept for a DST approach based on gestures. Porter (1986) proposed a model based on coordinative structures (gestures), but in which 'the speakers' intents may be best seen in the oscillatory 'modulations' of the vocal tract, rather than (or in addition to) being seen in the details of articulator positions or the vocal-tract shapes used' (p. 85). Porter indicated that the auditory system is sensitive to the amplitude modulations of the sort imprinted on the speech acoustic signal by these vocal tract modulations. In a more recent paper, Porter and Hogue (1998) elaborated on this notion, suggesting that next to relative phase as a measure of coupling between articulators and gestures, a second collective variable is needed, namely COP, which stands for constriction order parameter. This COP is an index of the relative degree of constriction relative to the rate of change in constriction. Thus it measures the degree and rate of vocal tract modulation, which according to the authors can capture the identity of both vowels and consonants (Porter and Hogue 1998). They summarize their claims in stating that 'We can propose that the non-linear, self-organized, perceptual processes which reveal modulations have control parameters tied to the broadband temporal structure of speech signals, and that the two emergent order parameters of *relative modulation phase*, and *modulation degree and rate* in perception are mirrored, respectively, by the two order parameters of *relative phase* and *COP* order parameters proposed for production' (Porter and Hogue 1998, p. 123). Obviously, such claims need further experimental verification, but the idea is clear. Do not concern yourselves about specific (articulatory or acoustic) static targets, but rather focus on the consistency in the way the vocal tract is modulated for given sound productions across variations in speech rate, and perhaps also (although this was not addressed) across anatomical and physiological changes in the vocal tract during maturation (cf. Callan *et al.* 2000). The interesting aspect of the claims of Porter and Hogue is the apparent seamless integration of oscillatory dynamics at the perceptual and production levels of speech, and the implicit natural adherence to oscillatory dynamics in self-organizing neural networks (e.g. Wuensche 2002). Porter and Hogue's view also emphasizes the role of the acoustic signal as the medium through which information is carried from talker to listener. The information carried by the vocal tract modulations is mirrored in the acoustic signal modulations, which, in turn, find easy access to the auditory system in the way the latter is sensitive to such modulations (e.g. Giraud *et al.* 2000). As such, this approach shares assumptions with the perception theory proposed by Carol Fowler (1986), which will be discussed next.

3.2.2 The direct perception theory

In 1986, Carol Fowler raised some eyebrows when she claimed that 'In speech perception, the distal event considered locally is the articulating vocal tract' (Fowler 1986, p. 5). Based on Gibson's notions of perception and affordance (Gibson 1966, 1979), Fowler argues that for speech perception, similar to other forms of perception, the target is a real world event, not the media through which it 'communicates' its presence. For example, in visual perception we perceive the object of interest directly, not through a cognitively mediated reconstruction of the light arrays that emanate from the object. The medium is structured by the event in such a way that it specifies the actual object or event to the senses, which allows the perceiver to pick up that information directly in a holistic way, if he or she is willing and able to do so (Fowler 1986).

To explain how listeners derive meaning from structured articulatory events, Fowler introduces the notion of a two-tier layered structure. One layer conveys information about the gestures themselves (phonetic tier) and the other layer specifies the way the talker has imposed constraints on the organization of gestures into words and syntactically formed sentences (linguistic tier). Fowler claims that 'Perceptual objects are not acoustic; they are not articulator movements. They are, minimally, gestures realized by coordinative structures' (Fowler and Rosenblum 1989, p. 153). In this, it resembles the (revised) motor theory of speech perception (Liberman and Mattingly 1985), but there is an important difference. The direct perception (DP) view assumes that information about gestures is immediately available to the listener (Fowler 1986), whereas in the motor theory a distinct (specific to humans) phonetic module is needed to recover the phonetic gesture from sound (Liberman and Mattingly 1985). In the latter view, it is perfectly logical to assume that phonetic and auditory percepts are processed independently from each other (Xu *et al.* 1997), in contrast to DP theory (Fowler and Rosenblum 1989).

Although listeners may experience some limitations in recovering the underlying gestures accurately under certain conditions of articulatory overlap, DP assumes that gestures as produced by overlapping vocal tract activities retain their identity (Fowler 1986). That is, unlike theories which assume that speech segments that are coarticulated change their identity by sharing or exchanging certain features, the gestural account assumes that gestures 'simply' overlap in time and space, without sacrificing their unique distinctiveness (cf. Fowler 1995). Obviously, overlap can at some point prevent a specific gesture from imprinting its presence on the structure of the acoustic signal, as shown by Löfqvist (1990), who aptly coined the phrase 'audible gestures' in the title of his paper.

It is important to realize that although information on gestures is available at the phonetic tier, listeners do not have to pick up (perceive) all the information that is provided. They can rely on a priori expectations for a given context and tune their perception towards identifying only those parts that (in some cases wrongly) confirm those expectations.

As mentioned, a central issue in DP is the claim that vocal-tract activities structure the acoustic medium, which carries that information to the listener. Fowler (1986) suggests that parsing the signal by acoustic segments to retrieve phonetic structure is difficult, as 'phonetic segments can be composed of any number of acoustic segments, ... and most acoustic segments reflect properties of more than one phonetic segment' (p. 12). For example, the presence of a /p/ followed by a vowel can be signalled by a number of acoustic cues, including voice onset time (VOT), spectral characteristics of burst, F1 + F2 transitions, and vowel duration. What cues are more relevant or how do listeners make a choice based on the signal that reaches their ears? In contrast, DP implies that gestures (the phonetic segment in DP) are recovered from the acoustic signal in a more or less holistic sense, provided this information is indeed represented in the acoustic signal. Support for the latter claim comes from a recent paper (Hogden *et al.* 1996), showing that details from vocal tract events could accurately be recovered from acoustic signals. Similarly, another study (Surprenant and Goldstein 1998) demonstrated a clear relationship between the amount of gestural overlap in consonant productions and the listener's ability to recover these gestures. These authors also found that the effect was different for bilabial and alveolar consonants, the latter being more vulnerable to the consequences of gestural overlap.

Indirect evidence for the claim that listeners have direct access to information about vocal tract activities comes from speech shadowing studies (Porter and Castellanos 1980; Porter and Lubker 1980; Small 1989), where people are found to be able to reproduce articulations from auditory stimuli at latencies that are not significantly different from simple motor reaction times for the same stimuli (both around 150 ms). The difference seems to be too small to include the involvement of a cognitive reconstruction process based on the analysis of isolated auditory cues, but since we do not know the exact time it would take to complete such an analysis, this remains speculative. Other studies (Tuller and Kelso 1990) have shown that listeners have access to gestural-based changes in relative phase values between lip articulation and vocal fold vibration, which were not associated with specific acoustic qualities. Further data that support a DP perspective can be found elsewhere (e.g. Fowler 1996).

3.2.3 Coordination dynamics

The revised TD model (Saltzman and Byrd 2000) incorporates situations of symmetry breaking in the coupling between gestures. Symmetry breaking in general terms refers to a difference in the intrinsic properties of coupled structures, but experimentally it is mostly defined in terms of differences in natural frequencies for the coupled effectors as, for example, between leg and arm movements during running (Jeka and Kelso 1995; Peper *et al.* 1995; Treffner and Turvey 1996; Sternad *et al.* 1999). Apart from inducing asymmetry in artificial ways (e.g. loading one arm with a weight), symmetry breaking can occur naturally in (mostly complex) tasks like piano playing, polyrhythmic tapping, juggling, or speech production where slower (quasi) cyclic events combine with faster cycles. An example of this can be found in the coordination between tongue body (TB) and bilabial closure (BC) gestures in a simple non-word like 'pipa' where the tongue moves at a slower rate than the lips (Fig. 3.3A). This is quite different from the more familiar symmetrical interlip coupling, where both lips move at the same cycle frequency (Fig. 3.3B).

A DST approach that deals with these and other phenomena in coordination is fittingly called coordination dynamics (CD). CD is probably best described as a dynamical systems approach in which the principles of coupling dynamics as originally defined in mathematics and physics (for a short historical review, see Kelso 1995) are applied to biological systems, *but* taking into account the unique nature of animate and adaptive complex systems as compared to inanimate physical systems (e.g. Turvey 1990; Kelso 1995). In essence, 'Coordination dynamics is not ordinary physics. It deals with the dynamics of informationally meaningful quan-

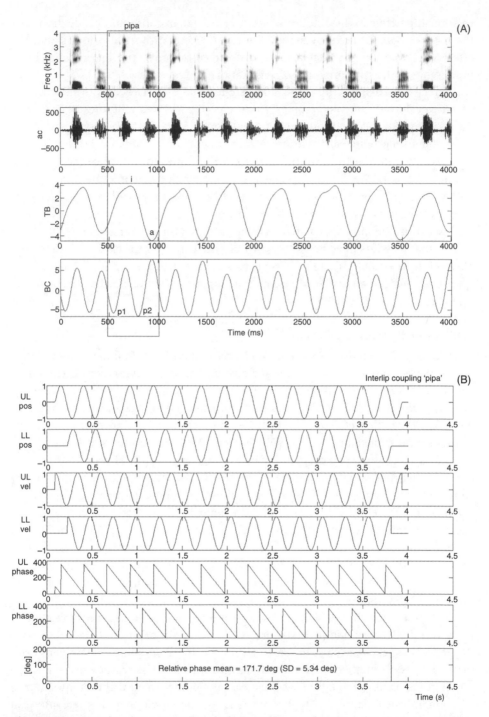

Fig. 3.3 Acoustic information (waveform and spectrogram) and position data for tongue body (TB) and bilabial closure (BC) gestures for the non-word /pipa/ (A); also, upper lip (UL) and lower lip (LL) data (position and velocity) and their relative phase values for the same utterance (B). (See the text for more details.)

tities. Coupling in biological systems must reflect functional, not merely mechanical constraints if behaviour is to be adaptive and successful' (Kelso 1995, p. 70).

Over recent years, CD has been very successful in many areas, including limb control (e.g. Jeka *et al.* 1993; Buchanan *et al.* 1996; Treffner and Turvey 1996; Kelso *et al.* 2001), brain pattern formation (e.g. Haken 1996; Jirsa *et al.* 1998; Fuchs *et al.* 2000; Bressler and Kelso 2001), motor learning (e.g. Zanone and Kelso 1997; Newell *et al.* 2001), motor development (Thelen 1995), the role of attention on movement control (e.g. Amazeen *et al.* 1997; Monno *et al.* 2000), and the role of feedback on coordination (e.g. Turvey 1998; Fink *et al.* 2000; Foo *et al.* 2000).

Work on speech production and perception originally started in the 1980s, with several publications on coupling dynamics, in particular for lip and jaw movements (e.g. Tuller and Munhall 1983; Kelso *et al.* 1985), which eventually cumulated in the formulation of the TD model discussed in Section 3.2.1 (Saltzman and Kelso 1987; Saltzman and Munhall 1989). In later years, when the CD approach was formulated more explicitly, speech moved out of focus. For example, in his brilliant book on dynamic patterns, Kelso (1995) dedicates one section, of fewer than three pages, to speech production and perception, embedded in a general chapter on coordination between organisms. In fact, apart from recent theoretically similarly inspired research efforts pertaining to the development of TD (e.g. McGowan and Saltzman 1995; Saltzman and Byrd 2000) speech production has been a bit on the back-burner in CD since the early/mid-1990s.

For perception, the story is a bit different and more encouraging. Recent studies in this area have led to unique and interesting findings regarding the potential underlying dynamical mechanisms in categorical perception and the verbal transformation effect (e.g. Tuller *et al.* 1994; Case *et al.* 1995; Ditzinger *et al.* 1997). There is also a small body of research on speech motor development from a CD perspective, in particular by Esther Thelen and her co-workers (Iverson and Thelen 1999).

A interesting application of CD principles can be found in recent studies on speech rhythm (Cummins and Port 1998; Port and Leary 2002), which finds its origin in similar work on polyrhythmic ratios in limb control (Treffner and Turvey 1993, 1995). In this view, rhythm is manifested as the 'temporal binding of events to specific and predictable phases of a superordinate cycle' (Cummins and Port 1998, p. 147). The events in this case relate to the interval between stress beats (the foot), and the superordinate cycle is defined by the repetition cycle of short phrases. In their experiment, Cummings and Port required subjects to align stress beats with a specific sequence of high and low tones, while continuously repeating simple short phrases such as 'beg for a dime' or 'big for a duck'. Whereas the interval between high and low tones was fixed, the interval between the low and the next high tone varied according to a specific phase relationship determined by the duration of that interval relative to the total duration of the high–high tone interval (phrase repetition cycle or PRC). The phase relationships were uniformly sampled in the range between 0.3 and 0.7 (108–252°). Instead of being able to achieve all target phase relationships as dictated by the tone stimuli, subjects showed only a small number of relatively stable phase relationships between the foot and PRC cycles. The authors interpreted their findings in terms of coordinative dynamics with specific attractor states for the hierarchical coupling between slower (PRC) and faster (foot) oscillators in the generation of speech rhythm. This corresponds to an asymmetric type of coupling as found in limb control (e.g. Jeka and Kelso 1995; Peper *et al.* 1995; Fuchs *et al.* 1996; Treffner and Turvey 1996), and the coordination between sucking and breathing in full-term and preterm infants (Goldfield *et al.* 1999).

The idea of rhythm as an organizing principle in speech is also echoed in the work of Eugene Buder, which focuses on the existence of different cyclic events in speech as crucial parts in a pattern formation process during dyadic interaction (Buder 1991, 1996). His work is aimed at an 'investigation of coordinated cycles in conversational speech data by regarding speech as physiologically generated by deterministic processes with fundamental cyclic dynamics' (Buder 1996, p. 307). Cross-spectral analysis on fundamental frequency data from two interacting speakers is used to identify and isolate shared (= coupled) cycles in conversation. A deterministic model (following the logistic map equation as described in Section 3.1) is used to demonstrate the effects of interpersonal differences in the rate of turn taking (similar to the control parameter r shown in Fig. 3.1) on the emergent pattern of interaction (Buder 1991). Although the model might be too limited in some of its details, it does provide an excellent background to assess the 'interaction dynamics between individuals with different amounts of motivation and different preferred levels of involvement' (Buder 1991, p. 192). Additional support for this type of higher-order coupling between interacting persons can be found in a recent study by McFarland (2001), who describes a consistent relationship between the kinematic patterns of breathing around conversational turn changes during speech. This parallels similar findings on visually entrained motions in limb control (e.g. Schmidt and Turvey 1994; Treffner 1999).

Finally, very recent work in our own lab at the University of Toronto has been inspired by coordination dynamics (van Lieshout 2001). Theoretically, our approach tries to address the following questions:

1. Are complex articulatory movements composed of motion primitives, which can be seen as elementary synergies in the generation of complex motor output? (For related views, see Bizzi *et al.* 1998; Sanguineti *et al.* 1998.)
2. If so, can the coupling between these motion primitives be interpreted in terms of a two-level model of coupling between central (neural pattern generators) and peripheral (effectors) systems, as suggested for limb control (Beek *et al.* 2002)? In particular, this addresses the potential influences of movement feedback on the stability of such couplings (e.g. Peper and Beek 1998; Williamson 1998; Fink *et al.* 2000).

These and other questions are addressed in oral motor control studies using kinematic data from articulators such as lips, jaw and tongue to assess the status of the coupling between frequency components of movement signals (the 'primitives'). This is similar to the approach taken by Buder (1991) for acoustic signals discussed above. It is hypothesized, that changes in coupling dynamics (e.g. instability) may arise due to changes in strength or phasing of feedback (e.g. Williamson 1998), or as a function of (intrinsic) differences between the coupled structures, captured in the notion of symmetry breaking discussed above. Regarding feedback, one potentially important source of change in feedback gains is the amplitude or relative strength of a primitive motion (cf. Peper and Beek 1998), and this forms a major topic in our studies.

An example from a normal speaker will be presented next to illustrate our approach. Movement signals are collected using the electro-magnetic midsagittal articulograph (EMMA) system (AG100; van Lieshout and Moussa 2000). Figure 3.4 shows a spectral coherence plot with a single dominant spectral component (the primitive) for upper lip (UL; second panel) and lower lip (LL; third panel) at 3.9 Hz in the interlip coupling for the same utterance as used in Fig. 3.3 ('pipa'). The spectral coherence panel in Fig. 3.4 shows a near perfect entrainment (spectral correlation value of 1.0) and a relative phase value of around 180° in the

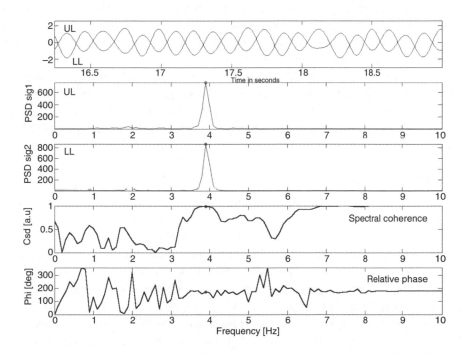

Fig. 3.4 Position data (upper panel) and spectral peaks for upper lip (UL) and lower lip (LL) and their spectral coherence (fourth panel) and relative phase (fifth panel) values (see text for more details).

relative phase panel at this value. The first panel shows the actual position signals for both lips.

These techniques allow us to assess the nature and stability of coordination within and between gestures. For example, Fig. 3.5A shows an example of intergestural coupling between bilabial closure (BILA cl) and tongue body constriction (TB con) gestures for a normal speaker producing the sequence 'tipa' at a preferred rate. Apart from the shared dominant primitive at 2.2 Hz, there is a secondary peak at 4.4 Hz, which was induced by jaw movements for word initial /t/ closure (panels 2 and 3, Fig. 3.5A). This in itself is not surprising, but what is unexpected is the fact that this jaw influence on lower lip movements was entrained by the upper lip during bilabial closure for the /p/ (not shown here). That is, although the presence of this spectral component in the lower lip signals a passive local event (lower lip riding on the jaw while the latter is moving upward for /t/), the coupling between both lips allows for entrainment and a relatively stable phase relationship (panel 5) at 103.5° (for 2.2 Hz) and 137.8° (for 4.4 Hz). Thus, the system avoids symmetry breaking in the coupling between the lips. In Fig. 3.5B, the same speaker produces the same utterance at a faster rate. This time the intergestural coupling shows only a single dominant spectral component at 3.1 Hz for both signals (panels 2 and 3, Fig. 3.5B). The passive interruption of the jaw movement on lower lip for /t/ closure has been neutralized. From a CD perspective, it can be argued that the faster rate makes movements more symmetrical and reduces coupling strength, thus attenuating the influence of the weaker (secondary) primitive (e.g. Peper and Beek 1998).

An example of applying this approach to data from a person who stutters (PWS) can be found elsewhere (Chapter 13, this volume), showing that a reduction in amplitude for underlying motion primitives had a direct influence on coupling stability, which, for this subject, was associated with a series of stutter blocks.

3.2.4 Chaos in speech

Chaos in speech is not a popular topic, with the exception of pure physical phenomena in airflow dynamics (turbulence). One potential source for this apparent anxiety in using the concept of Chaos in speech is related to the use of the word 'chaos', which (pardon the pun) has created chaos about Chaos. Chaos in layman terms means 'no order', as in 'your office is one big chaos' (which normally is not meant to be a compliment). However, in the mathematical definition of Chaos (I will use capital 'C' to indicate that I refer to the formal as opposed to the lay definition of the term), this is not correct. For example, in Fig. 3.1, looking at the panel displaying the logistic map data for $r = 3.99$, one might be under the impression that it shows 'random' behaviour. A formal description would be that randomness in a given system is a function of the way the probability of a behaviour to occur in time (i.e. its stochastic nature) is governed by a truly random

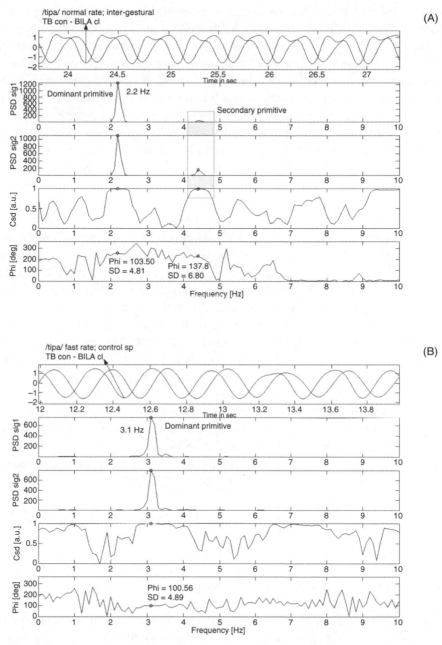

Fig. 3.5 Position data (upper panel) and spectral peaks for tongue body (TB con; second panel) and bilabial closure (BILA cl, third panel) gestures, and their spectral coherence (fourth panel) and relative phase (fifth panel) values at primary and secondary spectral peaks for /tipa/ (A). (B) Same information as in (A) but for a faster rate. (See text for more details.)

process (see Riley and Turvey 2002, for an excellent discussion on this topic). A popular term to denote this type of behaviour is white (neuromotor) noise. However, as already explained in Section 3.1, in the logistic map model any value at a given moment in time is a function of previous values, and therefore, by definition, reflects a deterministic process. Instead of white noise, we are dealing with a system displaying Chaos, that is 'the output of a deterministic system is so complex that it mimics the output generated by a random system. It does NOT mean that a system is driven by disorder, randomness, or chance' (Liebovitch 1998, p. 118). The process itself does not have to be complex, as shown for the logistic map, as long as the function relating input and output relationships is iterative.

As mentioned in Section 3.1, a typical feature of Chaos is divergence, that is the tendency for two trajectories that are part of a chaotic attractor and are very close to move away from each other (Abraham 1995). This is also referred to as sensitivity to initial conditions, and an example of this phenomenon is shown in Fig. 3.2. This means that predictability for such a system is limited, but not impossible. Order in Chaos can be found in the phase portrait of a system in the way it shows a clear and well-defined pattern, unlike a random system which has no structured pattern whatsoever (see figures in Liebovitch 1998, p. 123).

Is the concept of Chaos important for speech or human activities in general? The first place to look for Chaos is in systems with many highly interconnected nodes such as neural networks found in the brain (e.g. Wuensche 2002). There seems to be a growing confidence that Chaos is present in both normal (Mpitsos *et al.* 1988; Freeman 2000; Roberts *et al.* 2000) and pathological states of brain activity, such as found in epilepsy (e.g. Sarbadhikari and Chakrabarty 2001). However, several issues that have to do with methodology and the limitations of providing mathematical proof of Chaos with biological data need to be tackled before reaching firm conclusions on this matter (for potential ways of dealing with these problems, see, for example, Heath 2000; Faure and Korn 2001; Sarbadhikari and Chakrabarty 2001).

Another realm of potentially fruitful Chaos-based research is phonation. The complex nature of vocal fold oscillations in normal and pathological voice conditions make the laryngeal system almost an ideal setting to study typical aspects of non-linear dynamics, including Chaos. The latter approach is deemed important to determine whether the noisy parts of voice production are truly random, or if there is some sort of deterministic process going on, potentially allowing researchers to use that information to model these behaviours and gain a better understanding of the underlying mechanisms involved in normal and disordered voices (Mergell *et al.* 2000). Several studies have been published recently that used non-linear techniques and theories to model the behaviours of vocal folds in voicing (e.g. Herzel *et al.* 1995; Giovanni *et al.* 1999; Lucero 1999; Svec *et al.* 1999), including its interaction with vocal tract dynamics (Mergell and Herzel, 1997). Unlike the human articulatory system, the dynamics of vocal fold oscillations in humans can also be modelled using excised human or other mammal larynges (e.g. Giovanni *et al.* 1999; Svec *et al.* 1999). This provides more opportunities for experimental control than in living human beings.

A couple of studies have looked in the usefulness of concepts from Chaos theory as a way to classify voice irregularities. Whereas some report a limited success in using a specific non-linear measure (fractal dimension) to classify voice disorders (e.g. Boek *et al.* 1997; Hertrich *et al.* 1997), others are clearly more optimistic (e.g. Herzel *et al.* 1994). The same can be said for studies looking at Chaos in the acoustics of (vowel) speech sounds (e.g. Ouayoun *et al.* 1999; Chouard *et al.* 2001; Tokuda *et al.* 2001). Success in these areas is likely restricted due to aforementioned limitations in applying non-linear analysis techniques based in physics and theoretical mathematics to the type of short and non-stationary time series generated by complex living systems (e.g. Gregson and Pressing 2000).

Another application of Chaos theory to speech can be found in a paper by Skljarov (1999). This researcher used a logistic equation to model the generation of speech rhythm, in particular contrasting normal speech with stuttering. This is similar to the approach taken by Buder (1991), who used the logistic map as a model to study dyadic patterns. Speech is segmented in two sections, unvoiced and voiced, each with a specific duration parameter. Using two logistic maps, where the r parameter (the parameter that determines the rate of change in the system; see Section 3.1) of one system represents excitation, and the other r parameter represents inhibition, the normal situation shows a balance between the two, such that a change in excitation equals a change in inhibition (both r values are equal). Under these conditions, various rhythms can be generated, from simple alternating patterns of voiced and unvoiced segments with equal duration to more complex rhythms. In normal speech production, rhythms need to be flexible and therefore, by definition, complex, and in the model they are supposed to originate from the Chaotic region of the logistic map. In an unbalanced case, that is, where both r parameters are not equal, higher r-values are needed to bring a system in the preferred (because more flexible) Chaotic region. This forces the system through a series of bifurcations as is typical for logistic systems on route to Chaos (see Section 3.1). In such bifurcation zones, rhythms are cyclic oscillations (i.e. simple repetitions of voiced and unvoiced segments), and the author argues that stuttering arises when the unbalanced rhythm generating system is 'trapped' in these zones on its way to Chaos. In this theory, evolution (and perhaps development) of speech rhythm is characterized by moving the system from simple oscillations in bifurcation zones (like in babbling) to rhythms that are more complex as characteristic for Chaotic regions. In other words, stuttering is normal behaviour for these bifurcation zones. It is only abnormal that the system is unbalanced in terms of its r-values and, as a result, is forced to go through these bifurcation zones on its way to the preferred chaotic region, where rhythms are more adaptive to the demands of the communicative context (Skljarov 1999). How valid this approach will be, depends on future experimental verification of its assumptions, but it forms a refreshing departure from the more traditional approaches in stuttering.

3.3 What the future might bring

In this section, potential future lines of speech research from a DST perspective will be discussed briefly. A first topic that is likely to show major progress is work on brain network dynamics and its relationship to behavioural patterns. Exciting and pioneering work in this area has been published on limb control, in particular with respect to the coordination of hands (e.g. Jirsa *et al.* 1994; Fuchs *et al.*, 2000; Jirsa and Kelso 2000; Jantzen *et al.* 2001). In the area of speech, recent papers have emphasized the dynamics of self-organizing properties in (recurrent) neural networks with respect to the mapping of sound and motor representations (Morasso *et al.* 1998; Callan *et al.* 2000; Chapter 2, this volume). However, unlike limb control, a direct connection between the non-linear characteristics of neural networks (e.g. Mpitsos *et al.* 1988; Freeman 1994) and non-linear dynamics in speech movements has not yet been demonstrated. Eventually, future studies in speech also have to be linked to brain research on the dynamical aspects of language and cognition and their development (e.g. Carpenter and Grossberg 1991; Plunkett *et al.* 1997; van Gelder 1998) in order to gain a better understanding of the brain and its functions as a complex adaptive system in a more holistic sense (Kelso 2000).

A second topic of interest in recent publications deals with 'variability'. This is still a major source of controversy between DST and 'other' theories (Kelso 1997). This controversy focuses on the nature and relevance of (neuromotor) noise in motor control. Traditionally, noise is treated as a random source of variance that needs to be controlled or suppressed (e.g. van Gemmert and Van Galen 1997; Harris and Wolpert 1998). Alternatively, it can be seen as a mechanism to 'probe the stability of coordinative states and [to] allow the system to discover new coordinative states according to current environmental and task demands (Kelso 1997, p. 455,). Scott Kelso uses the term 'relative coordination' for expressing the adaptive nature of 'noisy' neuromotor signals (Kelso 1995) and its potential deterministic qualities (Kelso and Fuchs 1995; Newell and Slifkin 1998), in line with pioneering work by the German physiologist Erich von Holst. Von Holst discovered that in biological systems, coordination between components (e.g. between dorsal and pectoral fin movements in his studies) is driven by a competition between a tendency to remain coupled (magnet effect) and a tendency for the individual components to adhere to their intrinsic specific properties (the maintenance tendency). Kelso (1995) presents a nice illustration of relative coordination in his example of an adult walking along the beach with a small child (p. 98). The coupling between the two individuals is formed by the intention (!) to stay next to other (magnet effect), but given the intrinsic differences in their limb properties, both have to adjust their gait at an ongoing basis, leading to alternating moments of stable phase coupling and phase slippage during these adjustments. In other words, the coordination is stable, yet flexible.

Not every DST researcher shares Kelso's view on the role of noise in motor control. Some question the pure deterministic nature of noise (e.g. Riley and Turvey 2002), whereas others try to model variation in coordination as measured by relative phase in terms of constrained noise using pre-defined phase windows (Byrd and Saltzman 1998), where the boundaries of a window limit the extent of (otherwise) random variation. It is clear that the status of noise in the neuromotor system has changed from being an object of neglect to becoming a (if not THE) major topic of discussion and future research (see also Newell and Slifkin, 1998). It has to be, if we want take the concept of complex adaptive systems seriously (Kauffman 1995; Bar-Yam 1997; Kelso 2000). It will also have an impact on the way we understand the notion of variability in individuals with speech disorders, as discussed elsewhere (Chapter 13, this volume).

The third topic that warrants more attention in the near future is the general issue of timing control. An excellent review on the notion of timing in both stochastic (motor programming) and dynamical models can be found in a recent paper by Schöner (2002). It is argued that on a pure computational basis, the two classes of models are comparable (see also Pressing 1998). What seems to emerge from the current discussions on timing is a tendency to argue for the presence of multiple neural timers (pattern generators) underlying task execution, regardless whether this is based on an information processing perspective (e.g. Ivry and Richardson 2002; Rosenbaum 2002) or a dynamical systems perspective (Ding *et al.* 2002). In addition, the classic two-level model of clock and motor time (Wing and Kristofferson 1973) has found an equivalent in DST (Williamson 1998; Beek *et al.* 2002). As the information processing approach and DST start 'borrowing' certain concepts and techniques from each other, and at a more general mathematical level already share important assumptions (Pressing 1998), it seems likely that the once sharp boundary line between these theories on the notion of time keeping may gradually fade (on this issue, see, for example, Sternad 2000; Schöner 2002). Studies on the (combined) timing of speech and non-speech events (e.g. Hulstijn *et al.* 1992; Treffner and Peter 2002) will provide the kind of data that we need to address these issues in detail. In particular, the recent study by Treffner and Peter shows how hand and speech gestures are intimately related in the way their coordination (and variability therein) is governed by both dynamical (e.g. effects of rate and asymmetry) and informational (intention, attentional resources) constraints. Their data also show how the phasing between speech and hand gestures is determined by a coupling between a perceived centre of mandible movement relative to the hand movement cycle. The findings were nicely captured in an extended (asymmetric) version of the original Haken–Kelso–Bunz (HKB) model (Haken *et al.* 1985), thus transcending the traditional boundaries between limb and oral motor control.

3.4 Conclusions

This general and, due to space limitations, limited review of the dynamical systems theory as applied to speech can perhaps best be summarized in two overall statements:

1. DST in speech is still not very well represented compared to more traditional theories, with only a small group of researchers active in this specific area.
2. DST has powerful concepts and tools to offer to research in speech motor control, which deserve further attention and efforts as it provides a refreshing new view on notions of stability, flexibility, variability, and the relationship between brain activity and behavioural output.

Obviously, people have to make an effort to study and try to understand DST in its broader scope, as there are still a lot of misconceptions out there. On the other hand, researchers who work from a DST perspective will also need to do a better job to minimize the conceptual and practical barriers that thus far have kept others from entering the field and get a better understanding of the various aspects of the theory and its ramifications. This review was an attempt to do just that, and I hope that, at least, I have been able to raise some scientific curiosity in this type of work, and, at best, to see more studies reported in this area at future speech motor conferences. I am convinced that the DST approach will further our understanding of the nature of fluent and 'non-fluent' speech in speakers with and without a speech disorder (van Lieshout *et al.* 2002; Chapter 13, this volume), which, in turn, could lead to improved diagnostics and therapeutic interventions. The future will tell if I am too optimistic.

Acknowledgements

The author is grateful to the editors of this book and Drs Peter J. Alfonso, Kim Vicente, and Paul Treffner for comments and useful suggestions on earlier versions of this manuscript. The research presented in this paper was supported by the Natural Sciences and Engineering Research Council (NSERC) of Canada.

References

Abbs, J. H. and **Gracco, V. L.** (1984). Control of complex motor gestures: orofacial muscle responses to load perturbations of lip during speech. *J. Neurophysiol.*, 51, 705–723.

Abraham, F. D. (1995). Introduction to dynamics: A basic language; a basic meta-modeling strategy. In F.D. Abraham and A. R. Gilgen (Eds.), *Chaos theory in psychology* (pp. 31–49). Westport, CT: Praeger.

Alfonso, P. J. and **van Lieshout, P.** (1997). Spatial and temporal variability in obstruent gestural specification by stutterers and controls: Comparisons across sessions. In W. Hulstijn, H. F. Peters, and P. H. H. M. van Lieshout (Eds.), *Speech production: Motor control, brain research and fluency disorders* (pp. 151–160). Amsterdam: Elsevier Publishers.

Amazeen, E. L., Treffner, P. J., and **Turvey, M. T.** (1997). Attention and handedness in bimanual coordination dynamics. *J. Exp. Psychol.*, 23, 1552–1560.

Bar-Yam, Y. (1997). *Dynamics of complex systems.* Reading, MA: Perseus Books.

Bauer, A., Jancke, L., and **Kalveram, K. T.** (1995). Mechanical perturbation of jaw movements during speech: effects on articulation and phonation. *Percept. Motor Skills*, 80, 1108–1112.

Beek, P. J., Peper, C. E., and **Stegeman, D. F.** (1995). Dynamical models of movement coordination. *Human Movement Sci.*, 14, 573–608.

Beek, P. J., Peper, C. E., and **Daffertshofer, A.** (2002). Modeling rhythmic interlimb coordination: beyond the Haken–Kelso–Bunz model. *Brain Cogn*, 48, 149–165.

Bernstein, N. (1967). *The co-ordination and regulation of movements.* Oxford: Pergamon Press.

Bizzi, E., Saltiel, P., and **Tresch, M.** (1998). Modular organization of motor behavior. Zeitschrift fur Naturforschung C-A. *J. Biosci.*, 53, 510–517.

Boek, W., Wieneke, G. H., and **Dejonckere, P. H.** (1997). Clinical relevance of the fractal dimension of F0 perturbations computed by the box-counting method. *J. Voice*, 11, 437–442.

Bressler, S. L. and **Kelso, J. A.** (2001). Cortical coordination dynamics and cognition. *Trends Cogn. Sci.*, 5, 26–36.

Browman, C. P. and **Goldstein, L.** (1992). Articulatory phonology: an overview. *Phonetica*, 49, 155–180.

Buchanan, J. J., Kelso, J. A., and **Fuchs, A.** (1996). Coordination dynamics of trajectory formation. *Biol. Cybern.*, 74, 41–54.

Buder, E. H. (1991). A nonlinear dynamic model of social interaction. *Commun. Res.*, 18, 174–198.

Buder, E. H. (1996). Dynamics of speech processes in dyadic interaction. In J. H. Watt and C. A. Vanlear (Eds.), *Dynamic patterns in communication processes* (pp. 301–325). Thousand Oaks, CA: Sage.

Byrd, D. and **Saltzman, E.** (1998). Intragestural dynamics of multiple prosodic boundaries. *J. Phonetics*, 26, 173–199.

Callan, D. E., Kent, R. D., Guenther, F. H., and **Vorperian, H. K.** (2000). An auditory-feedback-based neural network model of speech production that is robust to developmental changes in the size and shape of the articulatory system. *J. Speech Lang. Hear. Res.*, 43, 721–736.

Carpenter, G. A. and **Grossberg, S.** (1991). *Pattern recognition by self-organizing neural networks.* Cambridge, MA: MIT Press.

Case, P., Tuller, B., Ding, M., and **Kelso, J. A.** (1995). Evaluation of a dynamical model of speech perception. *Percept. Psychophys.,* 57, 977–988.

Chouard, C. H., Pean, V., Ouayoun, M., and **Meyer, B.** (2001). A fractal approach to the features of speech consonants. *Acta Oto-laryngologica,* 121, 249–253.

Cummins, F. and **Port, R. F.** (1998). Rhythmic constraints on stress timing in English. *J. Phonetics,* 26, 145–171.

Diedrich, F. J. and **Warren, W. H.** (1995). Why Change Gaits—Dynamics of the Walk Run Transition. *J. Exp. Psychol.–Human Percept. Perform.,* 21, 183–202.

Ding, M., Chen, Y., and **Kelso, J. A. S.** (2002). Statistical analysis of timing errors. *Brain and Cognition.* Special Issue: Human movement timing and coordination, 48(1), 98–106.

Ditzinger, T., Tuller, B., Haken, H., and **Kelso, J. A.** (1997). A synergetic model for the verbal transformation effect. *Biol. Cybern.,* 77, 31–40.

Faure, P. and **Korn, H.** (2001). Is there chaos in the brain? I. Concepts of nonlinear dynamics and methods of investigation. *C. R. Acad. Sci III,* 324, 773–793.

Fink, P. W., Foo, P., Jirsa, V. K., and **Kelso, J. A.** (2000). Local and global stabilization of coordination by sensory information. *Exp. Brain Res.,* 134, 9–20.

Folkins, J. W. and **Zimmermann, G. N.** (1982). Lip and jaw interaction during speech: responses to perturbation of lower-lip movement prior to bilabial closure. *J. Acoust. Soc. Am.,* 71, 1225–1233.

Foo, P., Kelso, J. A., and **de Guzman, G. C.** (2000). Functional stabilization of unstable fixed points: human pole balancing using time-to-balance information. *J. Exp. Psychol. Hum. Percept. Perform.,* 26, 1281–1297.

Fowler, C. A. (1986). An event approach to the study of speech perception from a direct-realist perspective. *J. Phonetics,* 14, 3–28.

Fowler, C. A. (1995). Speech production. In J.L.Miller and P. D. Eimas (Eds.), *Speech, language, and communication* (pp. 29–61). San Diego, CA: Academic Press.

Fowler, C. A. (1996). Listeners do hear sounds, not tongues. *J. Acoust. Soc. Am.,* 99, 1730–1741.

Fowler, C. A. and **Rosenblum, L. D.** (1989). The perception of phonetic gestures. *Haskins Laboratories Status Report on Speech Research,* 100, 102–117.

Fowler, C. A., Rubin, P., Remez, R., and **Turvey, M. T.** (1980). Implications for speech production of a general theory of action. In B.Butterworth (Ed.), *Language Production, Volume 1: Speech and talk* (pp. 373–420). London: Academic Press.

Freeman, W. J. (1994). Neural networks and chaos. *J. Theor. Biol.,* 171, 13–18.

Freeman, W. J. (2000). A proposed name for aperiodic brain activity: stochastic chaos. *Neural Netw.,* 13, 11–13.

Fuchs, A., Jirsa, V. K., Haken, H., and **Kelso, J. A.** (1996). Extending the HKB model of coordinated movement to oscillators with different eigenfrequencies. *Biol. Cybern.*, 74, 21–30.

Fuchs, A., Jirsa, V. K., and **Kelso, J. A.** (2000). Issues in the coordination of human brain activity and motor behavior. *Neuroimage*, 11, 375–377.

Gibson, J. J. (1966). *The senses considered as perceptual systems.* Boston, MA: Houghton.

Gibson, J. J. (1979). *The ecological approach to visual perception.* Boston, MA: Houghton Mifflin.

Giovanni, A., Ouaknine, M., Guelfucci, B., Yu, P., Zanaret, M., and **Triglia, J. M.** (1999). Nonlinear behavior of vocal fold vibration: The role of coupling between the vocal folds. *J. Voice*, 13, 465–476.

Giraud, A. L., Lorenzi, C., Ashburner, J., Wable, J., Johnsrude, I., Frackowiak, R. *et al.* (2000). Representation of the temporal envelope of sounds in the human brain. *J. Neurophysiol.*, 84, 1588–1598.

Goldfield, E. C., Wolff, P. H., and **Schmidt, R. C.** (1999). Dynamics of oralrespiratory coordination in full-term and preterm infants: I. Comparisons at 38–40 weeks postconceptional age. *Develop. Sci.*, 2, 363–373.

Gregson, R. A. M. and **Pressing, J. L.** (2000). Dynamic modeling. In L.G.Tassinary, J. T. Cacioppo, and G. Berntson (Eds.), *Principles of Psychophysiology: Physical, Social, and Inferential Elements* (pp. 924–948). New York: Cambridge University Press.

Guastello, S. J. (2001). Nonlinear dynamics in psychology. *Discrete Dynamics in Nature and Society*, 6, 11–29.

Haken, H. (1983). *Synergetics, an introduction: Nonequilibrium Phase transitions and self-organization in physics, chemistry, and biology,* (3rd edn). Berlin: Springer Verlag.

Haken, H. (1996). Noise in the brain: a physical network model. *Int. J. Neural Syst.*, 7, 551–557.

Haken, H., Kelso, J. A., and **Bunz, H.** (1985). A theoretical model of phase transitions in human hand movements. *Biol. Cybern.*, 51, 347–356

Harris, C. M. and Wolpert, D. M. (1998). Signal-dependent noise determines motor planning. *Nature*, 394, 780–784.

Heath, R. A. (2000). *Nonlinear dynamics: Techniques and applications in psychology.* Mahwah, NJ: Lawrence Erlbaum Associates.

Hertrich, I., Lutzenberger, W., Spieker, S., and **Ackermann, H.** (1997). Fractal dimension of sustained vowel productions in neurological dysphonias: an acoustic and electroglottographic analysis. *J. Acoust. Soc. Am.*, 102, 652–654.

Herzel, H., Berry, D., Titze, I. R., and **Saleh, M.** (1994). Analysis of vocal disorders with methods from nonlinear dynamics. *J. Speech Hear. Res.*, 37, 1008–1019.

Herzel, H., Berry, D., Titze, I., and **Steinecke, I.** (1995). Nonlinear dynamics of the voice—signal analysis and biomechanical modeling. *Chaos*, 5, 30–34.

Hogden, J., Lofqvist, A., Gracco, V., Zlokarnik, I., Rubin, P., and Saltzman, E. (1996). Accurate recovery of articulator positions from acoustics: new conclusions based on human data. *J. Acoust. Soc. Am.*, 100, 1819–1834.

Hulstijn, W., Summers, J. J., Van Lieshout, P. H. M., and Peters, H. F. M. (1992). Timing in finger tapping and speech—a comparison between stutterers and fluent speakers. *Human Movement Sci.*, 11, 113–124.

Iverson J. M. and Thelen, E. (1999). Hand, mouth and brain. The dynamic emergence of speech and gesture. *J. Conscious. Studies*, 6, 19–40.

Ivry, R. B. and Richardson, T. C. (2002). Temporal control and coordination: The multiple timer model. *Brain and Cognition. Special Issue: Human movement timing and coordination*, 48(1), 117–132.

Jantzen, K. J., Fuchs, A., Mayville, J. M., Deecke, L., and Kelso, J. A. (2001). Neuromagnetic activity in alpha and beta bands reflect learning-induced increases in coordinative stability. *Clin. Neurophysiol.*, 112, 1685–1697.

Jeka, J. J. and Kelso, J. A. (1995). Manipulating symmetry in the coordination dynamics of human movement. *J. Exp. Psychol. Hum. Percept. Perform.*, 21, 360–374.

Jeka, J. J., Kelso, J. A. S., and Kiemel, T. (1993). Spontaneous transitions and symmetry: Pattern dynamics in human four-limb coordination. *Human Movement Sci.*, 12(6), 627–651.

Jirsa, V. K., Friedrich, R., Haken, H., and Kelso, J. A. (1994). A theoretical model of phase transitions in the human brain. *Biol. Cybern.*, 71, 27–35.

Jirsa, V. K., Fuchs, A., and Kelso, J. A. S. (1998). Connecting cortical and behavioral dynamics: bimanual coordination. *Neural Comput.*, 10, 2019–2045.

Jirsa, V. K. and Kelso, J. A. (2000). Spatiotemporal pattern formation in neural systems with heterogeneous connection topologies. *Phys. Rev. E Stat. Phys. Plasmas Fluids Relat. Interdiscip. Topics*, 62, 8462–8465.

Jordan, M. I. (1986). *Serial order: A parallel distributed processing approach (Rep. No. 8604)*. San Diego: University of California, Institute for Cognitive Science.

Kauffman, S. A. (1995). *At Home in the Universe: The Search for the Laws of Self-Organization and Complexity* . Oxford, UK: Oxford University Press.

Kelso, J. A. S. (1995). *Dynamic patterns. The self-organization of brain and behavior.* Cambridge, MA: MIT Press.

Kelso, J. A. S. (1997). Relative timing in brain and behavior: Some observations about the generalized motor program and self-organized coordination dynamics. *Human Movement Sci.*, 16, 453–460.

Kelso, J. A. S. (1998). From Bernstein's Physiology of activity to coordination dynamics. In M. L. Latash (Ed.), *Progress in motor control, volume 1: Bernstein's traditions in movement studies* (pp. 203–219). Champaign, IL: Human Kinetics.

Kelso, J. A. S. (2000). Principles of dynamic pattern formation and change for a science of human behavior. In L. Bergman, R. Cairns, L. Nilsson, and L. Nystedt (Eds.), *Developmental science and the holistic approach* (pp. 63–84). Mahway, NJ: Erlbaum.

Kelso, J. A. S. and **Fuchs, A.** (1995). Self-organizing dynamics of the human brain: Critical instabilities and Sil'nikov chaos. *Chaos*, 5, 64–69.

Kelso, J. A., Tuller, B., Vatikiotis-Bateson, E., and **Fowler, C. A.** (1984). Functionally specific articulatory cooperation following jaw perturbations during speech: evidence for coordinative structures. *J. Exp. Psychol. Hum. Percept. Perform.*, 10, 812–832.

Kelso, J. A., Vatikiotis-Bateson, E., Saltzman, E. L., and **Kay, B.** (1985). A qualitative dynamic analysis of reiterant speech production: phase portraits, kinematics, and dynamic modeling. *J. Acoust. Soc. Am.*, 77, 266–280.

Kelso, J. A. S., Saltzman, E., and **Tuller, B.** (1986). The dynamical theory in speech production: Data and theory. *J. Phonetics*, 14, 29–60.

Kelso, J. A. S., Fink, P. W., DeLaplain, C. R., and **Carson, R. G.** (2001). Haptic information stabilizes and destabilizes coordination dynamics. *Proc. R. Soc. Lond. B Biol. Sci*, 268, 1207–1213.

Kugler, P. N., Kelso, J. A. S., and **Turvey, M. T.** (1980). On the concept of coordinative structures as dissipative structures: I. Theoretical lines of convergence. In G. E. Stelmach and J. Requin (Eds.), *Tutorials in motor behavior* (pp. 3–47). New York: North-Holland.

Kugler, P. N., Kelso, J. A. S., and **Turvey, M. T.** (1982). On coordination and control in naturally developing systems. In J. A. S.Kelso and J. E. Clark (Eds.), *The development of movement control and coordination* (pp. 5–78). New York: Wiley.

Liberman, A. M. and **Mattingly, I. G.** (1985). The motor theory of speech perception revised. *Cognition*, 21, 1–36.

Liebovitch, L. (1998). *Fractals and chaos: Simplified for the life sciences*. New York: Oxford University Press.

Löfqvist, A. (1990). Speech as audible gestures. In W. J. Hardcastle and A. Marchal (Eds.), *Speech production and speech modelling* (pp. 289–322). Dordrecht, The Netherlands: Kluwer Academic Publishers.

Lucero, J. C. (1999). Theoretical study of the hysteresis phenomenon at vocal fold oscillation onset-offset. *J. Acoust. Soc. Am.*, 105, 423–431.

Maner, K. J., Smith, A., and **Grayson, L.** (2000). Influences of utterance length and complexity on speech motor performance in children and adults. *J. Speech Lang. Hear. Res.*, 43, 560–573.

McFarland, D. H. (2001). Respiratory markers of conversational interaction. *J. Speech Lang. Hear. Res.*, 44, 128–143.

McGowan, R. S. and **Saltzman, E. L.** (1995). Incorporating aerodynamic and laryngeal components into task dynamics. *J. Phonetics*, 23, 255–269.

Mergell, P. and **Herzel, H.** (1997). Modelling biphonation—The role of the vocal tract. *Speech Commun.*, 22, 141–154.

Mergell, P., Herzel, H., and **Titze, I. R.** (2000). Irregular vocal-fold vibration—High-speed observation and modeling. *J. Acoust. Soc. Am.*, 108, 2996–3002.

Michaels, C. F. and **Beek, P.** (1995). The state of ecological psychology. *Ecol. Psychol.* 7(4), 259–278.

Monno, A., Chardenon, A., Temprado, J. J., Zanone, P. G., and **Laurent, M.** (2000). Effects of attention on phase transitions between bimanual coordination patterns: a behavioral and cost analysis in humans. *Neurosci. Lett.*, 283, 93–96.

Morasso, P. G., Sanguineti, V., Frisone, F., and **Perico, L.** (1998). Coordinate-free sensorimotor processing: computer with population codes. *Neural Networks*, 11, 1417–1428.

Mpitsos, G. J., Burton, R. M., Creech, H. C., and **Soinila, S. O.** (1988). Evidence for chaos in spike trains of neurons that generate rhythmic motor patterns. *Brain Res. Bull.*, 21, 529–538.

Newell, K. M. and **Slifkin, A. B.** (1998). The nature of movement variability. In J. P. Piek (Ed.), *Motor behavior and human skill: A multidisciplinary approach* (pp. 143–160). Champaign, IL: Human Kinetics.

Newell, K. M., Liu, Y. T., and **Mayer-Kress, G.** (2001). Time scales in motor learning and development. *Psychol. Rev.*, 108, 57–82.

Ouayoun, M., Pean, V., Meyer, B., and **Chouard, C. H.** (1999). A study of speech fractal dimensions. *Acta Otolaryngol.*, 119, 261–266.

Peper, C. E. and **Beek, P. J.** (1998). Distinguishing between the effects of frequency and amplitude on interlimb coupling in tapping a 2:3 polyrhythm. *Exp. Brain Res.*, 118, 78–92.

Peper, C. E., Beek, P. J., and **Wieringen, P. C. W. V.** (1995). Multifrequency coordination in bimanual tapping: Asymmetrical coupling and signs of supercriticality. *J. Exp. Psychol.-Human Percept. Perform.*, 21, 1117–1138.

Plunkett, K., Karmiloff-Smith, A., Bates, E., Elman, J. L., and **Johnson, M. H.** (1997). Connectionism and developmental psychology. *J. Child Psychol. Psychiatry*, 38, 53–80.

Port, R. F. and **Leary, A. P.** (2002). Speech timing and linguistic theory. In C. Lorenzi and C. Drake (Eds.), *Le Temps en Audition [Hearing in Time]*. Louvain-la-Neuve, Belgium: De Boeck Université.

Port, R. F. and **van Gelder, T.** (1995). *Mind as motion: Explorations in the dynamics of cognition*. Cambridge, MA: MIT Press.

Porter, R. J. (1986). Speech messages, modulations and motions. *J. Phonetics*, 13, 193–197.

Porter, R. J. Jr and **Castellanos, F. X.** (1980). Speech-production measures of speech perception: rapid shadowing of VCV syllables. *J. Acoust. Soc. Am.*, 67, 1349–1356.

Porter, R. J. and **Hogue, D. M.** (1998). Nonlinear dynamical systems in speech perception and production. *Nonlinear Dynamics, Psychology, and Life Sciences*, 2, 95–131.

Porter, R. J. Jr and **Lubker, J. F.** (1980). Rapid reproduction of vowel–vowel sequences: evidence for a fast and direct acoustic-motoric linkage in speech. *J. Speech Hear. Res.*, 23, 593–602.

Pressing, J. L. (1998). Referential behaviour theory: A framework for multiple perspectives on motor control. In J. P. Piek (Ed.), *Motor control and human skill: A multidisciplinary approach* (pp. 357–384). Champaign, IL: Human Kinetics.

Riley, M. A. and Turvey, M. T. (2002). Variability of determinism in motor behavior. *J. Mot. Behav.*, 34, 99–125.

Roberts, S., Eykholt, R., and Thaut, M. H. (2000). Analysis of correlations and search for evidence of deterministic chaos in rhythmic motor control by the human brain. *Phys. Rev E Stat. Phys. Plasmas. Fluids Relat. Interdiscip. Topics*, 62, 2597–2607.

Rosenbaum, D. A. (2002). Time, space, and short-term memory. *Brain and Cognition*, 48, 52–65.

Saltzman, E. and Byrd, D. (2000). Task-dynamics of gestural timing: Phase windows and multifrequency rhythms. *Human Movement Sci.*, 19, 499–526.

Saltzman, E. and Kelso, J. A. (1987). Skilled actions: a task-dynamic approach. *Psychol. Rev.*, 94, 84–106.

Saltzman, E. L. and Munhall, K. (1989). A dynamical approach to gestural patterning in speech production'. *Ecol. Psychol.*, 1, 333–382.

Saltzman, E., Löfqvist, A., Kay, B., Kinsella-Shaw, J., and Rubin, P. (1998). Dynamics of intergestural timing: a perturbation study of lip–larynx coordination. *Exp. Brain Res.*, 123, 412–424.

Sanguineti, V., Laboissiere, R., and Ostry, D. J. (1998). Dynamic biomechanical model for neural control of speech production. *J. Acoust. Soc. Am.* 103, 1615–1627.

Sarbadhikari, S. N. and Chakrabarty, K. (2001). Chaos in the brain: a short review alluding to epilepsy, depression, exercise and lateralization. *Med. Eng. Phys.*, 23, 445–455.

Schmidt, R. C. and Turvey, M. T. (1994). Phase-entrainment dynamics of visually coupled rhythmic movements. *Biol.Cybern.*, 70, 369–376.

Schöner, G. (2002). Timing, clocks, and dynamical systems. *Brain Cogn.*, 48, 31–51.

Skljarov, O. P. (1999). Nonlinear neurodynamics in representation of a rhythm of speech. *J. Biol. Phys.*, 25, 223–234.

Small, L. H. (1989). Listeners' perceptual strategies in word recognition: shadowing misarticulated speech. *Percept. Motor Skills*, 69, 1211–1216.

Sternad, D. (2000). Debates in dynamics: A dynamical systems perspective on action and perception. *Human Movement Sci.*, 19, 407–423.

Sternad, D., Turvey, M. T., and Saltzman, E. L. (1999). Dynamics of 1:2 Coordination: Sources of Symmetry Breaking. *J. Motor Behav.*, 31, 224–235.

Summers, J. J. (1992). Movement behaviour: A field in crisis? In J.J. Summers (Ed.), *Approaches to the study of motor control and learning* (pp. 551–562). Amsterdam: Elsevier Science.

Surprenant, A. M. and Goldstein, L. (1998). The perception of speech gestures. *J. Acoust. Soc. Am.*, 104, 518–529.

Svec, J. G., Schutte, H. K., and Miller, D. G. (1999). On pitch jumps between chest and falsetto registers in voice: Data from living and excised human larynges. *J. Acoust. Soc. Am.*, 106, 1523–1531.

Thelen, E. (1995). Motor development. A new synthesis. *Am. Psychologist*, 50, 79–95.

Tokuda, I., Miyano, T., and Aihara, K. (2001). Surrogate analysis for detecting nonlinear dynamics in normal vowels. *J. Acoust. Soc. Am.*, 110, 3207–3217.

Treffner, P. J. (1999). Resonance contraints on between-person polyrhythms. In M.A.Grealy and J. A. Thomson (Eds.), *Studies in perception and action V* (pp. 165–169). Mahwah, NJ: Erlbaum.

Treffner, P. J. and Peter, M. (2002). Dynamics of speech–hand gestures. *Human Movement Sci.*, 21, 641–697.

Treffner, P. J. and Turvey, M. T. (1993). Resonance constraints on rhythmic movement. *J. Exp. Psychol-Human Percept Perform*, 19, 1221–1237.

Treffner, P. J. and Turvey, M. T. (1995). Handedness and the asymmetric dynamics of bimanual rhythmic coordination. *J. Exp. Psychol.-Human Percept. Perform.*, 21, 318–333.

Treffner, P. J. and Turvey, M. T. (1996). Symmetry, broken symmetry, and handedness in bimanual coordination dynamics. *Exp. Brain Res.*, 107, 463–478.

Tuller, B., Kelso, J. A., and Harris, K. S. (1983). Converging evidence for the role of relative timing in speech. *J. Exp. Psychol. Hum. Percept. Perform.*, 9, 829–833.

Tuller, B. and Kelso, J. A. S. (1990). Phase transitions in speech production and their perceptual consequences. In M. Jeannerod (Ed.), *Attention and performance XIII* (pp. 429–452). Hillsdale, NJ: Erlbaum.

Tuller, B., Case, P., Ding, M., and Kelso, J. A. (1994). The nonlinear dynamics of speech categorization. *J. Exp. Psychol. Hum. Percept. Perform.*, 20, 3–16.

Turvey, M. T. (1990). Coordination. *Am. Psychol.*, 45, 938–953.

Turvey, M. T. (1998). Dynamics of effortful touch and interlimb coordination. *J. Biomech.*, 31, 873–882.

van Gelder, T. (1998). The dynamical hypothesis in cognitive science. *Behav. Brain Sci.*, 21, 615–628.

van Gemmert, A. W. and Van Galen, G. P. (1997). Stress, neuromotor noise, and human performance: a theoretical perspective. *J. Exp. Psychol. Hum. Percept. Perform.*, 23, 1299–1313.

van Ingen Schenau, G. J., van Soest, A. J., Gabreels, F. J. M., and Horstink, M. W. I. M. (1995). The control of multi-joint movements relies on detailed internal reprsentations. *Human Movement Science. Special Issue: Coordination of multi-joint movements*, 14(4–5), 511–538.

van Lieshout, P. H. H. M. (2001). Coupling dynamics of motion primitives in speech movements and its potential relevance for fluency. *Soc. Chaos Theory Psychol. Life Sci. Newslett.* 8[4], 18.

van Lieshout, P. and **Moussa, W.** (2000). The assessment of speech motor behaviors using electromagnetic articulography. *The Phonetician*, 81, 9–22.

van Lieshout, P. H., Starkweather, C. W., Hulstijn, W., and **Peters, H. F.** (1995). Effects of linguistic correlates of stuttering on Emg activity in nonstuttering speakers. *J. Speech. Hear. Res.*, 38, 360–372.

van Lieshout, P. H. H. M., Hijl, M., and **Hulstijn, W.** (1999). Flexibility and stability in bilabial gestures: 2) Evidence from continuous syllable production. In J. J. Ohala, J. J. Hasegawa, M. Ohala, D. Granville, and A. C. Bailey (Eds.), *Proceedings XIVth International Congress of Phonetic Sciences* (pp. 45–48). San Francisco: American Institute of Physics.

van Lieshout, P. H. H. M., Rutjens, C. A. W., and **Spauwen, P. H. M.** (2002). The dynamics of interlip coupling in speakers with a repaired unilateral cleft-lip history. *J. Speech Lang. Hearing Res.*, 45, 5–19.

Williamson, M. M. (1998). Neural control of rhythmic arm movements. *Neural Networks*, 11, 1379–1394.

Wing, A. M. and **Kristofferson, A.** (1973). The timing of interresponse intervals. *Perception Psychophys.*, 14, 5–12.

Wuensche, A. (2002). Basins of attraction in network dynamics: A conceptual framework for biomolecular networks. In G.Schlosser and G. P. Wagner (Eds.), *Modularity in development and evolution.* Chicago: Chicago University Press.

Xu, Y., Liberman, A. M., and **Whalen, D. H.** (1997). On the immediacy of phonetic perception. *Psychol. Sci.*, 8, 358–362.

Zanone, P. G. and **Kelso, J. A.** (1997). Coordination dynamics of learning and transfer: collective and component levels. *J. Exp. Psychol. Hum. Percept. Perform.*, 23, 1454–1480.

PART 2

NEURAL PROCESSES

CHAPTER 4

FUNCTIONAL BRAIN IMAGING OF MOTOR ASPECTS OF SPEECH PRODUCTION

HERMANN ACKERMANN, AXEL RIECKER, AND DIRK WILDGRUBER

4.1 Introduction

As compared to other domains of motor control, e.g. locomotion or upper limb movements, rather sparse data on the cerebral organization of speech production are available so far. This discrepancy is due, among others, to the absence of a homologous animal model of human verbal communication and the biomechanical complexities of the vocal tract, concomitant with restricted opportunities for kinematic and electromyographic (EMG) measurements (Barlow and Farley 1989). Prior to the introduction of brain imaging techniques, analyses of the cerebral network subserving speech motor control predominantly had to rely on detailed perceptual and parametric analyses of dysarthric deficits in patients suffering from focal cerebral lesions or degenerative disorders bound to a distinct functional component of the central motor system, e.g. Parkinson's disease or cerebellar atrophy (see, for example, Kent 1997). Some further data on the cerebral organization of speech motor control have been obtained by means of electrophysiological recordings during brain surgery (craniotomy under local anesthesia) or preoperative diagnostic evaluation of epileptic subjects (subdural or depth electrodes; for a review, see Ojemann 1994). Functional brain imaging techniques such as positron emission tomography (PET) or functional magnetic resonance imaging (fMRI) provide a further approach to the investigation of the cerebral correlates of speech motor control. This chapter focuses on a series of recent fMRI studies of our group that address hypotheses, derived from clinical data, on functional lateralization effects at the level of cerebral cortex and the influence of various brain structures on syllable rate control.

4.2 Clinical aspects of speech motor control

4.2.1 Functional compartmentalization and lateralization at the level of dorsolateral frontal cortex

Speech production poses considerable demands on motor control mechanisms, requiring fast and accurate, i.e. skilled, execution of orofacial gestures properly adjusted in time to laryngeal and respiratory activities. Skilled motor tasks depend upon the integrity of the motor cortex and its projections to the cranial nerve nuclei (Brooks 1986). It has even been suggested that this cerebral component 'initially emerged to control the muscles of the face' in mammals performing manipulative behavior with orofacial and neck structures (Nudo *et al.* 1993). Since the brainstem motor neurons projecting to vocal tract muscles receive input from both cerebral hemispheres, apart from a few exceptions, such as the caudal component of the facial nerve nucleus, unilateral dysfunctions of the upper motor neuron (precentral gyrus and corticobulbar tracts) usually give rise to reduced strength of the lower facial muscles but, as a rule, fail to elicit significant and/or persistent dysarthria. By contrast, bilateral damage either at the cortical or subcortical level may result in the syndrome of spastic dysarthria, characterized, among others, by slowed speech tempo, reduced range of orofacial movements, and hyperadduction of the vocal folds (for a review, see Murdoch *et al.* 1997). In its extreme, anarthria and/or aphonia may develop (pseudobulbar palsy, Foix–Chavany–Marie syndrome).

Geschwind (1969) assumed left-hemisphere dominance of speech production to extend beyond cognitive aspects of language processing to the cortical representation of the orofacial and laryngeal muscle groups supporting articulation and phonation. On the basis of this model, the anterior language zone predominantly delivers its output via the ipsilateral primary motor cortex and the respective efferent corticobulbar tracts to the cranial nerve nuclei of both sides. Conceivably, this mode of innervation avoids lateral competition for the control of midline vocal tract musculature and, therefore, prevents mistiming of motor impulses (asynchronous input) to the relevant brainstem centers. Geschwind derived this concept from clinical data: damage to the left-sided corticobulbar tracts at the level of the internal capsule may give rise to (transient) dysarthria, whereas, in his view, the corresponding lesions at the opposite side fail to elicit speech motor deficits. Restitution of articulation in those instances should thus reflect compensatory activation of an alternative pathway projecting from the anterior language zone to the cranial nerve nuclei via corpus callosum, Broca-analogue of the non-dominant hemisphere and right Rolandic cortex. However, more recent data indicate that at least a subgroup of patients with right-sided damage to the upper motor neuron may exhibit transient speech motor deficits (Duffy and Folger 1996; Urban *et al.* 1997, 2000).

Electrical stimulation of the exposed cortex in awake subjects during brain surgery (intraoperative stimulation mapping) found excitation of the motor strip of either hemisphere to evoke sustained or interrupted 'vowel cries' (Penfield and Roberts

1959). Furthermore, electrical stimulation of left-sided inferior dorsolateral frontal structures rostral to motor cortex may elicit speech arrest as well as an inability to mimic single articulatory gestures (Ojemann 1994). The latter area, therefore, was assumed to represent a 'final motor pathway for speech'. In line with this suggestion, damage to the frontal operculum (Alexander *et al.* 1989) has been assumed to give rise to a variable set of speech motor deficits, including effortful and groping articulatory movements, dysprosody, inconsistent distortions of speech sounds across repeated productions, and obvious difficulties initiating verbal utterances, concomitant with unimpaired non-speech functions of laryngeal and orofacial muscles (apraxia of speech) (for a review, see McNeil *et al.* 1997; also Chapter 15, this volume). This syndrome is considered a higher-level dysfunction, reflecting 'inefficiencies in the translation of a well-formed and filled phonological frame to previously learned kinematic parameters'. More recent data indicate, however, that the clinical constellation referred to might be bound to dysfunctions of intrasylvian cortex rather than Broca's area or opercular precentral gyrus of the language-dominant hemisphere. Based on a large sample of patients, Dronkers (1996) found the anterior insula to represent the area of maximum overlap of lesion sites in apraxia of speech. Thus, conceivably, intrasylvian structures operate as a center of speech motor coordination.

4.2.2 The contribution of subcortical structures to articulation and phonation

Disorders both of the cerebellum and the basal ganglia may compromise vocal tract functions. Ataxic dysarthria of a cerebellar origin has been attributed to lesions of the paramedian aspects of the superior hemispheres. However, as concerns lateralization of speech motor functions within this domain, discrepant data are available so far (for a review, see Ackermann and Hertrich 2000). Cerebellar patients, as a group, exhibit a reduced speaking rate, both during syllable repetition and sentence production tasks. Kinematic recordings indicate this abnormality to reflect, at least within some limits, slowed movement execution of articulatory gestures. In contrast to spastic dysarthria (Ziegler and von Cramon 1986), speech tempo of cerebellar patients does not, however, seem to fall short of a syllable rate of about 3 Hz (Hertrich and Ackermann 1997). Most noteworthy, subjects with Parkinson's disease, a paradigm of basal ganglia disorders, show a mostly normal or even accelerated speech rate, eventually giving rise to speech freezing or hastening (Ackermann *et al.* 1997*a*; Konczak *et al.* 1997). Kinematic recordings revealed unimpaired lower lip excursions during production of sentence utterances in terms of velocity/displacement ratios (articulatory stiffness; Ackermann *et al.* 1997*b*).

4.2.3 Participation of mesiofrontal cortex in speech initiation (supplementary motor area; SMA)

Electrical stimulation of the upper mesiofrontal cortex in awake subjects during surgical interventions has been found to elicit speech arrest or involuntary vocal emissions (supplementary motor area; SMA) (Penfield and Roberts 1959). Neurophysiological investigations in epileptic patients using chronically implanted subdural electrodes were able to record movement-related potentials associated with self-paced tongue protrusions and vocalizations over left SMA (Ikeda *et al.* 1992; only left side explored). Damage to the mesiofrontal cortex may give rise to seizures in terms either of speech arrest or involuntary vocalizations, such as prolonged vocalic sounds or syllable repetitions (Ackermann *et al.* 1996*a*). Furthermore, a clinical syndrome resembling transcortical motor aphasia has been observed in patients suffering from left-sided SMA dysfunctions, characterized by reduced spontaneous verbal communication in the presence of unimpaired language comprehension, verbal repetition and speech articulation (Ackermann *et al.* 1996*b*). SMA, thus, might pertain to a 'starting mechanism of speech' (Botez and Barbeau 1971). Among others, this component of the mesiofrontal cortex shows reciprocal connections with anterior cingulate structures that seem to mediate motivational/attentional aspects of motor behaviour (Ackermann and Ziegler 1995).

4.2.4 Conclusions

Taken together, clinical observations and intraoperative stimulation mapping indicate, first, functional compartmentalization and distinct lateralization effects of speech motor control at the level of the frontal lobe, including the anterior insula, and the cerebellum. However, these data are not yet conclusive. Secondly, upper motor neurons, cerebellum and basal ganglia influence differentially syllable repetitions. For example, only rates above a threshold of about 3 Hz seem to depend critically upon the integrity of cerebellar circuits. Because of the sparse kinematic and EMG data available so far, any pathophysiological interpretation of these findings still faces considerable difficulties. With respect to both issues, functional brain imaging techniques might provide a further perspective for the analysis of the cerebral organization of speech motor control.

4.3 Methodological approaches to functional brain imaging

4.3.1 Electrophysiological procedures

Electro- (EEG) or magnetoencephalographic (MEG) recordings represent the most direct approach to the investigation of the neural correlates of distinct sensorimotor or cognitive tasks available in healthy humans. Given a multitude of adequately spaced channels as, for example, in whole-head MEG, functional brain maps can be computed on the basis of these data. Measurements of evoked electrical potentials or magnetic field strengths at the scalp are a widely used approach to the study of speech sound perception (see, for example, Hertrich *et al.* 2002). By contrast, few EEG and MEG analyses addressing cerebral speech motor control are available so far. Recordings of the readiness potential preceding word utterances revealed, for example, bilateral distribution of slow brain negativity, starting at about 1.5 s prior to the onset of speech (Deecke *et al.* 1986). A significant left-lateralization effect emerged only during a very late time interval of the foreperiod. Comparison of magnetic field changes bound to the production of visually triggered lexical items and vowel-like vocalizations, respectively, suggests preparation of verbal utterances to evolve across two steps that can be assigned tentaively to inferior dorsolateral frontal cortex (Broca's area and its right-emisphere analogue) and to sensorimotor representation areas (Sasaki *et al.* 1996). By contrast to the measurements of the readiness potential preceding self-paced verbal utterances, the latter study failed to document clear-cut lateralization effects.

4.3.2 PET and fMRI techniques

Based on experiments with laboratory animals, Roy and Sherrington (1890) first suggested an 'automatic' increase of regional cerebral blood flow (rCBF) in response to local variations of neural activity (neurovascular coupling; see Roland 1993). Thus, registration of hemodynamic changes should provide a feasible means for the identification of cerebral structures engaged in distinct sensorimotor or cognitive tasks. Early approaches used radioactive inert gases as rCBF tracers (e.g. Xenon clearance technique; see Ryding *et al.* 1987). At this time, PET and fMRI represent the two most important brain imaging techniques based on neurovascular coupling mechanisms. Alternatives such as near-infrared spectroscopy (NIRS) or optical imaging have not yet been applied to speech motor control issues, or are still restricted to animal experimentation. Besides rCBF, metabolic processes, for example, glucose consumption, show a strong correlation with the degree of neural activity. Using a feasible biological probe, PET technology allows for the calculation of local cerebral metabolic rates for glucose (lCMRGlc) within distinct brain structures. Because of a rather long delay (e.g. 30–75 min; Kluin *et al.* 1988) between administration of the tracer and subsequent PET measurements, this method is of limited relevance for the study of speech motor control in normal subjects. However, this procedure has been used to map hypometabolic areas in ataxic dysarthria (see below).

PET technology makes use of the unique radioactive decay characteristics of positrons, i.e. positively charged particles given off by the nucleus of unstable atoms such as ^{15}O (e.g. Toga and Mazziotta 1996). Emitted positrons lose their kinetic energy after traveling just a few millimeters in brain tissue and ultimately are attracted to the negative charge of electrons. Annihilation of these two particles creates two very powerful photons that leave the respective area in exactly opposite direction. Because of their high energy, the photons easily exit the brain at the speed of light. During PET scanning, the subject's head is placed within a corona of radiation detectors, electronically coupled by so-called coincidence circuits. Following the injection of a small amount of ^{15}O-labeled water, the radioactive substance accumulates at the level of the cerebral cortex in direct proportion to regional blood flow and, thus, local neural activity. If two detectors simultaneously record a photon, the respective annihilation event must have occurred on the respective connecting line. These simultaneous collisions are counted and the events converted into an image of blood flow in the brain during the 1 minute interval following injection.

As compared to PET, the more recent fMRI technology represents a completely non-invasive procedure, based on the detection of endogenous tissue contrasts associated with hemodynamic changes. Furthermore, this technique offers superior spatial resolution approximating that of anatomic MR imaging. Deoxygenated hemoglobin acts as a paramagnetic agent that compromises the T_2-weighted MRI signal. Neural activity within circumscribed brain areas gives rise to a transient local increase in rCBF and/or blood volume. The enhanced oxygen supply surpasses the respective metabolic demands. Fast MRI acquisition procedures allow for the monitoring of magnetic susceptibility effects subsequent to the shift in the balance between paramagnetic deoxyhemoglobin and its diamagnetic variant oxyhemoglobin. Thus, neural activity can be detected indirectly as an increase in the local T_2-weighted MRI signal (blood oxygen level dependent (BOLD) effect: more diamagnetic oxyhemoglobin = less paramagnetic deoxyhemoglobin = less distortion of T_2-weighted MRI). In summary, both PET, using radioactively labeled water as a tracer substance, and fMRI detect local changes of cerebral blood flow and, thus, represent indirect measures of neural activity.

4.4 PET studies of speech motor control in normal and dysarthric speakers

4.4.1 Hemodynamic PET investigations in normal subjects

4.4.1.1 Functional cerebral networks subserving motor aspects of speech production

Only a few PET investigations explicitly addressed the motor aspects of speech production. As a by-product, the seminal functional imaging data by Petersen and co-workers published in 1988 and 1989 provided the first systematic account of hemodynamic activation patterns associated with speech motor control. These studies were aimed at the delineation of the neural correlates of lexical operations during single-word processing. Subjects were confronted with a set of tasks of increasing complexity: (a) fixation of a sign appearing on a screen; (b) passive exposure to written or spoken English nouns; (c) spoken repetition of the auditorily or visually applied items; (d) generation of a verb semantically related to the presented noun (compound subtraction procedure or hierarchical design = paired-subtraction design comprising a set of tasks of increasing complexity). It was suggested that subtraction of the hemodynamic responses to the second level of performance, i.e. passive viewing of, or listening to, words, from the rCBF effects bound to the third level, i.e. loud repetition of the nouns, should isolate the brain areas related to motor aspects of speech production. This hierarchical paired-image subtraction procedure revealed bilateral hemodynamic responses at the level of sensorimotor cortex and anterior–superior portions of the cerebellum. Furthermore, activation of SMA, although of a rather faint degree, could be noted. Quite unexpected, finally, a spot 'buried' in the depth of the lateral sulcus emerged, whereas both Broca's area and basal ganglia failed any significant activation effects. In line with several sporadic observations (subjects 2–4 in McCarthy *et al.* 1993; Bookheimer *et al.* 1995), a recent PET study of the neural correlates of speech motor control (repetition of auditorily applied nouns versus stimulus anticipation) was able to attribute this intrasylvian hemodynamic response to the anterior insula (Wise *et al.* 1999; significant effect only at the left side). In accordance with the study by Petersen and co-workers referred to, bilateral activation of sensorimotor cortex and the rostral paravermal cerebellum could be noted. During single-word repetitions, furthermore, an increase of rCBF emerged within dorsal brainstem, anterior cingulate cortex and left posterior pallidum. Thus, the cerebral network of speech motor control as delineated by PET studies, based on the repetition of auditorily or visually displayed nouns as a probe of articulatory/phonatory functions, is in line with the available clinical data on dysarthric deficits (anterior insula, sensorimotor cortex, cerebellum, basal ganglia) and attentional/motivational aspects (anterior cingulate cortex, SMA) of verbal communication (see Introduction above). However, these findings do not corroborate the notion of functional lateralization of speech motor control at the level of Rolandic cortex and cerebellum.

4.4.1.2 *The role of frontal operculum and Broca's area during speech motor control*

A variety of PET studies attributed the subvocal rehearsal mechanism (articulatory loop) of verbal working memory to Broca's area (for a review, see Frackowiak *et al.* 1997). Indeed, articulatory and phonatory disorders had been reported in association with damage to the frontal operculum, i.e. those parts of the inferior frontal and precentral gyrus covering the insular cortex (Schiff *et al.* 1983; Alexander *et al.* 1989). In line with more recent investigations attributing speech apraxia to lesions of the anterior insula (Dronkers 1996), the PET studies on speech motor control referred to failed to detect any significant activation of opercular regions (Petersen *et al.* 1988, 1989; Wise *et al.* 1999). By contrast, hemodynamic responses of left inferior dorsolateral frontal cortex were observed in normal subjects during phonetic/phonological operations such as consonant rhyming or phoneme monitoring (Démonet *et al.* 1992; Zatorre *et al.* 1992) or processing of (difficult) syntactic structures (Caplan *et al.* 1998). Obviously, thus, the contribution of Broca's area to subvocal rehearsal mechanisms must be 'upstream' to the specification of sequenced articulatory gestures in terms of, for example, motor programs, and might be bound to short-term storage of phonetic/ phonological representations.

4.4.1.3 Differential activation patterns bound to orofacial and laryngeal processes during speech production

Petersen and co-workers (1988, 1989) used a compound subtraction procedure in order to separate cognitive (lexical retrieval) and motor aspects (articulation/phonation) of language processing (see above). As a test of the validity of this approach, a recent PET study applied the principles of decomposition logic on speech motor control itself (Sidtis *et al.* 1999). On these grounds, syllable repetitions might be conceived of as the 'sum' of lip closure movements and laryngeal activity. Thus, the activation pattern bound to phonation tasks (minus baseline) must be expected, for example, to equal the difference in hemodynamic responses to lip gestures and syllable repetitions. Besides a baseline condition, i.e. subjects being quiet and awake, three activation tasks were considered for analysis: (a) iteration of the syllables *pa, ta,* and *ka* as quickly as possible; (b) sustained production of the vowel *a*; and (c) repetitive lip closures. The PET measurements failed to document any task additivity under these conditions. Most noteworthy, the 'simpler' tasks of sustained phonation and lip closure movements yielded more pronounced activation foci (task versus baseline condition each) within several regions than the ostensibly more complex demands of syllable repetitions (see below, Section 4.5.4, for similar results). As concerns lateralization effects of speech motor control, visual inspection of Fig. 1 in Sidtis *et al.* (1999) indicates bilateral activation at the level of the cerebellum (left > right), superior temporal lobe, sensorimotor cortex, basal ganglia including thalamus, and SMA. Most noteworthy, phonation yielded predominant right-hemisphere activation at the level of pre- and postcentral as well as superior temporal gyrus (see below, Section 4.5.3.), whereas the two other tasks gave rise to a more symmetrical pattern of hemodynamic responses within these regions.

4.4.2 Metabolic and hemodynamic PET investigations in dysarthric speakers

Few PET studies explicitly tried to map metabolic or hemodynamic brain activity in dysarthric subjects. Kluin and co-workers (1988) studied the relationship between local glucose metabolism and perceptual dimensions of speech motor deficits in patients suffering from olivopontocerebellar atrophy. As its most important finding, this investigation documented a significant relationship between cerebellar hypometabolism and (a revised concept of) ataxic dysarthria. A further investigation conducted multiple linear regression analyses on PET measurements of rCBF and oral diadochokinesis data in normals and in subjects with hereditary ataxia (Sidtis *et al.* 1998). Most noteworthy, the various genotypes of the cerebellar disorder were characterized by different patterns of hemodynamic effects. In the majority of patients (molecular-genetic diagnoses: spinocerebellar atrophy 1 (SCA1) and 6 (SCA6), i.e. two variants of a progressive, autosomal-dominant cerebellar ataxia), a positive correlation between syllable repetition rate and left-frontal/right-cerebellar activity emerged. By contrast, behavioral performance in SCA5 could be predicted by a combined direct and inverse relationship with rCBF data obtained from SMA, thalamus, and cerebellum.

4.5 Cooperation of sensorimotor cortex, anterior insula, and cerebellum during speech production (word strings): fMRI investigations

4.5.1 Introduction

The following sections summarize recent work of our group on the functional compartmentalization and lateralization of speech motor control at the level of the central nervous system. Geschwind's suggestion (1969), that the anterior language zone of the left hemisphere delivers its output predominantly via the ipsilateral primary motor cortex and the respective efferent corticobulbar tracts to the cranial nerve nuclei of both sides, provided the vantage point of these investigations. PET studies on the cerebral correlates of speech motor control found, by contrast, repetition of auditorily or visually displayed nouns (Petersen *et al.* 1988, 1989; Wise *et al.* 1999) as well as syllable iterations (Sidtis *et al.* 1999) to yield rather symmetrical hemodynamic responses at the level of sensorimotor cortex. Sidtis and co-workers (1999) even found higher activation of the right hemisphere during sustained phonation. However, a series of PET experiments comprising various listening, repetition and reading conditions (single words each as test materials) reported unilateral left-sided responses of at least in a minority of the calculated contrasts (Price *et al.* 1996). Furthermore, production of different successive items resulted in more pronounced activation of the 'speech motor network' (SMA, motor cortex, subcortical grey matter, midline cerebellum) than continuous iteration of the same sensorimotor cortex word stimulus.

Conceivably, fMRI measurements provide a more sensitive tool for the evaluation of cerebral laterality effects. Since speaking aloud during fMRI may give rise to considerable motion artefacts (Birn *et al.* 1998), the early studies of language processing often favored 'silent' task paradigms (see, for example, Huang *et al.* 2001). Hemodynamic responses of motor cortex during silent word generation first were described in a fMRI study conducted by Rueckert and co-workers (1994; no explicit statement on laterality effects). Furthermore, several investigations found predominant engagement of left-hemisphere frontal structures, including sensorimotor cortex, during silent (covert) word generation (e.g. Yetkin *et al.* 1995). At a first glance, covert or inner speech, i.e. auditory verbal imagery, does not represent a feasible probe of speech motor control (Sidtis *et al.* 1998). However, EMG measurements found action potentials in vocal tract muscles during silent speaking (Sokolov 1972). Even passive listening to speech may specifically modulate the excitability of tongue musculature as determined by transcranial magnetic stimulation (Fadiga *et al.* 2002). It can be assumed, thus, that auditory verbal imagery recruits to some degree the central-motor system. Indeed, similar sensorimotor cortex activation patterns during covert and audible phonological fluency tasks have been observed (Yetkin *et al.* 1995).

To further elucidate cerebral lateralization effects of speech motor control, a series of fMRI studies was conducted using both auditory verbal imagery ('inner speech') and overt speech (word strings, utterances varying in phonetic complexity) as test materials. Silent and spoken production of tunes (melodies) as well as execution of non-speech orofacial movements served as control conditions. Furthermore, reorganization of activation patterns during follow-up in a patient with capsular dysarthria was studied. It turned out that the analyses of auditory imagery as well as singing, in addition to (overt) speech tasks, shed new light on the contribution of anterior insula and cerebellum to acoustic communication.

All functional imaging studies on peri-/intrasylvian and cerebellar laterality effects (Sections 4.5.2–4.5.5 below) were performed by means of a 1.5 Tesla whole-body scanner (Siemens Vision; Siemens, Germany) using an echoplanar imaging (EPI) sequence across complete brain volume. High-resolution images based on a T_1-weighted three-dimensional turbo-flash sequence served as an anatomic reference.

4.5.2 Functional compartmentalization and hemispheric lateralization at the level of sensorimotor cortex and cerebellum

4.5.2.1 Activation patterns of sensorimotor cortex during auditory imagery of speech and tunes

Experimental design

Considering the Geschwind model of speech production, left-lateralized hemodynamic responses of the motor strip in association with articulatory/phonatory processes must be expected. In contrast, a variety of clinical data indicated modulation of pitch to be controlled predominantly by the right precentral gyrus (for a review, see Wildgruber *et al.* 1996). To focus on segmental aspects of verbal utterances, and to avoid eventual confounding influences of intonational patterns, test materials were selected that should elicit a rather monotonous mode of speech production. Recitation of highly overlearned word strings such as the names of the months of the year might represent a feasible task in this regard (automatic speech; e.g. Ryding *et al.* 1987). Vertical non-speech tongue movements, the lips being closed, and singing of a well-known Christmas melody on the syllable /la/ served as control conditions. To avoid movement artefacts, the speaking and singing tasks had to be carried out in a silent mode (inner speech, auditory verbal imagery).

Ten healthy, right-handed subjects (five females, aged 20–36 years) participated in the fMRI investigation (Wildgruber *et al.* 1996). Each of the three tasks considered included eight successive groups of five measurements each, alternately performed during rest and activation (block design). Signal analysis relied on a region-of-interest (ROI) approach: several areas, among others, precentral gyrus and mesiofrontal cortex, were manually drawn on individual slices. Subsequently, the number of activated voxels was determined within each ROI.

Results and discussion

As an example, Fig. 4.1 displays the results obtained in a representative subject at the level of sensorimotor cortex: inner speech yielded predominant left-sided activation, whereas lateralization effects towards the contralateral hemisphere emerged during silent production of a tune. Hemodynamic responses of a rather symmetrical bilateral distribution could be observed in association with non-speech tongue movements. Since the activation spots obtained during speaking and singing were found localized within the area of tongue movement representation, significant contributions of Broca's area or its right-hemisphere analogue can be ruled out. These results provide the first functional imaging evidence for opposite lateralization effects within sensorimotor cortex during word generation and production of tunes, respectively.

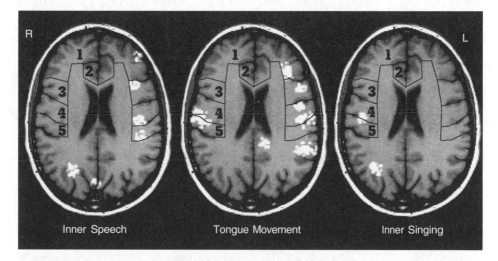

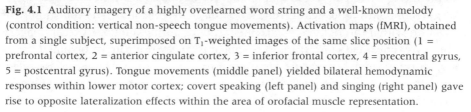

Fig. 4.1 Auditory imagery of a highly overlearned word string and a well-known melody (control condition: vertical non-speech tongue movements). Activation maps (fMRI), obtained from a single subject, superimposed on T_1-weighted images of the same slice position (1 = prefrontal cortex, 2 = anterior cingulate cortex, 3 = inferior frontal cortex, 4 = precentral gyrus, 5 = postcentral gyrus). Tongue movements (middle panel) yielded bilateral hemodynamic responses within lower motor cortex; covert speaking (left panel) and singing (right panel) gave rise to opposite lateralization effects within the area of orofacial muscle representation.

In spite of predominant left-sided activation of sensorimotor cortex at the group level during production of automatic speech, some interindividual variability of the elicited BOLD changes must be noted. For example, one participant exhibited a predominant right-hemisphere lateralization effect (see Wildgruber *et al.* 1996, Table 1, subject no.3). These observations are in accord with recent clinical studies reporting (at variance with the Geschwind model) (transient) dysarthria in a subgroup of patients with unilateral right-hemisphere upper motor neuron lesions (Urban *et al.* 2000; up to 24%).

4.5.2.2 *Cerebellar contributions to auditory verbal imagery (inner speech)*

Experimental design

Besides the neural correlates of speech motor control, Petersen and coworkers (1988, 1989) tried to identify the cerebral network supporting cognitive aspects of single-word processing, i.e. retrieval of lexical items. To these ends, activation maps obtained during reading or repetition of visually or auditorily displayed nouns were subtracted from the hemodynamic response patterns bound to verb genera-tion (see 4.4.1.1 for further details). Lexical operations were found to elicit a significant focal BOLD effect within the lateral parts of the right cerebellar hemi-sphere. Several subsequent investigations also documented focal right-cerebellar activation during semantic tasks (for a review, see Fiez and Raichle 1997). However, visual inspection of the activation maps obtained during the preceding investigation of auditory verbal imagery revealed a significant hemodynamic response of the lateral parts of the right cerebellar hemisphere as well. For the sake of better comparability with the PET data referred to, the previous study on 'inner speech' was replicated and extended (software for signal analysis: Statistical Parametric Mapping (SPM) system; Wellcome Institute of Cognitive Neuroscience, London, UK; see Frackowiak *et al.* 1997; anatomical localization of activation spots: coordinates of the 'Talairach-atlas'; see Talairach and Tournoux 1988). Eighteen subjects (ten of them had participated in experiment 4.5.2.1; eight females, aged 19–36 years) underwent fMRI measurements during continuous silent recitation of the names of the months of the year (Ackermann *et al.* 1998; the experimental design corresponded to that of study 4.5.2.1.).

Results and discussion

Signal analysis based on the SPM software package revealed four clusters of acti-vated voxels (corrected *P* value < 0.05): left sensorimotor cortex, left temporopari-etal junction, SMA, and right cerebellar hemisphere (Fig. 4.2). The topography of activation within the right cerebellar hemisphere during auditory verbal imagery of highly overlearned word strings resembled the response pattern obtained previ-ously during experiments addressing semantic operations (verbal response selec-tion), although the former task should not pose any significant demands on lexical search processes.

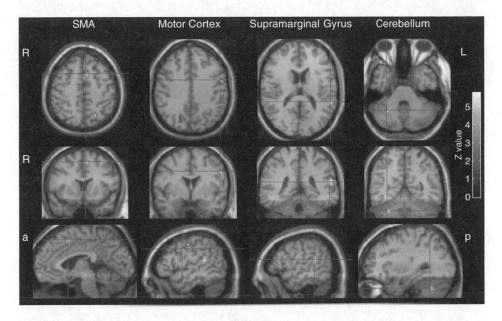

Fig. 4.2 Auditory verbal imagery (silent recitation of a highly overlearned word string): fMRI activation maps superimposed on the averaged T_1-weighted anatomical images (Talairach space) across subjects at the level of the supplementary motor area (SMA), motor cortex, temporoparietal junction, and cerebellum (upper row, transverse; middle row, coronal; lower row, sagittal slices). See also in colour, Plate 1.

Petersen and collaborators (1988, 1989) had compared repetition/reading tasks with verb generation. Indeed, both conditions include the same number and rate of target stimuli. It was assumed, therefore, that these two steps of single-word processing are comparable with respect to motor demands on speech production. Quite conceivably, however, the semantic task considered evokes involuntarily a plurality of subvocal representations of lexical items related to the target nouns, among which ultimately a single one is selected for response. Since silent speaking has been shown to activate the neural network subserving articulation and phonation, e.g. action potentials can be recorded from vocal tract muscles under these conditions, semantic tasks comprising lexical search processes, thus, can be expected to activate the speech motor system to a higher degree than repetition, reading and naming of single visually or auditorily displayed items. Thus, the hierarchical pair-wise subtraction approach might have failed to cancel articulatory processes, and the observed right-cerebellar response may reflect inner speech-based rehearsal mechanisms of working memory rather than lexical operations.

4.5.3 The contribution of the anterior insula to speech motor control: coordination of vocal tract musculature and/or processing of reafferent input

Experimental design

Based on neuroradiological data obtained in patients suffering from apraxia of speech, the anterior insula of the dominant hemisphere has been assumed to operate as a 'center' of speech motor coordination (Dronkers 1996). In accordance with this suggestion, PET studies documented predominantly left-sided activation of intrasylvian cortex during naming (line drawings depicting concrete objects), reading and repetition (auditorily or visually displayed nouns) tasks (Bookheimer *et al.* 1995; Wise *et al.* 1999; see, however, Price *et al.* 1996, p.926, for discrepant findings). Alongside spoken language, singing represents a second mode of acoustic (auditory-vocal) communication in mankind. Clinical observations as well as experimental studies provided some evidence that, at least within some limits, singing might critically depend upon right-hemisphere structures (for a review, see Riecker *et al.* 2000*a*). Since, first, the left intrasylvian cortex seems to mediate motor aspects of verbal utterances and since, second, silent speaking and silent singing had been found to elicit opposite lateralization effects at the level of the motor cortex (see Section 4.5.2.1), the right-hemisphere anterior insula can be expected to subserve coordination of vocal tract musculature during production of melodies (tunes).

Again, continuous recitation of the months of the year (automatic speech) served as a probe of speech motor control. Instead of syllabic singing of a well-known Christmas song (see Section 4.5.2.1, above), subjects were asked to reproduce a non-lyrical tune drawn from a serenade in order to avoid any retrieval of propositional materials. Both tasks were performed aloud and silently. Eighteen healthy, right-handed speakers of standard German (nine females, aged 22–63 years) underwent fMRI measurements during speech and melody production (Riecker *et al.* 2000*a*). Each task was applied 12 times in a counterbalanced order (onset-to-onset intervals between activation phases = 24 s). Subjects performed speaking and singing at their habitual tempo, and were asked to refrain from verbal thought during the intervening rest periods. Production rates of speaking and singing had been determined during the training phase (overt generation of the word string 'January–December': mean 5.6 s, standard deviation 1.3 s; overt production of a part of a serenade: mean 6.9 s, standard deviation 1.1 s). First, the data obtained during activation phases were compared to the respective baseline conditions. Secondly, in order to further enhance the hypothesized opposite hemispheric lateralization effects during speaking and singing, two cognitive subtraction approaches were added: (a) overt speech versus overt singing and vice versa; (b) overt versus covert speech as well as overt versus covert singing.

Results and discussion

Analysis of group data revealed exclusive activation of the right motor cortex/ posterior inferior frontal gyrus as well as the left cerebellar hemisphere during covert singing. Silent speech resulted in an opposite response pattern. Overt task performance yielded rather bilateral activation within these areas, concomitant, however, with moderate lateralization effects towards the same direction as the imagery conditions. Significant blood flow increase at the level of intrasylvian cortex was restricted to overt tasks (speaking aloud = left anterior insula; singing aloud = right anterior insula). This pattern of insular activation turned out to be preserved after subtraction of the respective hemodynamic responses obtained during the silent modes of speaking and singing (overt versus covert speech; overt versus covert singing; Fig. 4.3). Any differences between overt and covert performance, thus, do not just reflect threshold effects. Furthermore, the robust double dissociation at the level of the anterior insula was confirmed by the second cognitive subtraction procedure (i.e. singing aloud minus speaking aloud and vice versa).

As a new aspect of brain lateralization, these data point to two complementary cerebral networks subserving singing and speaking: reproduction of a non-lyrical tune predominantly elicited activation within the right motor cortex, the right anterior insula, and the left cerebellum, whereas the opposite response pattern emerged during a speech task. In contrast to the hemodynamic responses within motor cortex and cerebellum, activation of the intrasylvian cortex turned out to be bound to overt task performance. These findings, first, are compatible with the assumption that the left insula supports the coordination of speech articulation, and indicate, secondly, that the right insula might mediate, in a similar vein,

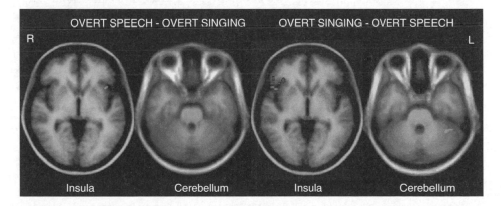

Fig. 4.3 Hemodynamic activation patterns at the level of the anterior insula during recitation of a highly overlearned word string (speaking) and reproduction of a non-lyrical tune (singing): cognitive subtraction approach (overt versus covert speaking, overt versus covert singing). See also in colour, Plate 2.

temporospatial control of vocal tract musculature during overt singing. Both speech and melody production require the integration of linguistic and melodic patterns, respectively, with a speaker's emotions and attitudes. Considering the widespread interconnections with premotor cortex, sensory areas, and limbic structures (Mesulam and Mufson 1985), the insula seems to be especially suited for this task. The physiological mechanisms of these opposite lateralization effects remain to be clarified. Behavioral as well as electrophysiological data indicate, for example, a higher proficiency of the right hemisphere for short-term storage of tonal information (Mathiak *et al.* 2002) as well as suprasegmental aspects of acoustic communication (e.g. Riecker *et al.* 2002*a*). Both these two side-differences in processing capabilities could contribute to predominant right-hemisphere support of melody production.

As an alternative to the suggestion that the anterior insula mediates the coordination of actual vocal tract innervation during speech production, the association of significant intrasylvian hemodynamic responses with overt speaking/singing might reflect the processing of reafferent auditory and/or somatosensory input arising during articulation and phonation. For example, activation of the insular cortex could be observed in response to passive listening to auditory stimuli (Ackermann *et al.* 2001). Although not yet conclusive, these data provide first support for the suggestion of insular processing of reafferent input arising during speech production.

4.5.4 Influence of the phonetic structure of verbal utterances on lateralization effects at the level of the sensorimotor cortex

Experimental design
In subjects with apraxia of speech, syllable repetition is often found to be less impaired than sentence production (Ackermann *et al.* 1997*c*). Thus, functional lateralization and compartmentalization of speech motor control might depend upon lexical status and/or phonological structure of the test materials considered. Based on these suggestions, hemodynamic responses were measured during reiteration of syllables differing in their demands on articulatory/phonetic sequencing (CV versus CCCV versus CVCVCV). Horizontal tongue movements and a polysyllabic lexical item served as control conditions.

Ten healthy, right-handed German subjects (five females, range 21–32 years) participated in the present study (Riecker *et al.* 2000*b*). Test materials comprised the monosyllables *ta* and *stra,* the syllable sequence *pataka,* the lexical item *Tagebau* ('strip mining') and horizontal tongue movements. All the nonsense-items considered, i.e. *ta, stra* and *pataka,* accord to the phonotactic rules of German but differ in articulatory/phonetic complexity. Subjects were asked to produce the syllables and words in a monotonous manner, i.e. without prosodic modulation, at a self-paced, comfortable speaking rate during the measurement periods (1 min each) and to refrain from verbal thought during the intervening rest periods. Similar to the CV and CCCV items, *pataka* and *Tagebau* had to be equally spaced during scanning (order of task administration randomized across participants). Subjects' utterances were recorded by means of a microphone during functional imaging in order to determine the number of syllables per minute. Since the rate of non-speech movements could not be determined during scanning, subjects were asked to perform with the mouth open horizontal tongue movements at a self-paced preferred tempo prior to the experiment. Tongue excursions from the left to the right side and back counted as a single gesture. Each task comprised 8 groups of 10 measurements, alternately performed during rest and activation (four groups of measurements each). Total scanning time per task thus amounted to 8 min (8 groups × 10 measurements of a duration of 6 s each).

Results and discussion
During the production of syllable strings, rCBF increase was found to be restricted to the anterior and posterior bank of the central sulcus. If at all, only horizontal tongue movements elicited activation spots extending to the rostral aspects of the precentral gyrus. Besides the latter task, bilateral hemodynamic responses also emerged during repetitions of *ta*, *stra*, and *Tagebau*. Under these conditions, however, a considerably reduced extent of the activation spots could be noted, both at the horizontal and coronal planes. As compared to the monosyllables *ta* and *stra*, the lexical item *Tagebau* yielded a more pronounced lateralization effect towards the dominant hemisphere, both in terms of the number of activated voxels as well as the maximum hemodynamic response. In contrast, the non-lexical polysyllables gave rise to an exclusively left-hemisphere response (at the given significance level of signal analysis) restricted to the sensorimotor region. There is neurophysiological evidence that the primary sensorimotor cortex mediates the 'fractionation of movements' (Brooks 1986). Assuming that the polysyllables considered are organized as coarticulated higher-order units, the observed restricted and lateralized cortical activation pattern, presumably, reflects a mode of 'non-individualized' motor control posing smaller demands on 'movement fractionation'. In line with this suggestion, non-speech orofacial movements yielded considerably larger activation spots than syllable strings (see Sidtis *et al.* 1999).

Production of syllable and word strings occurred at a rather low tempo (70–90 items per minute). Conceivably, the noisy environment and the supine position of the subjects during fMRI measurements account for these effects. The lessened repetition rates might explain the absence of significant insular activation as well as the missing hemodynamic responses, under most conditions, of the cerebellum. If at all, only horizontal tongue movements yielded a hemodynamic reaction extending beyond the sensorimotor cortex to rostral premotor areas. Since limbic projections target the inferior dorsolateral frontal lobe, the enlarged region of activation during horizontal tongue movements might reflect the increased attention or effort demands of this task.

4.5.5 Reorganization of cortical activation patterns after capsular dysarthria: a case study

Based on the Geschwind-model of speech production, restitution of articulation in cases of (transient) dysarthria subsequent to left-sided capsular lesions must be expected to reflect compensatory activation of an alternative pathway projecting from the anterior language zone to the cranial nerve nuclei via corpus callosum, Broca-analogue of the non-dominant hemisphere and right Rolandic cortex. In order to test this hypothesis, a follow-up fMRI study was performed in a 38-year-old male patient who had experienced sudden speech deterioration concomitant with right-sided weakness of the upper limb and face about 4 hours prior to admission to the Department of Neurology, University of Tübingen (Riecker *et al.* 2002*b*). Clinical evaluation of articulatory and phonatory functions on the same day revealed moderately slowed speech tempo, concomitant with impaired precision of consonant productions during conversation. Accordingly, syllable repetition tasks yielded reduced maximum performance as compared to control subjects. Besides hoarse and strained-strangled voice quality, a reduced range of pitch and loudness could be noted. These dysarthric signs completely recovered within the following 9 days. Computerized tomography and magnetic resonance imaging demonstrated an ischemic infarction, lacking any space-occupying effects, within the area of blood supply of the left lenticulostriate arteries, embracing the internal capsule and putamen.

Again, the subject was asked to continuously recite the names of the months of the year during fMRI measurements, a task that poses few, if any, demands on higher-order linguistic functions. Automatic speech had to be produced both aloud (overt speech) and in a silent mode (covert or inner speech). Each task was applied 12 times in a counterbalanced order. The subject had been instructed to produce the word strings at his habitual speech tempo and to refrain from verbal thought during the intervening rest periods. Distinct visual symbols displayed on a screen indicated the task to be performed. Functional imaging was performed both during the presence of dysarthria (4 days after onset) and after complete recovery from speech motor deficits (35 days after onset; measurement parameters corresponded to Section 4.5.3). At both sessions, speaking rate had been determined during a training phase prior to the experiment (4 days: mean time interval of overt production of the word string 'January–December' = 11.7 ms; 35 days: 6.3 s). Two levels of analysis were considered: (a) overt or covert speaking minus the respective baseline level, performed separately at both sessions; (b) activation at day 4 minus activation at day 35 and vice versa. The latter approach accentuates any signal changes in terms of reorganization across follow-up. Figure 4.4 demonstrates the mirror-like reversal of hemodynamic activation at the level of motor cortex and cerebellum both during overt and covert task performance.

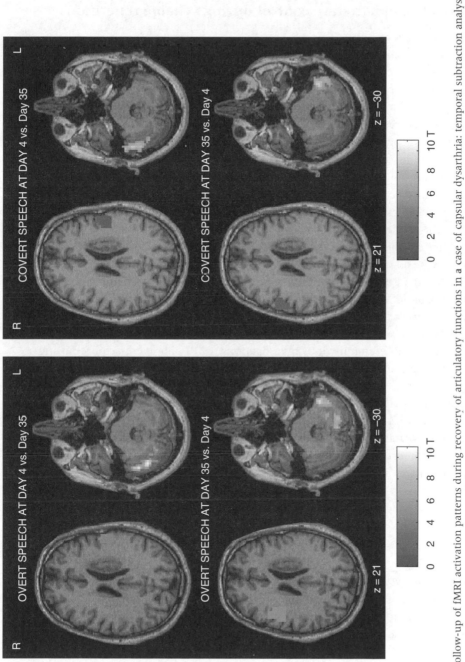

Fig. 4.4 Follow-up of fMRI activation patterns during recovery of articulatory functions in a case of capsular dysarthria: temporal subtraction analysis (measurements obtained during day 4 versus day 35 and vice versa) during overt and covert speech production. Significant hemodynamic responses within motor cortex and cerebellum are superimposed on transverse sections of the anatomical reference images (left half of a slice = right hemisphere and vice versa, z = distance to intercommisural plane, SPM99: $T > 4.70$, $P < 0.05$ corrected). See also in colour, Plate 3.

4.6 fMRI investigations on the contributions of the cerebellum and basal ganglia to rate control during syllable repetitions

Experimental design

Syllable repetitions performed as fast as possible (oral diadochokinesis) represent a valid probe of maximum speaking rate, being an important measure of articulatory performance (Kent *et al.* 1987). As a rule, patients with idiopathic Parkinson's disease (PD) show unimpaired oral diadochokinesis. By contrast, cerebellar dysarthria is characterized by a reduced maximum rate, which, nevertheless, does not seem to fall below 3 Hz (Hertrich and Ackermann 1997). Based on these clinical observations, a different contribution of motor cortex, basal ganglia, and cerebellum to the control of syllable iterations must be expected. To be more specific: only rates above a threshold of about 3 Hz seem to depend significantly upon the integrity of the cerebellum.

Ten right-handed, native German subjects (five females, aged 22–32 years) participated in the fMRI study on syllable repetitions (Wildgruber *et al.* 2001). Subjects were asked to produce repetitions of the syllable *ta* at three different rates (2.5, 4.0, and 5.5 Hz), performance being paced via earphones by recorded trains of the syllable *ta* at the respective repetition frequencies. In order to minimize movement artefacts, all tasks were carried out silently (covert or inner speech mode). This procedure had been proven valid as a means of evaluating speech motor control in several previous investigations. fMRI data were acquired using a multislice echoplanar imaging sequence (27 slices, thickness = 4 mm, gap = 1 mm, TR = 5 s, alpha = 90 deg, FOV = 192 × 192 mm, 64 × 64 matrix) implemented on a 1.5 Tesla whole-body scanner (Siemens Vision; Siemens, Germany). High-resolution images obtained with a T_1-weighted three-dimensional turbo-flash sequence served as an anatomical reference. The experiment was carried out in a block design: each session of continuous data acquisition comprised eight successive blocks of 10 measurements alternately carried out during rest and task administration. Statistical evaluation, comprising two different approaches of data analysis, i.e. categorical analysis and parametric evaluation of rate- and time-dependent effects, relied on the SPM software package (SPM99).

Results and discussion

Categorical analysis of group data revealed a significant hemodynamic response of the superior temporal gyrus and the precentral region across all task conditions. The activation cluster at the level of the motor cortex encompassed both the premotor area, i.e. lateral aspects of Brodmann area (BA) 6, as well as the primary motor region (BA 4). In contrast, cerebellar activation was restricted to 4.0 and 5.5 Hz. The latter two tasks elicited bilateral responses within superior paravermal regions extending symmetrically into the superior intermedio-lateral aspects of the posterior cerebellar lobe (lobulus simplex). As compared to 4.0 Hz repetitions, the

5.5 Hz responses showed a more pronounced extension in the caudal direction, whereas the cranial part of the activation clusters covered basically the same bilateral area within the cerebellar hemispheres. Analysis of activation differences via the subtraction approach corroborated the findings of frequency-dependent hemodynamic responses within the cerebellum.

Parametric analysis with respect to syllable production frequency yielded main effects across all tasks within bilateral motor cortex and cerebellum. In the absence of an extension threshold, additional clusters of activation emerged within SMA and left putamen. Considering the amplitudes of hemodynamic responses at local activation maxima within each cluster revealed an increase of response magnitude in parallel to syllable production rates at the level of SMA and bilateral motor cortex. In contrast, activation within the left putamen exhibited a maximum during 4.0 Hz, and a minimum during 5.5 Hz, repetitions. Cerebellar activation, in contrast, showed a threshold phenomenon with almost no signal increase during 2.5 Hz and basically similar response magnitudes during 4.0 and 5.5 Hz syllable productions. Thus, lower rates (2.5 and 4.0 Hz) gave rise to higher magnitudes of activation as compared to the 5.5 Hz condition within the left putamen, whereas cerebellar responses were restricted to fast performance (4.0 and 5.5 Hz) and exhibited a shift in caudal direction during 5.5 as compared to 4.0 Hz. These findings corroborate the suggestion of a differential impact of various cortical and subcortical areas on speech rate control.

Acoustic measurements had found reduced maximum syllable repetition rates in cerebellar disorders that, however, do not fall below 3 Hz (Hertrich and Ackermann 1997). In line with these data, significant cerebellar activation was restricted to repetition rates above 3 Hz. Thus, both acoustic and fMRI data indicate acceleration of syllable repetition rates beyond a threshold of about 3 Hz to depend upon the integrity of cerebellar circuitry. Furthermore, previous kinematic recordings of lower lip gestures in cerebellar patients had revealed a linear relationship between movement amplitude and peak velocity (Ackermann *et al.* 1995). By contrast to normal subjects, however, the slope of the calculated regression lines (articulatory stiffness) was significantly reduced, indicating reduced force generation. Thus, the impaired ability to accelerate syllable rates beyond a threshold of about 3 Hz might reflect compromised force generation of single articulatory gestures.

4.7 Summary: the contribution of cerebellum and anterior insula to speech motor control

A series of fMRI studies of our group investigated functional lateralization and compartmentalization of speech motor control at the level of the central nervous system. Spoken word strings (automatic speech) yielded bilateral hemodynamic activation of sensorimotor cortex and cerebellar hemispheres in association with the left anterior insula. By contrast, silent production of the same test materials (auditory verbal imagery, inner speech) resulted in a more limited response pattern encompassing left sensorimotor cortex and right cerebellum, but sparing intrasylvian cortex.

Jeannerod (1994) suggested motor imagery to provide a 'window' into the mechanisms of action planning, i.e. preparatory activities preceding actual performance of movement sequences. Considering the fMRI data obtained during inner speech, i.e. some kind of auditory verbal imagery, the left sensorimotor cortex and right cerebellar hemisphere—both structures are interconnected by reciprocal fiber systems— seem to support pre-articulatory motor control processes, at least at syllable rates above *c*. 3 Hz. By contrast, the anterior insula seems to operate 'downstream' to the cerebellum during production of verbal utterances. Conceivably, this region supports the transformation of a pre-articulatory speech code into an elaborated spatiotemporal pattern of motor commands driving vocal tract muscles. Alternatively, insular activation during overt task performance could reflect auditory and/or somatosensory reafferent input during speech production. For example, there is preliminary evidence for insular hemodynamic responses during passive listening to auditory input (Ackermann *et al*. 2001).

Inner speech is considered a pre-articulatory, but otherwise fully parsed and, thus, temporally organized, representation of sound structure (Levelt 1989). Clinical and experimental data indicate a contribution of the cerebellum to the sequencing both of motor and cognitive activities (for a review, see Schmahmann 1997). In line with these suggestions, a variety of acoustic and kinematic studies provided evidence for cerebellar participation in speech timing (Ackermann and Hertrich 2000). As a fully parsed representation of sound structure, inner speech must be expected to comprise a similar temporal syllabic organization as spoken verbal utterances. Thus, the cerebellum should also support the timing of the assumed pre-articulatory verbal code. Besides the timing of inner speech, the cerebellum contributes to motor execution. For example, previous kinematic studies reported evidence for compromised force generation in cerebellar disorders (Ackermann *et al*. 1995, 1997*b*). Participation in motor execution processes might explain the more widespread cerebellar activation pattern encroaching upon both hemispheres during overt speech production.

Whereas auditory verbal imagery in terms of the silent recitation of a highly overlearned word string yielded predominant activation of the left motor cortex concomitant with the right cerebellar hemisphere, reproduction of a non-lyrical tune resulted in a reversed pattern of cerebral activation, i.e. right precentral gyrus and left cerebellar hemisphere. Furthermore, overt speaking and singing gave rise to an opposite laterality effect at the level of anterior peri-/intrasylvian cortex. The physiological mechanisms of these functional asymmetries remain to be clarified. Conceivably, the right hemisphere possesses higher processing capabilities for short-term storage of tonal information (see Mathiak *et al*. 2002*a*) or, as an alternative, suprasegmental aspects of acoustic communication (see Riecker *et al*. 2002*a*).

References

Ackermann, H. and Hertrich, I. (2000). The contribution of the cerebellum to speech processing. *Journal of Neurolinguistics*, 13, 95–116.

Ackermann, H. and Ziegler, W. (1995). Akinetic mutism: a review. *Fortschritte der Neurologie und Psychiatrie*, 63, 59–67 (German).

Ackermann, H. and Hertrich, I. and **Scharf, G.** (1995). Kinematic analysis of lower lip movements in ataxic dysarthria. *Journal of Speech and Hearing Research*, 38, 1252–1259.

Ackermann, H., Daum, I., Schugens, M.M. and **Grodd, W.** (1996a). Impaired procedural learning following damage to the left supplementary motor area (SMA). *Journal of Neurology, Neurosurgery, and Psychiatry*, 60, 94–97.

Ackermann, H., Hertrich, I., Ziegler, W., Bitzer, M. and **Bien, S.** (1996b). Acquired dysfluencies following infarction of the left mesiofrontal cortex. *Aphasiology*, 10, 409–417.

Ackermann, H., Konczak, J. and **Hertrich, I.** (1997a). The temporal control of repetitive articulatory movements in Parkinson's disease. *Brain and Language*, 56, 312–319.

Ackermann, H., Hertrich, I., Daum, I., Scharf, G. and **Spieker, S.** (1997b). Kinematic analysis of articulatory movements in central motor disorders. *Movement Disorders*, 12, 1019–1027.

Ackermann, H., Scharf, G., Hertrich, I. and **Daum, I.** (1997c). Articulatory disorders in primary progressive aphasia: an acoustic and kinematic analysis. *Aphasiology*, 11, 1017–1030.

Ackermann, H., Wildgruber, D., Daum, I. and **Grodd, W.** (1998). Does the cerebellum contribute to cognitive aspects of speech production? A functional magnetic resonance imaging (fMRI) study in humans. *Neuroscience Letters*, 247, 187–190.

Ackermann, H., Riecker, A., Mathiak, K., Erb, M., Grodd, W. and **Wildgruber, D.** (2001). Rate-dependent activation of a prefrontal-insular-cerebellar network during passive listening to trains of click stimuli: an fMRI study. *NeuroReport*, 12, 4087–4092.

Alexander, M.P., Benson, D.F. and **Stuss, D.T.** (1989). Frontal lobes and language. *Brain and Language*, 37, 656–691.

Barlow, S.M. and **Farley, G.R.** (1989). Neurophysiology of speech. In D.P. Kuehn, M.L. Lemme and J.M. Baumgartner, eds. *Neural bases of speech, hearing, and language*, pp. 146–200. College-Hill Press, Boston, MA.

Birn, R.M., Bandettini, P.A., Cox, R.W., Jesmanowicz, A. and **Shaker, R.** (1998). Magnetic field changes in the human brain due to swallowing or speaking. *Magnetic Resonance in Medicine*, 40, 55–60.

Bookheimer, S.Y., Zeffiro, T.A., Blaxton, T., Gaillard, W. and **Theodore, W.** (1995). Regional cerebral blood flow during object naming and word reading. *Human Brain Mapping*, 3, 93–106.

Botez, M.I. and **Barbeau, A.** (1971). Role of subcortical structures, and particularly of the thalamus, in the mechanisms of speech and language: a review. *International Journal of Neurology,* 8, 300–320.

Brooks, V.B. (1986). *The neural basis of motor control.* Oxford Univ. Press, New York, NY.

Caplan, D., Alpert, N. and **Waters, G.** (1998). Effects of syntactic structure and propositional number on patterns of regional cerebral blood flow. *Journal of Cognitive Neuroscience,* 10, 541–552.

Deecke, L., Engel, M., Lang, W. and **Kornhuber, H.H.** (1986). Bereitschaftspotential preceding speech after holding breath. *Experimental Brain Research,* 65, 219–223.

Démonet, J.F., Chollet, F., Ramsay, S., Cardebat, D., Nespoulous, J.L., Wise, R., Rascol, A. and **Frackowiak, R.** (1992). The anatomy of phonological and semantic processing in normal subjects. *Brain,* 115, 1753–1768.

Dronkers, N.F. (1996). A new brain region for coordinating speech articulation. *Nature,* 384, 159–161.

Duffy, J.R. and **Folger, W.N.** (1996). Dysarthria associated with unilateral central nervous system lesions: a retrospective study. *Journal of Medical Speech-Language Pathology,* 4, 57–70.

Fadiga, L., Craighero, L., Buccino, G. and **Rizzolatti, G.** (2002). Speech listening specifically modulates the excitabilitiy of tongue muscles: a TMS study. *European Journal of Neuroscience,* 15, 399–402.

Fiez, J.A. and **Raichle, M.E.** (1997). Linguistic processing. In J.D. Schmahmann, ed. *The cerebellum and cognition,* pp. 233–254. Academic Press, San Diego, CA (International Review of Neurobiology, vol. 41).

Frackowiak, R.S.J., Friston, K.J., Frith, C.D., Dolan, R.J. and **Mazziotta, J.C.** (1997). *Human brain function.* Academic Press, San Diego, CA.

Geschwind, N. (1969). Problems in the anatomical understanding of the aphasias. In A.L. Benton, ed. *Contributions to clinical neuropsychology,* pp. 107–128. Aldine Press, Chicago, IL.

Hertrich, I. and **Ackermann, H.** (1997). Acoustic analysis of durational speech parameters in neurological dysarthrias. In Y. Lebrun, ed. *From the brain to the mouth: acquired dysarthria and dysfluency in adults,* pp. 11–47. Kluwer, Dordrecht.

Hertrich, I., Mathiak, K., Lutzenberger, W. and **Ackermann, H.** (2002). Hemispheric lateralization of the processing of consonant-vowel syllables (formant transitions): effects of stimulus characteristics and attentional demands on evoked magnetic fields. *Neuropsychologia,* 40, 1902–1917.

Huang, J., Carr, T.H. and **Cao, Y.** (2001). Comparing cortical activations for silent and overt speech using event-related fMRI. *Human Brain Mapping,* 15, 39–53.

Ikeda, A., Lüders, H.O., Burgess, R.C. and **Shibasaki, H.** (1992). Movement-related potentials recorded from supplementary motor area and primary motor area. *Brain,* 115, 1017–1043.

Jeannerod, M. (1994). The representing brain: neural correlates of motor intention and imagery. *Behavioral and Brain Sciences,* 17, 187–245.

Kent, R.D. (1997). *The speech sciences.* Singular Press, San Diego, CA.

Kent, R.D., Kent, J.F. and **Rosenbek, J.C.** (1987). Maximum performance tests of speech production. *Journal of Speech and Hearing Disorders,* 52, 367–387.

Kluin, K.J., Gilman, S., Markel, D.S., Koeppe, R.A., Rosenthal, G. and **Junck, L.** (1988). Speech disorders in olivopontocerebellar atrophy correlate with positron emission tomography findings. *Annals of Neurology,* 23, 547–554.

Konczak, J., Ackermann, H., Hertrich, I., Spieker, S. and **Dichgans, J.** (1997). Control of repetitive lip and finger movements in Parkinson's disease: influence of external timing signals and simultaneous execution on motor performance. *Movement Disorders,* 12, 665–676.

Levelt, W.J.M. (1989). *Speaking: from intention to articulation.* MIT Press, Cambridge, MA.

Mathiak, K., Hertrich, I., Lutzenberger, W. and **Ackermann, H.** (2002). Functional cerebral asymmetries of pitch processing during dichotic stimulus application: a whole-head magnetoencephalography study. *Neuropsychologia,* 40, 585–593.

McCarthy, G., Blamire, A.M., Rothman, D.L., Gruetter, R. and **Shulman, R.G.** (1993). Echo-planar magnetic resonance imaging studies of frontal cortex activation during word generation in humans. *Proceedings of the National Academy of Sciences USA,* 90, 4952–4956.

McNeil, M.R., Robin, D.A. and **Schmidt, R.A.** (1997). Apraxia of speech: definition, differentiation, and treatment. In M.R. McNeil, ed. *Clinical management of sensorimotor speech disorders,* pp. 311–344. Thieme Press, New York, NY.

Mesulam, M.-M. and **Mufson, E.F.** (1985). The insula of Reil in man and monkey: Architectonics, connectivity, and function. In A. Peters and E.G. Jones, eds. *Cerebral cortex,* vol. 4, pp. 179–226. Plenum Press, New York, NY.

Murdoch, B.E., Thompson, E.C. and **Theodoros, D.G.** (1997). Spastic dysarthria. In M.R. McNeil, ed. *Clinical management of sensorimotor speech disorders,* pp. 287–310. Thieme Press, New York, NY.

Nudo, R.J., Frost, S.B., Milliken, G.W. and **Masterton, R.B.** (1993). Somatosensory and motor representations in the gray short-tailed opossum (*Monodelphis domestica*). *Society of Neuroscience Abstracts,* 19, 1212.

Ojemann, G. A. (1994). Cortical stimulation and recording in language. In A. Kertesz, ed. *Localization and neuroimaging in neuropsychology,* pp. 35–55. Academic Press, San Diego, CA.

Penfield, W. and **Roberts, L.** (1959). *Speech and brain mechanisms.* Princeton Univ. Press, Princeton, NJ.

Petersen, S.E., Fox, P.T., Posner, M.I., Mintun, M. and **Raichle, M.E.** (1988). Positron emission tomographic studies of the cortical anatomy of single-word processing. *Nature,* 331, 585–589.

Petersen, S.E., Fox, P.T., Posner, M.I., Mintun, M. and **Raichle, M.E.** (1989). Positron emission tomographic studies of the processing of single words. *Journal of Cognitive Neuroscience,* 1, 153–170.

Price, C.J., Wise, R.J.S., Warburton, E.A., Moore, C.J., Howard, D., Patterson, K., Frackowiak, R.S.J. and **Friston, K.J.** (1996). Hearing and saying: the functional neuro-anatomy of auditory word processing. *Brain,* 119, 919–931.

Riecker, A., Ackermann, H., Wildgruber, D., Dogil, G. and **Grodd, W.** (2000*a*). Opposite hemispheric lateralization effects during speaking and singing at motor cortex, insula and cerebellum. *NeuroReport,* 11, 1997–2000.

Riecker, A., Ackermann, H., Wildgruber, D., Meyer, J., Dogil, G., Haider, H. and **Grodd, W.** (2000*b*). Articulatory/phonetic sequencing at the level of the anterior perisylvian cortex: a functional magnetic resonance imaging (fMRI) study. *Brain and Language,* 75, 259–276.

Riecker, A., Wildgruber, D., Dogil, G., Grodd, W. and **Ackermann, H.** (2002*a*). Hemispheric lateralization effects of rhythm implementation during syllable repetitions: an fMRI study. *NeuroImage,* 16, 169–176.

Riecker, A., Wildgruber, D., Grodd, W. and **Ackermann, H.** (2002*b*). Reorganization of speech production at the motor cortex and cerebellum following capsular infarction: a follow-up functional magnetic resonance imaging study. *Neurocase,* 8, 417–423.

Roland, P.E. (1993). *Brain activation.* Wiley-Liss Press, New York, NY.

Roy, C.S. and **Sherrington, C.S.** (1890). On the regulation of the blood-supply of the brain. *Journal of Physiology (London),* 11, 85–108.

Rueckert, L., Appollonio, I., Grafman, J., Jezzard, P., Johnson Jr., R., Le Bihan, D. and **Turner, R.** (1994). Magnetic resonance imaging functional activation of left frontal cortex during covert word production. *Journal of Neuroimaging,* 4, 67–70.

Ryding, E., Bradvik, B. and **Ingvar, D.H.** (1987). Changes of regional cerebral blood flow measured simultaneously in the right and left hemisphere during automatic speech and humming. *Brain,* 110, 1345–1358.

Sasaki, K., Nambu, A., Tsujimoto, T., Matsuzaki, R., Kyuhou, S. and **Gemba, H.** (1996). Studies on integrative functions of the human frontal association cortex with MEG. *Brain Research Cognitive Brain Research,* 5, 165–174.

Schiff, H.B., Alexander, M.P., Naeser, M.A. and **Galaburda, A.M.** (1983). Aphemia: clinical-anatomic correlations. *Archives of Neurology,* 40, 720–727.

Schmahmann, J.D., ed. (1997). *The cerebellum and cognition.* Academic Press, San Diego, CA (International Review of Neurobiology, vol. 41).

Sidtis, J.J., Gomez, C., Anderson, J.R., Strother, S.C. and **Rottenberg, D.A.** (1998). Predicting speech rate in normal and ataxic speakers from functional imaging data. *Brain and Language,* 65, 228–230.

Sidtis, J.J., Strother, S.C., Anderson, J.R. and **Rottenberg, D.A.** (1999). Are brain functions really additive? *NeuroImage,* 9, 490–496.

Sokolov, A.N. (1972). *Inner speech and thought.* Plenum Press, New York, NY.

Talairach, P. and **Tournoux, J.** (1988). *A stereotactic coplanar atlas of the human brain.* Thieme Verlag, Stuttgart.

Toga A.W. and **Mazziotta, J.C.** (1996). *Brain mapping: the methods.* Academic Press, San Diego, CA.

Urban, P.P., Hopf, H.C., Fleischer, S., Zorowka, P.G. and **Müller-Forell, W.** (1997). Impaired cortico-bulbar tract function in dysarthria due to hemispheric stroke: functional testing using transcranial magnetic stimulation. *Brain,* 120, 1077–1084.

Urban, P.P., Wicht, S., Fitzek, C., Vukurevic, G., Stoeter, P. and **Hopf, H.C.** (2000). Topodiagnostik ischämisch bedingter Dysarthrophonien. *Klinische Neuroradiologie,* 10, 35–45 (German).

Wildgruber, D., Ackermann, H., Klose, U., Kardatzki, B. and **Grodd, W.** (1996). Functional lateralization of speech production at primary motor cortex: a fMRI study. *NeuroReport,* 7, 2791–2795.

Wildgruber, D., Ackermann, H. and **Grodd, W.** (2001). Differential contributions of motor cortex, basal ganglia, and cerebellum to speech motor control: effects of syllable repetition rate evaluated by fMRI. *NeuroImage,* 13, 101–109.

Wise, R.S.J., Green, J., Büchel, C. and **Scott, S.K.** (1999). Brain regions involved in articulation. *Lancet,* 353, 1057–1061.

Yetkin, F.Z., Hammeke, T.A., Swanson, S.J., Morris, G.L., Mueller, W.M., McAuliffe, T.L. and **Haughton, V.M.** (1995). A comparison of functional MR activation patterns during silent and audible language tasks. *American Journal of Neuroradiology,* 16, 1087–1092.

Zatorre, R.J., Evans, A.C., Meyer, E. and **Gjedde, A.** (1992). Lateralization of phonetic and pitch discrimination in speech processing. *Science,* 256, 846–849.

Ziegler, W. and **von Cramon, D.** (1986). Spastic dysarthria after acquired brain injury: an acoustic study. *British Journal of Disorders of Communication,* 21, 173–187.

CHAPTER 5

RECENT DEVELOPMENTS IN BRAIN IMAGING RESEARCH IN STUTTERING

LUC F. DE NIL

5.1 Introduction

Ever since the formulation of the cerebral dominance theory (Orton 1928), researchers have speculated about potential involvement of aberrant neural processes in the onset and development of stuttering. Much of the earlier research into the nature of these hypothesized brain processes was based largely on the use of behavioural observations and electromyographical measures. Relevant observations included the relative slowness of laryngeal, respiratory, and articulatory reaction times in stuttering individuals (Bakker and Brutten 1989; Watson *et al.* 1991; Van Lieshout *et al.* 1993), the effects of auditory delayed feedback on the speech fluency of non-stuttering and stuttering speakers (Harrington 1987; Fukawa *et al.* 1988; Kalinowski *et al.* 1996), differences in dichotic listening and dual task interference performance between stuttering and non-stuttering speakers (Moore 1990; Forster and Webster 1991; Foundas *et al.* 1999), articulatory discoordinations during fluent and disfluent speech (Caruso *et al.* 1988; Peters *et al.* 1999), oral kinesthetic deficiencies (De Nil and Abbs 1991*a, b*; Loucks and De Nil 2001), and genetic influences in stuttering (Felsenfeld 1997; Yairi *et al.* 1996). These observations, among others, indirectly suggested to many researchers the presence of differences in neural processing between stuttering and non-stuttering individuals affecting the production of fluent speech. Support for the existence of neural systems or circuits involved in speech fluency also came from observations of acquired stuttering in adults without any previous history of speech fluency problems, who suffered neurological disease or insult (Helm *et al.* 1980; Lebrun *et al.* 1987; Ringo and Dietrich 1995). At the same time, the very fact that acquired stuttering did not seem to be associated with a well-circumscribed brain region, but rather seemed to follow disease or insult to a wide variety of regions, highlighted the fact that any neural system involved in speech fluency is likely complex and involves many different cortical and subcortical structures.

More recently, the use of evoked potentials and other electrophysiological measures of brain activation has provided the means to obtain more direct measures of task-related neural processes (Moore and Lang 1977; Moore 1986; Wells and Moore 1990). These techniques have proven to be powerful tools for the study of brain function in healthy children, even infants, and adults (Molfese and Searock, 1986; Molfese *et al.* 1996), as well as those with a variety of developmental or acquired disorders (Sandson *et al.* 1994). Electrophysiological techniques are ideally suited to track very fast neural processes such as those involved in cognitive and language tasks. However, these techniques are more limited in their ability to probe activation below the cortical surfaces, or in detecting cortical areas for which the sources of magnetic flux are oriented perpendicular to the head surface (Papanicolaou 1998). These and other inherent problems restrict the use of electrophysiological measures for the precise localization of neural activation throughout the brain. Consequently, this research approach, while powerful in its own right, limits investigators in their ability to formulate theoretical frameworks regarding the involvement of specific neural systems or brain regions in people with disordered speech fluency.

Over the past two decades, the rapid development and refinement of functional neuroimaging techniques, such as positron emission tomography (PET) and functional magnetic resonance imaging (fMRI), has provided neuroscientists with another powerful tool in their search for understanding the role of the brain in seemingly disparate human activities, such as memory, vision, language, and consciousness, to name only a few. The landmark paper by Petersen *et al.* (1988) is often identified as the publication that marked the start of the exponential growth of functional imaging research. Using PET to study the production of single words, Petersen and his colleagues outlined many of the basic paradigms, such as the subtraction paradigm, used in subsequent studies. Since the publication of this paper, only 14 years ago, the number of peer-reviewed functional imaging publications has witnessed an unbelievable growth, reaching approximately 15 000 papers (which is probably still an underestimate) at the end of 2001.

One of the important advantages of PET and fMRI imaging techniques is their ability to localize neural activation in healthy and disordered individuals with a reasonable degree of spatial resolution, both at cortical and subcortical levels. As such, they provide researchers with the tools needed to investigate distributed neural systems involved in various sensory, motor, and cognitive processes that underlie human behaviour. These techniques, obviously, also have their own specific limitations that will be discussed in some detail later in this chapter.

In this chapter I first discuss briefly a number of theoretical models of brain function in stuttering that have been proposed by researchers during the past century. Following this, I will provide a short description of the principles behind the most frequently used functional neuroimaging techniques, followed by a summary and attempted integration of the main findings of functional imaging research in stuttering. Finally, I will propose how the various findings can be integrated in a comprehensive view of stuttering and provide an outline of some future research needs.

5.2 Models of brain function in stuttering

The earliest scientific attempt to formulate a model of brain function in stuttering was proposed by Orton (1928) and Travis (1931), although Van Riper (1971) traces its roots back to earlier publications by Stier (1911) and Sachs (1924). In their cerebral dominance theory of stuttering, Orton and Travis proposed that stuttering results from the lack of an appropriately developed dominance of hemispheric function. This lack of proper lateral dominance results in central asynchronization of motor impulses to the bilaterally paired speech musculature. The hypothesized mistimings of muscle actions resulting from this asynchronization were thought to lead behaviourally to the disfluencies that characterize stuttering. The cerebral dominance theory speculated about a link between the lack of dominance and forced right-handedness of naturally left-handed individuals. As a result, most of the early attempts to test the theory scientifically were based on investigating the incidence of left-handedness in stuttering subjects. In addition, electromyographical recordings of muscle activity were used to document the presence of neural firing mistiming. Given the status of technology available to study brain functions and the relatively unsophisticated nature of neuroscience at that time, these early attempts to link a complex behaviour such as stuttering with abnormal brain lateralization largely failed to find any convincing evidence. The early work of Orton, Travis, and their students unfortunately did taint many of the subsequent theoretical efforts to study the role of brain processes in stuttering, and paved the way for attempts to find a socio-cultural or psychological explanation of stuttering (Johnson and Leutenegger 1955; Travis 1978). In addition, initial failures to link brain lateralization to stuttering cast a shadow for many years over research into brain laterality and stuttering, leading Van Riper to talk about the 'old boneyard of laterality research on stuttering' (Van Riper 1982, p. 335).

More recently, Moore and his colleagues 'resurrected' the idea that stuttering could be linked to atypical lateralization of speech and language processes (Moore 1990). They based the interpretation of their results on a model of differential hemispheric specialization proposed by Bradshaw and Nettleton (1981). According to this model, the left hemisphere is best equipped to handle time-sensitive, sequential tasks, such as those involved in the phonetic sequencing of speech, while the right hemisphere is best equipped to handle tasks that rely on more global, time-insensitive processes. Moore and his colleagues, based on the results from dichotic listening, tachistoscopic, and evoked potential studies as well as early blood flow studies, hypothesized that stutterers showed increased right hemisphere activation for perceptual and motor processes involved in speech production. According to their model, stuttering speakers use right hemisphere processes, which are best suited for the handling of time-independent, non-segmental information, and for the processing of time-dependent and segmental language tasks. The use of a less appropriate processor is thought to result in the stuttered speech observed by listeners. The reason for the right hemisphere control over speech and language in stutterers was left open, but, importantly, Moore (1984) viewed this dependency on right hemisphere function as a 'manipulable process, rather than as a static disorder resulting from CNS disfunction'(p. 49).

A third model speculating about the role of atypical brain lateralization in stuttering speakers has been proposed by Webster (Webster 1985, 1986; Forster and Webster 2001). His two-factor model of stuttering is based on the assumption that stuttering speakers, just like non-stuttering speakers, demonstrate normal left hemisphere lateralization of neural mechanisms for speech production. However, stuttering speakers are thought to differ from non-stutterers because the former show left hemisphere functions that are inefficient or fragile and more easily susceptible to inferences from ongoing neural activities, of both intra- and inter-hemispheric origin. In his model, Webster particularly identifies the supplementary motor area (SMA) in the left hemisphere as a cortical area crucially involved in stuttering. Furthermore, according to the model, stuttering individuals lack the normal left hemisphere activation bias normally seen in non-stuttering, right-handed individuals. Instead, stuttering individuals, similar to left-handed non-stuttering individuals, show a bilateral activation bias. This leads to temporary overactivation of the right hemisphere, which in turn, can interfere with normal functioning in the fragile left hemisphere, resulting in stuttering.

The three neural theories of stuttering reviewed so far are all focused primarily on atypical lateralization of neural functions in persons who stutter. Not all neural models of stuttering, however, have focused on such atypical hemispheric lateralization. Zimmermann (1980), for instance, suggested that stuttering might result from abnormally altered gains of brainstem reflexes, triggered when speech structures operate outside their 'normal' ranges influenced by emotional, perceptual, and/or physiological events. The altered reflex gains, subsequently, are thought to lead to a breakdown of fluent speech as a result of the ensuing imbalance of the articulatory system. Caruso (1991) suggested that the articulatory discoordinations, more specifically the aberrant timing and sequencing of orofacial movements, observed in stutterers' speech even when perceptually fluent, could point to a deficiency at the levels of the SMA and basal ganglia. Based on the rich interconnections of the basal ganglia with the motor system, Molt (1999) also speculated on the possible involvement of these subcortical nuclei in stuttering. In support for his hypothesis, Molt pointed to a number of similarities between stuttering and other disorders involving basal ganglia disfunction, such as dystonia and Tourette's syndrome.

5.3 Functional neuroimaging and stuttering

In the previous section, some of the experimental and theoretical literature on neural processes and their role in stuttering has been reviewed very briefly. I now want to turn to the more recent functional neuroimaging studies which are the focus of this chapter. As has been pointed out before, behavioural and electro-physiological studies of the neurology of stuttering, while powerful in their own right, fail to provide direct evidence of involvement of specific neural substrates in stuttering. The development of functional imaging techniques, such as positron emission tomography and functional magnetic resonance imaging, has provided researchers with powerful tools to look inside a stuttering person's functioning brain and to compare the observed patterns of activation directly with those of non-stuttering individuals engaged in the same experimental task. As I hope will become evident from the review of the existing literature, the data from this research have yielded a number of interesting observations that may throw new light on the role of specific brain regions in stuttering. However, before reviewing the studies on stuttering done to date, I believe it is important to review very briefly some of the basic principles and assumptions underlying both positron emission tomography and functional magnetic resonance imaging. For a more detailed review, the reader is referred to Chapter 4 in this volume. Rugg (1999) also provides an accessible review of imaging techniques used in cognitive neuro-science. In order to provide a framework for the interpretation of the results from studies in stuttering, I will also review very briefly some of the more salient neuroimaging findings in the study of language formulation and speech production.

5.3.1 Functional neuroimaging: basic principles

Much of the early neuroimaging studies in language and speech, and most published studies in stuttering at the time of this writing, are based on measures of neural activation using positron emission tomography, or PET. Imaging the brain with PET is based on the principle that increased neural activation is accompanied by increased metabolism of glucose or oxygen, among other elements. In order to allow researchers to measure the relative distribution of these elements in the brain during an experimental or baseline task, the elements are radioactively labelled prior to injection in the bloodstream. The denser the concentration of the used radioisotope in a given region of the brain, as a result of increased blood flow associated with higher metabolic demand, the higher the emission of positrons which can be registered by the PET scanner's detector cameras. In this way, researchers are able to construct a detailed map of increased and decreased activations in various parts of the brain as the subject is engaged in a given task.

While PET scanning has proven to be a powerful tool in neuroscience, it never-theless has a number of drawbacks, which are important to understand when evaluating and comparing published studies in stuttering. Obviously, one of them is the need to inject radioactive isotopes during the experiment, thereby limiting the number of scans a single person can undergo. This is especially important for studies requiring multiple scans, such as when investigating treatment effects. The use of radioactive isotopes places restrictions on the use of PET scanning for the study of neural processes in children, which is an important limitation for the study of developmental stuttering. Finally, PET signals generated from increased cognitive activation, amidst all other activation happening simultaneously in the brain, typically only represent a local signal increase of about 4–6% (Kapur *et al.* 1995). As such, to improve the signal-to-noise ratio and increase the chances of reliably detecting the signal of interest, the neural activation maps for several individuals are typically averaged across task repetitions and/or across several subjects. As a result, imaging activation patterns in single individuals can be difficult, putting limits on the study of inter-individual variability in stuttering.

Recently, a rapidly increasing number of functional imaging studies have used functional magnetic resonance imaging (fMRI) rather than PET, undoubtedly stimulated by the growing availability of MRI facilities with functional imaging capabilities, and the ability to obtain functional brain images without the need to inject a radioisotope. Another major advantage of fMRI is the opportunity to investigate inter-individual differences in performance, and to obtain repeated scans from the same subjects.

Functional MRI is based on the inherent magnetic properties of hydrogen protons and the changes and resulting energy emissions that can be inflicted on these properties by manipulating the magnetic properties of the environment in the MRI scanner. As with PET, fMRI images rely on the increases and decreases in metabolic activity associated with changes in neural activation. An important factor in fMRI, especially as it relates to investigations of speech and stuttering, is the significant noise level that is generated by the pulsating magnetic field in the scanner. This noise level obviously influences such things as the ability to record speech output and introduces possible masking effects on speech fluency. Another important limiting factor in fMRI is its sensitivity to body movement. Even very slight movements of the head, for instance as a result of jaw movements during speech, can introduce significant artefacts and noise in the functional image. Researchers have developed sophisticated movement-correction algorithms and event-related experimental designs to reduce or eliminate movement artefacts, but the possible influence of such artefacts still poses serious limitations on researchers' abilities to investigate natural speech production.

5.3.2 Functional neuroimaging: normal language and speech processes

The intent of this section is to provide a brief overview of some of the main findings from the functional imaging research on normal language and speech processes. The scope of this chapter precludes a more detailed, and probably more balanced, discussion of the vast literature available on this topic. However, some discussion is important to provide a broader framework in which we can interpret the results from studies on stuttering.

The two language processes that have received most attention in the functional neuroimaging research are phonological and semantic processing. In their landmark 1988 study, Petersen and his colleagues, using single-word reading and verb-generation tasks, identified phonological processing with activation in the temporo-parietal cortex, while semantic processing appeared to involve more anterior inferior frontal regions. Since that initial study, a more complete and differentiated picture of the neural basis of these two cognitive language processes has emerged. Phonological processing, which deals with the segmentation of speech into its sound-based components, as well as the generation of the sound-based codes required for speech production, seems to involve the following areas primarily (Neville and Bavelier 1998; Binder 1999):

(1) Broca's area, especially the pars opercularis, especially during tasks involving more automatic speech processing;
(2) the temporal cortex, in particular Wernicke's area for acoustic processing and the computation of abstract representations of speech sounds; and
(3) the supramarginal cortex, for articulatory recoding in association with frontal cortical regions.

Semantic processing, which involves the storing, retrieving, and manipulation of knowledge about the world, seems to activate primarily: (1) the temporal and parietal cortex, related to the storage of the information; and (2) the prefrontal cortex, which seems to be involved primarily with the manipulation and usage of that information in the speech context. A number of recent studies (Gabrieli *et al.* 1998; Tyler *et al.* 2001) have suggested that the inferior lateral prefrontal cortex activation may be more readily present in tasks requiring more complex, effortful processing. To date, most studies of phonological and semantic processing have used comprehension rather than production task. One reason for this, other than the movement artefact problems alluded to before, is that oral speech production not only activates the neural substrates involved in the cognitive processes underlying the linguistic task, but also activates areas involved in sensorimotor control of speech and auditory processing tasks. Nevertheless, the distinction between production and comprehension is an important one, with potential implications for the identification of differential neural processes involved in each of these tasks. A detailed overview of the increasing body of neuroimaging literature that addresses these and related issue is outside the scope of this chapter, but the interested reader can find an excellent review in a recent paper by Price (2000).

Fewer studies have been published on the use of functional imaging to study other components of language processing, such as discourse and syntactic processing. In a PET study of discourse (generation of autobiographical narratives in both spoken language and American Sign Language), Braun *et al.* (2001), perhaps not surprisingly, found widespread cortical activation. However, an interesting observation was that the level of lateralization varied, based on the stage of language formulation, with earlier conceptual stages being represented more bilaterally while a more unilateral (left) lateralization was observed during articulatory–motor processing. Selective right and left lateral involvement was also involved in a recent fMRI study of grammatical encoding (Cooke *et al.* 2001), with right posterior superior temporal activation involved in passive short-term memory processes during grammatical processing and more left lateralized inferior frontal activation being engaged for cognitive processing of grammatical dependencies.

Of particular importance to the study of stuttering are investigations of activation patterns associated with speech articulation. In general, these studies have shown widespread involvement of sensorimotor areas, both cortically and subcortically. These areas include motor cortex, both primary and premotor, insular cortex, supplementary motor area, cerebellum, and basal ganglia nuclei. These activations can be bilateral or left-lateralized, depending on the complexity and length of the produced linguistic or non-linguistic stimuli (Riecker *et al.*, 2000*b*). In addition to these classical speech motor areas, functional imaging has revealed the potential involvement of other areas. For instance, Riecker *et al.* (2000*a*) have provided evidence that the anterior insula may be an important area for the control of the motor execution of articulatory movements. In addition, it is becoming increasingly clear that brain regions may have functions that are immensely more complex than previously thought. For instance, Huang *et al.* (2002) have suggested that Broca's area may be involved in complex phonological processing, especially as it relates to direct retrieval of stored phonological codes. Consequently, Keller *et al.* (2001) have proposed that one of the outcomes of recent functional imaging research may be a better appreciation that:

(1) language is represented by a widespread network of cortical and subcortical areas;
(2) a single area may serve multiple functions, depending on task requirements; and
(3) complex cognitive processes, such as language formulation, may involve extensive collaborative interactions among various areas of the brain.

5.3.3 Functional neuroimaging: stuttering

In general, the functional neuroimaging studies in stuttering done to date reflect on two main questions:

(1) are there differences in neural processes between stuttering and non-stuttering speakers during the execution of various speech, language, and non-speech tasks?; and

(2) are there differences in neural processes between fluent and disfluent speech?

As we will see, both of these questions can cautiously be answered affirmatively.

5.3.3.1 Differences between stuttering and non-stuttering speakers

Most functional imaging studies have compared neural activation of stuttering and non-stuttering speakers with the individuals involved in some type of speech or language task. In what was probably the first study using blood-flow-based functional imaging, Wood et al. (1980) observed asymmetrical blood flow during stuttering in Broca's (right > left) and Wernicke's (left > right) area. However, the very coarse time and spatial resolution offered by the imaging technology available at that time, as well as the lack of proper control conditions, in addition to other methodological issues, calls for caution in the interpretation of these initial results. Nevertheless, as we will see, the overall brain activation pattern observed by Wood and his colleagues foreshadowed more recent findings.

More recently, Wu et al. (1995) used fluorodeoxyglucose (FDG) in a PET study of continuous reading in stuttering and non-stuttering adults. When comparing four stuttering adults to a group of normally fluent subjects, they observed decreased regional glucose metabolism on the left in Broca's and Wernicke's area, higher-order frontal association areas, and the deep frontal cortex. Other areas of decreased metabolism were observed in the bilateral posterior cingulate cortex and right cerebellum. While the observed deactivation in these areas was found to vary depending on the level of fluency in the speech of the stuttering individuals, relatively constant decreased activation in the left caudate metabolism led them to hypothesize that stuttering may be due, in part, to a permanent hypometabolism in the basal ganglia, particularly in the left caudate nucleus.

The studies of both Wood et al. (1980) and Wu et al. (1995) used extended continuous reading (>30 min) to obtain functional images of brain activation averaged over that time window. It is possible that such long time windows may have introduced uncontrolled-for variables, such as fatigue, changes in speech behaviour, attentional shifts, etc. In an attempt to increase temporal resolution, and better control such, and other, variables, recent PET studies have used radioactively labelled water ($^{15}H_2O$) rather than FDG as the radiotracer. $^{15}H_2O$ has a half-life of approximately 2 min, which allows for scans averaged over a time window of 45 s to 1 min. In general, and despite significant differences in methodology and experimental tasks, the results from these studies have provided evidence of increased right lateralized or bilateral activation of cortical and subcortical areas involved in motor control in stuttering speakers. In a study using natural and choral speech, Fox et al. (1996) observed proportionally greater right hemisphere activation, especially in primary motor and premotor cortex, and sharply decreased activation in the posterior temporal cortex and the superior temporal and left inferior frontal cortex. They interpreted their results as suggesting that neural activation in stuttering adults during natural reading is characterized by a general overactivation of the motor system, a deactivation of the fronto-temporal fluency circuit, and a lack of the phonological self-monitoring processes seen in non-stuttering speakers. A lack of left hemisphere lateralization of neural activation during language tasks was also observed in a study by Braun *et al.* (1997). Using natural language tasks (spontaneous narrative speech and sentence construction), they observed that stuttering subjects had more frequent bilateral or right lateralized activation compared to non-stuttering controls, especially in the frontal brain regions. Similar to Fox, *et al.* (1996), Braun and his colleagues found deactivation in the left temporal posterior and superior temporal cortex, and suggested that this may point to a disordered activation of neocortical language areas in stuttering adults. More recently, we have studied natural single-word reading, both silently and orally, in stuttering and non-stuttering adults (De Nil *et al.* 2000). Significant differences were observed between the two subject groups during both silent and oral reading, pointing to increased bilateral or right-lateralized activation primarily in frontal regions. Activation patterns in the stuttering subjects were also characterized by increased left hemisphere activation in premotor cortex, in particular the insula, during silent reading. However, one of the areas that differentiated most significantly between the two groups was the anterior cingulate. Proportionally higher activation in this medial region also has been reported by Braun *et al.* (1997). The functional involvement of this medial cortical region in human behaviour is highly complex (Devinsky *et al.* 1995; Bush *et al.* 2000), but it appears to be involved mainly in tasks that require a relatively high degree of attention and decision-making regarding response selection (Peterson *et al.* 1999). It has also been speculated that the anterior cingulate may be involved in articulatory rehearsal and motor learning (Raichle *et al.* 1994; Jueptner *et al.* 1997). We have suggested that the increased cingulate activation may be linked to the higher likelihood of anticipatory scanning behaviour in the stuttering subjects. This interpretation seems to fit our observation that stuttering speakers, even during silent reading, engage more intensely areas typically associated with articulatory planning and execution.

Of particular importance, in a number of these studies, is the finding of significantly increased activation of the cerebellum of stuttering speakers (Fox *et al.* 1996, 2000; Braun *et al.* 1997; De Nil *et al.* 2001). The cerebellum is known to have an important role in the timing and error correction of movement (Ivry and Keele 1989; Ghez 1991). Increased cerebellar activation typically is seen during the early stages of motor learning, when movements are not yet highly automatized, or when there is a stronger demand to integrate motor patterns with their sensory consequences. The involvement of the cerebellum may not be limited to motor tasks, as there is growing evidence that its role may extend to cognitive tasks as well (Thach 1987; Fiez and Raichle 1997). The differences observed in cerebellar activation pattern in stuttering speakers may support a difference in the level of automaticity attained in speech production. Such a link is supported by the observation of increased cerebellar activation immediately following treatment (see below).

An important question is whether differences observed between stuttering and non-stuttering speakers reflect the speech motor or cognitive language formulation processes involved in speech. We have attempted to differentiate between patterns of activation associated with these two processes in stuttering adults (De Nil *et al.* 2003), using a verb-generation task and contrasting the results obtained during this task with those obtained during overt reading of single words. Because both tasks result in the subjects saying single words out loud, it was assumed that they were similar in terms of motor processing demands, but differed primarily with regard to the differential involvement of semantic and phonological processes. In order to compare the neural maps from these two tasks, the functional activation during word reading was subtracted from that obtained during the verb-generation task. The resulting subtraction map revealed minimal activation differences between the stuttering and the non-stuttering speakers pretreatment. Moreover, the functional maps obtained in the stuttering subjects showed minimal changes before and after treatment and at the 1-year follow-up. This finding is in sharp contrast with the significant activation differences found between the two subject groups during oral reading and seems to suggest that the neural differences observed between the stuttering and non-stuttering speakers reflect primarily the sensorimotor processes involved in speech production. As such, these findings do not support a linguistic explanation of stuttering. However, further research is clearly needed in this area. Indeed, data from a recent study completed in our laboratory, investigating phonological and semantic decision tasks in stuttering speakers, have suggested that stuttering speakers may have greater difficulty performing these tasks optimally during dual-task conditions than non-stuttering speakers (De Nil and Bosshardt 2001).

5.3.3.2 *Functional imaging of language and speech in stutterers: a preliminary synthesis*

When reading the various functional neuroimaging studies of stuttering speakers, initially one is struck, or maybe bewildered, by the many differences in activation patterns that are reported in the published reports. Of course, many of these differences are influenced by differences between the studies in either imaging methods, subject characteristics, experimental or baseline tasks, temporal resolution, etc. However, when one analyzes the results in greater detail, it becomes apparent that, despite all the differences, a rather consistent pattern seems to emerge. Figure 5.1 shows anatomical brain images with the various locations of activations and deactivations, as reported in four studies, superimposed. The anatomical localizations shown in this figure are based on the reported stereotaxic coordinates reported in these studies or, when such coordinates were not available, are estimated from the anatomical descriptions or Brodmann areas provided in the papers. As such, while Fig. 5.1 demonstrates an overall and rather general pattern, the reader needs to be

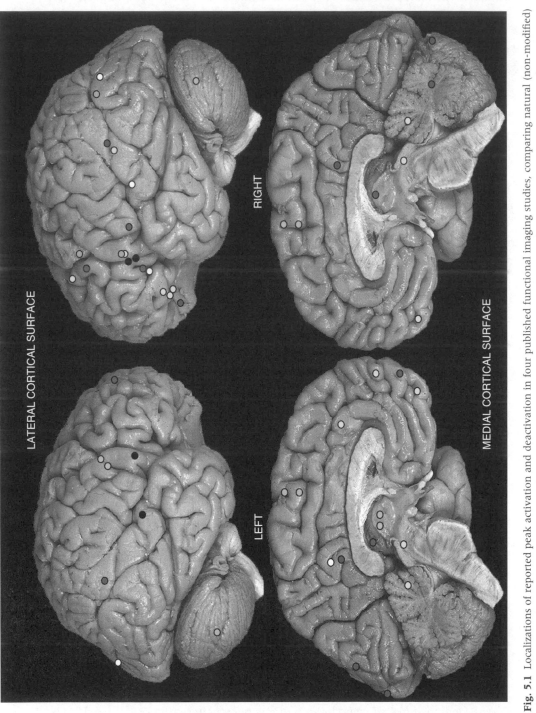

Fig. 5.1 Localizations of reported peak activation and deactivation in four published functional imaging studies, comparing natural (non-modified) overt speech of stuttering and non-stuttering adults. Localization of activations was determined based on reported stereotactic coordinates or Brodmann areas. Peak activation coding: yellow, Braun *et al.* (1997); red, De Nil *et al.* (2000); pink, Fox *et al.* (1996). Peak deactivation coding: green,

cautioned against using this figure to draw conclusions with regard to detailed localization of activation differences between stuttering and non-stuttering speakers.

The top two brain images show the lateral cortical surfaces of the right and left hemispheres. As is immediately evident from this figure, differences in cortical activation between the stuttering and the non-stuttering speakers are not confined to either one of the two halves of the brain. Both left and right hemispheres show regions of increased or decreased activation in stuttering speakers when compared to non-stuttering individuals. A second observation is that the location of increased activation in the stuttering adults is concentrated primarily in the lateral–frontal cortex, especially the primary motor and premotor cortex, and in the cerebellum. Activation in the inferior lateral frontal region (which includes Broca's area) is characterized primarily by increased activation in the right hemisphere and decreased activation in the left hemisphere. Thirdly, while increases and decreases in activation can be observed in both hemispheres, most of the areas of increased activation seem to be located in the right hemisphere, while most of the areas of decreased activation are on the left, especially in the inferior lateral cortex, as mentioned before, and in the superior temporal region. Additional areas of deactivation can be seen in the occipital region.

The bottom two brain images show the medial cortical surfaces of the right and the left hemispheres. While it appears that most of the differences in activation between the stuttering and the non-stuttering speakers are located in the left hemisphere, it is important to note that the coordinates only indicate activation peaks, and that several of the areas of activation involved both the left and right medial surfaces. Nevertheless, the peak activations tended to be concentrated primarily in the anterior part of the cingulate cortex, the supplementary motor cortex and subcortically in the thalamic and basal ganglia regions.

The overall picture that is revealed by this synthesis of (de-)activation sites from these four studies is one of primary involvement of cortical and subcortical areas that have a role in the sensorimotor planning and execution of speech. These include primary and premotor cortices, insula, SMA, inferior lateral frontal regions, anterior cingulate, cerebellum, thalamus and basal ganglia. In addition, consistent and significant differences can be observed in the auditory cortex. The latter observation suggests that any differences between stuttering and non-stuttering speakers involve not only brain regions involved in motor planning and execution, but also those areas important for processing of sensory feedback.

5.3.3.3 Differences between fluent and disfluent speech

In the functional imaging studies discussed so far, the speech of stuttering participants included both stuttered and fluent utterances. Obviously, another important question is whether neural activation patterns change, depending on the level of speech fluency. A number of researchers have attempted to address this issue by manipulating the fluency of stuttering speakers. Both Fox *et al.* (1996) and Wu *et al.* (1995) manipulated fluency by introducing a choral reading condition, known to increase fluency in stuttering speakers. In the study by Fox *et al.* (1996) choral reading resulted in a marked reduction or elimination of the previously discussed overactivation observed during natural reading. The increased right hemisphere bias in primary motor and SMA activation did not change. Normalization of the activation pattern following choral speech, with the exception of the caudate nucleus and the substantia nigra, was also observed in the study by Wu *et al.* (1995). Interestingly, Ingham *et al.* (2000) reported a similar pattern of activation changes during covert (imagined) speech. They took their results to suggest that the presence of overt speech may not be required to reveal these differences between stuttered and fluent speech. However, it needs to be pointed out that a number of potentially important activation differences were observed during covert speech, especially in the primary motor cortex, basal ganglia, and cerebellum, among others. This caution against the use of covert speech as an analogy for overt speech is also evident in a recent study by Huang *et al.* (2002), who reported important differences between the two speech conditions.

Braun *et al.* (1997) used either paced or automatic speech tasks to induce fluency in stuttering adults. Increased fluency resulted in higher activation bilaterally in post-rolandic sensory areas and the insular cortex. In addition, increased activation was seen in the right supramarginal gyrus, as well as in right primary and association auditory cortex. In our own studies, fluency level was manipulated using an intensive 3-week treatment programme based on the Precision Fluency Shaping Program (Webster 1974), in which stuttering subjects acquired fluency-enhancing speech motor skills (Kroll *et al.* 1997; Kroll and De Nil 1998). Immediately following treatment, the stuttering subjects showed a significant increase in activation in the left hemisphere motor and premotor areas, and cerebellar cortex. Overactivation of the anterior cingulate cortex was reduced significantly. One year later, the overall level of activation in the stuttering subjects, who had been able to maintain their post-treatment fluency, was greatly normalized.

A different approach to the study of the relationship between stuttering and brain activation was used by Braun *et al.* (1997) and Fox *et al.* (2000), who correlated levels of brain activation with observed frequency of disfluency. Braun *et al.* observed a positive correlation between disfluency scores and primarily left lateralized activation in anterior brain regions, anterior and posterior cingulate, subcortical motor areas and frontal association regions. Negative correlations were found between disfluency and right hemisphere activation in primary and association auditory cortex, primary somatosensory areas and supramarginal gyrus, insular cortex and frontal operculum, among other areas. On the other hand, Fox *et al.* (2000) found a strong relationship (both positive and negative) between stuttering scores and right cortical motor areas, including primary motor cortex, supplementary motor area, right homologous of Broca's area, anterior insula, and left cere-bellar activation. While discrepancies between these two studies may be partly related to differences in speech tasks or to the method used to count disfluency rate, the reported results clearly point to the need for further investigations into this relationship.

5.3.3.4 Differences between stuttering and non-stuttering speakers during non-speech tasks

The studies discussed so far have compared neural activation patterns between stuttering and non-stuttering individuals during various speech and language tasks. Moore (1984) suggested that differences in brain lateralization might be specific for linguistic tasks. The question thus arises whether the observed differ-ences during functional imaging tasks are limited to speech or language tasks, or whether they reflect differences in brain organization that can be seen in non-linguistic tasks as well. To date, only a few studies have addressed this question. Braun *et al.* (1997), as part of a larger study, compared stutterers and non-stutter-ers during the production of non-speech articulatory–laryngeal movement sequences. In general, the stuttering and non-stuttering speakers demonstrated highly similar bilateral neural activation patterns during this non-linguistic motor task. However, a few differences were observed. Stuttering individuals showed somewhat greater activation in left premotor and primary sensorimotor cortex, and right primary and association auditory cortex. The activation in the primary left sensorimotor cortex also was found to be more variable in the stuttering subjects. In addition, while the overall pattern of activation was similar between the two groups, the level of activation observed in the stuttering speakers tended to be somewhat stronger. Braun and co-workers also compared neural activation during a rest condition in which subjects were not actively involved in an experi-mentally controlled overt or covert task. No differences were found between the two groups during the rest condition. The absence of functional activation differ-ences during rest was confirmed in a study by Ingham *et al.* (1996). Findings from these two studies are in contrast with those obtained in an earlier study by Pool *et al.* (1991), who reported global decreases in blood flow in stuttering versus non-stuttering individuals, with focal reductions in the anterior cingulate and temporal cortex. The fact that these two areas appeared to differentiate between the two subject groups is interesting in light of the observation that these same areas also have been found to differentiate strongly between stuttering and non-stuttering speakers during speech tasks.

5.4 An attempted synthesis

An important observation in several functional imaging studies in stuttering is that the increased right hemisphere activation often appears to be part of a general overactivation of the motor system. As such, the data do not necessarily support some of the earlier lateralization models, such as the one proposed by Moore (1984). In his model, increased right hemisphere activation was thought to replace or compensate for the normally observed left lateralized processes for speech and language, which in stutterers were somehow insufficient or deficient. In contrast, one could argue that what seems to be emerging from the functional imaging studies to date is that neural activation in stuttering adults is characterized by a more generalized bilateral recruitment of cortical and subcortical neural resources involved in language formulation in general, and speech production in specific. Our data on effects of treatment seem to suggest that behavioural treatment initially results in an even further increase in recruitment of resources after an intensive 3-week treatment period, followed by a significant reduction in the overall amount of activation after 1 year. At the 1 year mark, the overall activation pattern observed in the stuttering speakers was more similar to that observed in the normally fluent speakers. We have interpreted this finding as signalling increased automaticity in the application of learned speech motor skills.

This more generalized recruitment of resources, and the subsequent reduction in activation, is not unlike the overall pattern of activation that emerges from studies on skill acquisition and automaticity. In an early PET study on skill acquisition, Raichle *et al.* (1994) asked subjects to repeatedly generate verbs when presented with the same list of nouns. They found that the process of verb generation during the initial presentation of the list was characterized primarily by activation of the anterior cingulate, left prefrontal and left posterior temporal cortex, and right cerebellum. Following practice, activation in these areas decreased significantly, while increased activation could be observed in the bilateral sylvian–insular cortex and left medial extrastriate cortex. Similar changes in activation have been reported more recently by Balslev *et al.* (2002) during a motor mirror tracing task. They identified a total of six functional clusters, three of which showed task-related changes in activation. Two of these clusters, which included premotor, parietal and cerebellar regions, showed decreased activation with task practice. Similar reductions in activation as a result of increased automaticity have been reported in numerous other studies (Jenkins *et al.* 1994; Deiber *et al.* 1997; Van Mier *et al.* 1998).

The observation of increased recruitment of cortical and subcortical neural resources during natural (i.e. non-manipulated) speech in stuttering adults may suggest that they execute speech control in a much less automatic manner compared to non-stuttering individuals, even during relatively simple speech, such as single-word reading. I have suggested elsewhere that the overt manifestation of stuttering may be linked, in part, to the speaker's attempt to control separately the many degrees of freedom in speech production (De Nil 1999). Such attempts to control intrinsically complex motor behaviours can be readily observed during the relatively clumsy performance typical of the initial stages of motor learning. The increased attention and effort often associated with task performance during those initial stages is associated with more widely distributed and more intense bilateral cortical and subcortical activation. Within this framework, successful stuttering treatment may result from the increased ability of stuttering speakers to reduce the number of degrees of freedom they need to control during speech. In turn, successful maintenance may follow when clients are able to practise this control to a relatively high degree of automaticity. If true, relapse could then be related to the failure to develop a sufficiently high level of automaticity, perhaps because of either inappropriate practice or some innate limitation in neural plasticity.

5.5 Conclusion and some remaining questions

Earlier in this chapter, it was stated that current functional imaging research in stuttering is driven primarily by the search for differences in neural processes underlying speech and language formulation between stutterers and non-stutterers and between fluent and disfluent speech. Based on the evidence reviewed here, such differences can be said to exist, although with some caution. From the evidence available to date, it is clear that the functional maps of neural activation during speech and language tasks differ between stuttering and non-stuttering individuals. In general, when not speaking under fluency-enhancing conditions, stuttering subjects show increased bilateral activation, primarily of frontal motor cortex, although increased activation also is seen in other cortical and subcortical regions involved in motor planning and execution. Under fluency-enhancing conditions, the activation pattern seen in stuttering speakers starts to resemble that normally observed in non-stuttering speakers, possibly as a result of a reduction in the general overactivation of the neural system, although a number of potentially significant differences, especially in primary sensorimotor cortex, continue to be observed, possibly suggesting a differentiation between learned and inherent aspects of stuttering (see below).

As stated, the current functional imaging results, while very promising, need to be approached with some caution. First of all, the total number of functional imaging studies in stuttering is still small, providing little opportunity to check the replicability of findings within or across laboratories. Secondly, all of these studies have been carried out on adult speakers, which leaves open the question of whether the observed differences reflect acquired characteristics of compensatory or otherwise learned strategies, or whether they reflect truly inherent differences in neural processes. It could be argued that the ease with which the observed neural patterns can be changed suggests that at least some of the observed activations reflect transient (learned) rather than innate characteristics. In this regard, more focused studies of those areas that remain consistently hyperactivated or deactivated in stuttering subjects, despite changes in fluency, may be a promising approach to help differentiate between transient and 'hard-wired' differences in neural processing. In addition, linking research in stuttering to other investigations into neural plasticity and learning (Neville and Bavelier 1998; Hallett 2000) will provide further insight into what is learned and what is not.

The effects of specific task requirements on observed activation patterns are in need of further exploration. It is well known that variations in task requirements and subject instruction can have a significant influence on observed functional activation maps. In our studies, we have found significant lateralization differences in functional activation maps between stuttering and non-stuttering speakers during single-word reading but not during verb-generation tasks (De Nil *et al.* 2003). These differences in observed activation maps, despite the fact that both word-reading and verb-generation tasks result in the generation of a single word, highlights the need for more focused research into the effects of task characteristics on observed activation. Alternatively, the observed activation differences between word or paragraph reading and a more cognitive–linguistic task such as verb generation, with a more 'normal' activation pattern seen in the latter, may suggest that the disfluencies seen in stuttering reflect a deficit in motor, rather than linguistic, processing.

One of the main shortcomings of current functional imaging studies used in stuttering is the limited temporal resolution of PET and fMRI. This is especially crucial for the study of speech and language processes, during which processing takes place in a matter of milliseconds rather than seconds or minutes. A very promising approach here would be to combine PET or fMRI techniques, which have good spatial resolution, with electrophysiological measures such as magnetoencephalography (MEG), which has excellent temporal resolution (Salmelin *et al.* 2000). Such approaches are increasingly available to researchers (Ilmoniemi and Aronen 1999) and, undoubtedly, studies in stuttering using combined imaging technique will be forthcoming. Ideally, such techniques will allow researchers to differentiate not only between generally fluent or disfluent speech, but also between individual instances of fluent and disfluent utterances.

The availability of functional imaging tools has provided a wonderful opportunity to study, in great detail, neural processes underlying stuttering. Despite the current limitations in terms of cost, subject selection, and task characteristics, these investigations have already provided exciting new insights into possible relationships between brain processes and speech disfluencies. Undoubtedly, the current findings also will raise many new questions that will engage researchers for years to come, with some of these questions probably needing to wait future technological developments before they can be answered.

Acknowledgements

The preparation of this chapter was supported by grants from the Canadian Institutes of Health Research (former Medical Research Council of Canada) and the

Natural Sciences and Engineering Research Council of Canada. My thanks to my co-investigators, Dr Kroll and Dr Houle, and lab members Dr Torrey Loucks, Jayanthi Sasisekaran and Sophie Lafaille, for many insightful discussions of the material presented here and contributions to the preparation of the chapter. I would also like to thank Dr Raymond Kent and Dr Ben Maassen for their thoughtful and very helpful comments on an earlier version of this chapter.

References

Bakker, K. and **Brutten, G. J.** (1989). A comparative investigation of the laryngeal premotor, adjustment, and reaction times of stutterers and nonstutterers. *Journal of Speech and Hearing Research, 32,* 239–244.

Balslev, D., Nielsen, F. A., Frutiger, S. A., Sidtis, J. J., Christiansen, T. B., Svarer, C., Strother, S. C., Rottenberg, D. A., Hansen, L. K., Paulson, O. B., and **Law, I.** (2002). Cluster analysis of activity-time series in motor learning. *Human Brain Mapping, 15,* 135–145.

Binder, J. R. (1999). Functional MRI of the language system. In C.T.W.Moonen and P. A. Bandettini (Eds.), *Functional MRI* (pp. 407–419). New York: Springer-Verlag.

Bradshaw, J. and **Nettleton, N.** (1981). The nature of hemispheric specialization in man. *Behavioral and Brain Sciences, 4,* 51–91.

Braun, A. R., Varga, M., Stager, S., Schulz, G., Selbie, S., Maisog, J. M., Carson, R. E., and **Ludlow, C. L.** (1997). Altered patterns of cerebral activity during speech and language production in developmental stuttering: An $H_2^{15}O$ positron emission tomography study. *Brain, 120,* 761–784.

Braun, A. R., Guillemin, A., Hosey, L., and **Varga, M.** (2001). The neural organization of discourse. An $H_2^{15}O$-PET study of narrative production in English and American sign language. *Brain, 124,* 2028–2044.

Bush, G., Luu, P., and **Posner, M. I.** (2000). Cognitive and emotional influences in anterior cingulate cortex. *Trends in Cognitive Sciences, 4,* 215–222.

Caruso, A. J. (1991). Neuromotor processes underlying stuttering. In H. F. M.Peters, W. Hulstijn, and C. W. Starkweather (Eds.), *Speech Motor Control and Stuttering* (pp. 101–116). New York: Elsevier Science Publishers.

Caruso, A. J., Abbs, J. H., and **Gracco, V. L.** (1988). Kinematic analysis of multiple movement coordination during speech in stutterers. *Brain, 111,* 439–456.

Cooke, A., Zurif, E. B., DeVita, C., Alsop, D., Koenig, P., Detre, J., Gee, J., Pinango, M., Balogh, J., and **Grossman, M.** (2001). Neural basis for sentence comprehension: Grammatical and short- term memory components. *Human Brain Mapping, 15,* 80–94.

Deiber, M. P., Wise, S. P., Honda, M., Catalan, M. J., Grafman, J., and **Hallett, M.** (1997). Frontal and parietal networks for conditional motor-learning: A positron emission tomography study. *Journal of Neurophysiology, 78,* 977–991.

De Nil, L. F. (1999). Stuttering: A neurophysiological perspective. In N. Bernstein Ratner and C. Healey (Eds.), *Stuttering Research and Practice: Bridging the Gap* (pp. 85–102). Mahwah, NJ: Erlbaum.

De Nil, L. F. and **Abbs, J. H.** (1991a). Kinaesthetic acuity of stutterers and non-stutterers for oral and non-oral movements. *Brain, 114,* 2145–2158.

De Nil, L. F. and **Abbs, J. H.** (1991b). Oral and finger kinesthetic thresholds in stuttering. In H. F. M. Peters, W. Hulstijn, and C. W. Starkweather (Eds.), *Speech Motor Control and Stuttering* (pp. 123–130). New York: Elsevier.

De Nil, L. F. and **Bosshardt, H. G.** (2001). Studying stuttering from a neurological and cognitive information processing perspective. In H. G. Bosshardt, J. S. Yaruss, and H. F. M. Peters (Eds.), *Stuttering: Research, Therapy and Self-Help. Proceedings of the Third World Congress on Fluency Disorders* (pp. 53–58). Nijmegen: Nijmegen University Press.

De Nil, L. F., Kroll, R. M., Kapur, S. and **Houle, S.** (2000). A positron emission tomography study of silent and oral reading of single words in stuttering and nonstuttering adults. *Journal of Speech, Language, and Hearing Research, 43,* 1038–1053.

De Nil, L. F., Kroll, R. M., and **Houle, S.** (2001). Functional neuroimaging of cerebellar activation during single word reading and verb generation in stuttering and nonstuttering adults. *Neuroscience Letters, 302,* 77–80.

De Nil, L. F., Kroll, R. M., Lafaille, S. J. and **Houle, S.** (2003). A positron emission tomography study of short- and long-term treatment effects on functional brain activation in adults who stutter. *Journal of Fluency Disorders, 28,* in press.

Devinsky, O., Morrell, M. J., and **Vogt, B. A.** (1995). Contributions of anterior cingulate cortex to behavior. *Brain, 118,* 279–306.

Felsenfeld, S. (1997). Epidemiology and genetics of stuttering. In R. F.Curlee and G. M. Siegel (Eds.), *Nature and Treatment of Stuttering: New Directions* (2nd edn), (pp. 3–23). Boston: Allyn and Bacon.

Fiez, J. A. and **Raichle, M. E.** (1997). Linguistic processing. *International Review Of Neurobiology, 41,* 233–254.

Forster, D. C. and **Webster, W. G.** (1991). Concurrent task interference in stutterers: Dissociating hemispheric specialization and activation. *Canadian Journal of Psychology, 45,* 321–335.

Forster, D. C. and **Webster, W. G.** (2001). Speech-motor control and interhemispheric relations in recovered and persistent stuttering. *Developmental Neuropsychology, 19,* 125–145.

Foundas, A. L., Hurley, M. M. and **Browning, C. A.** (1999). Anomalous auditory processing in adults with persistent developmental stuttering: Dichotic listening measures of free recall and directed attention. *Neurology, 52,* A489–A490.

Fox, P. T., Ingham, R. J., Ingham, J. C., Hirsch, T. B., Downs, J. H., Martin, C., Jerabek, P., Glass, Th., Lancaster, J. L., and **Glass, T.** (1996). A PET study of the neural systems of stuttering. *Nature, 382,* 158–162.

Fox, P. T., Ingham, R. J., Ingham, J. C., Zamarripa, F., Xiong, J. H., and **Lancaster, J. L.** (2000). Brain correlates of stuttering and syllable production. A PET performance-correlation analysis. *Brain, 123,* 1985–2004.

Fukawa, T., Yoshioka, H., Ozawa, E., and **Yoshida, S.** (1988). Difference of susceptibility to delayed auditory feedback between stutterers and nonstutterers. *Journal of Speech and Hearing Research, 31,* 475–479.

Gabrieli, J. D. E., Poldrack, R. A., and **Desmond, J. E.** (1998). The role of left prefrontal cortex in language and memory. *Proceedings of the National Academy of Sciences of the United States of America, 95,* 906–913.

Ghez, C. (1991). The cerebellum. In E. R. Kandel, J. H. Schwartz, and T. M. Jessell (Eds.), *The Principles of Neural Science* (pp. 626–646). New York: Elsevier.

Hallett, M. (2000). Plasticity. In J. C. Mazziotta, A. W. Toga, and R. S. J. Frackowiak (Eds.), *Brain Mapping. The Disorders* (pp. 569–585). San Diego: Academic Press.

Harrington, J. (1987). A model of stuttering and the production of speech under delayed auditory feedback conditions. In H. F. M.Peters and W. Hulstijn (Eds.), *Speech Motor Dynamics in Stuttering* (pp. 353–359). New York: Springer-Verlag.

Helm, N. A., Butler, R. B., and **Canter, G. J.** (1980). Neurogenic acquired stuttering. *Journal of Fluency Disorders, 5,* 269–279.

Huang, J., Carr, T. H., and **Cao, Y.** (2002). Comparing cortical activations for silent and overt speech using event-related fMRI. *Human Brain Mapping, 15,* 39 53.

Ilmoniemi, R. J. and **Aronen, H. J.** (1999). Cortical excitability and connectivity reflected in fMRI, MEG, EEG, and TMS. In C. T. W. Moonen and P. A. Bandettini (Eds.), *Functional MRI* (pp. 453–464). Berlin: Springer.

Ingham, R. J., Fox, P. T., Ingham, J. C., Zamarripa, F., Martin, C., Jerabek, P. and **Cotton, J.** (1996). Functional lesion investigation of developmental stuttering with positron emission tomography. *Journal of Speech and Hearing Research, 39,* 1208–1227.

Ingham, R. J., Fox, P. T., Ingham, J. C. and **Zamarripa, F.** (2000). Is overt stuttered speech a prerequisite for the neural activations associated with chronic developmental stuttering? *Brain and Language, 75,* 163–194.

Ivry, R. B. and **Keele, S. W.** (1989). Timing functions of the cerebellum. *Journal of Cognitive Neuroscience, 1,* 136–152.

Jenkins, I. H., Brooks, D. J., Nixon, P. D., Frackowiak, R. S. J., and **Passingham, R. E.** (1994). Motor sequence learning—A study with positron emission tomography. *Journal of Neuroscience, 14,* 3775–3790.

Johnson, W. and **Leutenegger, R. R.** (1955). *Stuttering in Children and Adults.* Minneapolis: University of Minnesota Press.

Jueptner, M., Frith, C. D., Brooks, D. J., Frackowiak, R. S. J., and **Passingham, R. E.** (1997). Anatomy of motor learning. 2. Subcortical structures and learning by trial and error. *Journal of Neurophysiology, 77,* 1325–1337.

Kalinowski, J., Stuart, A., Sark, S., and **Armson, J.** (1996). Stuttering amelioration at various auditory feedback delays and speech rates. *European Journal of Disorders of Communication, 31,* 259–269.

Kapur, S., Hussey, D., Wilson, D., and **Houle, S.** (1995). The statistical power of [^{15}O]-water PET activation studies of cognitive processes. *Nuclear Medicine Communications, 16,* 779–784.

Keller, T. A., Carpenter, P. A., and **Just, M. A.** (2001). The neural bases of sentence comprehension: a fMRI examination of syntactic and lexical processing. *Cerebral Cortex, 11,* 223–237.

Kroll, R. M. and **De Nil, L. F.** (1998). Positron emission tomography studies of stuttering: Their relationship to our theoretical and clinical understanding of the disorder. *Journal of Speech-Language Pathology and Audiology, 22,* 261–270.

Kroll, R. M., De Nil, L. F., Kapur, S., and **Houle, S.** (1997). A positron emission tomography investigation of post-treatment brain activation in stutterers. In H. F. M.Peters, W. Hulstijn, and P. H. H. M. Van Lieshout (Eds.), *Speech Production: Motor Control, Brain Research and Fluency Disorders* (pp. 307–320). Amsterdam: Elsevier Science Publishers.

Lebrun, Y., Leleux, C. and **Retif, J.** (1987). Neurogenic stuttering. *Acta Neurochirurgica, 85,* 103–109.

Loucks, T. M. J. and **De Nil, L. F.** (2001). Oral kinesthetic deficit in stuttering evaluated by movement accuracy and tendon vibration. In B. Maassen, W. Hulstijn, R. Kent, H. F. M. Peters, and P. H. H. M. Van Lieshout (Eds.), *Speech Motor Control in Normal and Disordered Speech. Proceedings of the Fourth International Speech Motor Conference,* Nijmegen: Uitgeverij Vantilt.

Molfese, D. L. and **Searock, K. J.** (1986). The use of auditory evoked responses at one-year-of-age to predict language skills at 3-years. *Australian Journal of Human Communication Disorders, 14,* 35–46.

Molfese, D. L., Burger-Judisch, L. M., Gill, L. A., Golinkoff, R. M., and **Hirsch-Pasek, K. A.** (1996). Electrophysiological correlates of noun–verb processing in adults. *Brain and Language, 54,* 388–413.

Molt, L. (1999). The basal ganglia's possible role in stuttering: An examination of similarities between Stuttering, Tourette Syndrome, Dystonia, and other neurological-based disorders of movement. ISAD Online Conference http://www.mankato.msus.edu/dept/comdis/isad2/isadcon2.html

Moore, W. H. (1984). Hemispheric alpha asymmetries during an electromyographic biofeedback procedure for stuttering: A single-subject experimental design. *Journal of Fluency Disorders, 9,* 143–162.

Moore, W. H. (1986). Hemispheric alpha asymmetries of stutterers and nonstutterers for the recall and recognition of words and connected reading passages: Some relationships to severity of stuttering. *Journal of Fluency Disorders, 11,* 71–89.

Moore, W. H. (1990). Pathophysiology of stuttering: Cerebral activation differences in stutterers vs. nonstutterers. *ASHA Reports, 18,* 72–80.

Moore, W. H. and **Lang, M. K.** (1977). Alpha asymmetry over the right and left hemispheres of stutterers and control subjects preceding massed oral readings: A preliminary investigation. *Perceptual and Motor Skills, 44,* 223–230.

Neville, H. J. and **Bavelier, D.** (1998). Neural organization and plasticity of language. *Current Opinion in Neurobiology, 8,* 254–258.

Orton, S. T. (1928). A physiological theory of reading disability and stuttering in children. *New England Journal of Medicine, 199,* 1045–1052.

Papanicolaou, A. C. (1998). *Fundamentals of Functional Brain Imaging.* Lisse, The Netherlands: Swets and Zeitlinger.

Peters, H. F. M., Hulstijn, W., and **Van Lieshout, P. H. H. M.** (1999). Recent developments in speech motor research into stuttering. *Folia Phoniatrica et Logopaedica, 52,* 103–119.

Petersen, S. E., Fox, P. T., Posner, M. I., Mintun, M., and **Raichle, M. E.** (1988). Positron emission tomographic studies of the cortical anatomy of single-word processing. *Nature, 331,* 585–589.

Peterson, B. S., Skudlarski, P., Gatenby, J. C., Zhang, H. P., Anderson, A. W., and **Gore, J. C.** (1999). An fMRI study of Stroop word–color interference: Evidence for cingulate subregions subserving multiple distributed attentional systems. *Biological Psychiatry, 45,* 1237–1258.

Pool, K. D., Devous, M. D., Freeman, F. J., Watson, B. C., and **Finitzo, T.** (1991). Regional cerebral blood flow in developmental stutterers. *Archives of Neurology, 48,* 509–512.

Price, C. J. (2000). The anatomy of language: Contributions from functional neuroimaging. *Anatomy of Language, 197,* 335–357.

Raichle, M. E., Fiez, J. A., Videen, T. O., Macleod, A. M. K., Pardo, J. V., Fox, P. T., and **Petersen, S. E.** (1994). Practice-related changes in human brain functional anatomy during nonmotor learning. *Cerebral Cortex, 4,* 8–26.

Riecker, A., Ackermann, H., Wildgruber, D., Dogil, G., and **Grodd, W.** (2000a). Opposite hemispheric lateralization effects during speaking and singing at motor cortex, insula and cerebellum. *Neuroreport, 11,* 1997–2000.

Riecker, A., Ackermann, H., Wildgruber, D., Meyer, J., Dogil, G., Haider, H., and **Grodd, W.** (2000b). Articulatory/phonetic sequencing at the level of the anterior perisylvian cortex: A functional magnetic resonance imaging (fMRI) study. *Brain and Language, 75,* 259–276.

Ringo, C. and **Dietrich, S.** (1995). Neurogenic stuttering: an analysis and critique. *Journal of Medical Speech-Language Pathology, 3,* 111–122.

Rugg, M. D. (1999). Functional neuroimaging in cognitive neuroscience. In: C. M. Brown and P. Hagoort (Eds.), *The Neurocognition of Language* (pp. 15–36). Oxford: Oxford University Press.

Sachs, M. W. (1924). Zur aetiologie des stotterns. *Klinische Wochenschrift, 37,* 113–115.

Salmelin, R., Schnitzler, A., Schmitz, F., and **Freund, H. J.** (2000). Single word reading in development stutterers and fluent speakers. *Brain, 123,* 1184–1202.

Sandson, T. A., Manoach, D. S., Price, B. H., Rentz, D., and **Weintraub, S.** (1994). Right hemisphere learning disability associated with left hemisphere dysfunction: anomalous dominance and development. *Journal of Neurology, Neurosurgery and Psychiatry, 57,* 1129–1132.

Stier, E. (1911). *Untersuchen über linkshändigkeit und die funktionellen differenzen der hirn-hälften.* Jena: Fischer.

Thach, W. (1987). Cerebellar inputs to motor cortex. In Ciba Foundation (Ed.), *Motor Areas of the Cerebral Cortex* (pp. 201–220). Toronto: Wiley & Sons.

Travis, L. E. (1931). *Speech Pathology.* New York: Appleton-Century.

Travis, L. E. (1978). The cerebral dominance theory of stuttering: 1931–1978. *Journal of Speech and Hearing Disorders, 43,* 278–281.

Tyler, L. K., Russell, R., Fadili, J., and **Moss, H. E.** (2001). The neural representation of nouns and verbs: PET studies. *Brain, 124,* 1619–1634.

Van Lieshout, P. H., Peters, H. F., Starkweather, C. W., and **Hulstijn, W.** (1993). Physiological differences between stutterers and nonstutterers in perceptually fluent speech: EMG amplitude and duration. *Journal of Speech and Hearing Research, 36,* 55–63.

van Mier, H., Tempel, L. W., Perlmutter, J. S., Raichle, M. E. and **Petersen, S. E.** (1998). Changes in brain activity during motor learning measured with PET: Effects of hand of performance and practice. *Journal of Neurophysiology, 80,* 2177–2199.

Van Riper, C. (1971). *The Nature of Stuttering.* Englewood Cliffs, NJ: Prentice-Hall.

Van Riper, C. (1982). *The Nature of Stuttering* (2nd edn). Englewood Cliffs: Prentice-Hall.

Watson, B. C., Freeman, F. J., Chapman, S. B., Miller, S., Finitzo, T., Pool, K. D., and **Devous, M. D.** (1991). Linguistic performance deficits in stutterers: Relation to laryngeal reaction time profiles. *Journal of Fluency Disorders, 16,* 85–100.

Webster, R. L. (1974). A behavioral analysis of stuttering: Treatment and theory. In K. S. Calhoun, H. E. Adams, and K. M. Mitchell (Eds.), *Innovative Treatment Methods in Psychopathology* (2nd edn), (p. 61). New York: Wiley.

Webster, W. G. (1985). Neuropsychological models of stuttering: I. Representation of sequential response mechanisms. *Neuropsychologia, 23,* 263–267.

Webster, W. G. (1986). Neuropsychological models of stuttering. II. Interhemispheric interference. *Neuropsychologia, 24,* 737–741.

Wells, B. G. and **Moore, W. H. Jr** (1990). EEG alpha asymmetries in stutterers and non-stutterers: effects of linguistic variables on hemispheric processing and fluency. *Neuropsychologia, 28,* 1295–1305.

Wood, F., Stump, D., McKeehan, A. B., Sheldon, S., and **Proctor, J.** (1980). Patterns of regional cerebral blood flow during attempted reading aloud by stutterers both on and off haloperidol medication: Evidence for inadequate left frontal activation during stuttering. *Brain and Language, 9,* 141–144.

Wu, J. C., Maguire, G., Riley, G., Fallon, J., LaCasse, L., Chin, S., Klein, E., Tang, C., Cadwell, S., and **Lottenberg, S.** (1995). A positron emission tomography [18F]deoxyglucose study of developmental stuttering. *Neuroreport, 6,* 501–505.

Yairi, E., Ambrose, N., and **Cox, N.** (1996). Genetics of stuttering: A critical review. *Journal of Speech and Hearing Research, 39,* 771–784.

Zimmermann, G. (1980). Articulatory behaviors associated with stuttering: A cinefluorographic analysis. *Journal of Speech and Hearing Research, 23,* 108–121.

CHAPTER 6

SUBCORTICAL BRAIN MECHANISMS IN SPEECH MOTOR CONTROL

BRUCE E. MURDOCH

6.1 Introduction

Speech production requires smooth coordination of orofacial, laryngeal, and respiratory muscles. Clinical data indicate that initiation and precise execution of articulatory movements depend upon the integrity of various neural subsystems involving both cortical and subcortical structures, such as the primary motor cortex, supplementary motor area, the basal ganglia, and the cerebellum.

It is well established that neurological disorders considered to be attributable primarily to lesions involving subcortical structures such as the basal ganglia and cerebellum are frequently associated with the occurrence of motor speech disorders (Darley *et al.* 1975; Murdoch 1998). For instance, hypokinetic dysarthria—a motor speech disorder characterized by features such as monotony of pitch and loudness; decreased use of all vocal parameters for effecting stress and emphasis; breathy and harsh vocal quality; reduced vocal intensity; variable speech rate, including short rushes of speech or accelerated speech; consonant imprecision; impaired breath support for speech; reduction in phonation time; difficulty in the initiation of speech activities; and inappropriate silences—has been reported to occur in association with Parkinson's disease, a condition caused by nerve cell loss in the pigmented brainstem nuclei, most markedly the pars compacta of the substantia nigra (Darley *et al.* 1969a, b; Theodoros and Murdoch 1998a). Likewise, a variety of motor speech disorders collectively referred to as 'hyperkinetic dysarthria' may occur in association with the abnormal involuntary movements encountered in a range of other neurological conditions caused by neuropathological changes in the basal ganglia system, including chorea, dystonia, etc. (Darley *et al.* 1975). Further, lesions to, or diseases of, the cerebellum or its afferent or efferent connections may disrupt the motor components of speech production at the segmental and suprasegmental level, giving rise to 'ataxic dysarthria', a motor speech disorder characterized by articulatory inaccuracy (imprecision of consonant production, irregular articulatory breakdowns and distorted vowels), prosodic excess (excess and equal stress, prolonged phonemes, prolonged intervals and slow rate), and phonatory–prosodic insufficiency (harshness, monopitch and monoloudness) (Murdoch and Theodoros 1998).

The occurrence of motor speech disorders in association with lesions to the basal ganglia and/or cerebellum implies that these subcortical brain structures have a role in the normal regulation of the motor functioning of the speech musculature. Unfortunately, the precise nature of this role remains elusive. In recent years, several models have been proposed in an attempt to further elucidate the possible contribution of subcortical structures to motor control, and to explain the occurrence of movement disorders subsequent to basal ganglia and cerebellar lesions. These models, which are discussed more fully later in this chapter, have served a valuable role by providing testable hypotheses and, in some cases, have guided the development of new pharmacological and neurosurgical treatments for movement disorders of subcortical origin.

The basal ganglia and cerebellum are two groups of subcortical nuclei that have classically been regarded as motor structures. In addition to their role in motor functions, anatomical studies and clinical research conducted over the past 10–15 years have increasingly implicated the basal ganglia and cerebellum in a range of behavioural functions, including several different types of cognitive and limbic functions. Consequently, the traditional view that the basal ganglia and cerebellum are only involved in motor functions has been challenged. A major reason for this reappraisal has been new information regarding basal ganglia and cerebellar connections with the cerebral cortex. Recently reported anatomical studies have noted that these connections are organized into discrete circuits or 'loops'. Rather than simply enabling widespread cortical areas to gain access to the motor system, these loops reciprocally interconnect a large and diverse set of cerebral cortical areas with the basal ganglia and cerebellum, enabling the latter structures to influence a range of cognitive functions in addition to their more traditional motor roles. For example, Alexander *et al.* (1986) proposed that the output of the basal ganglia targeted not only the primary motor cortex, but also specific areas of premotor and prefrontal cortex, thereby suggesting that the basal ganglia have the ability to influence not only motor control, but also several different types of cognitive and limbic (e.g. memory) functions. Similarly, it has been hypothesized that output from the lateral deep cerebellar nucleus (the dentate) influences not only motor areas of the cerebral cortex but also areas of the prefrontal cortex involved in language and cognition (Leiner *et al.* 1993). Evidence to support this functional diversity of the basal ganglia and cerebellum comes from several sources, including: neuroanatomical studies documenting the presence of extensive connections between the basal ganglia and cerebral cortex; animal studies reporting a range of behavioural correlates documented by single-cell recordings from basal ganglia neurons; observations of the behavioural effects of disease-induced lesions in the basal ganglia; clinico-neuroradiological studies documenting the presence of speech disorders and other behavioural deficits in association with subcortical lesions; the findings of studies based on functional neuroimaging, including positron emission tomography (PET) and functional magnetic resonance imaging (fMRI), and, more recently, observations of the behavioural effects of deep brain stimulation and surgically induced lesions in the globus palllidus (pallidotomy), thalamus (thalamotomy) and subthalamic nucleus, carried out as part of the treatment for Parkinson's disease and other basal ganglia syndromes.

Although it is acknowledged that subcortical structures such as the basal ganglia and cerebellum may have functions extending beyond motor activities, the present chapter will focus on their possible role in motor control, with particular emphasis on speech motor control. Both the macrostructure of the basal ganglia and cerebellum, including their connections with other brain structures, and the microstructural aspects, including details of neurotransmitter types, will be briefly summarized as an essential precursor to discussion of the functional role of these structures. Contemporary models and theories of subcortical participation in motor control will be described and discussed, with particular emphasis given to how these models may explain the occurrence of motor speech disorders such as hyperkinetic, hypokinetic and ataxic dysarthria subsequent to neuropathology involving the basal ganglia or cerebellum. However, in so doing, it is acknowledged that other subcortical pathologies, such as damage to the corticobulbar tracts as they course through the subcortical white matter, may also be associated with dysarthria.

6.2 Functional neuroanatomy of the basal ganglia and cerebellum

Damage to the basal ganglia and cerebellum produces well-described alterations in motor function, such as tremor, rigidity, akinesia or dysmetria, which may affect the speech production mechanism. It is thought that many of these symptoms may be due to disruption of basal ganglia or cerebellar outputs to areas of the cerebral cortex involved in the control of movement. Models of basal ganglia–thalamocortical and cerebellar–cortical circuits, have, therefore, become central to research and theoretical approaches aimed at understanding the role of the basal ganglia and cerebellum in speech motor functions. Consequently, central to any attempt to understand the role of these subcortical structures in speech motor control is a knowledge of their basic neuroanatomy.

6.2.1 Functional neuroanatomy of the basal ganglia

Although the connections of the basal ganglia are not yet fully understood. with new findings continuing to be made, the basic anatomy of the circuitry connecting these structures was clearly described by Alexander *et al.* (1986). Essentially, according to their description, information originating in the cerebral cortex passes through the basal ganglia and returns via the thalamus to specific areas of the frontal lobe, this feedback circuit often being referred to as the cortico-striato-pallido-thalamo-cortical loop.

The major components of the basal ganglia include: the putamen and caudate nucleus (CN), collectively known as the neostriatum (NS); the globus pallidus (GP); the substantia nigra pars compacta (SNPC) and pars reticulata (SNPR); and the subthalamic nucleus (STN). In general, the basal ganglia can be considered to be comprised of a group of 'input'structures (the CN, putamen and ventral striatum), which receive direct input essentially from areas of the cerebral cortex, and 'output' structures (the internal segment of the GP (GPi), the SNPR and the ventral pallidum), which project back to the cerebral cortex via the thalamus. Over the past two decades, notions of the organization of the basal ganglia, the thalamus and connections with various cortical regions have been revised. Originally, the NS was considered to serve primarily to integrate diverse inputs from the entire cerebral cortex and to 'funnel' these influences via the ventrolateral thalamus to the primary motor cortex alone. Consistent with the view held at the time, that they functioned primarily in the domain of motor control, the basal ganglia were thus seen as a mechanism for 'funnelling' information into the motor system. Based on recent research, it is now clear that output from the basal ganglia terminates in thalamic regions that gain access to a wider region of the frontal lobe than just the primary motor cortex. Rather, these subcortical nuclei appear to project to many or most of the same cortical areas that send efferents to them. Consequently, the original notion of the basal ganglia acting as a mechanism to 'funnel' information to the motor cortex has been superseded by the view of the NS as a 'multi-laned throughway', which forms part of a series of multi-segregated circuits connecting the cortex, the basal ganglia and the thalamus (Alexander *et al.* 1986; Graybiel and Kimura 1995; Middleton and Strick 2000). Thus the anatomy of the basal ganglia is characterized by their participation in multiple 'loops' with the cerebral cortex, each of which follows the basic route of cortex→striatum→globus pallidus/substantia nigra→thalamus→cortex in a unidirectional fashion.

Alexander *et al.* (1986) identified at least five separate, parallel cortico-basal ganglia circuits according to the specific region of the frontal lobe that serves as a target for their thalamocortical projections. One of these cortico-basal ganglia circuits projected to the skeletomotor areas of the frontal cortex, while another projected to the oculomotor areas. The three remaining circuits projected to non-motor areas of the frontal cortex, including the dorsolateral prefrontal area (area 46), the lateral orbitofrontal cortex (area 12), and the anterior cingulate/medial orbitofrontal cortices (areas 24 and 13). Importantly, these circuits appear to be, to a large extent, functionally segregated (Alexander *et al.* 1986), suggesting that structural convergence and functional integration occur within, rather than between, each of the identified circuits. Given the segregated nature of the cortico-basal ganglia circuits, collectively they may be viewed as having a unified role in modulating the operations of the entire frontal lobe, thereby influencing such diverse frontal lobe processes as motor activities, behavioural, cognitive, language, and even limbic, processes. This anatomical arrangement, whereby the output from the basal ganglia gains access to multiple areas of the frontal lobe, including non-motor areas, has profound consequences for the possible functional roles of the basal ganglia system and provides a basic neuroanatomical mechanism whereby these subcortical structures can influence aspects of behaviour, cognition and language, as well as motor function.

The cortico-basal ganglia circuit that has received the greatest attention in the literature, and which is of greatest relevance to movement disorders associated with motor speech impairments, is the 'skeletomotor circuit'. At the cortical level this circuit is comprised of the pre- and postcentral sensorimotor areas, while at the subcortical level it is comprised of sensorimotor areas in the basal ganglia and the ventral anterior and ventrolateral thalamus. Cortical projections of the motor circuit terminate largely in the putamen. According to current models of the organization of the basal ganglia, putaminal output is directed over two separate projection systems, the so-called 'direct' and 'indirect' pathways. The direct pathway originates from striatal neurons that contain γ-aminobutyric acid (GABA) plus the peptide substance P and/or dynorphin, and conveys activity from the NS monosynaptically to the GPi and SNPR. In contrast, the indirect pathway arises from striatal neurons that contain GABA and enkephalin and conveys activity to the GPi and SNPR polysynaptically via a sequence of connections involving the external segment of the globus pallidus (GPe) and the STN. In both cases the returning thalamocortical connections seem to reach precisely the regions of the frontal cortex that contribute as inputs to the NS (Strick *et al.* 1995). A diagramatic representation of the basic circuitry of the basal ganglia is presented in Fig. 6.1.

Imbalance between the activity in the direct and indirect pathways and the resulting alterations in the activity of the GPi and SNPR are thought to account for the hypo- and hyperkinetic features of basal ganglia disorders, including hypo- and hyperkinetic dysarthria. The possible roles of the direct and indirect pathways to the development of hypo- and hyperkinetic movement disorders are discussed further below. However, it is noteworthy that, based on the findings of single-axon training studies in primates, the simple dual (direct/indirect) division of basal ganglia circuitry has recently been challenged (Parent *et al.* 2001). Using a single-cell labelling procedure, Parent *et al.* (2001) showed that striatal axons are highly collateralized, suggesting that the basal ganglia should not be regarded as a simple dual (direct/indirect) neuronal system but rather should be viewed as a widely distributed network.

The nature of the neurotransmitters utilized by the neurons that comprise the cortico-basal ganglia circuits provides further insight as to the possible functional

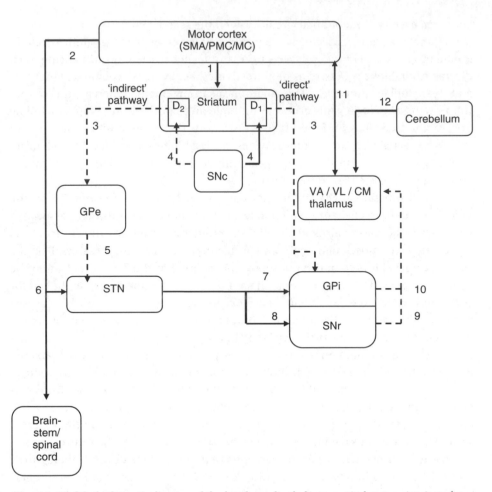

Fig. 6.1 Modified schematic diagram of the basal ganglia thalamo-cortical motor circuit under normal conditions based on DeLong (1990). SMA, supplementary motor area; PMC, pre-motor cortex; MC, motor cortex; D_1, striatal output neuron receptor type D_1; D_2, striatal output receptor type D_2; SNc, substantia nigra compacta; GPe, globus pallidus externus; STN, subthalamic nucleus; GPi, globus pallidus internus; SNr, substantia nigra reticulata; VA, ventral anterior nucleus of thalamus; VL, ventral lateral nucleus of thalamus; CM, centrum medianum; ⟶, excitatory pathway; ┄┄▶, inhibitory pathway. 1, cortico-striatal pathway; 2, cortico-bulbar and cortico-spinal pathways; 3, striato-pallidal pathways; 4, nigro-striatal pathways; 5, pallido-subthalamic pathway, 6, cortico-subthalamic pathway; 7, subthalamo-pallidal pathway; 8, subthalamo-nigral pathway; 9, nigro-thalamic pathway; 10, pallido-thalamic pathway; 11, thalamo-cortical and cortico-thalamic pathways; 12, cerebello-thalamic pathway.

roles of these circuits. The cerebral cortex is connected to the NS by way of excitatory neurons that use glutamate as a transmitter. In contrast, as noted above, the neurons connecting the NS to GP use GABA, which exerts an inhibitory effect on targets in the medial and lateral GP and in the SNPR, although these neurons also contain neuropeptides such as substance P and enkephalin. The GP neurons are themselves inhibitory and, consequently, there are two inhibitory synapses in series between the NS and the thalamus. In effect, these two inhibitory synapses in series act as an excitation. When the NS is active, the GP neurons disinhibit the thalamocortical projection via the direct pathway and thus presumably facilitate the initiation of movement (or some other frontal lobe activity). Briefly, the suggested mechanism for this initiation of movement is as follows: corticostriatal activation of the direct pathway produces a GABA-mediated inhibition of GPi/SNPR neurons, leading in turn to disinhibition of their thalamic target, thereby facilitating the thalamic projection to the precentral motor fields. The overall effect of this sequence is positive feedback for cortically initiated movements. Suppression of unwanted movements (activities) probably ensues through inhibition of the thalamocortical projections via the indirect pathway (Wichmann *et al.* 1994), because projections from the STN to the GPi are excitatory. Put simply, corticostriatal stimulation of the GABA-enkephalin neurons in the indirect pathway inhibits the GPi and secondarily facilitiates the STN. The latter results in increased excitatory drive on to the GPi/SNPR, which respond by increasing their output, thereby further inhibiting their thalamic and brainstem targets. The overall effect of this sequence is to provide negative feedback for movement, thereby acting to inhibit undesired movements or to signal a halt to movements in progress.

Thus both excitatory and inhibitory influences converge on the GP, and their balance probably determines the activity in the thalamocortical projections. The most important neuromodulator of the balance between the activity of the direct and indirect pathways at the level of the NS is dopamine. The dopaminergic input to the NS is provided by the nigrostriatal projections from the SNPC. Release of dopamine from terminals of the nigrostriatal projections appears to facilitate transmission over the direct pathway and to inhibit transmission over the indirect pathway via dopamine subtype D_1 and D_2 receptors respectively (Gerfen 1995) (see Fig. 6.1). Consequently, reduced basal ganglia output from the GPi/SNPR leading to increased activity of thalamocortical projection neurons is the outcome of striatal dopamine release. The role of abnormal striatal dopamine release in the occurrence of hypo- and hyperkinetic speech disorders is discussed below in the section dealing with subcortical models of hypo- and hyperkinetic dysarthria.

6.2.2 Functional neuroanatomy of the cerebellum

The cerebellum is comprised of two large cerebellar hemispheres, which are connected by a mid-portion called the vermis. As in the case of the cerebral hemispheres, the cerebellar hemispheres are covered by a layer of grey matter or cortex. Unlike the cerebral cortex, however, the cerebellar cortex tends to be uniform in structure throughout its extent. The cerebellar cortex is highly folded into thin transverse folds, or folia. A series of deep and definite fissures divides the cerebellum into a number of lobes. Although the lobe system of the cerebellum is classified differently by different authors, three lobes are commonly recognized: the anterior lobe, the posterior lobe and the flocculonodular lobe. The posterior lobe, also referred to as the neocerebellum, lies between the other two lobes and is the largest portion of the cerebellum. Phylogenetically it is the newest portion of the cerebellum and is most concerned with the regulation of voluntary movements. In particular, it plays an essential role in the coordination of phasic movements and is the most important part of the cerebellum for the coordination of speech movements.

The central core of the cerebellum, like that of the cerebral hemispheres, is made up of white matter. Located within the white matter, on either side of the midline, are four grey masses called the cerebellar or deep nuclei. These are the dentate nucleus, the globose and emboliform nuclei (collectively referred to as the interpositus), and the fastigial nucleus. The majority of the Purkinje cell axons, which carry impulses away from the cerebellar cortex, terminate in these nuclei.

In order to be able to perform its primary function of synergistic coordination of muscular activity, the cerebellum requires extensive connections with other parts of the nervous system. Damage to the pathways making up these connections can cause cerebellar dysfunction and possible ataxic dysarthria, in the same way as damage to the cerebellum itself. Briefly, the cerebellum functions in part by comparing input from the motor cortex with information concerning the momentary status of muscle contraction, degree of tension of the muscle tendons, positions of parts of the body, and forces acting on the surfaces of the body originating from muscle spindles, Golgi tendon organs, etc., and then sending appropriate messages back to the motor cortex to ensure smooth, co-ordinated muscle function. Consequently, the cerebellum requires input from the motor cortex, muscle and joint receptors, receptors in the internal ear detecting changes in the position and rate of rotation in the head, skin receptors, etc. Conversely, pathways carrying signals from the cerebellum back to the cortex are also required to complete the cerebrocerebellar loop.

The traditional view of cerebrocerebellar loops is that they receive information from widespread cortical areas in the frontal, parietal, and temporal lobes, with the major afferent pathway connecting the cerebral cortex and the cerebellum being the corticopontine–cerebellar pathway. This pathway originates primarily from the motor cortex and projects to the ipsilateral pontine nuclei, from where secondary fibres project mainly to the cortex of the neocerebellum. Other afferent pathways project to the cerebellum from structures in the brainstem, such as the olive (olivo-cerebellar tracts), the red nucleus (rubro-cerebellar tracts), the reticular formation (reticulo-cerebellar tract), the midbrain (tectocerebellar tract), and the cuneate nucleus (cuneocerebellar tract), as well as from the spinal cord (spinocerebellar tracts).

Efferent pathways from the cerebellum originate almost entirely from the deep nuclei and project to many parts of the central nervous system, including the cerebral cortex (via the thalamus), basal ganglia, red nucleus, brainstem reticular formation, and vestibular nuclei. Traditionally, the output of cerebellar processing is thought to be directed at only a single cortical area, namely the primary motor cortex, consistent with the belief the corticocerebellar circuits function primarily in the domain of motor control. In recent years, however, this point of view has been challenged. For instance, anatomical evidence is now available that demonstrates that the site of termination of cerebellar efferents is not restricted to only the subdivisions of the ventrolateral thalamus that innervate the primary motor cortex. Rather, the regions of the thalamus that receive cerebellar input are now recognized as including those regions that project to many motor, as well as non-motor, areas of the cerebral cortex (Middleton and Strick 1997, 2001). In support of the anatomical evidence, functional neuroimaging studies have demonstrated that, in addition to motor activities, the cerebellum is involved in functions that include higher cognitive functions such as language and attention (Schmahmann 2001). As yet, clinical data on the cerebellar representations of speech motor control do not provide a coherent picture. Although some studies have emphasized the importance of medial cerebellar structures to speech, others suggest a predominant contribution from the lateral parts of the cerebellum (Ackermann and Hertrich 2000). Several investigations have linked ataxic dysarthria to bilateral damage to the cerebellum, while others have reported dysarthria in association with unilateral lesions (Ackermann and Ziegler 1992). Although Lechtenberg and Gilman (1978) observed a significantly higher prevalence of dysarthria in patients with left cerebellar lesions, Ackermann *et al.* (1992), in a study of speech deficits associated with ischaemic cerebellar lesions, reported that three of their four dysarthric subjects had unilateral right-sided ischaemia. The findings of these latter authors demonstrated that lesions of the cerebellar cortex without involvement of the dentate nucleus can cause dysarthria.

6.3 Hypokinetic, hyperkinetic, and ataxic dysarthria

Research into the motor functions of the basal ganglia, thalamus, and cerebellum has primarily focused on the role of these structures in regulating the activity of limb and trunk muscles. Very little attention has been paid to the possible role that these subcortical structures may play in regulating the functioning of craniofacial muscles, especially the muscles of the speech production apparatus. However, the occurrence of motor speech disorders in association with neurological conditions caused by pathological changes in the basal ganglia (e.g. Parkinson's disease) and cerebellum has been regarded as indicative of a role for these structures in the motor control of the speech-production mechanism.

6.3.1 Hypo- and hyperkinetic dysarthria

As in the case of movement disorders of basal ganglia origin affecting limb and trunk muscles, motor speech disorders associated with lesions in the basal ganglia take the form of hypo- or hyperkinetic movement disorders. In general, hypokinetic disorders such as Parkinson's disease are associated with increased basal ganglia output, whereas hyperkinetic movement disorders such as Huntington's disease are associated with decreased output. Hypokinetic disorders are characterized by significant impairments in movement initiation (akinesia) and reduction in the velocity of voluntary movements (bradykinesia), and are usually accompanied by muscular rigidity and tremor at rest. By contrast, hyperkinetic disorders are characterized by excessive motor activity in the form of involuntary movements (dyskinesias) and varying degrees of hypotonia. With regard to their effect on the speech-production mechanism, these disorders manifest as hypokinetic dysarthria (classically associated with Parkinson's disease) and hyperkinetic dysarthria (seen in association with a range of hyperkinetic conditions, such as Huntington's disease, dystonia, etc.).

The speech characteristics associated with hypokinetic dysarthria follow largely from the generalized pattern of hypokinetic motor disorder, which includes marked reduction in the amplitude of voluntary movements, slowness of movement, initiation difficulties, muscular rigidity, loss of the automatic (associated) aspects of movement, and tremor at rest. For example, a pervading feature of articulatory impairment in persons with Parkinson's disease includes a reduction in the amplitude of displacement of the articulators and a decrease in the velocity of movement (Forrest and Weismer 1995). Hunker and Abbs (1984) suggested that tremor of the orofacial structures in persons with Parkinson's disease may have a significant effect on their reaction times during speech, such that the patient may be unable to initiate a muscle contraction until it coincides with a tremor oscillation. Furthermore, Hunker and Abbs (1984) suggested that movement times of the articulators may be prolonged because of the superimposition of a number of tremor-related muscle inhibitions. The abnormal speech breathing characteristics of persons with Parkinson's disease have largely been attributed to rigidity of the respiratory muscles, which imposes limitations on the movements of the chest wall, resulting in reduced respiratory capacity and incoordination of the rib cage and abdomen during respiration (Murdoch *et al.* 1989; Solomon and Hixon 1993).

Extensive perceptual, acoustic, and physiological analyses of hypokinetic dysarthria have been conducted in an attempt to produce a definitive description of the speech disorder and provide a basis for treatment programming (for a review, see Theodoros and Murdoch 1998*a*). Although various studies have identified impairment in all aspects of speech production (respiration, phonation, resonance, articulation, and prosody) involving the various subsystems of the speech-production mechanism, the individual with Parkinson's disease is most likely to exhibit disturbances of prosody, phonation, and articulation (Darley *et al.*

1975; Chenery *et al.* 1988; Zwirner and Barnes 1992). However, the findings of these studies have not always been consistent with respect to the type of disturbance, the frequency of occurrence, and the degree of severity of the abnormal perceptual, acoustic, and physiological speech features present in the speech of hypokinetic dysarthric speakers. These inconsistencies reflect the extensive variability in the presentation of the hypokinetic dysarthria associated with Parkinson's disease, which may in itself be related to the progressive nature of the disease and/or factors such as individual responses to anti-Parkinsonian medication.

Hyperkinetic dysarthria is a collective name for a diverse group of speech disorders in which the deviant speech characteristics are the product of abnormal involuntary movements that disturb the rhythm and rate of motor activities, including those involved in speech production. These involuntary movements, which may involve the limbs, trunk, neck, face, etc., may be rhythmic or irregular and unpredictable, rapid, or slow. The abnormal involuntary movements involved vary considerably in their form and locus across the different diseases of the basal ganglia. Consequently, there is considerable heterogeneity in the deviant speech dimensions manifest in the speech disorders encompassed under the term 'hyperkinetic dysarthria'. Any or all of the major subcomponents of the speech production apparatus may be involved, including the respiratory system, phonatory valve, resonatory valve, and articulatory valve. Disturbances in prosody are also often present. Darley *et al.* (1975) distinguished between two categories of hyperkinetic disorders: quick hyperkinesias and slow hyperkinesias. Quick hyperkinesias include myoclonic jerks (e.g. palatopharyngolaryngeal myoclonus), tics, chorea, and ballism, and are characterized by rapid, abnormal, involuntary movements that are either unsustained or sustained only very briefly, and are random in occurrence with respect to the particular body part affected. In contrast, the abnormal involuntary movements seen in slow hyperkinesias build up to a peak slowly and are sustained for at least 1 second or longer. In some instances the abnormal muscle contractions seen in association with slow hyperkinesias are sustained for many seconds or even minutes, with muscle tone waxing and waning to produce a variety of distorted postures. The three major conditions included in the category of slow hyperkinesias are athetosis, dyskinesia (lingual–facial–buccal dyskinesia), and dystonia. The clinical characteristics of the speech disorder associated with these conditions have been reviewed by Theodoros and Murdoch (1998*b*); however, by way of example, the clinical speech characteristics of one quick (chorea) and one slow (dystonia) hyperkinetic condition are presented briefly here. The most prevalent abnormalities reported in the speech of persons with chorea are prosodic disturbances which are thought to reflect the interruption of speech flow by the choreiform movements, as well as the speaker's tendency to compensate for sudden, unpredictable arrests of respiratory, phonatory, resonatory, or articulatory function. Specifically, the speech of persons with chorea is characterized by prosodic excess (prolonged intervals, inappropriate silences, prolonged phonemes and excess, and equal stress), prosodic insufficiency (monopitch, monoloudness, reduced stress, and short phrases), and variable rate (Murdoch 1990; Theodoros and Murdoch 1998b). Dystonias affecting the speech mechanism may result in motor speech deficits that predominantly involve articulation, phonation, and prosody (Zraick *et al.* 1993), and, to some extent, respiration (La Blance and Rutherford 1991). The main effects of dystonia on speech production include delays in the initiation of voluntary movements necessary for speech, due to prolonged dystonic movements, and slowness and restricted range of voluntary speech movements once initiated (Murdoch 1990). Dystonias affecting the speech mechanism may result in respiratory irregularities and/or abnormal movement and bizarre posturing of the jaw (mouth opening and closing), lips (pursing and retraction), tongue (involuntary protrusion and rotation), face (facial spasm and grimacing), and neck (elevation of larynx, torsion of the neck, and alteration of the vocal tract) (Theodoros and Murdoch 1998b).

In describing hypo- and hyperkinetic speech disorders, it has generally been assumed that the speech musculature is affected by subcortical lesions in the same way as limb muscles, implying that the role of the basal ganglia in the motor control of limb and craniofacial muscles is the same. Recently, however, evidence arising from investigations into the effects of stereotactic neurosurgically induced lesions in the GP or thalamus on speech production has suggested that the role of the basal ganglia in controlling the speech-production muscles may not be the same as their role in regulating limb muscle function. Specifically, some reports have suggested that, although surgically induced lesions of the GP may be effective in relieving symptoms such as akinesia in limb muscles, they do not produce a concomitant improvement in the functioning of the speech musculature; in some cases speech intelligibility actually declines following such surgery (Johannson *et al.* 1997; Lang *et al.* 1998; Samuels *et al.* 1998; Theodoros and Murdoch 1998a). However, prior to examining this evidence further, there is a need to study models of the pathophysiological mechanisms that underly such diverse symptomatology as the hypokinesia in Parkinson's disease and the involuntary movements associated with hyperkinetic disorders.

6.3.2 Subcortical models of motor control applicable to hypo- and hyperkinetic dysarthria

Hypo- and hyperkinetic movement disorders represent the extreme ends of the clinical spectrum of basal-ganglia-associated motor disturbances. Parkinsonism is characterized by a reduction in striatal dopaminergic transmission leading to increased basal ganglia output to the thalamus. In contrast, the major hyperkinetic syndromes such as chorea, athetosis, dystonia, etc. are all characterized by reduced basal ganglia output to the thalamus, leading to disinhibition of the thalamocortical neurons which in turn leads to the development of involuntary movements. DeLong (1990) suggested that hypo- and hyperkinetic movement disorders can be explained using a functional model of the basal ganglia–thalamocortical circuit derived from findings of experiments involving monitoring of the neuronal activity of various basal ganglia sites in primates treated with MPTP (1-methyl-4-phenyl-1,2,3,6 tetra-hydropyridine). In primates treated with MPTP, the dopaminergic cells in the SNPC degenerate, and the animals subsequently develop a clinical syndrome that closely resembles human parkinsonism (Miller and DeLong 1987). What the findings of these studies suggest is that the hypokinetic movement disorders associated with Parkinson's disease may result from increased inhibition of the thalamocortical neurons, which renders the cortical projection areas less responsive to other inputs normally involved in initiating movements. Briefly, according to the model of hypokinetic movement disorders proposed by DeLong (1990) (see Fig. 6.2), loss of striatal dopamine leads to excessive inhibition of the GPe, leading to disinhibition of the STN which, in turn, provides excessive excitatory drive to the basal ganglia output nuclei (i.e. the GPi and SNPR) via the indirect pathway leading to thalamic inhibition. This effect is reinforced by reduced inhibitory input to the basal ganglia output nuclei through the direct pathway, also leading to inhibition of thalamocortical neurons. According to DeLong (1990), these effects are postulated to result in a reduction in the usual reinforcing influence of the subcortical motor circuit upon cortically initiated movements, leading to symptoms such as akinesia and bradykinesia. The model proposed by DeLong (1990) is supported by data based on microelectrode recordings of basal ganglia neuron activity in MPTP-treated primates (Filion *et al.* 1988; Filion and Tremblay 1991), which have shown that neurons in the STN and GPi of these primates have higher discharge rates and show prominent changes in their discharge patterns, including a greater tendancy to discharge in bursts. Further support has been derived from metabolic studies based on positron emission tomography (PET), which have demonstrated that the changes in basal ganglia discharge that results from dopamine depletion alter the neuronal activity in the thalamus and brainstem as well as cortical metabolic activity, consistent with the hypokinetic model (Brooks 1991; Eidelberg 1992; Calne and Snow 1993; Leenders 1997). Given that, according to the above hypokinetic model, motor disturbances in Parkinson's disease are postulated to result, in large part, from increased thalamic inhibition due to excess excitatory drive from the STN to the output nuclei of the basal ganglia, it has been speculated that induced lesions in the STN would ameliorate symptoms such as bradykinesia and akinesia (DeLong 1990). Experiments involving selective lesioning of the STN with ibotenate (a fibre-sparing neurotoxin) in MPTP-treated monkeys have confirmed this hypothesis (DeLong 1990).

In addition to the model of hypokinetic movement disorders, DeLong (1990) also proposed a functional model to explain hyperkinetic movement disorders. Evidence is available to suggest that a common mechanism underlies the various hyperkinetic movement disorders, such as the choreiform movement in Huntington's disease and the dyskinetic movements seen in hemiballismus. In fact,

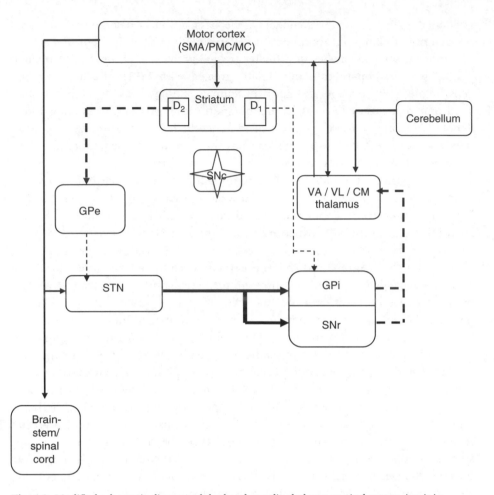

Fig. 6.2 Modified schematic diagram of the basal ganglia thalamo-cortical motor circuit in Parkinson's disease, based on DeLong (1990). SMA, supplementary motor area; PMC, pre-motor cortex; MC, motor cortex; D_1, striatal output neuron receptor type D_1; D_2, striatal output receptor type D_2; SNc, substantia nigra compacta; GPe, globus pallidus externus; STN, subthalamic nucleus; GPi, globus pallidus internus; SNr, substantia nigra reticulata; VA, ventral anterior nucleus of thalamus; VL, ventral lateral nucleus of thalamus; CM, centrum medianum; ⟶, excitatory pathway; ·····➤, inhibitory pathway.; ◇, lesion site.

it has been suggested that these dyskinesias differ only by the intensity and amplitude of the movements. It is known that, early in the course of Huntington's disease, there is a selective loss of striatal GABA/enkephalin neurons that give rise to the indirect pathway. Experiments involving neurotoxin (ibotenate) induced lesions in the STN of monkeys suggest that ballismus is associated with disinhibition of the thalamus as a result of STN lesions. According to the model of hyperki-

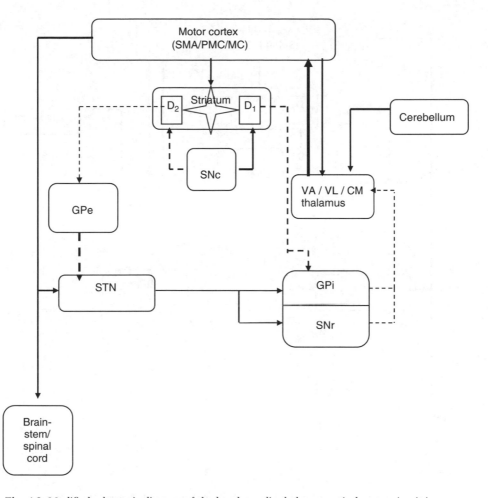

Fig. 6.3 Modified schematic diagram of the basal ganglia thalamo-cortical motor circuit in Huntington's disease based on DeLong (1990). SMA, supplementary motor area; PMC, pre-motor cortex; MC, motor cortex; D_1, striatal output neuron receptor type D_1; D_2, striatal output receptor type D_2; SNc, substantia nigra compacta; GPe, globus pallidus externus; STN, subthalamic nucleus; GPi, globus pallidus internus; SNr, substantia nigra reticulata; VA, ventral anterior nucleus of thalamus; VL, ventral lateral nucleus of thalamus; CM, centrum medianum; ⟶, excitatory pathway; ┄┄▶, inhibitory pathway.; ◇, lesion site.

netic movement disorders preposed by DeLong (1990), reduced excitatory projec-tions from the STN to the GPi, due to either STN lesions (as in ballismus) or reduced striatopallidal inhibitory influences along the indirect pathway (as in Huntington's disease) (see Fig. 6.3), lead to reduced inhibitory outflow from the GPi/SNPR and excessive disinhibition of the thalamus. In the case of L-dopa induced dyskinesias, disinhibition of the thalamus is thought to result from exces-

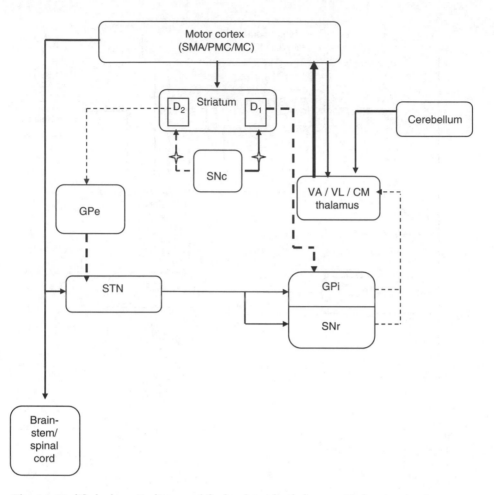

Fig. 6.4 Modified schematic diagram of the basal ganglia thalamo-cortical motor circuit subserving drug-induced dyskinesias based on DeLong (1990). SMA, supplementary motor area; PMC, pre-motor cortex; MC, motor cortex; D_1, striatal output neuron receptor type D_1; D_2, striatal output receptor type D_2; SNc, substantia nigra compacta; GPe, globus pallidus externus; STN, subthalamic nucleus; GPi, globus pallidus internus; SNr, substantia nigra reticulata; VA, ventral anterior nucleus of thalamus; VL, ventral lateral nucleus of thalamus; CM, centrum medianum; ——▶, excitatory pathway; ·····▶, inhibitory pathway.; ✧, excessive dopaminergic stimulation of GABA/substance P neurons.

sive dopaminergic stimulation of the striatal GABA/substance P neurons that send inhibitory projections to the output nuclei of the basal ganglia via the direct pathway (see Fig. 6.4). The proposed overall effect is that of excessive positive feedback to the precentral motor fields engaged by the 'skeletomotor' circuit resulting in hyperkinetic movements (DeLong 1990).

Although the above models serve to explain the basic pathophysiological mechanisms underlying hypo- and hyperkinetic movement disorders, they do not account for a number of clinical and experimental observations. For example, the above models do not provide a satisfactory explanation for the lack of dyskinesias after pallidotomy, the lack of parkinsonian signs after thalamotomy and the failure of experimental GPe lesions to abolish drug-induced dyskinesias. Although predicted by the model, according to Bathia and Marsden (1994) lesions of the thalamus are not associated with parkinsonism, even though such lesions could be expected to reduce or interrupt thalamocortical drive. Likewise, lesions of the GPi in normal monkeys or humans do not induce dyskinesias, as would be predicted by the model (Baron *et al.* 1997). Despite these limitations, the primate-based models proposed by DeLong (1990) provide an ideal context for looking further at the role of the basal ganglia in speech motor control based on evidence provided by the study of patients with circumscribed, surgically induced lesions in specific nuclei of the basal ganglia system.

6.3.3 Ataxic dysarthria

Ataxic dysarthria is a motor speech disorder classically associated with brain lesions involving the cerebellum or its connections. The clinical features of ataxic dysarthria follow on from the neuromotor abnormalities associated with damage to the cerebellum, in particular ataxia. In contemporary neurological literature, the term 'ataxia' is used to define motor disturbances of cerebellar origin associated with a variety of clinical symptoms, including dysmetria–hypermetria, asynergia, postural and gait instability, intention tremor and space–time motor incoordination. Dysmetria is a condition in which there is improper measuring of distance in muscular acts. The presence of dysmetria is evidenced by the patient's inability to stop a movement at the desired point. For example, when reaching for an object, the patient's hand may over-reach the intended point (hypermetria) or under-reach the intended point (hypometria). Dyssynergia represents a breakdown in the 'cooperative action of muscles' and is reflected in patients with cerebellar lesions in the separation of a series of voluntary movements that normally flow smoothly and in sequence into a succession of mechanical or puppet-like movements (decomposition of movement). It may also be manifest as movement abnormalities such as delayed starting or stopping of movements. Disturbances of posture and gait may be very pronounced, the patient possibly being unable to maintain an upright posture, or walking in a staggering fashion with a broad base of support. Tremor is another feature of cerebellar disease and refers to the presence of an involuntary, rhythmic oscillatory movement of a body part. The tremor of cerebellar disease is typically exaggerated by goal-oriented movements (intention tremor) and is consequently seen during movement of a body part but is absent at rest. This is in contrast to the muscle tremor seen in Parkinson's disease, which is most obvious during rest and is reduced during movement.

The predominant features of ataxic dysarthria are a breakdown in the articulatory and prosodic aspects of speech. Unlike some forms of dysarthria (e.g. flaccid dysarthria), where the speech disorder can be linked to deficits in individual muscles, ataxic dysarthria is associated with decomposition of complex movements arising from a breakdown in the coordinated action of the muscles of the speech production apparatus to produce speech. Consequently, individual and repetitive movements of parts of the speech mechanism contain errors of force, range, timing and direction, and tend to be slow, leading to irregularity of motor performance and to impaired coordination of simultaneous and sequenced movements. Increased variability in both limb and speech movement direction, force, velocity, amplitude, rate, movement onsets and terminations have been noted subsequent to cerebellar damage (Kent *et al.* 1979; Schonle *et al.* 1990; Hallett *et al.* 1991; Ackermann and Hertrich 1994, 2000). In particular, inaccuracy of movement, irregular rhythm of repetitive movement, discoordination, slowness of both individual and repetitive movements and hypotonia of affected muscles appear to be the principal neuromuscular deficits associated with cerebellar damage that underlie ataxic dysarthria.

As noted above, movement-timing disorders account for the majority of the reported movement disorders following cerebellar damage. The major speech production timing deficit identified in cases of cerebellar disease has been increased durations for sentences, words, syllables and phonemes (Kent *et al.* 1979, 1997; Schonle *et al.* 1990; Ackermann and Hertrich 1994). Other speech timing deficits reported following cerebellar lesions include abnormal transitions from consonants to vowels, an inability to increase speech rate, reduced velocities and reduced speech movement acceleration (Kent and Netsell 1975; Ackermann *et al.* 1995; Kent *et al.* 1997). It would appear, however, that not all aspects of timing control are impaired in persons with cerebellar damage, with some individuals being able to preplan certain aspects of limb and utterance timing. For instance, some individuals with cerebellar damage have been observed to reduce initial limb movement and utterance segment duration as more segments are added to the movement, in a manner similar to normal controls (Kent *et al.* 1979; Bell-Barti and Chevrie-Muller 1991). In addition, not all speech durations are abnormally long in these patients, with voice onset time and tense vowel duration being reported to be less susceptible to lengthening (Kent and Netsall 1975; Kent *et al.* 1997). Further, recent evidence suggests that the timing dysregulation affects longer utterances in cerebellar pathology more than single word productions (Kent *et al.* 1997), suggesting that patients with cerebellar disorders are able to compensate for movement-timing disorders during production of single words.

In addition to its role in coordination of muscular activity, the cerebellum has also been shown to participate in motor learning (Sanes *et al.* 1990; Topka *et al.* 1993). The majority of evidence to support such a role in motor learning comes from simple motor learning paradigms, such as reflex adaptation and classical conditioning (Lisberger 1988), with both animals and humans with cerebellar lesions demonstrating deficits in the acquisition, learning and relearning of classically conditioned sensorimotor responses. A number of PET studies have also demonstrated cerebellar involvement during complex motor learning tasks, with normal controls demonstrating increased cerebellar metabolism during motor learning (Grafton *et al.* 1992; Jenkins and Frackowiak 1993). Interestingly, the cerebellum has also been shown to increase in activation during a verbal learning task (Raichle *et al.* 1994).

In that stuttering has been characterized as a disorder of temporal coordination of the sensorimotor and/or cognitive–linguistic processes involved in speech, De Nil *et al.* (2001) have recently questioned the role of the cerebellum in the genesis of articulatory disruptions seen in stuttered speech. Based on the findings of a PET investigation of cerebellar activation during single-word reading and verb generation in stuttering and nonstuttering adults, De Nil *et al.* (2001) concluded that there is a need to consider cerebellar processes in investigations of the neural bases of stuttering (see also Chapter 5, this volume).

Therefore, although the central contribution of the cerebellum to timing and coordination of sensorimotor actions is well established, and the link between cerebellar damage and the occurrence of ataxic dysarthria well recognized, the exact contribution of the cerebellum to speech motor control is not fully understood. In particular, the potential roles of the cerebellum in speech and oral learning and to the genesis of articulatory disturbances in stuttering has yet to be determined. As a further complication, based on the findings of a functional magnetic resonance imaging (fMRI) study, Wildgruber *et al.* (2001) confirmed a differential contribution of various cortical and subcortical structures, including the cerebellum and basal ganglia, to speech motor control, depending on syllable production rate. In particular, they found that cerebellar responses as determined by fMRI were primarily restricted to fast performance of silent repetitions. They suggested that, in order to further characterize the specific role of the various cortical and subcortical areas involved in speech, motor control production of different articulatory gestures at different frequencies and rhythm patterns must be evaluated via functional neuroimaging.

6.4 Subcortical structures in speech motor control: Evidence from neurosurgical studies

The rationale behind neurosurgical procedures used in the treatment of motor disturbances associated with Parkinson's disease lies in the findings of MPTP primate studies that increased basal ganglia output is a major pathophysiological step in the development of parkinsonian motor signs. Neurological procedures such as pallidotomy, involving thermo-lesioning of the GPi, and thalamotomy, involving thermo-ablation of the ventral intermedius (VIM) of the ventrolateral thalamus, therefore represent attempts to reduce basal ganglia output surgically. Although the feasibility of this approach was first demonstrated with lesions involving the STN in MPTP-treated primates (Wichmann *et al.* 1994), STN lesions in humans have been considered potentially hazardous because of the risk of development of persistent dyskinesias. Consequently, neurosurgical procedures for the treatment of Parkinson's disease in humans have involved primarily pallido-tomy and thalamotomy. More recently, non-destructive neurosurgical procedures involving implantation of deep-brain stimulators have been utilized to control basal ganglia output.

6.4.1 Pallidotomy, thalamotomy, and deep-brain stimulation

Although relatively common in the 1960s (Svennilson *et al.* 1960; Allan *et al.* 1966), at that time pallidotomy and thalamotomy were only supported by rela-tively primitive neuroradiological procedures to confirm the precise location of the lesion. Not unexpectedly, therefore, these techniques were associated with some complications. Subsequently, the introduction of L-dopa as an effective anti-kinetic treatment for Parkinson's disease in 1967 led to a major reduction in the use of pallidotomy and thalamotomy in the treatment of this condition. However, for a number of reasons, recent years have witnessed a renaissance in the neurosurgical treatment of movement disorders associated with Parkinson's disease. These include: enhanced understanding of basal ganglia circuitry, function, and patho-physiology, based largely on experiments conducted on the MPTP primate model; advances in neuroimaging and neurosurgical techniques, making lesion localiza-tion more accurate; a degree of disillusionment with drug treatment for movement disorders, with a large number of patients remaining disabled despite optimal medical therapy; and positive reports of clinical studies suggesting that neurosur-gical procedures are effective in improving a number of movement disorders, including akinesia, dyskinesia, dystonia, tremor and rigidity (Iacono *et al.* 1995; Kelly 1995).

For patients with Parkinson's disease, in whom tremor is the dominant feature, the VIM of the thalamus or its afferent projections is still the most commonly chosen surgical target. Thalamotomies have been shown to be particularly effective in patients with significant tremor, rigidity, or drug-induced dyskinesias, but they have not been shown to be effective in patients with akinesia or bradykinesia (Selby 1967). However, patients with tremor-dominant Parkinson's disease consti-tute a small minority. More common are patients with akinetic/rigid Parkinson's disease with fluctuating on/off periods. For this latter group of patients, the GPi is considered to be a more appropriate surgical target. Consequently, most neurosur-gical procedures involving lesions of the basal ganglia output structures have focused on reduction of the activity of the GPi by stereotactic lesioning. Pallidotomy has been shown to be effective against akinesia/bradykinesia, rigidity, and tremor, as well as dyskinesia/dystonia and motor fluctuations (Laitinen 1995; Baron *et al.* 1996). Other symptoms, such as postural disequilibrium, gait abnormalities, and freezing episodes, respond less well.

In recent years, an increased understanding of the pathophysiology of Parkinson's disease has led to the development of new approaches to the treatment of motor disturbance associated with this condition. These approaches include non-destructive neurosurgical techniques that involve the implantation of chronic, high-frequency stimulation devices into various deep-brain structures. Chronic electrical stimulation was first developed as a treatment for tremor, using stimulation of the VIM nucleus of the thalamus; however, this has since been applied to other deep-brain structures, including the GPi and, more recently, the STN.

High-frequency stimulation of the VIM has been observed to have the same effect in reducing parkinsonian tremor as thermo-ablation of the VIM (Hirai *et al.* 1983), with some authors recommending the implantation of high-frequency thalamic stimulators as the surgical procedure of choice for the treatment of tremor disorders. Stated advantages of thalamic stimulation over thermo-lesioning of the thalamus include its reversibility and the ability to perform bilateral operations without causing permanent dysarthria (Koller and Hristova 1996). Although the precise mechanism of action of implanted thalamic stimulators is unknown, neuronal jamming leading to deactivation of cyclic neuronal phenomena (Benabid *et al.* 1994) and decreased activity in the cerebellum (Dieber *et al.* 1993) have been proposed as possible mechanisms.

Stimulation of the GPi has been reported to reduce akinesia, rigidity, tremor and levodopa-induced dyskinesias (Gross *et al.* 1997) in a similar way to GPi ablation. Likewise, preliminary studies suggest that STN stimulation improves all of the cardinal features of Parkinson's disease, with the further suggestion that these improvements are superior to those achieved with pallidal stimulation (Limousin *et al.* 1997; Krack *et al.* 1998). It is suggested that these positive effects are the outcome of the electrical stimulation of the STN counteracting the inhibitory effects on the thalamus arising from the globus pallidus, thereby increasing thalamocortical activation (Limousin *et al.* 1995). The reduction in bradykinesia and tremor associated with stimulation of the GPi has been shown to be paralleled by increased activity (as measured by PET as increased regional blood flow) in the medial frontal cortex anterior to the supplementary motor area (Grafton and DeLong 1997). These findings suggest that electrical stimulation alters inhibitory GPi output, resulting in increased activity in brain areas controlling movement, in a manner analogous to surgical ablation.

6.4.2 Effect of pallidotomy, thalamotomy, and deep-brain stimulation on speech

Although the beneficial effects of pallidotomy, thalamotomy and deep-brain stimulation on general motor function in patients with Parkinson's disease have been well documented (Hirai *et al.* 1983; Dieber *et al.* 1993; Benabid *et al.* 1994; Iacono *et al.* 1995; Kelly 1995; Limousin *et al.* 1995), specific clinical evaluation of the effects of these surgical procedures on speech motor function has been limited. Of the studies that have reported the effects of pallidotomy, thalamotomy, and deep-brain stimulation on speech, the majority of the data collected has been subjective, unsophisticated and perceptually based. Further, the results of those studies that have investigated the effects of these procedures on speech are equivocal, with some studies reporting improvements in speech and/or voice (Iacono *et al.* 1995; Legg and Sonnenberg 1998) and others reporting either no changes or a worsening of speech (Scott *et al.* 1998; Schneider *et al.* 1999) after procedures such as pallidotomy.

Iacono *et al.* (1995) investigated the effects of pallidotomy on speech production in a group of 62 patients with Parkinson's disease who underwent posteroventral pallidotomy. Based on one question taken from the Unified Parkinson's Disease Rating Scale (UPDRS) conducted pre- and post-surgery, they noted a decline in the severity of the speech impairment experienced by the patients post-surgery. However, although significant improvements in speech were reported in the total group performance, the subjects continued to exhibit residual speech deficits post-surgery. Although these findings suggest that pallidotomy has a positive effect on speech production in patients with Parkinson's disease, they provide very little information regarding the specific improvements observed post-surgery. Indeed, Iacono *et al.* (1995) did not evaluate the speech abilities of their subjects using a comprehensive perceptual and/or physiological assessment battery, and consequently were unable to provide specific information as to the characteristics of the speech disorder remaining post-operatively. In contrast to the findings of Iacono *et al.* (1995), a number of other studies have reported a lack of improvement in speech abilities post-pallidotomy, as measured by the UPDRS (Richards *et al.* 1994; Johannson *et al.* 1997; Barlow *et al.* 1998). These equivocal findings may, at least in part, be due to poor inter-rater reliability of the UPDRS (Scott *et al.* 1998).

Scott *et al.* (1998) used a more specific measure of speech function to investigate the effects of pallidotomy on the speech abilities of 20 post-pallidotomy patients with Parkinson's disease. Specifically, changes in the motor speech abilities were evaluated by the number of correct pronunciations of 'mama', 'papa', 'thanks', 'pitter-patter' and 'pataka' in 5 seconds, with eight subjects exhibiting reduced articulation rates following bilateral pallidotomy. Although unable to specify the quality or aetiology of these changes, the authors reinforced the need for more detailed and specialized investigation of the motor speech mechanism post-pallidotomy.

The Frenchay Dysarthria Assessment (FDA) was used by Legg and Sonnenburg (1998) to demonstrate improved speech abilities in a single case post-pallidotomy. In particular, the subject exhibited increased laryngeal modulation (evident in fewer audible pitch breaks), improved intonation, loudness and tongue function post-operatively. However, involuntary movements and asymmetrical distortions of lips and jaw remained unchanged, and although overall speech was improved, the subject remained dysarthric. The speech changes observed in this case were attributed to relief of tremor in the thoracic regions of the body.

To date, only three studies reported in the literature, involving very small numbers of subjects, have used objective physiological or acoustic measures to evaluate the effects of neurosurgical treatment for Parkinson's disease on motor speech function (Barlow *et al.* 1998; Shulz *et al.* 1999; Theodoros *et al.* 2000). Barlow *et al.* (1998) investigated perioral force and control and laryngeal aerodynamics immediately before and 48–144 hours post-pallidotomy in 11 subjects with Parkinson's disease. They reported a significant reduction in laryngeal airway resistance post-pallidotomy, while mean vocalic airflows were observed to increase to within normal limits. Other speech changes following pallidotomy included more consistent syllable production rates, reduced voice onset variability, and improved force control of the perioral apparatus. However, a number of factors relating to the design of the study reported by Barlow *et al.* (1998) are the source of some concern. It is generally thought that assessment of motor function should occur when the neurological system is stable. Acutely, the lesion itself causes a core of neuronal death surrounded by an area of damaged cells (Samuels *et al.* 1998). Additionally, perilesional oedema may become evident from 36 h onwards and may last up to 3–4 weeks post-operatively. The early effects of surgery observed by Barlow *et al.* (1998) may, therefore, be a result of sublethal neuronal perilesional damage and, due to the effects of oedema, an assessment carried out in the acute stage post-surgery may provide an inaccurate indication of the long-term effects of pallidotomy on speech production.

In a preliminary study conducted in the author's own laboratory, involving a perceptual and physiological analysis of the effects of pallidotomy on motor speech function in persons with Parkinson's disease, a group of 12 subjects was found to have a significant reduction in speech intelligibility post-pallidotomy compared to pre-pallidotomy (Theodoros *et al.* 2000). Physiological analysis of a subgroup of four subjects, using a range of assessment techniques covering respiratory, laryngeal, velopharyngeal and articulatory function, revealed that physiological changes in motor speech function following pallidotomy were either negative or non-existent in the majority of speech subsystems, with improvements in function noted in only few components of the speech production mechanism (Theodoros *et al.* 2000). Intersubject variability was apparent across the four cases, even in those subjects who were closely matched for age, stage of disease, and surgical procedure. Intrasubject variability was present in the form of differential subsystem impairment/improvement with respect to the specific subsystem affected and type of change that occurred. It was suggested that the observed negative effects of pallidotomy on motor speech function may be related to impaired muscle force generation (Barlow *et al.* 1998) and movement preparation/motor set associated with lesioning of the motor circuit, the GPi (Alexander *et al.* 1990) and/or to lesioning of specific neuronal fibres in the adjacent internal capsule. The positive effects demonstrated post-pallidotomy may be associated with improvements in general motor function, resulting in more stable postural and speech musculature (Barlow *et al.* 1998; Theodoros *et al.* 2000).

Acoustic analysis of specific speech and voice parameters in six patients with Parkinson's disease following unilateral pallidotomy identified considerable variability amongst the subjects with respect to measures of phonation and articulation (Schulz *et al.* 1999). Four of the six patients were reported to demonstrate positive changes post-pallidotomy in either phonatory or both phonatory and articulatory measures, with some subjects showing greater intensity, more syllables per second and longer extended vowel duration post-surgery (Schulz *et al.* 1999).

As in the case of pallidotomy, few studies have documented the effects of thalamotomy on speech motor function. The few perceptual studies that have been reported suggest that in most instances thalamotomy has deleterious effects on speech. Tasker *et al.* (1983) reported that speech deteriorates post-operatively after VIM thalamotomy. In addition, operations involving the thalamus in the dominant hemisphere have been observed to be more likely to produce speech disturbances than equivalent neurosurgical procedures involving the non-dominant thalamus, including dysarthria, monotonous voice, slow speech (Jenkins 1968), and decreased loudness and articulation difficulties (Quaglieri and Celesia 1977). Aspects of speech production, including initiation of speech, maintenance and control of speech, fluency and vocal loudness, have been reported to be disturbed in VIM thalamotomy involving either hemisphere (Petrovici 1980). Diminished loudness, dysarthria and dysphasia have been reported to be disturbed in VIM thalamotomy involving either hemisphere (Petrovici 1980). Diminished loudness, dysarthria and dysphasia have been observed subsequent to lesioning of the ventral lateral thalamus (Bell 1968).

Although chronic high-frequency unilateral thalamic stimulation is effective in reducing both essential and parkinsonian tremor (Koller *et al.* 1997), the effect of stimulation of the thalamus on speech remains uncertain. Stimulation of the thalamus has been reported to produce silencing and slowing of speech (Schaltenbrand 1975), while stimulation of the left ventrolateral thalamus causes alterations in object naming in the form of agnosia, perseveration, and anomia (Ojemann and Ward 1971). Several studies have recently reported the effects of thalamic stimulation for essential tremor on speech (Carpenter *et al.* 1998; Pahwa *et al.* 1999; Taha *et al.* 1999). Carpenter *et al.* (1998) reported that VIM stimulation that successfully controls hand tremor can also reduce the severity of vocal tremor, but with a less dramatic effect on the voice. Pahwa *et al.* (1999) noted that the speech deficits exhibited by some patients who become dysarthric following bilateral thalamic stimulation can often be ameliorated by adjusting stimulator settings, although this also frequently reduces the control of the tremor. In a study of 23 patients with thalamic stimulation, Taha *et al.* (1999) reported their perception that vocal tremor improved; however, no objective speech data were provided.

As yet, little is known of the effect of STN stimulation on speech. Dromey *et al.* (2000) examined the vocal performance of seven patients with Parkinson's disease fitted with deep-brain stimulators to provide chronic electrical stimulation to the subthalamic nucleus bilaterally. Although significant improvements in limb motor performance in response to medication before surgery and when the STN was stimulated after surgery were noted, only small, but statistically significant, increases in sound pressure level and fundamental frequency variability were reported in response to stimulation in the medication on condition, with no other significant speech changes being observed. These authors concluded that their findings are consistent with other studies that have reported a disparity between limb and speech movements after neurosurgical intervention for Parkinson's disease. Gentil *et al.* (1999*a*) reported improvements in UPDRS speech scores with STN stimulation, but did not report any instrumental speech data. These latter authors also reported improvements in lip and tongue force regulation in non-speech tasks. In a similar study, Gentil *et al.* (1999*h*) observed that the bilateral STN stimulation improved oral control and speech intelligibility in a single patient with Parkinson's disease, in contrast to L-dopa therapy, which showed a poor effect.

In summary, although the beneficial effects of neurosurgical treatments for Parkinson's disease and other basal ganglia disorders on various aspects of general motor function are well documented, the effects of lesions induced by these proce-dures on the control of the speech musculature remains largely unknown. As a consequence, the potential of procedures such as pallidotomy, thalamotomy, and deep-brain stimulation to yield new information regarding the role of specific subcortical structures in speech motor control has yet to be fully realized. However, based on the preliminary evidence available to date, it would appear that proce-dures such as pallidotomy do not always have the positive effects on speech production as seen in the muscles in other parts of the body, such as the limbs. To the contrary, in many instances speech intelligibility has been noted to decline post-pallidotomy. This difference may, at least in part, be an outcome of the segre-gated nature of the neuronal circuits that connect the cerebral cortex, basal ganglia, and thalamus, with specific independent circuits subserving specific anatomical structures, such as the oro-facial structures versus the limb muscles (Alexander *et al.* 1990). Therefore, small inconsistencies in the site and volume of the lesions induced by sterotactic neurosurgery could variably affect the function-ing of the skeletal muscles in different regions of the body, consistent with the case-to-case variability noted by several authors in their neurosurgical subjects. Another possible reason for the observed disparity between limb musculature and speech musculature is that subcortical modulation of the speech-production muscles involves primarily non-dopaminergic subcortical pathways (Agid 1998). Among these are neuronal systems originating in subcortical areas, such as the cholinergic, serotoninergic, and noradrenergic systems. This suggestion is based on the observation that although treatment of Parkinson's disease with levodopa results in improvements in symptoms such as bradykinesia, rigidity, and tremor, which arise from degeneration of the nigrostriatal system (Bonnet *et al.* 1987), other symptoms, such as abnormal gait/postural instability, dysarthria and cognitive impairment, considered to be produced by non-dopaminergic lesions, do not (Agid 1998). This hypothesis is supported by the knowledge that the effects of levodopa therapy on speech production is less effective than on limb function in patients with Parkinson's disease (Wolfe *et al.* 1975; Kompoliti *et al.* 2000). Kompoliti *et al.* (2000) examined the effect of central dopaminergic stimulation with apomorphine on speech in individuals with Parkinson's disease and reported that no index of laryngeal or articulatory function improved significantly after apomorphine stimulation. They concluded that laryngeal function and articulation are not under predominant dopaminergic control in Parkinson's disease, leading them to suggest that treatment for dysarthria in Parkinson's disease should focus on non-dopaminergic pharmacology and other therapies. Bonnet *et al.* (1987) suggested that aggravation of Parkinson's disease following chronic levodopa therapy (e.g. increased involuntary abnormal movements, gait disorders, and dysarthria) mainly results from increasing severity of cerebral non-dopaminergic lesions. Further research, involving the investigation of larger numbers of neurosurgical cases using a range of quantifiable physiological and acoustic assessments, is required if we are to achieve a greater understanding of the role of various subcortical structures in motor speech control.

Although the dysarthria associated with Parkinson's disease shows little or no improvement in response to dopamine replacement therapy, or indeed to standard speech pathology techniques, the short- and long-term efficacy of a behavioral intervention known as the Lee Silverman Voice Treatment (LSVT) has been documented (Ramig *et al.* 1995). The LSVT aims to rescale the magnitude of speech-motor output through sustained phonation, increased loudness, and continuous feedback on performance. Based on a PET study of three patients with Parkinson's disease, Liotti *et al.* (1999) reported that treatment with the LSVT was followed by functional reorganization of the speech-motor areas of the brain. Specifically, the LSVT was reported to reduce baseline GP overactivity at rest but, at the same time, increase GP activity during sustained vocalization. Liotti *et al.* (1999) suggested that the increased GP activity post-LVST may represent a 'normalization' of pretreatment abnormality. Although the findings of Liotti *et al.* (1999) can only be regarded as preliminary until confirmed by investigations based on larger subject numbers, they do provide evidence to suggest that further investigations of the effects of behavioral intervention, such as the LSVT, on brain reorganization are warranted. In particular, their findings indicate that investigations of this type, using functional imaging techniques, have the potential to further elucidate the role of subcortical structures in normal and abnormal speech motor control.

6.5 Summary

Although it has long been recognized that brain lesions involving subcortical structures may disrupt speech production, the precise role of subcortical structures such as the basal ganglia, thalamus, and cerebellum in speech motor control remains elusive. To determine the basis of subcortical motor disorders, in recent years a number of theoretical models have been developed in an attempt to explain the roles of subcortical structures such as the basal ganglia, thalamus, and cerebellum in speech motor control. Central to the development of these theoretical models has been experimentation based primarily on MPTP-treated primate models and functional neuroimaging studies, which has led to a greater understanding of the basal ganglia–thalamocortical circuitry and cerebello-thalamocortical circuits, which are now recognized as being comprised of a series of parallel, multi-segregated circuits or 'loops'. Models developed that have incorporated this new knowledge of the neuroanatomy of the subcortical circuitry include those aimed at explaining the development of both hypo-, hyperkinetic, and ataxic movement disorders subsequent to basal ganglia pathology and cerebellar pathology. In recent years, renewed interest in the use of stereotactic neurosurgical procedures and deep-brain stimulation in the treatment of Parkinson's disease and other basal ganglia disorders has provided the potential for examining the effects of discrete circumscribed lesions in the globus pallidus and thalamus, and electrical stimulation of the STN and thalamus, on motor speech function. The preliminary data from this line of research suggest that the use of these techniques, combined with functional neuroimaging based on PET and fMRI, has the potential to further inform debate regarding the hypothesized roles of subcortical structures in speech motor control. In particular, when combined with functional neuroimaging such as PET and fMRI, deep-brain stimulation has the potential to be a powerful technique for assessing the effect of discrete perturbations at different nodes of the basal ganglia-thalamocortical and cerebello-thalamocortical circuits (including the substantia nigra, GP, putamen, caudate nucleus, thalamus, subthalamic nucleus, and cerebellum). Utilization of such a combined approach would enable testing of contemporary models of subcortical functional organization through comparison of expected responses predicted by the models with specific changes in brain activity as identified by the functional neuroimaging. Such comparisons, based on a range of task-specific speech production activities, would enable further determination of the differential contributions of various subcortical structures to speech motor control.

References

Ackermann, H. and **Hertrich, I.** (1994). Speech rate and rhythm in cerebellar dysarthria: An acoustic analysis of syllabic timing. *Folia Phoniatrica*, **46**, 70–78.

Ackermann, H. and **Hertrich, I.** (2000). The contribution of the cerebellum to speech processing. *Journal of Neurolinguistics,* **13**, 95–116.

Ackermann, H. and **Ziegler, W.** (1992). Cerebellar dysarthria: A review. *Fortsch Neurology Psychiatry,* **60**, 28–40.

Ackermann, H., Vogel, M., Petersen, D. and **Poremba, M.** (1992). Speech deficits in ischaemic cerebellar lesions. *Journal of Neurology,* **239**, 223–227.

Ackermann, H., Hertrich, I. and **Scharf, G.** (1995). Kinematic analysis of lower lip movements in ataxic dysarthria. *Journal of Speech and Hearing Research,* **38**, 1252–1259.

Agid, Y. (1998). Levodopa: is toxicology a myth? *Neurology,* **50**, 858–863.

Alexander, G.E., DeLong, M.R. and **Strick, P.L.** (1986). Parallel organization of functionally segregated circuits linking basal ganglia and cortex. *Annual Review of Neuroscience,* **9**, 357–381.

Alexander, G.E., Crutcher, M.D. and **DeLong, M.R.** (1990). Basal ganglia–thalamocortical circuits: Parallel substrates for motor, oculomotor, prefrontal and limbic functions. In HBM Uylings, CG Van Eden, JPC De Bruin, MA Corner and MGP Feenstra, eds. *Progress in brain research,* Vol 85, pp. 119–146. Elsevier Science Publishers, The Netherlands.

Allan, C.M., Turner, J.W. and **Gadea-Ciria, M.** (1966). Investigations into speech disturbance following stereotaxic surgery for Parkinsonism. *British Journal of Disorders of Communication,* **1**, 55–59.

Barlow, S.H., Iacono, R.P., Paseman, L.A., Biswas, A. and **D'Antonio, L.** (1998). The effects of posteroventral pallidotomy on force and speech aerodynamics in Parkinson's disease. In MP Cannito, CM Yorkston and DR Beukelman, eds. *Neuromotor speech disorders: Nature, assessment and management,* pp. 117–155. Paul Brookes Publishing Co., Baltimore.

Baron, M.S., Jerrold, L., Vitek, J., Roy, A.E., Bakay, R. and **Green, J.** (1996). Treatment of advanced Parkinson's disease by GPi pallidotomy: 1 year pilot study results. *Annals of Neurology,* **40**, 355–366.

Bathia, K.P. and **Marsden, C.D.** (1994). The behavioural and motor consequences of focal lesions of the basal ganglia in man. *Brain,* **117**, 859–876.

Bell, D.S. (1968). Speech functions of the thalamus inferred from the effects of thalamotomy. *Brain,* **91**, 619–638.

Bell-Barti, F. and **Chevrie-Muller, C.** (1991). Motor levels of speech timing: Evidence from studies of ataxia. *Haskins Laboratories Status Report on Speech Research,* SR-107/108, 87–92.

Benabid, A.L., Pollak, P., Gross, C. *et al.* (1994). Acute and long-term effects of subthalamic nucleus stimulation in Parkinson's disease. *Stereotactic Functional Neurosurgery,* **62**, 76–84.

Bonnet, A.M., Loria, Y., Saint-Hilaire, M.H., Lhermitte, F. and **Agid, Y.** (1987). Does long-term aggravation of Parkinson's disease result from non-dopaminergic lesions. *Neurology,* **37**, 1539–1542.

Brooks, D.J. (1991). Detection of preclinical Parkinson's disease with PET. *Neurology*, **41** (suppl. 2), 24.

Calne, D. and **Snow, B.J.** (1993). PET imaging in Parkinsonism. *Advances in Neurology*, **60**, 484.

Carpenter, M.A., Pahwa, R., Miyawaki, K.L., Wilkinson, S.B., Searl, J.P. and **Koller, W.C.** (1998). Reduction in voice tremor under thalamic stimulation. *Neurology*, **50**, 796–798.

Chenery, H.J., Murdoch, B.E. and **Ingram, J.C.L.** (1988). Studies in Parkinson's disease: 1. Perceptual speech analysis. *Australian Journal of Human Communication Disorders*, **16**, 17–29.

Darley, F.L., Aronson, A.E. and **Brown, J.R.** (1969*a*). Differential diagnostic patterns of dysarthria. *Journal of Speech and Hearing Research*, **12**, 246–269.

Darley, F.L., Aronson, A.E. and **Brown, J.R.** (1969*b*). Clusters of deviant speech dimensions in the dysarthrias. *Journal of Speech and Hearing Research*, **12**, 462–496.

Darley, F.L., Aronson, A.E. and **Brown, J.R.** (1975). *Motor speech disorders*. W.B. Saunders, Philadelphia.

DeLong, M.R. (1990). Primate models of movement disorders of basal ganglia origin. *TINS*, **13**, 281–285.

DeNil, L.F., Kroll, R.M. and **Houle, S.** (2001). Functional neuroimaging of cerebellar activation during single word reading and verb generation in stuttering and nonstuttering adults. *Neuroscience Letters*, **302**, 77–80.

Dieber, M.P., Pollak, P. and **Passingham, R.** (1993). Thalamic stimulation and suppression of parkinsonian tremor: Evidence of cerebellar deactivation using position emission tomography. *Brain*, **116**, 267–279.

Dromey, C., Kumar, R., Lang, A.E. and **Lozano, A.M.** (2000). An investigation of the effects of subthalamic nucleus stimulation on acoustic measures of voice. *Movement Disorders*, **15**, 1132–1138.

Eidelberg, D. (1992). Positron emission tomography studies in Parkinsonism. *Neurology Clinics*, **10**, 421.

Filion, M. and **Tremblay, L.** (1991). Abnormal spontaneous activity of globus pallidus neurons in monkeys with MPTP-induced Parkinsonism. *Brain Research*, **547**, 142.

Filion, M., Tremblay, L. and **Bedard, P.J.** (1988). Abnormal influences of passive limb movement on the activity of globus pallidus neurons in parkinsonian monkeys. *Brain Research*, **444**, 165.

Forrest, K. and **Weismer, G.** (1995). Dynamic aspects of lower lip movement in parkinsonian and neurologically normal geriatric speakers' production of stress. *Journal of Speech and Hearing Research*, **38**, 260–272.

Gentil, M., Garcia-Ruiz, P., Pollak, P. and **Benabid, A.L.** (1999*a*). Effects of stimulation of the subthalamic nucleus on oral control of patients with parkinsonism. *Journal of Neurology, Neurosurgery and Psychiatry*, **67**, 329–333.

Gentil, M., Tournier, C.L., Pollak, P. and **Benabid, A.L.** (1999*b*). Effect of bilateral subthalamic nucleus stimulation and dopatherapy on oral control in Parkinson's disease. *European Neurology*, **42**, 136–140.

Gerfen, C.R. (1995). Dopamine receptor function in the basal ganglia. *Clinical Neuropharmacology*, **18**, S162.

Grafton, S.T. and **DeLong, M.** (1997). Tracing the brain's circuitry with functional imaging. *Nature Medicine*, **3**, 602–603.

Grafton, S.T., Mazziotta, J.C., Presty, S., Friston, K.J., Frackowiak, R.S. and **Phelps, M.E.** (1992). Functional anatomy of human procedural learning determined with regional cerebral blood flow and PET. *Journal of Neuroscience*, **12**, 2542–2548.

Graybiel, A.M. and **Kimura, M.** (1995). Adaptive neural networks in the basal ganglia. In JD Houk, JL Davis and DG Beiser, eds. *Models of information processing in the basal ganglia*, pp. 103–116. MIT Press, Cambridge MA.

Gross, C., Rougier, A., Guehl, D., Boraud, T., Julien, J. and **Bioulac, B.** (1997). High-frequency stimulation of the globus pallidus internalis in Parkinson's disease: A study of seven cases. *Journal of Neurosurgery*, **87**, 491–498.

Hallett, M., Berardelli, A., Matheson, J., Rothwell, J. and **Marsden, C.D.** (1991). Physiological analysis of simple rapid movements in patients with cerebellar deficits. *Journal of Neurology, Neurosurgery and Psychiatry*, **53**, 124–133.

Hirai, T., Miyazaki, M., Nakajima, H., Shibazaki, T. and **Ohye, C.** (1983). The correlation between tremor characteristics and the predicted volume of effective lesions in the stereotaxic nucleus ventralis intermedius thalamotomy. *Brain*, **106**, 1001–1018.

Hunker, C.J. and **Abbs, J.H.** (1984). Physiological analyses of parkinsonian tremors in the orofacial system. In MR McNeil, JC Rosenbek and AE Aronson, eds. *The dysarthrias: Physiology, acoustics, perception, management*, pp. 69–100. College-Hill Press, San Diego CA.

Iacono, R.P., Shima, F., Lonser, R., Kuniyoshi, S., Maeda, G. and **Yamada, S.** (1995). The results, indications and physiology of posteroventral pallidotomy for patients with Parkinson's disease. *Neurosurgery*, **36**, 1118–1124.

Jenkins, A.C. (1968). Speech defects following stereotaxic operations for the relief of tremor and rigidity in Parkinsonism. *The Medical Journal of Australia*, **7**, 585–588.

Jenkins, I.H. and **Frackowiak, R.S.** (1993). Functional studies in human cerebellum with positron emission tomography. *Review Neurology Paris*, **149**, 647–653.

Johannson, F., Malm, J., Nordh, E. and **Hariz, M.** (1997). Usefulness of pallidotomy for advanced Parkinson's disease. *Journal of Neurology, Neurosurgery and Psychiatry*, **62**, 125–132.

Kelly, P. (1995). Pallidotomy in Parkinson's disease. *Neurosurgery*, **36**, 1154–1157.

Kent, R.D. and **Netsell, R.** (1975). A case study of an ataxic dysarthric: Cineradiographic and spectrographic observations. *Journal of Speech and Hearing Disorders*, **40**, 115–134.

Kent, R.D., Netsell, R. and **Abbs, J.** (1979). Acoustic characteristics of dysarthria associated with cerebellar disease. *Journal of Speech and Hearing Research,* **22**, 627–648.

Kent, R.D., Kent, J.F., Rosenbek, J.C., Vorperian, H.K. and **Weismer, G.** (1997). A speaking task analysis of the dysarthria in cerebellar disease. *Folia Phoniatrica and Logopedica,* **49**, 63–82.

Koller, W. and **Hristova, A.** (1996). Efficacy and safety of stereotaxic surgical treatment of tremor disorders. *European Journal of Neurology,* **3**, 507–514.

Koller, W., Pahwa, R., Busenbark, K., Hubble, S., Wilkinson, S.B. and **Lang, A.E.** (1997). High frequency unilateral thalamic stimulation in the treatment of essential and parkinsonian tremor. *Annals of Neurology,* **42**, 292–299.

Kompoliti, K., Wang, Q.E., Goetz, C.F., Leurgans, S. and **Raman, R.** (2000). Effects of central dopaminergic stimulation by apomorphine on speech in Parkinson's disease. *Neurology,* **54**, 458–462.

Krack, P., Pollak, P. and **Limousin, P.** (1998). Subthalamic nucleus or internal pallidal stimulation in young-onset Parkinson's disease. *Brain,* **121**, 451–457.

LaBlance, G.R. and **Rutherford, D.R.** (1991). Respiratory dynamics and speech intelligibility in speakers with generalized dystonia. *Journal of Communication Disorders,* **24**, 141–156.

Laitinen, L.V. (1995). Pallidotomy for Parkinson's disease. *Neurosurgery Clinics North America,* **6**, 105.

Lang A.E., Lozano, A.M. Montgomery, E., Duffy, J., Tasker, R. and **Hutchinson, W.** (1998). Posteroventral medial pallidotomy in advanced Parkinson's disease. *New England Journal of Medicine,* **338**, 262–263.

Lechtenberg, R. and **Gilman, S.** (1978). Speech disorders in cerebellar disease. *Annals of Neurology,* **3**, 285–290.

Leenders, K.L. (1997). Pathophysiology of movement disorders studied using PET. *Journal of Neural Transmission,* (suppl. 50), 39.

Legg, C.F. and **Sonnenberg, B.R.** (1998). Changes in aspects of speech and language functioning following unilateral pallidotomy. *Aphasiology,* **12**, 257–266.

Leiner, H.C., Leiner, A.L. and **Dow, R.S.** (1993). Cognitive and language functions in the human cerebellum. *Trends in Neuroscience,* **16**, 444–447.

Limousin, P., Greene, J., Pollak, P., Rothwell, J., Benabid, A.L. and **Frackowiak, R.** (1997). Changes in cerebral activity pattern due to subthalamic nucleus or internal pallidum stimulation in Parkinson's disease. *Annals of Neurology,* **42**, 283–291.

Limousin, P., Pollack, P., Benazzouz, A. *et al.* (1995). Effect of parkinsonian signs and symptoms of bilateral subthalamic nucleus stimulation. *The Lancet,* **345**, 91–95.

Liotti, M., Vogel, D., New, P., Ramig, L., Mayberg, H.S., Cook, C.I. and **Fox, P.T.** (1999). A PET study of functional reorganization of premotor regions in Parkinson's disease following intensive speech and voice treatment (LSVT). *Neurology,* **52** (suppl. 2), 4.

Lisberger, S.G. (1988). The neural basis for learning of simple motor skills. *Science*, **242**, 728–735.

Middleton, F.A. and **Strick, P.L.** (1997). Dentate output channels: motor and cognitive components. *Progress in Brain Research*, **114**, 555–568.

Middleton, F.A. and **Strick, P.L.** (2000). Basal ganglia output and cognition: Evidence from anatomical, behavioural and clinical studies. *Brain and Cognition*, **42**, 183–200.

Middleton, F.A. and **Strick, P.L.** (2001). Cerebellar projections to the prefrontal cortex of the primate. *The Journal of Neuroscience*, **21**, 700–712.

Miller, W.C. and **DeLong, M.R.** (1987). Altered tonic activity of neurons in the globus pallidus and subthalamic nucleus in the primate MPTP model of parkinsonism. In MB Carpenter and A Jayaraman, eds. *The basal ganglia II*, p. 415. Plenum, New York.

Murdoch, B.E. (1990). *Acquired speech and language disorders: A neuroanatomical and functional neurological approach*. Chapman and Hall, London.

Murdoch, B.E. (1998). *Dysarthria: A physiological approach to assessment and treatment*. Stanley Thornes Publishers, Cheltenham, UK.

Murdoch, B.E. and **Theodoros, D.G.** (1998). Ataxic dysarthria. In BE Murdoch, ed. *Dysarthria: A physiological approach to assessment and treatment*, pp. 242–265. Stanley Thornes Publishers, Cheltenham, UK.

Murdoch, B.E., Chenery, H.J., Bowler, S. and **Ingram, J.C.L.** (1989). Respiratory function in Parkinson's subjects exhibiting a perceptible speech deficit: A kinematic and spirometric analysis. *Journal of Speech and Hearing Disorders*, **54**, 610–626.

Ojemann, G.A. and **Ward, A.A.** (1971). Speech representation in ventrolateral thalamus. *Brain*, **94**, 669–680.

Pahwa, R., Lyons, K. and **Wilkinson, S.B.** (1999). Bilateral thalamic stimulation for the treatment of essential tremor. *Neurology*, **53**, 1147–1450.

Parent, A., Lévesque, M. and **Parent, M.** (2001). A re-evaluation of the current model of the basal ganglia. *Parkinsonism and Related Disorders*, **7**, 193–198.

Petrovici, J.N. (1980). Speech disturbances following stereotaxic surgery in ventrolateral thalamus. *Neurosurgical Review*, **3**, 189–195.

Quaglieri, C.E. and **Celesia, G.G.** (1977). Effects of thalamotomy and levadopa therapy on the speech of Parkinson patients. *European Neurology*, **15**, 34–39.

Raichle, M.E., Fiez, J.A., Videen, T.O. *et al.* (1994). Practice-related changes in human brain functional anatomy during nonmotor learning. *Cerebral Cortex*, **4**, 8–26.

Ramig, L.O., Countryman, S., Thompson, L.L. and **Harii, Y.** (1995). A comparison of two forms of intensive speech treatment for Parkinson's disease. *Journal of Speech and Hearing Research*, **38**, 1232–1251.

Richards, M., Marder, K., Cote, L. and **Mayeux, R.** (1994). Interrater reliability of the Unified Parkinson's Disease Rating Scale motor examination. *Movement Disorders*, **9**, 89–91.

Samuels, M., Caputo, E., Brooks, D.J., *et al.* (1998). A study of medial pallidotomy for Parkinson's disease: Clinical outcome, MRI location and complications. *Brain,* **121**, 59–75.

Sanes, J.N., Dimitrov, B. and **Hallett, M.** (1990). Motor learning in patients with cerebellar dysfunction. *Brain,* **113**, 103–120.

Schaltenbrand, G. (1975). The effects on speech and language of stereotactical stimulation in thalamus and corpus callosum. *Brain and Language,* **2**, 70–77.

Schmahmann, J.D. (2001). The cerebrocerebellar system: Anatomic substrates of the cerebellar contribution to cognition and emotion. *International Review of Psychiatry,* **13**, 247–260.

Schneider, S.L., Duffy, J.R. and **Uitti, R.J.** (1999). Motor speech changes following pallidotomy in patients with Parkinson's disease. Paper presented at the American-Speech-Language-Hearing Association Annual Convention, San Francisco.

Schonle, P.W., Dressler, D. and **Conrad, B.** (1990). Orofacial movement impairments in cerebellar dysarthria: A kinematic analysis with electromagnetic articulography. In A Beradelli, R Benecke, M Manfredi and CD Marsden, eds. *Motor disturbances II,* pp. 249–259. Academic Press, New York.

Schulz, G.M., Peterson, T., Sapienza, C.M., Greer, M. and **Friedman, W.** (1999). Voice and speech characteristics of persons with Parkinson's disease pre- and post-pallidotomy surgery: Preliminary findings. *Journal of Speech, Language and Hearing Research,* **42**, 1176–1194.

Scott, R., Gregory, R., Hines, N. *et al.* (1998). Neuropsychological, neurological and functional outcome following pallidotomy for Parkinson's disease: A consecutive series of eight simultaneous bilateral and twelve unilateral procedures. *Brain,* **121**, 659–675.

Selby, G. (1967). Stereotactic surgery for the relief of Parkinson's disease. 1. A critical review. *Journal of Neurological Science,* **5**, 315.

Solomon, N.P. and **Hixon, T.J.** (1993). Speech breathing in Parkinson's disease. *Journal of Speech and Hearing Research,* **36**, 294–310.

Strick, P.L., Dunn, R.P. and **Picard, N.** (1995). Macro-organization of the circuits connecting the basal ganglia with the cortical motor areas. In JC Houk, JL Davis and DG Beiser, eds. *Models of information processing in the basal ganglia,* pp. 117–130. MIT Press, Cambridge, MA.

Svennilson, E., Torvik, A. and **Lowe, R.** (1960). Treatment of Parkinsonism by stereotactic thermolesions in the pallidal region. *Acta Psychiatry Neurology Sandinavia,* **35**, 358–377.

Taha, J.M., Janszen, M.A. and **Favre, J.** (1999). Thalamic deep brain stimulation for the treatment of head, voice and bilateral limb tremor. *Journal of Neurosurgery,* **91**, 68–72.

Tasker, R.R., Siqueira, J. and **Hawrylyshyn, L.W.O.** (1983). What happened to VIM thalamotomy for Parkinson's disease? *Applied Neurophysiology,* **46**, 68–83.

Theodoros, D.G. and Murdoch, B.E. (1998*a*). Hypokinetic dysarthria. In BE Murdoch, ed. *Dysarthria: A physiological approach to assessment and treatment*, pp. 266–313. Stanley Thornes Publishers, Cheltenham, UK.

Theodoros, D.G. and Murdoch, B.E. (1998*b*). Hyperkinetic dysarthria. In BE Murdoch, ed. *Dysarthria: A physiological approach to assessment and treatment*, pp. 314–336. Stanley Thornes Publishers, Cheltenham, UK.

Theodoros, D.G., Ward, E.C., Murdoch, B.E., Silburn, P. and Lethlean, J. (2000). Impact of pallidotomy on motor speech function in Parkinson's disease: Preliminary perceptual and physiological findings. *Journal of Medical Speech-Language Pathology*, **8**, 315–322.

Topka, H., Valls-Sole, J., Massaquoi, S.G. and Hallett, M. (1993). Deficits in classical conditioning in patients with cerebellar degeneration. *Brain*, **116**, 961–969.

Wichmann, T., Bergman, H. and DeLong, M.R. (1994). The primate subthalamic nucleus. 1. Functional properties in intact animals. *Journal of Neurophysiology*, **72**, 494.

Wildgruber, D., Ackermann, H. and Grodd, W. (2001). Differential contributions of motor cortex, basal ganglia and cerebellum to speech motor control: Effects of syllable repetition rate evaluated by fMRI. *Neuroimage*, **13**, 101–109.

Wolfe, V.I., Garvin, J.S., Bacon, M. and Waldrop, W. (1975). Speech changes in Parkinson's disease during treatment with L-dopa. *Journal of Communication Disorders*, **8**, 271–279.

Zraick, R.I., LaPointe, L.L., Case, J.L. and Duane, D.D. (1993). Acoustic correlates of vocal quality in individuals with spasmodic torticolis. *Journal of Medical Speech-Language Pathology*, **1**, 261–269.

Zwirner, P. and Barnes, G.J. (1992). Vocal tract steadiness: A measure of phonatory upper airway motor control during phonation in dysarthria. *Journal of Speech and Hearing Research*, **35**, 761–768.

PART 3

SPEECH MOTOR DEVELOPMENT

CHAPTER 7

HOW DO INFANTS COME TO CONTROL THE ORGANS OF SPEECH?

JOHN L. LOCKE

7.1 Introduction

Speaking involves the production of syllables. The most typical of these begin with a labial or lingual constriction, which starts to relax with the onset of vocalization and mandibular descent. The perceptible result is a consonant-vowel syllable.

In development, the organs involved in this activity are operative at birth in sucking, and later in the year, in chewing and babbling. These activities usually antedate, by several months, movements of the same organs in replication of sounds heard in spoken words. Thus, a theory of the development of speech-motor control must address the infant's initial attempts to achieve speech sounds with structures that already have long histories of vegetative and vocal service.

I will begin by discussing the concept of 'antecedent activities of the vocal tract' from the standpoint of evolution and development, then speculate about the processes by which infants first appropriate these systems for the new purpose of linguistic sound making.

7.2 Evolution

Obviously one must move one's jaw to eat, and lower it to perform high-volume vocal signaling. But what can we assume, more specifically, about any *social* uses of mandibular activity, during phonation, in our evolutionary ancestors?

The only line of empirical inquiry available requires us to reach past *Homo habilis* about 2 million years ago, to the ancestral stock shared with other primates. Although less voluble than humans, most primate species call to each other, and also vocalize quietly in more relaxed social settings.

It is the second category of quiet sound-making that concerns us here, for it includes two classes of behavior that bear faint resemblance to speech, both in form and function. The first, lipsmacking, is an oral behavior that is effected by mandibular oscillations. It is sometimes called tongue smacking, for the sound is thought to result from repeated lingual contact with the palate in a way so vigorous that it generates local air pressure (Anthoney 1968; Redican 1975).

Lipsmacking appears to function affiliatively since it frequently accompanies social grooming, greeting, and copulating, and may be offered as a gesture of pacification or appeasement. In some primate species there is an incidence of lipsmacking in infancy. Kenney *et al.* (1979) found that in socially reared rhesus monkeys, lipsmacking was present at birth, increased in frequency over the succeeding month, and subsequently declined.

Although lipsmacking is a purely aspirate sound, there is a second class of oral activity that has some of the phonatory properties of speech: the girney. In vervet and rhesus macaque monkeys, girneys seem to originate behind closed lips and, perhaps for that reason, tend to sound nasal. They resemble the subdued murmur of conversational speech (Hauser 1992). Although girneys begin just after birth, they are most frequently emitted by mothers who are interacting with other mothers or juvenile females. Males rarely girney, although young males entering a new social group may girney to high-ranking males. Significantly, girneys may be intermixed with tongue-smacks.

Lipsmacking is well entrenched in the motoric capabilities of nonhuman primates, is present early in development, arises in particular social situations, and functions as a social signal. But how did this audible activity of the vocal tract become available for the purposes to which it is presently put?

7.3 Emancipation

It has been speculated that lipsmacking originated in the oral movements associated with nursing (Redican 1975) or the ingestion of ectoparasites and other foreign particles removed during grooming (Marler and Tenaza 1977), but it became a social display, thus at some stage became separated from its original function. If our hominid ancestors had been able to combine the laryngeal activity of girneys with the articulatory activity of lip- and tongue-smacking, they might have been able to produce vocal pulses resembling syllables, possibly with contrasting points of oral closure.

The act of combining separate maneuvers requires flexibility, an attribute that one sees in the evolution of facial signaling systems. When primates were generally nocturnal, it is assumed that auditory signals were critically important; nocturnal primates can be prolific vocalizers, as studies of 'night monkeys' reveal (Moynihan 1964). When primates became diurnal, there were interesting changes in motor control. For example, contraction of the orbicularis oris occurs during many different types of primate vocalization, but at some point silent contraction of this muscle came to function as a visual signal (Andrew 1963). Thus in evolution, primates extended their capability for visuofacial communication while retaining earlier vocal displays.

If we are to understand how the infant comes to control the organs of speech, we may need to consider the processes by which pre-existing movements—that is, actions that are linked in evolution and development to an 'original' function— become available for other uses. These processes have been of considerable interest in ethology ever since Julian Huxley described the stereotyped activities of great crested grebes in 1914. Now there is a small body of evidence on the nature and functions of social displays, the specifies-specific signaling functions that attract, repel, threaten, appease, and otherwise regulate the activities of group-living species (cf. Huxley 1966; Smith 1977).

Displays are highly informative, but they need not be issued *in order* to inform. The motivation to signal was already worked out in evolution, when signaling behaviors increased fitness and thus made their way into the genome (Fitch and Hauser 2002). Examples of displays include the 'dances' of bees and great crested grebes, the howls of dogs and wolves, and the blushes of humans (cf. Smith 1977).

At the heart of displays are fixed or modal action patterns, species-specific motor behaviors that are relatively unaffected by experience. Most species, according to the meta-analysis conducted by Moynihan (1970), have between 15 and 35 displays. These fixed action patterns often consist of conspicuously visible movements that make sounds or that co-occur with vocalizations.

Our own species has a large number of displays, a fact that did not escape Darwin's (1872) notice. Having read descriptions of the seemingly conventional facial and bodily gestures of a deaf and blind girl, Laura Bridgeman (Lieber 1850), he asked colleagues in various cultures about the circumstances giving rise to frowns, smiles, shrugs, and other visible expressions of emotion. Their responses satisfied Darwin that humans have a more or less fixed repertoire of social displays. This was confirmed, a century later, in a small group of deaf–blind children (Eibl-Eibesfeldt 1973; see also Goldin-Meadow 1999). I will discuss the developmental significance of these displays later.

In the meanwhile, we need to ask how species-typical, experience-independent behaviors can come to be used flexibly, and modified, for other, perhaps more social, purposes. According to Tinbergen (1952), when a natural act—a behavior with a unique evolutionary history—is displaced, or used in a new way, it does not lose its original function but is usually modified to some extent. This is largely due to the fact that displacement activities are signals. Frequently, they arise when conspecific observers sense the significance of a movement before the movement is completed. When the ensuing reactions are processed by the actor, the original movement may be simultaneously truncated and exaggerated. Since subsequent generations learn the displaced activity as a social signal, additional variation creeps in. At this point, the displaced behavior is governed by its own rules, and one assumes that the mechanisms used to control and process the derived behavior are also different.

Tinbergen referred to this schematization of behavior, whereby contextualized movements become decontextualized signals, as 'ritualization'. He saw all such changes as serving one functional end, 'adaptation to the responsive capacities of the reacting individual' (Tinbergen 1952, p. 24). Sympathetically, Guilford and Dawkins (1991) argued 40 years later that signals evolve largely under the influence of 'receiver psychology', that is, the perceptions of other animals.

When a behavior is subsumed under a new drive, such as threat avoidance, it is submitted to a different set of controlling mechanisms. Recognizing this, Tinbergen referred to the 'neurophysiological emancipation' of behavior. For when ritualization removes behaviors from the 'executive motor pattern' of the original drive, they '"get away" from the synchronizing influences of the central nervous system, "allowing" them, so to speak, to have their own tempo independent of those of the other elements' (Tinbergen 1952, p. 28).

In evolution, then, displays were ritualized and smaller bits of behavior emancipated. The process began with the recognition that other animals were reacting to those smaller elements. Through ritualization, inherently expressive movements become intentional and willful as they are redeployed from their original contexts to new ones.

7.4 Function

From the foregoing, it might seem that my intention here is to argue that the movements of speech emerged from a set of pre-existing vegetative movements. But my purpose is to ask about the function of the sound-making activity one associates with babbling, and then to explore the possibility that principles such as displacement and emancipation could contribute to the development of speech-motor control.

The standard ethological approach would be to examine the circumstances under which babbling occurs, but infant sound-making has not been studied in such a framework. Consequently, very little is known about the circumstances in which babies babble. But there is one observation, that may be reliable. It is that infants vocalize more alone than in the company of an adult (Jones and Moss 1971), the effect beginning to grow in strength at 18 weeks, reaching a maximum at 38 weeks—when 90% of infants have begun to babble (Koopmans-van Beinum and van der Stelt 1986)—and declining to 48 weeks, when vocalization in solitary situations continues to exceed vocalization in the presence of the mother or a stranger (Delack 1976).

I suggested recently that the evolutionary function of babbling may have been the elicitation of care (Locke 2001, in press). The suggestion was stimulated by speculation that the vocalizations of a particular primate species have this effect. Elowson and Snowdon and their colleagues have found that, in the first weeks of life, the calls of dependent pygmy marmoset infants include infantile elements as well as adult-like sounds. Since these sounds are repeated with unusual frequency, Snowdon's group has compared these calls to the reduplicated babbling of human infants. Significantly, context analyses indicate that calling infants were more likely than silent ones to be picked up or cared for (Snowdon *et al.* 1997; Elowson *et al.* 1998*a*, *b*). After 8 weeks, the proportion of time when solitary marmoset infants called began to decline.

Human infants, of course, remain dependent for several years. But it is interesting that between 6 and 9 months, when nearly all babbling onsets occur, there is a near-total increase in crawling. Between the ages of 7 and 10 months, there is a sharp increase in chewing (Sheppard and Mysak 1984). Thus, one might speculate that during the period in which babbling begins there is both an increasing need to attract the mother and the mandibular means to do so.

Although we currently have no evidence that human babbling elicits approach or engagement, there is at least one reason to suppose that it may. Babble is far more pleasing to the ear than cries, or even nonsyllabic vocalizations. Bloom and her colleagues have reported that infants who produce syllabic utterances are adjudged, from audiotapes, to be more pleasant, friendly, and likeable than infants who use simpler forms of vocalization (Bloom and Lo 1990; Bloom *et al.* 1993). This could have operated in pre-linguistic history, before [dada] was considered 'speech-like' (Locke 2001).

7.5 Development

The title of this chapter refers to 'organs of speech' but this should not be construed to mean that there are organs that are exclusively dedicated to speech. When the infant *appropriates* for speech the organs that are conventionally used for that purpose, they have already spent several months in the service of nonspeech goals, the mandible and tongue in eating, the respiratory system in breathing, and the larynx in signaling. These systems work perfectly well in individuals who cannot speak, regardless of whether the inability is because they received too little of the relevant perceptual and social experience or lack the cognitive capacity to benefit from that experience.

Even after speaking for several decades, there is little reason to suppose that many of the basic closures, especially those associated with the stops, nasals, and glides, strike the ear differently than they do in infancy. That they may be *willfully* produced in late infancy and early childhood is a more significant development than any change in their physical form.

For the most part, our knowledge of speech-like movements rests, inferentially, on the sounds that we hear infants making. These speech-like sounds usually begin between the ages of 7 and 10 months in normally hearing infants with no physical or cognitive impairments. It is thus during this period that infants initially prevail upon the moveable parts of the mouth—the lips, tongue, jaw, and velum—for sound making.

The consonant-like sounds that are made in the pre-speech period, and are still available when speech begins, resemble the stops, nasals, and glides that exist in standard languages. Babbling analyses also reveal a preference for voiced stops, anterior closures, and syllables that begin with an obstruent. These core movements are like fixed or modal action patterns (Barlow 1977). Hearing and learning are not responsible for their 'selection'.

As relatively fixed action patterns, of course, the characteristic movement sequences associated with babbling might be less modifiable than the products of more open behavior programs. A decade ago, Dawn Pearson and I offered a biological hypothesis, according to which 'universal' phonemes—ones showing up frequently in babbling and languages—should assume *fewer* different forms of expression than 'non-universal' ones (Locke and Pearson 1992). We tested this assumption with two English consonants that seemed to qualify, /m/ and /r/, the former occurring in 97% of the documented languages, the latter in just 5% (UCLA Phonological Segment Inventory Database 1981). On purely statistical grounds, one would expect the more universal /m/ to have about 20 times as many variants as the less frequent /r/. In strong support of the biological hypothesis, however, we found only *half* as many types of bilabial nasals as /r/-like liquids.

At the population level, the jaw movements of babbling begin at about the same time as the jaw movements of chewing. What do we know about the timing of the transition from sucking to chewing in relation to the onset of babbling? What processes are needed to appropriate these pre-existing systems for speech?

To be sure, the means of shifting from prelexical sound making to speech was worked out evolutionarily, leaving the human infant with an endowment adequate to the task, but it is possible to question the nature of this endowment and its mode of activation. When infants speak, do they initially do so with a 'non-speech' jaw-, tongue-, and lip-control system, achieving later a more specialized and dedicated system for the coordination of speech? Do some nonlinguistic properties remain to influence the speech of children and adults, influencing the speed with which the jaw is elevated and lowered, and the tongue exercised? To what degree might these parameters be predicted by measurements of the individual's physical machinery?

As for the sounds themselves, the 'user-friendly' structure of baby words—for example, 'da-da,' 'moo-moo' and 'wa-wa'–indicates that adults want extant movement sequences to be useable. These are extreme examples, but phonological systems are very accepting. They take much of what the infant already has. In our interest in the *development* of control over the movements needed for speech, we are thus tempted to ignore the fact that linguistic sound systems were pre-engineered to admit the vocal–motor dispositions of learners. What looks like 'precocity' may be phonological naturalness, a point I will return to shortly.

Of course, languages are not limited to the sounds made by infants, and so there is a period of several years during which the developing child's repertoire of sound movements must expand. Will this reflect maturation? It would seem not, at least in any obvious way. For there is evidence that infants who are born deaf and remain effectively unaided produce few sounds beyond those heard in the babbling of hearing infants in the first year of life, even at the age of 3–6 years (Sykes 1940). Thus it is tempting, in the first instance, to link expansions of the child's repertoire of speech-like movements to perceptual experience. On this view, the older infant is driven by a desire to mimic ambient sounds and, in the process, performs movements that are specific to speech, therefore less naturally a part of its prelexical phonetic repertoire. Some of these less natural sounds (e.g. fricatives, affricates, liquids) have a protracted course of development, relative to core movements, and it is predictable that they should.

Work on phonological universals has produced a sense of the kinds of movement patterns that are the most likely to be used in speaking. Consonant-vowel syllables, beginning with a voiced stop, nasal or glide, are relatively more frequent than other elements. By inspecting these details, as I first did 20 years ago (Locke 1983), one quickly develops the impression that human adults, left to their own devices, would prefer to lower the mandible and close it rather firmly without interrupting or delaying phonation.

This suggests, ironically, that the most natural attributes of *speech* are the product of movements that are not specific to speech, but to a nonlinguistic sound-making system that operates in accordance with physical principles. If so, we would not expect infants' first articulate sounds to undergo a lengthy course of development, and it appears that they do not. In normative studies, it is not unusual for some consonants to meet adult standards at the beginning, that is, to be said 'correctly' by even the youngest children evaluated. In one study, [n] was produced accurately by so many 2-year-olds that it was assumed to have already 'been there' earlier (Prather *et al.* 1975). If this alveolar nasal owes its existence to a developmental process, the investigators missed it.

Studies of babbling and early speech refer to sounds, with the implication that the sounds were supported by movements, but listeners who hear [dada] or [baba] at 7 months must be careful not to conclude that the closures were the result of *intraoral* activity. It seems more likely that the movements are mandibular, with little more than passive posturing within the mouth. If the apex of the tongue is flat, the closure will be *passively* labial (Green *et al.* 2000, 2002); if the tongue happens to be bunched, the closure will be *passively* lingual.

The substantive continuity between babble and speech applies at the level of the species (MacNeilage and Davis 2000), but there is also phonetic continuity at the level of the individual. In several studies, Vihman and her associates (cf. Vihman 1996) have observed a significant degree of overlap between the preferences evident in babbling and the sounds present in the speech of the same children.

Continuity can suggest that babbling prepares infants for speech. At the neurological level, this is almost certainly the case, as we will see shortly. But one must be careful to avoid confounding factors. For it appears that infants who begin to babble on time are more likely to be in good health, and more likely to learn spoken language apace.

Support has been produced by Kim Oller and his colleagues. They found that infants who begin to babble after 10–12 months evince far more developmental problems, including sensory, cognitive, and linguistic disorders, than infants who begin to babble earlier (Oller *et al.* 1998). They also found that in a high-risk population (as indexed by low birthweight, socio-economic status, and exposure to illness or drugs), late babblers had significantly lower expressive vocabulary scores at 18, 24, and 30 months than those who began to babble on time (Oller *et al.* 1999).

These findings suggest that the neuro-vocal systems required for babbling and speech may be largely shared, at least initially. If so, the normal onset of babbling may indicate that, other things being equal, speech is just around the corner.

The use of similar movements in babbling and speaking also reflects the codification of human sound-making properties in languages. That is, language may have taken its form from oral movements that, as it so happens, are expressed audibly in babbling. As interchangeable movements with no inherent meaning, these behaviors could become 'units' in a codifiable system that also values the transparent and therefore 'honest' signals that imply emotional state and social intentions.

Babbling was the missing piece, for it involves movements that are manipulable, thus eligible for sequential deployment and recombination, into patterns of behavior. These patterns, because the articulators are so few, and their range of motion so limited, must be constantly repeated, giving them the properties of a system in which the behavioral units can have no significance of their own.

7.6 Control

Whatever its antecedents in the initial state, speech activity becomes increasingly adult-like over developmental time. It is assumed that control functions must also develop. If speech is like other motor skills in this respect, development occurs in response to experience and maturation. As for maturation, at 5–6 months postnatally, there is evidence of greater dendritic branching in manual and vocal-motor areas of the left hemisphere than in homologous areas in the right hemisphere (Simonds and Scheibel 1989).

This could be taken to suggest that syllabic sound making is *enabled* by such developments. While activity depends on maturation, it is also the case that activity fosters the neural advances that control it in mammals (Johnson *et al.* 1972; Greenough *et al.* 1985), including humans (Elbert *et al.* 1995). Thus use of the 'vocal tract' for a variety of functions, whether vegetative or vocal, may foster precision and control in the use of this system for sound making. Improved sound production also undoubtedly reflects developing powers of perception. Thus while there may be improvement in skills responsible for motor implementation, there is also enrichment of the representations that inform the relevant motor plans.

This is not to say that infants, in babbling, are *practicing* the movements that will be needed for speech. There is no evidence that 7-month-old infants are able to anticipate or prepare for their future linguistic needs (Locke 1996). This invites questions as to the immediate or proximal function of babbling, and this is the context for my suggestion that babbling may have been selected, in evolution, by nurturant parents.

Although babbling is audible, its onset is co-timed with a host of other behaviors, such as crawling, that do not make a sound (Koopmans-van Beinum and van der Stelt 1986). This is even more dramatically evident in two classes of manual behavior. One, rhythmic hand movements, emerges at about 27 weeks (Thelen 1981), that is, within a week of the usual onset of babbling. The second manual behavior is one-handed reaching, which occurs within a week of reduplicated babbling, at 6.7 months (Ramsay 1984). There also is evidence of longer right-hand grasping when toys are placed equally often in right and left hands at approximately the same age (Caplan and Kinsbourne 1976; Hawn and Harris 1983).

If babbling is 'turned on' by the activation of vocal-motor systems that must first reach a certain level of maturation, one might ask if babies ever babble silently. The answer is that they do. Meier and his colleagues at the University of Texas have found that infants often carry out jaw openings and closings silently (Meier *et al.* 1997). Periods of peak activity of these 'jaw wags' occurred between 7 and 9 months for three deaf infants, slightly later for the one hearing infant in their study. Most of the wags consisted of one or two cycles, the equivalent of [da] and [dada], with far fewer three-cycle openings and closings.

This study did not determine whether the deaf produce as many jaw wags as the hearing, but it does challenge the assumption that infants babble only for the sound. What, then, is to be made of the fact that in many cultures infants seem to enjoy various kinds of noisemakers? If self-produced sound is the attraction of rattles, why not activate the vocal tract and achieve similar effects?

Several years ago, my colleagues and I put into the hands of 60 infants of different ages a normal rattle and a rattle that had been silenced (Locke *et al.* 1995). We recorded more shakes per second when the rattle was placed in the right than the left hand, and there was a sharp increase in shakes per second during the period in which babbling began, regardless of whether the rattle made a noise or not. We also obtained a weak advantage for the audible over the silent rattle. In a similar study conducted a few years later by Ejiri (1998), a significant audibility effect was obtained.

These findings suggest that reduplicated babbling, also a repetitive activity, may be controlled by mechanisms in the left cerebral hemisphere. This conclusion is supported by a recent finding that infants produce syllables, but not nonsyllabic vocalizations, with asymmetrical mouth postures suggestive of left hemisphere control (Holowka and Petitto 2002). The authors concluded that 'language functions' are lateralized from an early age, but it is less adventurous to suppose that the motor activity underlying speech-like sounds 'awakens' some months before it is *appropriated* for lexical use.

In any case, one sees in these studies additional reasons why infants who begin to babble during the normal interval are likely to proceed to more complex vocal behaviors and speech. Indeed, EMG measurements of the mandible have shown that variegated babbling is more similar to speech than it is to chewing (Moore and Ruark 1996). It makes less sense to think of this alteration as a change in local demands associated with food processing than sensory and social goals that promote, and respond to, 'neurophysiological emancipation'.

7.6.1 Developmental emancipation?

All this leads us to a recapitulatory question—whether parental response to incidental vocalization can produce vocal emancipation in the young. This may seem a strange thing to wonder about, but consider the case of smiling. Infants, as we know, smile in the first few weeks of life. Vision plays little or no role in this, since blind infants smile in similar circumstances (Freedman 1964). At some point, however, infants begin to smile instrumentally (Wolff 1963). That is, they *use* this pre-existing, unlearned, action pattern *for effect*. One would naturally like to know how, at the level of the brain, the first instrumental smile differs from a non-instrumental smile produced on the same day. But the larger question is, how are species-specific behaviors changed by intentionality and decontextualization?

In the case of speech, one can witness parental reactions to, and reinforcement of, pre-existing vocal behaviors. Pawlby (1977) studied eight mother–infant dyads, in which the infants were 17–43 weeks of age, looking at the incidence of mother-to-infant and infant-to-mother imitation. She commented that 'babies do pay special attention (in that they laugh and smile and appear to be pleased) when the mothers themselves imitate an action that the child has just performed. The infant's action is thus "highlighted" or "marked out" as something special' (p. 220). She also thought that 'in kind' maternal responses 'may be what leads to the infant's more deliberate production of the action. Because the mother has repeatedly reflected back an event which he himself has just performed and since he finds this pleasing and attractive, the same action is produced by the child on a different occasion *in order that* his mother does likewise' (p. 220).

Veneziano (1988) found that contingent responding, in which mothers echo their infants' prelexical forms, encourages the infant to reproduce the original utterance and, in some cases, to accommodate to the mother's pronunciation. In other work, a significant correlation has been obtained between mothers' frequency of contingent responding and the communicative development of their infant at 1 year (Hardy-Brown *et al.* 1981).

It is thus possible that in development, as in evolution, selective social response causes vocal behaviors that are pre-existing, owing to relatively closed behavioral programs, to become more available to the individual. In that sense, these behaviors may be said to be 'emancipated.'

7.7 Motor patterns of phonology

If there are movement sequences, not just articulatory configurations, that are unusually natural or easy to produce, these will presumably show up in the statistics of sound systems. But phonological archives will not be of much help here, for they usually just list all the languages that have the various phonemes, offering less detail about sound sequences. Fortunately, there are a few studies in which investigators, for one reason or another, have chosen to count up all the different words in the lexicon, or the total words in conversations, having certain sequences. Similar analyses have also been performed on the speech of young children.

Several patterns of movement that are evident in babble are preserved in the statistics of established phonologies (Locke 2000). Some years ago, I pointed to an 'anterior-to-posterior progression' in the utterances of children and the vocabularies of English and French (Locke 1983). Lip-to-tongue words like 'pat' and 'mad' surpassed reverse-order items like 'tap' and 'dam'. I also reported data indicating that the 'fronting' pattern is far more common when velar consonants appear in word-initial than in word-final position. Whether this pattern somehow reflects more basic patterns of movement associated with feeding, as I suspected at the time, is unclear. But MacNeilage and Davis (2000) found this 'labial-coronal' effect, as they term it, in several other languages besides English. Clearly, the human vocal tract has preferred patterns of movement, and many of these are carried over into speech and stabilized in phonological structure.

It has also been discovered that infants produce *sequences* of sounds that commonly occur in established languages. In the babbled syllables of prelexical infants and the speech of very young children, consonants and vowels tend to travel together. When the tongue tip is positioned for a consonant-like sound, the positioning tends to carry-over into the following vowel (Stoel-Gammon 1983). A few years ago, my colleagues and I recorded sounds produced spontaneously by 9- to 18-month-old American infants in their homes, and tabulated all the syllables in which alveolars preceded front vowels, labials preceded mid-vowels, and velars preceded back vowels (Locke *et al.* 1997; also see Locke 2001). These sums were then divided by the total frequency with which segments of these places of articulation preceded all vowels. In the labial and velar distributions, there was a regular progression whereby back vowels exceeded mid vowels, which exceeded front vowels. In the alveolar distributions, the pattern was reversed. It appeared that the tongue movement associated with consonant-like sounds such as /d/ dragged the vowel along with it, making [di] syllables more frequent than [da] or [du] syllables. A similar, though seemingly stronger, effect was reported later by MacNeilage and Davis (2000).

7.8 Final comment

I have raised a number of questions about the transition from prespeech vocal and nonvocal activities to the movements used in speech. There are two specific issues on which further work seems especially important.

The first has to do with the 'original' function served by movements that, due to their audibility, are noticed and responded to by key figures in the infant's environment, movements that through social and perceptual reaction become available for 'other' uses. If we are to have a complete explanation of the development of speech-motor control in the human infant, I believe we will need to know how this happens both at the cognitive and neural levels of analysis, and we will need to monitor any changes in vocal morphology or control that occur at that time.

The second, related question is candidly mechanistic. It asks how the developing, socially reared human brain assumes the ability to isolate from larger action patterns constituent elements that can be interchanged with other elements. Where the patterns are vocal and the elements phonetic, this process apparently enables the infant to operationalize the phonological principle (cf. Abler 1989) and, we might suppose, to use modified patterns of control for the production of sounds that will be heard as speech.

Acknowledgement

I am indebted to Michael Studdert-Kennedy for helpful conversations, and for comments on an earlier draft.

References

Abler, W. L. (1989). On the particulate principle of self-diversifying systems. *Journal of Social and Biological Structure, 12,* 1–13.

Andrew, R. J. (1963). Evolution of facial expression. *Science, 141,* 1034–1041.

Anthoney, T. R. (1968). The ontogeny of greeting, grooming and sexual motor patterns in captive baboons (superspecies *Papio cynocephalus*). *Behaviour, 31,* 358–372.

Barlow, G. W. (1977). Modal action patterns. In Sebeok, T. A. (Ed.), *How animals communicate*. Bloomington, IN: Indiana University Press.

Bloom, K. and **Lo, E.** (1990). Adult perceptions of vocalizing infants. *Infant Behavior and Development, 13,* 209–219.

Bloom, K., D'Odorico, L., and **Beaumont, S.** (1993). Adult preferences for syllabic vocalizations: generalizations to parity and native language. *Infant Behavior and Development, 16,* 109–120.

Caplan, P. and **Kinsbourne, M.** (1976). Baby drops the rattle: asymmetry in duration of grasp by infants. *Child Development, 47,* 532–534.

Darwin, C. (1872/1965). *The expression of the emotions in man and animals.* Chicago, IL: University of Chicago Press.

Delack, J. B. (1976). Aspects of infant speech development in the first year of life. *Canadian Journal of Linguistics, 21,* 17–37.

Eibl-Eibesfeldt, I. (1973). The expressive behavior of the deaf-and-blind-born. In von Cranach, M. and Vine, I. (Eds.), *Social communication and movement: studies of interaction and expression in man and chimpanzee.* London: Academic Press.

Ejiri, K. (1998). Relationship between rhythmic behavior and canonical babbling in infant vocal development. *Phonetica, 55,* 226–237.

Elbert, T., Pantev, C., Wienbruch, C., Rockstroh, B., and **Taub, E.** (1995). Increased cortical representation of the fingers of the left hand in string players. *Science, 270,* 305–307.

Elowson, A. M., Snowdon, C. T., and **Lazaro-Perea, C.** (1998a). 'Babbling' and social context in infant monkeys: parallels to human infants. *Trends in Cognitive Sciences, 2,* 31–37.

Elowson, A. M., Snowdon, C. T., and **Lazaro-Perea, C.** (1998b). Infant 'babbling' in a nonhuman primate: complex vocal sequences with repeated call types. *Behaviour, 135,* 643–664.

Fitch, W. T. and **Hauser, M. D.** (2002). Unpacking 'honesty': vertebrate vocal production and the evolution of acoustic signals. In Fay, R. R. and Popper, A. N. (Eds.), *Acoustic communication.* New York: Springer.

Freedman, D. G. (1964). Smiling in blind infants and the issue of innate vs. acquired. *Journal of Child Psychology and Psychiatry, 5,* 171–184.

Goldin-Meadow, S. (1999). The role of gesture in communicating and thinking. *Trends in Cognitive Sciences, 3,* 419–429.

Green, J. R., Moore, C. A., Higashikawa, M., and **Steeve, R. W.** (2000). The physiologic development of speech motor control: lip and jaw coordination. *Journal of Speech, Language, and Hearing Research, 43,* 239–255.

Green, J. R., Moore, C. A., and **Reilly, K. J.** (2002). The sequential development of jaw and lip control for speech. *Journal of Speech, Language, and Hearing Research, 45,* 66–79.

Greenough, W. T., Larson, J. R., and **Withers, G. S.** (1985). Effects of unilateral and bilateral training in a reaching task on dendritic branching of neurons in the rat motor-sensory forelimb cortex. *Behavioral and Neural Biology, 44,* 301–314.

Guilford, T. and **Dawkins, M. S.** (1991). Receiver psychology and the evolution of animal signals. *Animal Behaviour, 42,* 1–14.

Hardy-Brown, K., Plomin, R., and **DeFries, J.** (1981. Genetic and environmental influences on the rate of communicative development in the first year of life. *Developmental Psychology, 17,* 704–717.

Hauser, M. D. (1992). A mechanism guiding conversational turn-taking in vervet monkeys and rhesus macaques. *Topics in primatology. Vol. 1. Human origins.* Tokyo: Tokyo University Press.

Hawn, P. R. and **Harris, L. J.** (1983). Hand differences in grasp duration and reaching in two- and five-month-old infants. In Young, G., Segalowitz, S. J., Corter, C. M., and Trehub, S. E. (Eds.), *Manual specialization and the developing brain.* New York: Academic Press.

Holowka, S. and **Petitto, L. A.** (2002). Left hemisphere cerebral specialization for babies while babbling. *Science, 297,* 1515.

Huxley, J. (1966). Introduction. In Huxley, J. (Ed.), A discussion on ritualization of behaviour in animals and man. *Philosophical Transactions of the Royal Society of Britain, 251,* 249–271.

Johnson, J. I., Hamilton, T. C., Hsung, J-C., and **Ulinski, P. S.** (1972). Gracile nucleus absent in adult opossums after leg removal in infancy. *Brain Research, 38,* 421–424.

Jones, S. J. and **Moss, H. A.** (1971). Age, state, and maternal behavior associated with infant vocalizations. *Child Development, 42,* 1039–1051.

Kenney, M. D., Mason, W. A., and **Hill, S. D.** (1979). Effects of age, objects, and visual experience on affective responses of rhesus monkeys to strangers. *Developmental Psychology, 15,* 176–184.

Koopmans-van Beinum, F. J. and **van der Stelt, J. M.** (1986). Early stages in the development of speech movements. In Lindblom, B. and Zetterstrom, R. (Eds.), *Precursors of early speech.* New York: Stockton Press.

Lieber, F. (1850). A paper on the vocal sounds of Laura Bridgeman, the blind deaf-mute at Boston; compared with the elements of phonetic language. *Smithsonian Contributions to Knowledge, Volume II, Article 2.*

Locke, J. L. (1983). *Phonological acquisition and change.* New York: Academic Press.

Locke, J. L. (1996). Why do infants begin to talk? Language as an unintended consequence. *Journal of Child Language, 23,* 251–268.

Locke, J. L. (2000). Movement patterns in spoken language. *Science, 288,* 449–450.

Locke, J. L. (2001). The benefits of babbling in the infant and the species: from sound-making to speech. In Hewlett, N., Kelly, L., and Windsor, F. (Eds.), *Themes in clinical linguistics and phonetics.* Lawrence Erlbaum.

Locke, J. L. (in press) Parental selection of vocal behaviors in the evolution of spoken language. In Tallerman, M. (Ed.), *Evolutionary prerequisites for language.* Oxford: Oxford University Press.

Locke, J. L. and **Pearson, D. M.** (1992). Vocal learning and the emergence of phonological capacity: a neurobiological approach. In Ferguson, C., Menn, L., and Stoel-Gammon, C. (Eds.), *Phonological development: models, research, implications*. Parkton, MD: York Press.

Locke, J. L., Bekken, K. E., McMinn-Larson, L., and **Wein, D.** (1995). Emergent control of manual and vocal-motor activity in relation to the development of speech. *Brain and Language, 51,* 498–508.

Locke, J. L., Hodgson, J., Macaruso, P., Roberts, J., Lambrecht-Smith, S., and **Guttentag, C.** (1997). The development of developmental dyslexia. In Hulme, C. and Snowling, M. (Eds.), *Dyslexia: biological bases, identification and intervention*. London: Whurr Publishers.

MacNeilage, P. F. and **Davis, B. L.** (2000). On the origin of internal structure of word forms. *Science, 288,* 527–531.

Marler, P. and **Tenaza, R.** (1977). Signaling behavior of apes with special reference to vocalization. In Sebeok, T. A. (Ed.), *How animals communicate*. Bloomington, IN: Indiana University Press.

Meier, R. P., McGarvin, L., Zakia, R. A. E., and **Willerman, R.** (1997). Silent mandibular oscillations in vocal babbling. *Phonetica, 54,* 153–171.

Moore, C. A. and **Ruark, J. L.** (1996). Does speech emerge from earlier appearing oral motor behaviors? *Journal of Speech and Hearing Research, 39,* 1034–1047.

Moynihan, M. H. (1964). Some behavior patterns of platyrrhine monkeys. I. The night monkey (*Aotus trivargatus*). *Smithsonian Miscellaneous Collections, 146,* 1–84.

Moynihan, M. (1970). The control, suppression, decay, disappearance and replacement of displays. *Journal of Theoretical Biology, 29,* 85–112.

Oller, D. K., Eilers, R. E., Neal, A. R., and **Cobo-Lewis, A. B.** (1998). Late onset canonical babbling: a possible early marker of abnormal development. *American Journal on Mental Retardation, 103,* 249–263.

Oller, D. K., Eilers, R. E., Neal, A. R., and **Schwartz, H. K.** (1999). Precursors to speech in infancy: the prediction of speech and language disorders. *Journal of Communication Disorders, 32,* 223–245.

Pawlby, S. J. (1977). Imitative interaction. In Schaffer, H. R. (Ed.), *Studies in mother–infant interaction*. New York: Academic Press.

Prather, E. M., Hedrick, D. L., and **Kern, C. A.** (1975). Articulation development in children aged two to four years. *Journal of Speech and Hearing Disorders, 40,* 179–191.

Ramsay, D. S. (1984). Onset of duplicated syllable babbling and unimanual handedness in infancy: evidence for developmental change in hemispheric specialization? *Developmental Psychology, 20,* 64–71.

Redican, W. K. (1975). Facial expressions in nonhuman primates. In Rosenblum, L. A. (Ed.), *Primate behavior: developments in field and laboratory research*. New York: Academic Press.

Sheppard, J. J. and **Mysak, E. D.** (1984). Ontogeny of infantile oral reflexes and emerging chewing. *Child Development, 55*, 831–843.

Simonds, R. J. and **Scheibel, A. B.** (1989). The postnatal development of the motor speech area: a preliminary study. *Brain and Language, 37*, 42–58.

Smith, W. J. (1977). *The behavior of communicating: an ethological approach*. Cambridge, MA: Harvard University Press.

Snowdon, C. T., Elowson, A. M., and **Roush, R. S.** (1997). Social influences on vocal development in New World primates. In Snowdon, C. and Hausberger, M. (Eds.), *Social influences on vocal development*. Cambridge: Cambridge University Press.

Stoel-Gammon, C. (1983). Constraints on consonant-vowel sequences in early words. *Journal of Child Language, 10*, 455–457.

Sykes, J. L. (1940). A study of the spontaneous vocalizations of young deaf children. *Psychological Monographs, 52*, 104–123.

Thelen, E. (1981). Rhythmical behavior in infancy: an ethological perspective. *Developmental Psychology, 17*, 237–257.

Tinbergen, N. (1952). 'Derived' activities; their causation, biological significance, origin, and emancipation during evolution. *Quarterly Review of Biology, 27*, 1–32.

UCLA Phonological Segment Inventory Database: Data and Index 1981. *UCLA Working Papers in Phonetics, 53*, 1–243.

Veneziano, E. (1988). Vocal–verbal interaction and the construction of early lexical knowledge. In Smith, M. D. and Locke, J. L. (Eds.), *The emergent lexicon: the child's development of a linguistic vocabulary*. New York: Academic Press.

Vihman, M. M. (1996). *Phonological development: the origins of language in the child*. Cambridge, MA: Blackwell.

Wolff, P. (1963). Observations on the early development of smiling. In Foss, B. M. (Ed.), *Determinants of infant behavior II*. London: Methuen.

CHAPTER 8

PHYSIOLOGIC DEVELOPMENT OF SPEECH PRODUCTION

CHRISTOPHER A. MOORE

8.1 Introduction

The emergence of speech production in infants signifies the attainment of a broad range of developmental capacities, including, among others, cognitive, perceptual, social, linguistic, and physiologic proficiencies. Among these areas of speech development, perhaps physiologic development remains least described and understood, primarily for reasons of experimental challenge; achieving experimental control and maintaining accurate physiologic measures in a toddler obviously present a host of difficulties. Unfortunately, this lack of uniformity in our understanding of the essential capacities underlying speech development precludes a complete model of communicative development. Moreover, most theoretical approaches are then forced to posit specific, though empirically unsupported, assumptions regarding the motor infrastructure upon which developing speech is built.

As the product of emergent, interdependent skills, speech development is probably constrained at any given age by the least-developed component, which then acts as the rate-limiting factor in development. Not all skills develop in parallel. A common suggestion is that a typically developing child may have the perceptual and cognitive capacity to distinguish among perceived phonetic contrasts, but will, for a period, lack the motor capacity to generate those contrasts. The identity of this rate-limiting skill may vary with age, as development across capacities may be dissociated, with any one area (e.g. motor control) lagging behind the rest and deterministically constraining the overall capabilities of the speech production system. Speech motor development appears to be the likely rate-limiter during the initial periods of the emergence of true words, as the coordination of respiratory, phonatory, and articulatory systems presents a challenge that the child may not have encountered previously. Although a wide range of vocal and non-vocal oral motor behaviors is exhibited by the typical 11-month-old, none entails the temporal and spatial specifications on the order of those typical of speech production.

In addition to this specific goal of understanding the constraints and specific capacities underlying speech development, it is also apparent that a clear representation of physiologic development is essential both to models of mature speech production and to models of speech impairment. The processes evident during early speech development are likely subsumed under later-developing speech production, but probably reveal the essential organization of mature speech. For example, the timing of expiratory support of phonation must emerge early in speech development, with subsequent refinement of timing and amplitude modulation. As the infant learns to modulate vocal fundamental frequency and intensity, the respiratory system will have to function in novel, previously unobserved ways. With respect to disruptions in development of speech motor control, a basic tenet of epidemiology is that systems do not fail randomly; developmental aberrations are not uniformly distributed among speech systems and behaviors. Failures can identify system vulnerabilities and may also expose underlying capacities. Diagnosis, treatment, and theoretical representations of speech impairment must be approached with a clear model of the typical developmental process.

Although no dominant representation of speech development has yet emerged, a conceptual framework for physiologic development of speech production can be built from several compelling approaches. A dynamic systems perspective, for example would lead empiricists to seek developmental periods of marked stability demarcated by intervals of marked instability. Alternatively, one might assume a biologic systems perspective, focusing on periods of neural and musculoskeletal growth and the presumed consequential development in motor control capacities. Additional theoretical structure should also accommodate observations of universals in phonetic development (Locke; MacNeilage and Davis 2000) and animal models of oral motor control (Luschei and Goldberg 1981). Each of these approaches predicts rather specific, testable patterns of development, such that empirical work can be focused productively on evaluating these predictions.

Evaluation of the dynamic systems perspective on speech development is especially sensitive to decisions of quantification and levels of observation. Within an observational domain (e.g. mandibular kinematics) one must seek developmental periods or stages during which a measure exhibits comparatively reduced stability (i.e. increased variability), followed or preceded by periods of increased stability. Among the rapidly emerging speech production systems of the infant/toddler, these stabilities might be expected to be especially apparent, given appropriate metrics. The mandibular system presents an appealing focus of this approach for several reasons: the role of the jaw in most speech development models is seen as being disproportionately important during babbling and early speech; the position and muscle activation patterns of the jaw are readily accessible to noninvasive observation; the mandible has an obvious role in other oral motor behaviors; and the well-researched function of the mandible in ingestive cyclicities (e.g. mastication) has been advanced as essential in the emergence of speech production (MacNeilage and Davis 2000). The coordinative organization of mandibular movement afforded by the putative central pattern generator for mastication can be represented as providing the stability upon which more complex speech movements can be established. Subsequent instabilities might be expected to emerge as speech movements are adapted to movement patterns that are more complex than can be accommodated by the organization for mastication. Though no physiologic data have been shown to support this model, this conceptualization has obvious intuitive appeal.

Another especially intriguing aspect of the physiologic development of speech is the rapidly changing biologic context in which it occurs. Many of the characteristics, properties, and capacities incorporated into the adult model are simply not present in, nor attainable by, young children. The mass of the mandible, for example, increases very rapidly during the period of initial speech acquisition, requiring the child to generate new speech behaviors without the benefit of a known, constant sensorimotor system. Similarly, the vocal folds appear to lack the essential biomechanical properties that would permit modulation of fundamental frequency (f_0) and intensity using adult-like strategies. Whereas the elasticity of the vocal ligament in the mature system imbues it with the capacity to generate a wide range of tensions, the immature vocal folds have no such capacity. Modulation of f_0 and intensity then requires the use of a poorly understood, immature control mechanism. Finally, the respiratory system of the adult is dramatically different from that of the infant. This difference is attributable primarily to the lack of elasticity in the infant's rib cage and to the more horizontal orientation of the infant's ribs. Consequently, infants are generally 'obligate belly-breathers', relying on active muscular forces to regulate airflow and lung volume. This assortment of physiologic differences between the speech systems of adults and children further complicates the problem of establishing a framework for studying speech development. More significantly, these differences reinforce the notion that speech is developed using a mechanism that is fundamentally different from that of the mature, target system.

This chapter describes a range of physiologic measures obtained from young children during speech development. The orientation underlying physiologic measures, including those described here, entails the implicit assumption that the output of controlled elements of developing motor control can be observed in the movement and physiologic modulations of speech systems. Beyond this more general assumption are much more specific hypotheses of how controlled variables are manifest and specifically quantified. For example, peak movement amplitude of a single articulator is commonly used as a dependent measure of speech motor performance. The tacit assumption, of course, is that this value reflects the underlying modulations of the motor control systems. Comparable alternative measures include movement duration, peak movement velocities, time-to-peak movement amplitude, and a host of others.

The experimental results described here are based on an approach of sampling broad portions of physiologic signals to extract the preponderant relationships using time series analyses (e.g. variability across repetitions of normalized or warped signals, cross-correlational analyses, spectral analysis, coherence measures). This approach has the appeal of distilling from each sample the general amplitude and temporal tendencies of the whole behavior, avoiding any reliance on single-point measures (e.g. onset, offset, peak). Point measures are especially susceptible to systematic and random variability introduced by signal processing decisions, point-selection criteria, and intrinsic factors relating to the original phenomenon (e.g. variability in the actual movement). Systematic reduction in peak measures, for example, will arise from lowpass filtering; similarly, sample rates that are relatively low with respect to the observed phenomenon will yield lowered and more variable peak values, as the probability of sampling the actual peak decreases with sample rate. By including the entire signal in an analysis, these point-specific weaknesses can be avoided. Similarly, sampling a broad range of naturally occurring or elicited behaviors reduces experimental control, but enhances the opportunity to observe more general principles of behavior. The challenge then shifts from the choice of appropriate stimuli to the design of sufficient analytic techniques to extract general tendencies from the entire range of observed behaviors. The study of infant and toddler vocalizations requires such an approach and is evident in the studies described here.

8.2 The relationship of speech and nonspeech behaviors

One prevailing challenge in describing the physiologic development of speech is formulating a frame of reference, including the range of behaviors and the inherent constraints associated with each speech system. How do speech behaviors fit in the context of the full range of motor behaviors, especially those involving systems used in speech production? This frame of reference problem has consistently been underestimated, as scientists and clinicians have presupposed, without empirical support, that nonspeech behaviors are precursors to speech development. Darley *et al.* (1975) stated this assumption most explicitly, noting that 'As the baby progresses to soft and then to solid food... jaw movements are modified for chewing ... The motor control of these nutritional movements *must be adapted for speech production* ... It is readily apparent that the pursing of the lips for sucking may be adapted to produce the phoneme /oo/ ... opening of the jaws is necessary for the phoneme /o/ ... ' (p. 65, italics added).

Evaluation of this assumption empirically has been a major focus in establishing a descriptive framework for these systems. Control of mandibular movement has been evaluated with respect to mastication, sucking, swallowing, and jaw oscillation, a behavior seen in infants wherein the child voluntarily raises and depresses the mandible. Lip muscle activity has also been studied for a comparable range of behaviors (Ruark and Moore 1997). Similarly, breathing for speech purposes has been investigated in the context of rest breathing and a wide range of other behaviors involving respiratory drive (e.g. cough, cry, laugh; Moore *et al.* 2001). Speech vocalization has been compared to cry and, in animals, to a range of electrically stimulated vocal behaviors.

Comparisons of speech and nonspeech behaviors bear on several diverse areas of interest to speech researchers. For example, the neural mechanisms underlying many nonspeech behaviors are well-understood in animal and human models, and may be extensible to speech production. Behavioral commonalities across speech and nonspeech behaviors (e.g. similar kinematic properties) can be taken to suggest that these specific neural mechanisms are shared across behaviors. These commonalities may also be taken to suggest shared ontogenetic and phylogenetic pathways across behaviors. The most frequently invoked of these mechanisms are the central pattern generators for mastication (e.g. Grillner, 1981) and respiration (Bellingham 1998), but comparable parallels exist for vocalization (e.g. Jürgens 1995).

Clinically, the presumption of shared behavioral properties has led to the expectation that treatment in a specific domain (e.g. oral motor control) will generalize across a wide range of behaviors, including speech. Although published data are lacking, clinicians have often reasoned that training nonspeech behaviors in children with speech impairment will capitalize on the shared control properties among behaviors, and will facilitate speech by the transfer of developing skills to impaired, related behaviors. Although empirical data addressing this question do not exist for speech development, there is an abundance of treatment programs devoted to the notion that nonspeech skills transfer to and support the development of speech motor control. The results described in the current experiments, although they were not designed to test this hypothesis, might generally be taken to support an opposing view, that speech and nonspeech behaviors are sufficiently distinct in their developmental time lines and in their observable properties, that the idea of transfer across behaviors lacks the essential parsimony and effectiveness claimed.

8.3 Physiologic observations

Physiologic observations of speech production have focused primarily on the most accessible systems (e.g. mandible, lips, respiratory system) in adult subjects, although continuing technical developments have made lingual tracking more commonly available. These observations of mature speech production are probably not extensible to the developing system, however, which therefore requires direct observations of infants and toddlers. We have completed a range of physiologic studies of young children, including studies of mandibular (Moore and Ruark 1996; Green et al. 1997) and labial (Ruark and Moore 1997) movement, respiratory coordination (Moore et al. 2001), phonation, bilabial closure (Green et al. 2000, 2002), and velopharyngeal valving. By employing measurement and analytic techniques that are noninvasive and can be generalized beyond controlled utterances, it may be possible to represent general properties or tendencies in very early speech production.

8.3.1 Studies of mandibular and labial movement

The mandible has been implicated repeatedly as the primary articulator supporting early speech and nonspeech vocalizations. Clinical and theoretical (MacNeilage and Davis 2000) approaches have been built on a cornerstone of mandibular motor control as the essential element of developing speech articulation. For example, Prompt therapy, a current approach to articulatory impairment, stresses mandibular stability as a prerequisite for later differentiation of speech sounds (Chumpelik (Hayden) 1984). Others have held that the influence of mandibular movement dictates placement of the tongue, yielding universal articulatory preferences for specific sound sequences (consonant-vowel) produced by parallel movement of the tongue and jaw (MacNeilage and Davis 2000). These hypotheses, and the accessibility of the jaw to experimental observation, have made it an obvious focus for quantification of developing speech production.

Comparison of muscle activation patterns (electromyograms, EMGs) for speech and other early-appearing oral motor behaviors revealed in 15-month-old children that emergent speech exhibits greater stability (i.e. predictability and consistency of EMG activation) than behaviors such as chewing, sucking, or other jaw movements (Moore and Ruark 1996). Whereas the EMG signals associated with chewing exhibited relatively high variability across cycles, and lacked consistent activation across muscles, vocalizations were associated with EMG signals that were statistically more predictable in time and across muscles. Moreover, the patterns across behaviors were categorically distinct: chewing in these toddlers was characterized by weakly phasic activation of varying jaw elevators against more tonic activation of jaw depressors. Vocalization, in contrast, exhibited significantly more consistent phasic activity, with relatively rigid coupling across muscles, with frequent synchronous, phasic coactivation of mandibular antagonists. This latter observation was rarely observed during chewing or other mandibular cyclicities, and suggests distinct coordinative infrastructures for chewing and vocalization, even at this very early age of speech development. Moreover, individual children appeared to exhibit idiosyncratic muscle groupings during vocalization, and more general activation of all mandibular muscles during chewing. This finding fails to support hypotheses built upon the presumed role of ingestive cyclicities (e.g. for chewing or jaw wagging) as the ontogenetic and phylogenetic antecedents of early babbling and speech (MacNeilage and Davis 2000); significant differences across speech and nonspeech tasks even at this very early age are consistent with parallel, independent developmental paths.

Figure 8.1 illustrates the dramatic changes in the coordinative organization exhibited by children at 1 and 4 years of age. Chewing at 1 year was characterized by highly variable periodicity, poorly defined patterns of muscle activation, and weakly established muscle synergies. The temporal overlap of muscle activity in antagonistic muscles was significant in these younger children. In contrast, 4-year-olds generate a very stable (i.e. consistent and predictable within an observation) pattern of muscle activation, exhibiting well-defined synergies among muscles (i.e. coactivation of synergistic muscles, reciprocal activation of antagonistic muscles). Synchronous activation of antagonists, which occurred primarily during the reversal from jaw elevation to jaw depression, decreased significantly with age. Quantitative analyses of these characteristics in four children, observed longitudinally at intervals of 3 months from 1 to 4 years of age, were compelling, demonstrating that coupling among muscles becomes progressively stronger with development, and that the reciprocal activation pattern of antagonistic muscles becomes more strictly defined (Green *et al.* 1997). Most surprisingly, with respect to speech development, it appears that development of mastication actually lags slightly behind the establishment of muscle activation patterns associated with vocalization, including babbling and production of true words. These results provide further support for the idea that speech development relies on a motor control structure that is independent from that of other oral motor behaviors, and that it may emerge quite rapidly.

Figure 8.2 illustrates mandibular muscle activation associated with babbling by a 9-month-old child. Although no single example can typify EMG patterns during babbling by 9-month-old children, these records do illustrate the coupling among

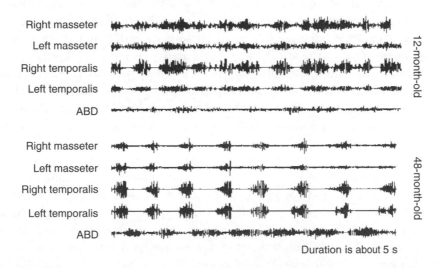

Fig. 8.1 Comparison of mandibular electromyographic activity during chewing by a 1-year-old with that by a 4-year-old. The top four traces in each panel are derived from mandibular elevators; the bottom trace, labeled 'ABD', is derived from jaw-lowering muscles. The increased predictability and consistency seen in the EMG patterns of the 4-year-old were typical of the developmental trend seen in these groups.

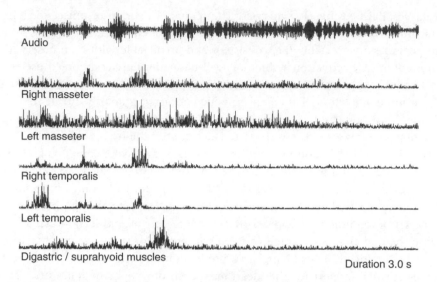

Audio

Right masseter

Left masseter

Right temporalis

Left temporalis

Digastric / suprahyoid muscles

Duration 3.0 s

Fig. 8.2 An example of babbling by a 9-month-old child. Evident in this figure is the close synchrony of activity in the mandibular elevators (seen in the middle four traces, with the exception of left masseter), and the reciprocal modulation of this activity with that of the jaw depressor muscles (bottom trace).

jaw muscles that was seen in these subjects. For example, the tonic activation of left masseter and deeply modulated, high-level phasic activity in left temporalis is atypical of chewing or any other oromandibular behavior seen in these children. Variability within each child was qualitatively seen to be significantly less than that observed either across children during vocalization or within and across children during sucking or chewing at this age (in preparation). Figure 8.2 illustrates reciprocity of activity among antagonistic muscles (i.e. digastric activity was generally reciprocal with the activity of the jaw-closing muscles), which was another general observation among these activities. Although reciprocity among mandibular antagonists is characteristic of mature chewing, it was not observed in the chewing patterns of these young children.

In a related investigation of the development of articulatory kinematics, Green *et al.* (2000) quantified the relative kinematic contributions of the mandible and the upper and lower lips in achieving oral closure, demonstrating clearly that the role of the jaw is particularly prominent in early speech production, diminishing slightly with development, but still maintaining its relative importance in this closing gesture. Figure 8.3 illustrates the developmental progression in the kinematic pattern used to achieve bilabial closure. Several aspects of these data are immediately apparent: the jaw is initially the primary articulator responsible for oral closure, but by adulthood, displacement of the lower lip (i.e. displacement of the lip in excess of that caused by mandibular displacement) is comparable to that of the mandible. The contribution of the upper lip increases initially, following the

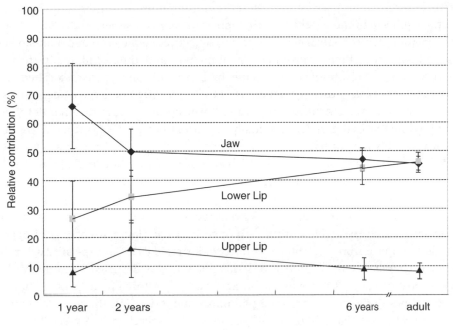

Fig. 8.3 Developmental change in the relative contributions of upper lip, lower lip, and jaw to the achievement of bilabial closure for production of the syllable /ba/. Elevation of the mandible was most predominant at 1 year of age, decreasing as the contribution of lower lip elevation increased. The contribution of the upper lip exhibited a non-monotonic change, increasing initially, then diminishing to the mature form. (After Green *et al.* 2000.)

increased role of the lower lip, but then upper lip movement dissociates from that of the lower lip, falling by 6 years to nearly half of its peak contribution. Variability also decreases dramatically with development as these mechanisms presumably become more established. The lack of uniformity in the developmental course of these articulators might be taken to suggest that universal tendencies in acquisition of phonemes may have a basis in constraints of oromandibular motor control. For example, production of bilabial sounds is facilitated by the jaw-dominated patterns of early development, whereas sounds requiring differentiated output of lips and the jaw (e.g. labiodental fricatives) would be precluded by such a pattern. Continued evaluation of this relationship of developmental universals and motor development may be able to provide the evidence necessary to implicate motor constraints as rate-limiting with respect to phoneme acquisition and speech development.

Analyses of lip movement revealed the clearest evidence of a non-monotonic developmental function. Displacement of the upper and lower lips became differentiated with development, such that children progress initially through a period during which lip displacement is the passive consequence of mandibular move-ment (e.g. even to the extent that the upper lip is driven superiorly by mandibu-lar elevation during bilabial closure), to a period during which the upper and lower lips mirror each other's movement in amplitude and time, and finally to the mature form in which movements of the lips are significantly more dissociated and independent of each other (Green *et al.* 2000). These differences are evident in Fig. 8.3, which shows the contribution of the lower lip to increase through develop-ment, while that of the upper lip initially increases through 2 years, then decreases for 6-year-olds and adults.

Electromyographic observations of labial movement (Ruark and Moore 1997) provide further explication of these findings. Although the displacement of the lips is far less than that of the mandible during bilabial closure (Fig. 8.3), lip muscle activation by 2-year-olds during speech production overall suggests that these articulators are very active during early speech. A correlational analysis of upper and lower lip electromyographic records demonstrated clear task specificity during speech, chewing, and lip protrusion. This analysis was designed to evaluate the synchrony of upper and lower lip muscle activity. Although most observations revealed positively correlated activity in upper and lower lips, the tasks for which these structures appeared most weakly coupled were speech tasks, especially for lip rounding and for speech tokens that did not involve labial articulation (Ruark and Moore 1997). In these analyses, highly correlated activity in upper and lower lips was interpreted to suggest that the lips were coordinated as a single unit, possibly exhibiting sphincteric movement. Weakly correlated movement was taken to support the suggestion that the activity of the upper and lower lips could be modu-lated individually. Thus, even though bilabial closure was shown in kinematic observations to rely most heavily on mandibular elevation (i.e. with the mandible essentially 'carrying' the lower lip to the point of closure; Fig. 8.3), there is significant, task-specific, independent labial muscle activity observed throughout periods of speech and vocalization in 2 year olds. This level of differentiated activ-ity across articulators is especially significant with respect to the potential degrees of freedom afforded by this system and, conversely, with respect to the range of controlled movement parameters that is apparent. With reference to the burgeon-ing phonetic inventory of the typically developing 2 year old, it may be reasoned that the emergence of independent upper and lower lip movement supports, or even allows, production of phonemes requiring this facility.

8.3.2 Studies of phonatory and respiratory movement

The development of phonation for speech vocalization is observed in changes in respiratory support as well as in control of specific parameters of voice (e.g. onset, offset, fundamental frequency and intensity modulation). As voicing is quite obvi-ously present at birth for typical infants, developmental investigations can focus on the changing characteristics of voicing throughout infancy. Parameters of interest have included fundamental frequency (f_0) characteristics (e.g. range, mean, variability), f_0 contour shapes (Fernald and Kuhl 1987), voice onset time, and voicing duration and intensity (Smith and Kenney 1998). These studies, though primarily descriptive, provide a basis for estimating the phonatory control capacities of the infant. Similarly, respiratory kinematics have been described in detail in a large group of infants and toddlers by Boliek *et al.* (1996, 1997). These highly detailed investigations provide a description of the variation in respiratory drive associated with production of the full range of an infant's vocal capabilities. We have sought to combine these observational domains, quantifying modulation of f_0 and vocal intensity with respect to changes in respiratory kinematics.

Inferring the underlying control structures for modulation of phonation requires descriptive methods with temporal resolution that approximates the modulation seen in the corresponding vocal output. These methodological requirements far exceed the resolution offered by such measures as peak f_0 or end expiratory levels, which carry a single value as representing a behavior lasting as long as 10 s or more. Rather, we have sought to develop methods by which momentary changes in respiratory drive can be registered with concomitant changes in phonatory intensity and f_0. Figure 8.4 illustrates the first stage in the comparison of adults and 6-month-old children during vocalization. This figure includes the averaged respiratory kinematic records for 10 infants and 13 adults during rest breathing (left panels) and vocalization (right panels). Within each panel, each horizontal band represents the averaged data for one subject (e.g. the yellow band at the bottom of the lower left panel represents the time-normalized average of all inspiratory phases during rest breathing for one subject; that subject's expiratory phase is shown as the blue continuation of the bottom horizontal bar). Inspiratory and expiratory phases are shown to the left and right respectively of the center dividing line in each of the four panels. All records have been time-normalized to the mean duration for each phase, task, and subject group (e.g. the left side of the upper left panel is time-normalized to the mean duration for the inspiratory phase of rest breathing by all 6 month olds), which served to emphasize relative changes within each phase of respiratory behavior. The colors of the bands represent the relative phase of the changes in ribcage and abdomen over time (following phase angles described by Hoit and Hixon 1986). The color key shown in the upper right corner of the figure is oriented according to the motion–motion plots typical of graphics of respiratory kinematics. Rib-cage expansion is represented by vertical increases; abdominal expansion is represented by increases toward the right. Translation of the angles associated with combined displacement is shown with colors toward the vertical (i.e. red and magenta) being associated with rib-cage changes, upward (red) being expansive, downward (magenta) being compressive. Similarly, colors toward the horizontal (cyan and green) represent changes in abdominal circumference with leftward (cyan) being compressive and rightward (green) being expansive. Colors on the rising diagonal (blue and yellow) reflect equally balanced compression (blue) or expansion (yellow) of the ribcage and abdomen; colors on the falling diagonal (white and gray) reflect paradoxing with either the ribcage expanding (white) or the abdomen expanding (gray).

As might be expected, Fig. 8.4 shows that rest breathing and speech breathing in adults are heavily dominated by ribcage expansion and compression. Infants show much greater variability both within and across subjects. Generalizations of belly-breathing (i.e. predominance of abdominal displacement) or rib-cage dominance are unwarranted by these data. Nevertheless, each infant appears to use a single breathing pattern for speech and rest breathing. For example, the bottom three bands in each of the top two panels are for three subjects who exhibited a predominance of abdominal displacement for expiration and inspiration, and for speech and rest breathing. Adults, even with a greatly shortened inspiratory phase for speech breathing, still rely predominantly on rib cage displacement. These results might be somewhat unexpected, given the consistent findings among the articulators that speech exhibits coordinative differences that are distinct from other behaviors. Analyses of respiratory kinematics have consistently revealed across-subject variability that is significantly larger than within-subject, across-task vari-

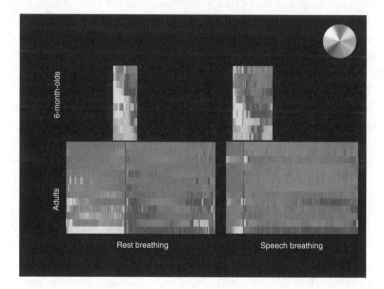

Fig. 8.4 Graphic comparisons of rest breathing and speech breathing in 6-month-old infants and adults. Relative durations are shown for inspiratory and expiratory phases, and for adult versus infant productions. Compared with rest breathing by infants, rest breathing by adults was much longer in inspiratory and expiratory duration, and vocalization by infants or adults exhibited a much longer expiratory phase. Adults were seen to rely heavily on rib-cage displacement (indicated by the predominance of red in the inspiratory phase and magenta in the expiratory phase), whereas infants were more variable across subjects, with some children showing a predominance of abdominal displacement (green in the inspiratory phase, cyan in the expiratory phase). See also in colour, Plate 5.

ability, suggesting that individual factors outweigh task demands. Ongoing analyses of these data are focused on evaluating the statistical strength of these observations that respiratory kinematics are determined less by task-specific adjustments (e.g. speech versus rest breathing) than by individual differences. Additional observations have shown subject-specific kinematic characteristics for production of lexical stress. Current efforts are focused on quantifying these adjustments and correlating them across systems to identify the physiologic mechanisms underlying short- and long-term speech modulation.

8.3.3 Studies of timing across systems

In the hierarchy of investigation of speech development, the next level that remains relatively unexplored is the coordination of activity across systems (i.e. spatiotemporal relationships among the respiratory, phonatory, and articulatory systems). Development of cross-system coordination for speech production is especially intriguing as the uniqueness of speech production is most evident in the timing of events across systems; comparable demands across the involved structures are not as apparent as in the consideration of isolated structures. For example, coordination of lip and jaw movement has been discussed in the context of extant behaviors such as chewing and sucking, and speech phonation has been described with reference to other types of vocalization such as cry and cooing. However, the demands of speech are uniquely manifest in such sequences as in the generation of appropriate voice onset time: closure of the velopharyngeal port, graded expiratory pressure, adduction of the vocal folds, compression and plosive release of the lips, and depression of the mandible. Sequences such as this entail graded, timed output from each speech system. Recent technical and analytic capabilities have made these descriptions and comparisons feasible even in very young children.

Figure 8.5 illustrates the multidimensional data stream for production of /ba'ba/ by a 6-year-old child. The audio signal (top trace) and the extracted f_0 contour (second trace from top) are consistent with observations of adult stress production. The lips appear to move synchronously in opposition to each other, and lead the movement of the mandible quite substantially in achieving oral closure for the second /b/ in this token. Fundamental frequency modulation does not appear to follow respiratory drive, which is a more likely possibility in much younger children. These records can be combined across repetitions, conditions, and speakers to yield more general properties of development. High temporal resolution indications of respiratory dynamics can be seen in the bottom bar, which indicates that for this token, the subject performed an isovolume adjustment prior to voice initiation (i.e. indicated by the white portion of the bar at the far left), possibly to adjust his respiratory posture to a configuration more appropriate to speech initiation and production. Observations such as these will help to elucidate the coordinative properties across systems and across observational domains in developing speech.

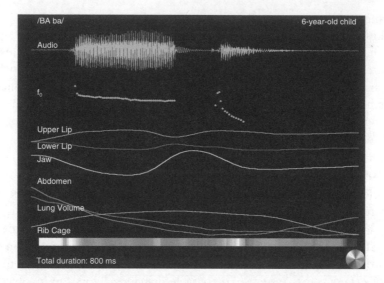

Fig. 8.5 Multidimensional observation of speech production by a 6-year-old child. From top to bottom, waveforms include: the child's audio, the extracted vocal fundamental frequency, position of the upper lip (orange), lower lip (red), and jaw (yellow), abdominal circumference (green), derived lung volume (blue), rib cage circumference (light green), and a graphic representation of relative motion of the rib cage and abdomen. See also in colour, Plate 6.

Multidimensional analyses of speech production have helped to obviate some of the problems of more focused observations. One pervasive difficulty has been the *level of analysis* problem, which is not unique to speech research, but has been especially challenging (Stetson 1951; Stetson *et al.* 1988). Analysis at one level of observation weakly predicts observations at another level (e.g. acoustic output is not isomorphic with vocal-tract configuration or muscle activation pattern), even though, paradoxically, processes at one level are causal for behaviors at other levels (e.g. vocal-tract shape is deterministic for acoustic output). Observations of speech development across domains are intended to provide a means for formalizing these complex relationships in a model of speech acquisition.

Multidimensional observations also provide a methodology for evaluating speech production relative to complex behaviors in other species. For example, the rich framework provided by animal models of vocalization offers another specific motivation for studying speech development across systems. Unlike other applications of animal models to speech development (e.g. mastication, swallowing, ventilation), nonhuman vocalization systems can be conceptually extended almost directly to speech vocalization. The parameters of vocalization—duration, intensity, fundamental frequency modulation, offset/onset—can be seen in both speech and nonspeech productions. Nonspeech vocalization by nonhuman primates, the neural circuitry of which has been studied and mapped (Jürgens 1995), includes most of the elements that are similarly modulated for speech vocalizations by

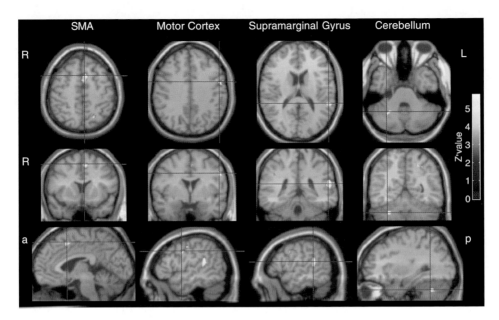

Plate 1 Auditory verbal imagery (silent recitation of a highly overlearned word string): fMRI activation maps superimposed on the averaged T_1-weighted anatomical images (Talairach space) across subjects at the level of the supplementary motor area (SMA), motor cortex, temporoparietal junction, and cerebellum (upper row, transverse; middle row, coronal; lower row, sagittal slices). (Fig. 4.2 in text.)

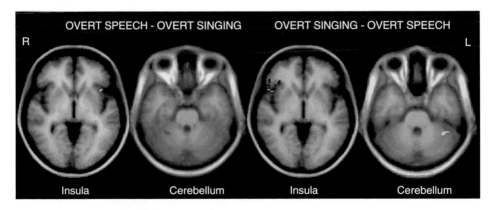

Plate 2 Hemodynamic activation patterns at the level of the anterior insula during recitation of a highly overlearned word string (speaking) and reproduction of a non-lyrical tune (singing): cognitive subtraction approach (overt versus covert speaking, overt versus covert singing). (Fig. 4.3 in text.)

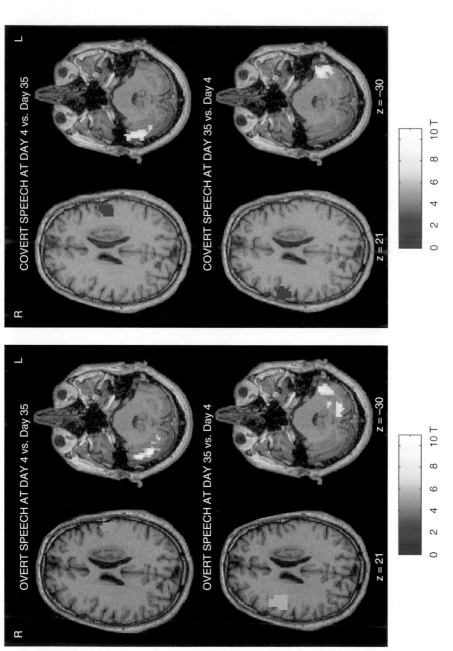

Plate 3 Follow-up of fMRI activation patterns during recovery of articulatory functions in a case of capsular dysarthria: Temporal subtraction analysis (measurements obtained during day 4 versus day 35 and vice versa) during overt and covert speech production. Significant hemodynamic responses within motor cortex and cerebellum are superimposed on transverse sections of the anatomical reference images (left half of a slice = right hemisphere and vice versa. z = distance to intercommisural plane, SPM99: T > 4.70, P < 0.05 corrected). (Fig. 4.4 in text.)

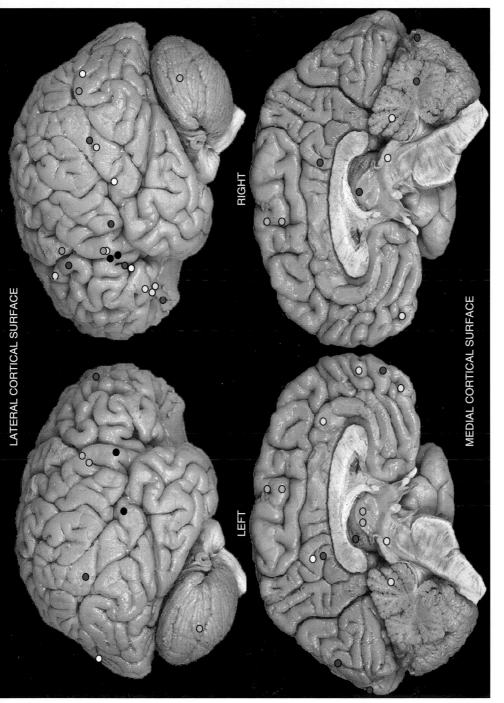

Plate 4 Localizations of reported peak activation and deactivation in four published functional imaging studies, comparing natural (non-modified) overt speech of stuttering and non-stuttering adults. Localization of activations was determined based on reported stereotactic coordinates or Brodmann areas. Peak activation coding: yellow, Braun *et al.* (1997); red, De Nil *et al.* (2000); pink, Fox *et al.* (1996). Peak deactivation coding: green, Braun *et al.* (1997); white, De Nil *et al.* (2000); light blue, Fox *et al.* (1996); dark blue, Wu *et al.* (1995). (Fig. 5.1 in text.)

LATERAL CORTICAL SURFACE

MEDIAL CORTICAL SURFACE

RIGHT

LEFT

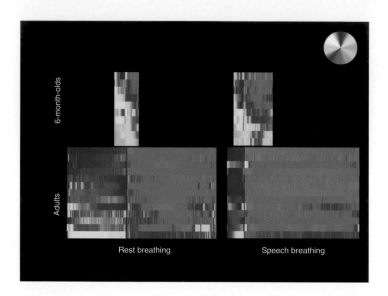

Plate 5 Graphic comparisons of rest breathing and speech breathing in 6-month-old infants and adults. Relative durations are shown for inspiratory and expiratory phases, and for adult versus infant productions. Compared with rest breathing by infants, rest breathing by adults was much longer in inspiratory and expiratory duration, and vocalization by infants or adults exhibited a much longer expiratory phase. Adults were seen to rely heavily on rib-cage displacement (indicated by the predominance of red in the inspiratory phase and magenta in the expiratory phase), whereas infants were more variable across subjects, with some children showing a predominance of abdominal displacement (green in the inspiratory phase, cyan in the expiratory phase). (Fig. 8.4 in text.)

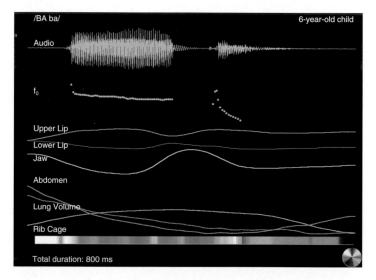

Plate 6 Multidimensional observation of speech production by a 6-year-old child. From top to bottom, waveforms include: the child's audio, the extracted vocal fundamental frequency, position of the upper lip (orange), lower lip (red), and jaw (yellow), abdominal circumference (green), derived lung volume (blue), rib cage circumference (light green), and a graphic representation of relative motion of the rib cage and abdomen. (Fig. 8.5 in text.)

humans: expiratory force, laryngeal adduction, dilation of the supraglottal spaces, and positioning of supraglottal articulators (i.e. lips, tongue, jaw, velopharynx). From both developmental and evolutionary perspectives, it is important to evaluate the neurophysiologic redundancy of these various behaviors.

8.4 Studies of populations with speech disorders

Speech disorders present a clear opportunity to identify the limitations and capacities, the vulnerabilities and stabilities, and the antecedents and mature abilities, of speech motor control. Are there physiologic factors that predispose some speech sounds to developmental delay or to disruption secondary to neuropathology? How do phonological encoding and motor planning interact with the physiologic capacities of the motor control system? Prior observations of adults with Parkinson's syndrome have shown that electromyographic measures can distinguish subclinical disruptions of speech coordination that persist following effective treatment of dysarthria (Moore and Scudder 1989). This investigation of adults with dysarthria demonstrated markedly aberrant muscle activation patters underlying speech production (e.g. tonic activation of one muscle coincident with phasic activation of its contralateral homologous muscle) that was completely intelligible and perceptually only mildly disrupted. These findings suggest that the mature speech motor control system has remarkable compensatory capacities, redundant means to generate a given acoustic target, and the ability to redistribute movement patterns across differentially impaired systems.

While the 'ubiquitous variability' (MacNeilage 1970) of speech, and the capacity of speech production systems to exhibit motor equivalence (Hebb 1949; Hughes and Abbs 1976) are well known in mature, and even disordered, systems, the appearance of these characteristics in children is unknown. One plausible hypothesis is that children rely on movement templates initially, gradually introducing meaningful variations in these templates to produce an expanding phonetic and lexical repertoire. In fact, our initial observations would suggest that variability among very young children is resultant primarily from unsystematic error rather than from any sort of trading relationship among articulators. Thus, the hallmark variability of mature speech production may be a very different phenomenon in young children. This question awaits empirical study. These studies capitalize not only on the predictable ways in which systems break down, but also on the observation that disruption reveals not only intrinsic weaknesses in the system, but also brings other organizational characteristics to an observable level.

Another aspect of developmental speech impairment that frequently receives attention is the consideration of whether impairment represents a simple delay of the typical acquisition process or an aberration of typical development. We are continuing to amass observations supporting the idea that idiopathic speech delay is not a simple delay of a typical process; rather, observations of these systems

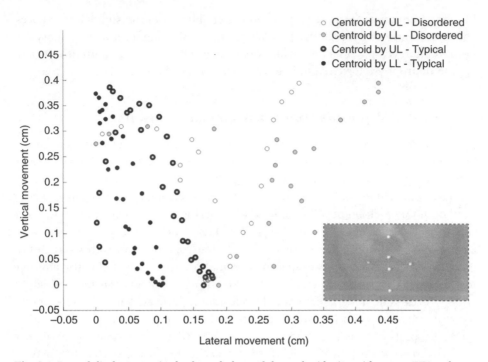

Fig. 8.6 Lateral displacement in the frontal plane of the oral midpoint with upper (UL) or lower lip (LL) position. The midpoint was defined as the intersection of the lines connecting the lateral markers and the vertical lip markers. Whereas the upper and lower lip movements of the typically developing child (darker points) are seen to remain with 2 mm of the midline, those of the child with articulatory impairment (lighter points) deviate as much as 4.5 mm from midline. The inset photograph shows the positions of the lip markers at the corners and midlines of the lips, as well as the nose marker (used for calibration) and the mandibular marker (not included in these analyses).

demonstrate aberrant patterns across the systems observed. For example, Fig. 8.6 provides an example of atypical lip movement obtained during an opening–closing gesture by a 6-year-old child with moderate articulatory impairment. The lateral deviation of the oral centroid by this child, though subclinical with respect to speech impairment, was quite atypical and might reasonably be taken as a positive clinical finding for disrupted speech motor control. These observational methods are currently being extended to children recovering from traumatic brain injury and to young children with nonspecific speech delay.

8.5 Discussion

Research into the physiologic development of speech production continues to yield a range of consistent findings that will help to guide future research and applications. The development of speech production does not appear to follow a continuous, monotonic progression from infancy to adulthood, but rather is seen to exhibit intermediate discontinuities in the developing coordinative relationships among articulators. These discontinuities are consistent with a dynamic systems perspective, although to be useful, the sources of contextual determinants of stabilities and instabilities must be identified among a large field of potential influences. For example, the dominance of the mandible in generating early appearing articulatory movements is well supported by the current results and by numerous empirical and anecdotal observations. This role is subsequently augmented by the emerging independent movements of the upper and lower lips (and probably the tongue), though the mandible persists as the primary articulator for oral closure. Initially, movement of the lips appears to be a consequence of mandibular movement, with the jaw 'carrying' the lower lip and 'pushing' the upper lip upward in creating oral closure. Such a system presents the stability afforded by the jaw's bilaterally hinged joint, a proportionately large mass, and biomechanical coupling to the tongue and lips, such that movement of the entire system can be generated by control of this single articulator. The potential phonetic limitations associated with this gross level of control become more apparent as the child's lexicon expands, requiring the dissociation of lip and tongue movement from that of the mandible.

The consistent finding of task-specific differences across articulators and across the ages studied suggests that speech emerges from a motor control structure that is unique among oral motor behaviors, and that speech development is not a consequence of earlier appearing nonspeech behaviors. This suggestion immediately brings into question theories and treatments based on the assumption that speech emerges from earlier appearing behaviors. The hypotheses that infants capitalize on extant coordinative organization to generate new behaviors (e.g. adapting the motor organization of chewing and sucking to babbling) is not supported by these physiologic findings. However, these opposing views can be reconciled by noting that most early appearing oral motor behaviors rely most significantly on jaw movement, yielding grossly similar movements, but having significantly different muscle activation patterns and kinematic characteristics. For example, large, multilanguage inventories of phonetic propensities and developmental tendencies in consonant-vowel combinations suggest a biological influence on lexical and phonetic acquisition (MacNeilage and Davis 2000). This influence has been purported to be derived from ingestive cyclicities, such as chewing, but might also simply reflect parallel, but separate, effects of the dominance of mandibular movement in each of these tasks. The weight of the current findings suggests that this shared primacy of mandibular movement in speech and nonspeech tasks is nonetheless imposed by different coordinative mechanisms. This determination further supports a representation of developing speech as arising as a distinct, separable behavior.

Future investigations will extend these observations to larger populations of typical speakers and to speakers with disordered speech. A sample of 260 young children with nonspecific speech impairment and 40 typically developing 4 year olds is currently being acquired. One objective of this current investigation is to map the range of ways in which speech development can be disrupted. A similar investigation is under way to evaluate the impairment and the recovery path for speech in children who have suffered traumatic brain injury. This expanding framework of physiologic development of speech production and related behaviors will provide a context in which to understand the mechanisms underlying typical and impaired speech.

Acknowledgments

The work cited here was supported by grants from the National Institutes of Health, National Institute on Deafness and Other Communication Disorders (R01 DC00822), the University of Pittsburgh, and the University of Washington. The author gratefully acknowledges the invaluable assistance of Kathryn Connaghan, Jordan Green, Kevin Reilly, and Roger Steeve.

References

Bellingham, M.C. (1998). Driving respiration: The respiratory central pattern generator. *Clinical and Experimental Pharmacology and Physiology, 25,* 847–856.

Boliek, C.A., Hixon, T.J., Watson, P.J., and **Morgan, W.J.** (1996). Vocalization and breathing during the first year of life. *Journal of Voice, 10,* 1–22.

Boliek, C.A., Hixon, T.J., Watson, P.J., and **Morgan, W.J.** (1997). Vocalization and breathing during the second and third years of life. *Journal of Voice, 11,* 373–390.

Chumpelik (Hayden), D. (1984). The PROMPT system of therapy: Theoretical framework and applications for developmental apraxia of speech. *Seminars in Speech and Language, 5,* 139–156.

Darley, F.L., Aronson, A.E., and **Brown, J.R.** (1975). *Motor Speech Disorders.* W.B. Saunders, Philadelphia.

Fernald, A. and **Kuhl, P.K.** (1987). Acoustic determinants of infant preference for motherese speech. *Infant Behavior and Development, 10,* 279–293.

Green, J.R., Moore, C.A., Ruark, J.L., Rodda, P.R., Morvée, W.T., and **VanWitzenburg, M.J.** (1997). Development of chewing in children from 12 to 48 months: Longitudinal study of EMG patterns. *Journal of Neurophysiology, 77,* 2704–2716.

Green, J.R., Moore, C.A., Higashikawa, M., and **Steeve, R.W.** (2000). The physiologic development of speech motor control: Lip and jaw coordination. *Journal of Speech, Language, and Hearing Research, 43,* 239–255.

Green, J.R., Moore, C.A., and **Reilly, K.J.** (2002). The sequential development of lip and jaw control for speech. *Journal of Speech, Language, and Hearing Research, 45,* 66–79.

Grillner, S. (1981). Possible analogies in the control of innate motor acts and the production of sound in speech. In S. Grillner, B. Lindblom, J. Lubker, and A. person (Eds.), *Speech motor control* (pp. 217–230). Pergamon Press, New York.

Hoit, J. and **Hixon, T.J.** (1986). Body type and speech breathing. *Journal of Speech and Hearing Research, 29,* 313–324.

Hughes, O. and **Abbs, J.H.** (1976). Labial–mandibular coordination in the production of speech: Implication for the operation of motor equivalence. *Phonetica, 33,* 199–221.

Kelso, J.A.S. and **Munhall, K.G.** (Eds.) (1988). *R.H. Stetson's Motor Phonetics: A retrospective edition.* College-Hill/Little, Brown and Co., Boston.

Jürgens, U. (1995). Neuronal control of vocalization in non-human and human primates. In E. Zimmerman, J.D. Newman, and U. Jürgens (Eds.), *Current topics in primate vocal communication,* pp. 199–206. New York: Plenum.

Luschei, E.S. and **Goldberg, L.J.** (1981). Neural mechanisms of mandibular control: Mastication and voluntary biting. In V.B. Brooks (Ed.), *Handbook of physiology— section I: The nervous system, volume II, motor control* (pp. 1237–1274). American Physiological Society, Bethesda, MD.

MacNeilage, P.F. (1970). Motor control of serial ordering of speech. *Psychological Review, 77,* 182–196.

MacNeilage, P.F. and **Davis, B.** (2000). On the origin of internal structure of word forms. *Science, 288,* 527–531.

Moore, C.A. (1993). Symmetry of mandibular muscle activity as an index of coordinative strategy. *Journal of Speech and Hearing Research, 36,* 1145–1157.

Moore, C.A. and **Ruark, J.L.** (1996). Does speech emerge from earlier appearing motor behaviors? *Journal of Speech and Hearing Research, 39,* 1034–1047.

Moore, C.A. and **Scudder, R.R.** (1989). Coordination of jaw muscle activity in parkinsonian movement: Description and response to traditional treatment. In: K. Yorkston and D. Beukelman (Eds.), *Clinical dysarthria.* College-Hill: Boston.

Moore, C.A., Smith, A., and **Ringel, R.L.** (1988). Task-specific organization of activity in human jaw muscles. *Journal of Speech and Hearing Research, 31,* 670–680.

Moore, C.A., Cohn, J.F., and **Katz, G.S.** (1994). Quantitative description and differentiation of fundamental frequency (f_o) contours. *Computer Speech and Language, 8,* 385–4044.

Moore, C.A., Caulfield, T.J., and **Green, J.R.** (2001). Relative kinematics of the rib cage and abdomen during speech and nonspeech behaviors by 15-month-old children. *Journal of Speech, Language, and Hearing Research, 44,* 80–94.

Ruark, J.L. and **Moore, C.A.** (1997). Coordination of lip muscle activity by two-year-old children during speech and nonspeech tasks. *Journal of Speech, Language, and Hearing Research, 40,* 1373–1385.

Stetson, R.H. (1951). *Motor Phonetics,* North Holland, Amsterdam.

CHAPTER 9

SENSORIMOTOR ENTRAINMENT OF RESPIRATORY AND OROFACIAL SYSTEMS IN HUMANS

STEVEN M. BARLOW, DONALD S. FINAN, AND
SO-YOUNG PARK

9.1 Introduction

The motor system is regarded as part of the infrastructure of the body, enabling the organism to locomote, feed, fly, respire, and, in humans, produce speech. The assembly of the neuronal machinery in a number of animal species has shown that motor behavior evolves from dynamic changes that take place at the molecular, cellular, and network level (Grillner 2001). Some motor behaviors are mediated by central neuronal circuits known as central pattern generators (CPGs). Numerous CPGs have been analyzed, and it is clear that a wide variety of cellular, synaptic, and network properties are involved in modulating the output characteristics of these local networks (Pearson and Gordon 2000).

There are notable challenges facing scientists interested in exploring mechanisms of sensorimotor integration among pattern-generating networks (Rossignol *et al.* 1988). The first is the issue of experimental accessibility of the neuronal network. Jeffrey Smith and colleagues have developed an elegant *in vitro* brain slice preparation from the ventrolateral medulla of the rat brainstem. Using whole-cell patch–clamp recording techniques, they have been able to isolate and study the respiratory pattern generator located in the pre-Bötzinger complex (Smith *et al.* 1991, 1992; Butera, *et al.* 1999; Koshiya and Smith 1999). An additional concern is persistence of motor network activity, and, finally, conservation of proprioceptive and mechanoreceptor feedback pathways vital to the operation of the pattern-generating neuronal circuits.

Three basic forms of neural circuits that produce patterned output have been identified (Westberg *et al.* 1998). *Dedicated circuits* generate only one pattern and, when triggered by sensory input, may suppress other ongoing behaviors. *Distributed circuits* consist of a single population of neurons to pattern all variations in the pattern of movement. For example, neurons in primate motor cortex that control the shoulder muscles seem to perform as a distributed circuit during arm reaching. Each fires maximally during movement in a particular direction. A population response vector reflecting the composite neuronal response determines the trajectory of the arm (Georgopoulos *et al.* 1988; Kalaska and Crammond 1992). *Reorganizing circuits* generate different patterns when the effectiveness of synaptic connections between members of the total population of neurons changes. The key feature of this form is that some neurons do not take part in the full repertory of behaviors generated by the whole population.

There are a number of features that characterize CPGs. They are primarily composed of *interneurons* that act or direct output to lower motor neurons. These internuncial circuits are found in the cerebral cortex, brainstem, and spinal cord. CPGs *develop* and *change* with ontogenesis. The locomotor CPG in mouse has been well documented in this regard. At embryonic stage E12–E14, the mouse locomotor CPG produces bilateral synchronous inputs to lower motor neurons (LMNs) (Branchereau *et al.* 2000). As crossed inhibitory neurons are added to the basic CPG locomotor circuit during E15–17, the alternating pattern of limb muscle activation among ipsilateral and contralateral structures becomes apparent until the mature form is stabilized at E18–P2, manifesting reciprocal activation between ipsilateral and contralateral muscle systems. *Experience* plays a significant role in modulating sensory mechanisms that impinge on CPGs. Moreover, there are several potent mechanisms that serve to modify the structure and function and modulate the activity patterns of CPGs. *Descending inputs* from the primary somatosensory cortex (SI) play a part in modulating the mastication CPG (Lin *et al.* 1998).

For some CPGs a rhythmic motor pattern can be produced in the absence of any sensory feedback (Delcomyn 1980). However, the majority of reports in the literature clearly indicate that modulation of sensory input and changes in task dynamics lead to dynamic reassembly of the neuronal networks that compose the CPG, thus producing new forms. An excellent example has been observed in the lobster, in which changes in the activity patterns of a single mechanoreceptor located in the lobster gastric mill will fractionate CPG outputs (Combes *et al.* 1999), generating two distinct motor patterns. Centrally generated motor patterns in mammals can be strongly influenced by phasic signals from peripheral receptors (Rossignol *et al.*, 1988). These sensory signals are important for normal motor patterning in intact behaving animals and they contribute to the generation and maintenance of rhythmic activity. Phasic sensory signals also initiate major phase transitions in intact motor systems. For example, in the mammalian respiratory system, elongation of pulmonary stretch receptors and diaphragmatic proprioceptors contribute to the termination of the inspiratory phase of the Hering–Breuer reflex (Speck *et al.* 1993). Sensory signals serve to regulate the magnitude of ongoing motor activity and dynamically adjust the sensitivity of somatic reflexes, thereby providing an adaptive and flexible neural substrate with changes in task dynamics and environmental conditions. As will be shown later in this report, phasic sensory inputs can produce entrainment responses to an already active human suck CPG.

Qualitative changes in neurotransmitter types and concentration levels among neuromodulators can have profound effects on the operational dynamics of a CPG. A clever set of experiments in the crab has demonstrated systematic fractionation of pyloric CPGs with changes in neuromodulator type as well as neuromodulator concentration levels. Neuromodulatory substances can alter the cellular and synaptic properties of neurons in CPG pathways (Swensen and Marder 2001) to regulate phase switching, reflex reversal, and reflex gain. For the respiratory CPG circuitry, serotonin, cholecystokinin, somatostatin, acetylcholine (ACh), endorphins, substance P, and thyrotropin-releasing hormone (TRH) have been shown to affect the membrane properties of neurons located within the nucleus tractus solitarius. Dopamine can modify the sensitivity of peripheral chemoreceptors. Moreover, afferent feedback can reconfigure the function of a CPG and even recruit additional neurons into the system generating the motor pattern.

There are a variety of sensorimotor processes that either drive or provide evidence of this elaboration in structure and function of central neural networks capable of patterned output. Entrainment is one such phenomenon, defined as the synchronization of an endogenous oscillator to external periodic events (Pavlidis 1973; Glass and Mackey 1988; Kriellaars *et al.* 1994). For a given stimulus with fixed amplitude and period, a stable phase relationship between the stimulus and oscillator must exist to satisfy the conditions for entrainment. One such endogenous oscillator in the human neonate is the non-nutritive suck rhythm generator and the associated motor output. An external periodic event representing a periodic orofacial input, and considered in detail in the present chapter, is the pulsating surface of a pneumatically controlled pacifier baglet (nipple). The ability of an oscillator to synchronize to an external periodic signal provides adaptive and predictive control that allows fast and reliable responses to external changes (Pavlidis 1973). This type of control would aid in adapting the suck rate set by higher brain centers to variations in pacifier compliance and physical characteristics. The ability of a peripheral signal to entrain suck requires an integration of those signals into the suck rhythm generating circuitry. Entrainment techniques have been effective in a variety of animal preparations to regulate and modify the rhythm of central pattern generators involved in the control of cyclic motor behaviors such as stepping and locomotion (Conway *et al.* 1987; Pearson *et al.* 1992; Pearson 2000), and mastication (Rossignol *et al.* 1988). Stimulation of intraoral tissues is also effective in modulating the masticatory cycle in humans (Hannam and Lund 1981).

Entrainment in the chest wall implies a resetting of the respiratory rhythm such that a fixed temporal relationship exists between the onset of the inspiratory activity and the onset of the mechanical breath. Mechanical ventilation of the human chest wall produces respiratory entrainment, especially during a wakeful state

(Baconnier *et al.* 1993; Simon *et al.* 1999, 2000). In another study, respiratory–abdominal movements were recorded while neonates (*n* = 18) were manually rocked at varying rates between 30 and 60 cycles per minute (Sammon and Darnall 1994). Coherence analysis between respiratory movements and rocker signals demonstrated strong entrainment to rocking (coherence spectra >0.85). Natural stimulation associated with rocking a newborn provides a phasic input to its respiratory pattern generator that is capable of resetting the system's oscillation and entraining its rhythm (Sammon and Darnall 1994). Infants >35 weeks post-conceptional age exhibited greater coherence to rocking than infants <35 weeks.

Medullary respiratory pattern generators (mRGs) can be driven by periodic electrical stimulation to the ventral part of the spinal grey at the C5 level in newborn rats (Dubayle and Viala 1996). These authors developed phase–response curves to determine the parameters of phase resetting for predicting the limits of a stable 1:1 harmonic entrainment. The authors concluded that ascending neural connections from the C5 segment of the spinal cord in rat might be involved in locomotor–respiratory coupling.

Another line of study that has shown the potency of entraining inputs involves a 'breathing' teddy bear (BrBr), which provides an irregularly breathing neonate with a source of optional rhythmic stimulation (Ingersoll and Thoman 1994). At post conceptual age 33 weeks (CA), 19 premature infants were given a BrBr and 17 premature infants were given a nonbreathing bear to serve as a control. Respiratory patterning was sampled at 35 and 45 weeks in both groups. BrBr babies showed significantly more quiet sleep, less active sleep, and increased respiratory regularity. The authors suggested that BrBr entrainment facilitates neurobehavioral development of one of the infant's own biological rhythms. This study also demonstrated clearly that a premature infant with an irregular oscillator will entrain to that of a breathing bear (a regular oscillator, or *zeitgeber*) under the conditions that the BrBr's rate of breathing reflects that of the individual infant.

In the context of neonatal oromotor control, the development and application of an entrainment paradigm suitable for reorganizing a disordered motor control system is appealing. In neonatal guinea-pigs, the CPG for sucking is located in the periaqueductal gray of the brainstem and is thought to be regulated in part by a neocortical region known as the cortical sucking area (CSA) (Nozaki *et al.* 1986; Iriki *et al.* 1988). The use of 'natural' forms of stimulation is preferred to preserve the physiologic nature of recruitment pattern in the hopes of synthesizing a sensory experience that can be reinforced through motor learning. The application of entrainment as a habilitation strategy, utilizing natural mechanical stimulation, has ecological validity in assisting the infant to produce an appropriate motor output. Moreover, this approach is consistent with contemporary ideas on the role of sensory-driven neural activity (Penn and Shatz 1999) and Bosma's (1970) contention that appropriate oral experiences may be critical in the final weeks of gestation in the formation of functional central neural circuits. Use of a mechanical entrainment stimulus also has the distinct advantage of being safe and comfortable for the neonate.

9.2 The actifier and orofacial stimulation

Our research team has developed a new instrument and paradigm for studies of oromotor entrainment and electrophysiological recordings of perioral sensorimotor integration during non-nutritive sucking in preterm and term neonates and infants. Known as the actifier (Finan and Barlow 1996), the design consists of an array of linear servo motors interfaced to the housing of a pacifier equipped with eight miniature Ag/AgCl surface electrodes (Fig. 9.1). This electrode array allows noninvasive sampling of four EMG channels from muscle sites around the oral opening. The linear motors are strategically located for independent stimulation of the upper and lower lip margin. An additional linear motor is pneumatically coupled to the baglet (nipple) via polyethylene tubing. This allows the shape and intraluminal pressure of the baglet to be modulated dynamically by an external controller (digital computer). Based on our experience with non-nutritive suck

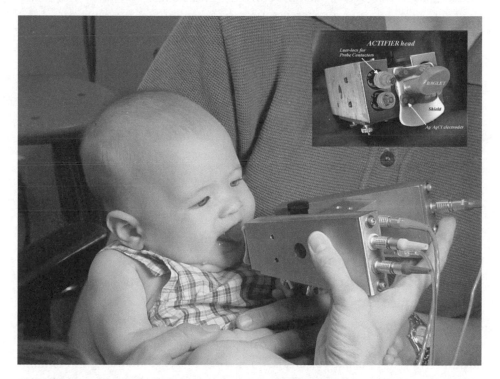

Fig. 9.1 Orientation of the actifier to an attentive infant. The inset figure shows the oral surface of the actifier unit, including the electrode array, pneumatically coupled baglet, and cutaneous probe contactor extending from one of the servo-controlled linear motors.

dynamics in healthy term infants, we have been able to digitally synthesize control (input) signals to drive the baglet and produce a spectrally salient mechanical stimulus that produces 1:1 oromotor entrainment during non-nutritive suck. This control feature essentially transforms the pacifier into an active orofacial stimulator, thus the term actifier. The electromechanical system of the pneumatically coupled linear motor and baglet yields a nearly flat frequency response from DC–20 Hz with a pure time delay (~8 ms) through the pass band. This is adequate to satisfy the spectral dynamics of the non-nutritive suck that is concentrated from DC–4 Hz.

Recent studies (Finan and Barlow 1996, 1998; Barlow *et al.* 1997, 2001; Barlow 1998; Finan 1998) demonstrated the range of possibilities of the entrainment and reflex modulation paradigm in awake neonates using the actifier. Thus far, the actifier has been used to investigate the responsiveness of the suck CPG to cyclic mechanical stimulation of the intraoral and perioral mechanoreceptors in 15 term human neonates.

An excellent example of 1:1 entrainment is shown in Fig. 9.2. The data were sampled from a 3-week-old baby girl. The sequence of signals includes integrated electromyograms (IEMGs) from the left and right divisions of the orbicularis oris inferior, jaw strain gage, intraluminal pressure of the baglet (nipple), linear motor shaft displacement, and a coherence suck cycle period plot, to demonstrate the degree of mechanically induced entrainment. As shown, jaw movements and lip EMGs became synchronized to the entraining input signal throughout the duration of the stimulus burst. The neonate modified her suck cycle period from 500–600 ms to the 400 ms period of the entraining input for the duration of the stimulus. These findings provide positive evidence that the temporal characteristics of the suck CPG can be modified by afferent feedback. The fact that phase entrainment was achieved quickly over a time period as short as a single suck cycle is evidence of strong oscillator coupling to the external mechanical input provided by the actifier (Zacksenhouse 2001). The richness of the somatic sensory experience offered by the dynamic baglet of the actifier affords some exciting possibilities for the habilitation of an aberrant suck pattern generator.

9.3 Orofacial entrainment and phase-dependent mechanosensory modulation of non-nutritive sucking in human infants

Finan (1998) used a synthesis technique to deliver a rhythmic mechanical stimulus train (2.5 Hz AC-coupled square wave, 4 s in duration) during non-nutritive sucking (NNS) to 16 babies (mean age = 1 month, 28 days), producing 155 entrainment stimulation burst trials. To evaluate potential entrainment responses to stimulation, Finan (1998) constructed frequency ratio/phase polar plots for all stimulated NNS bursts with more than 2 cycles concurrent with stimulation (*n* = 145 bursts), following procedures outlined in Kriellaars *et al.* (1994). Briefly,

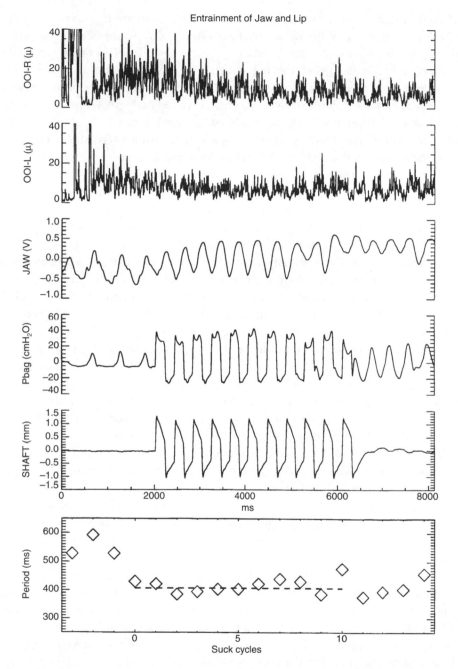

Fig. 9.2 An example of 1:1 non-nutritive suck entrainment to an externally delivered mechanical signal delivered through a pacifier baglet. The data were sampled from a 3-week-old baby girl. The sequence of signals includes IEMGs from the left and right divisions of the orbicularis oris inferior, jaw strain gage, intraluminal pressure of the baglet (nipple), linear motor shaft displacement, and a coherence suck cycle period plot, to demonstrate the degree of mechanically induced entrainment (adapted from Finan and Barlow, 1996).

a frequency ratio was calculated for each NNS cycle concurrent with the stimulus waveform, consisting of the period of the NNS cycle (in ms) divided by the period of the stimulus waveform. The resultant quotient was multiplied by 100 to obtain a percentage. Angular phase (polar plot azimuth) was defined as the start of the NNS cycle (start = NNS cycle onset subtracted from stimulus cycle onset) divided by the period of the stimulus waveform and converted to degrees. The onset of the first suck cycle to be measured in each burst occurred prior to stimulus onset and was therefore represented by negative phase angle values. For the polar plots, frequency ratio corresponds to the radius, and phase angle represents azimuth (circumference). Harmonic entrainment (1:1 relationship between stimulus cycles and NNS cycles) is evidenced by a grouping of the data points near the 100% frequency ratio radius and a restricted phase angle range. Subharmonic entrainment is evidenced by grouping of data points near a radius corresponding to an integer submultiple of the stimulus frequency (i.e. 50%).

Frequency ratio/polar plot analyses of NNS bursts sampled from two babies (age 1.7 and 1.3 months) demonstrating harmonic entrainment are shown in Figs 9.3a and b. A metric showing absolute deviation scores of frequency ratio data points around the 100% radius (equivalent to MD_{100}) was used to categorize the entrainment characteristics of suck bursts. The frequency ratio/phase polar plot shown in Fig. 9.3a has an equivalent MD of 1.99, whereas the polar plot in Fig. 9.3b has an MD of 2.68. The initial stimulated cycle of the burst is designated by the triangle symbol; subsequent cycles are connected by lines. [MD = mean deviation 100 based on absolute deviation scores of frequency ratio data points around the 100% radius (Finan 1998). Therefore, a MD_{100} score of '0%' represents perfect harmonic entrainment (all NNS cycles equal to stimulus period)].

These results indicated: (1) decreased suck cycle temporal variability; (2) reduced mean cycle period values; and (3) harmonic entrainment for cycles concurrent with stimulation. Mean NNS cycle period values for the later cycles of stimulated bursts were nearly equal to the period of the stimulus waveform. Therefore, the typical pattern of intraburst cycle period change observed during normal NNS was altered following stimulation and was characterized by a more gradual increase of cycle period throughout the initial cycles of a burst. Harmonic entrainment of the NNS behavior to the mechanical stimulus train is shown clearly in frequency ratio/phase polar plots (results from the two different babies shown above). The rhythmic stimulus waveform likely acted as a fixed timing signal, thereby reducing one source of variability inherent to the suck system. These data provide another line of evidence that the NNS system in human infants resets the pattern, based on rapid feedback mechanisms conveying information about the orofacial sensorium. Reduction of temporal variability and entrainment of sucking motor patterns suggests that mechanosensitive afferents from circumoral and/or intraoral areas are integral components of the rhythm generating circuitry for sucking and, quite possibly, for other rhythmic oromotor patterns, including mastication and speech.

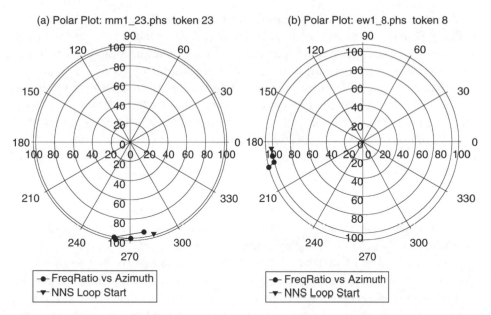

Fig. 9.3 (a) and (b) Frequency ratio/polar plots of non-nutritive suck bursts from two infants (ages 1.7 months and 1.3 months, respectively) during harmonic entrainment to an externally delivered mechanical input to the baglet of the actifier. A metric showing absolute deviation scores of frequency ratio data points around the 100% radius (equivalent to MD_{100}) was used to categorize the entrainment characteristics of suck bursts. The initial stimulated cycle of the burst is designated by the triangle symbol, subsequent cycles are connected by lines. MD = mean deviation 100 based on absolute deviation scores of frequency ratio data points around the 100% radius. (Adapted from Finan 1998.)

9.4 Discussion

Central pattern-generating circuits in the brain include complex assemblies of neurons that are closely involved in the production of motor behaviors, including locomotion, escape/struggle, flight, respiration, swallowing, mastication, sucking, and quite possibly vocalization and call production. The role of CPGs in the production of speech and voice remains unknown; however, a rudimentary understanding of the pattern-generating circuitry for respiration, suck, and mastication suggests multiple loci in brainstem and motor cortex with a significant role for integration among subsystems within the periaqueductal gray (PAG). Clearly, this provokes some intriguing options for the dynamic assembly of CPGs from relatively early appearing motor behaviors into the ontogeny of speech production. Moreover, there are components or segments of speech that include repetitious sequences of alternating movements among synergists which could benefit from dynamically assembled composite pattern-generating circuits involving trigeminal, facial, hypoglossal, and vagal pre-motor internuncial circuits. The possibility that speech and vocalization may utilize such a scheme for motor control has been entertained by notable neuroscientists, including Keir Pearson (2000) and Sten Grillner (1981). Consistent with their findings from spinal motor mechanisms, synergist movement pattern modules or unit burst generators located in the brain-stem would be activated largely by control signals from the cortex. A real-time stream of sensory cues from cutaneous and deep afferents may serve to refine the timing and magnitude of the efferent code delivered to LMNs. One possible advan-tage of CPG subcircuits for speech motor control is to reduce the computational load on motor cortex to the selection and sequencing of synergist patterns located in brainstem (PAG) and spinal cord. Motor cortex is thus programmed to select patterns of synergies residing in component CPGs in the brainstem and spinal cord.

Clearly, Grillner's (2001) contention that the assembly of the neuronal machin-ery evolves from dynamic changes that take place at the molecular, cellular, and network level is applicable to a number of patterned motor outputs. But what about human speech? At first glance, speech does not appear to be a patterned or repetitious sequence of alternating movements in the same way that bipedal loco-motion, swimming, locust flight, respiration, or suck are characterized, yet the neuroanatomy of speech abounds with numerous pattern generators subserving suck, mastication, and respiration. But speech does incorporate repeated sequences that occur at natural frequencies ranging from 2 to 6 Hz. For example, the popular test phrase used in many studies of speech motor control and speech acoustics 'Buy Bobby a puppy' includes an inventory of bilabial articulatory synergies (i.e. lip opening/closure) that is an expression of coupling and coordination by an undefined central pattern generator in the nervous system. As suggested by Marder and Bucher (2001), a given circuit of interconnected neurons can produce a whole range of different outputs with respect to frequency and phase relation-ships under the influence of different neuromodulators and/or neuromodulator concentration levels.

The existence of these neuronal assemblies in the brainstem has been implicated in a number of animal models of vocalization. Larson's (1985) microstimulation work in the PAG of the primate brainstem demonstrated the presence of pattern-generating circuits, resulting in controlled vocalizations with coordinated outputs from orofacial, laryngeal, and respiratory subsystems. The complex neuronal circuitry within the PAG is known to influence several loci of the brainstem, including trigeminal, facial, vagal, and hypoglossal motor nuclei. The functional capacity of the brainstem to produce a wide range of patterned motor behaviors, involving coordinated activity among four major cranial motor nuclear systems (cranial nerves V, VII, X, XII), in response to localized electrical microstimulation of the PAG, is truly remarkable and leaves little doubt about the existence of specialized neuronal networks in the brainstem. Several other reports support the existence of coordinated synergies for vocalization and orofacial control in both cat (Larson *et al.* 1983; Garrett and Luschei 1987; Farley *et al.* 1992*a, b*) and monkey (Larson and Kistler 1984; Larson 1985; DeRosier *et al.* 1987, 1988). The challenge remains in determining the extent to which CPGs located throughout the brainstem and spinal cord are modulated and dynamically reassembled for the purposes of vocalization/speech production. In this scenario, it is likely that different central pattern-generating networks in the brainstem are selected or modulated by suprabulbar inputs, are coordinated with one another with respect to phase and frequency, undergo repeated cycles of assembly and reconfiguration in response to task demands and local environment, and are continuously modified by experience. As suggested by Marder and Bucher (2001), similar circuit reconfigurations involving many of the same neuronal elements may allow a large circuit to produce a number of related behaviors. For the respiratory system, this could mean breathing, coughing, gasping, sighing, vomiting, vocalization, and speech.

References

Baconnier, P.F., Benchetrit, G., Pachot, P., and Demongeot, J. (1993). Entrainment of the respiratory rhythm: A new approach. *Journal Theoretical Biology*, 164, 149–162.

Barlow, S.M. (1998). Real-time modulation of speech–orofacial motor performance by means of motion sense. *Journal of Communicative Disorders*, 31 (6), 511–534.

Barlow, S.M., Finan, D.S., and Andreatta, R. (1997). Neuronal group selection and emergent orofacial motor control: Towards a unifying theory of speech development. In W. Hulstijn, H.F.M. Peters, and P.H.H.M. van Lieshout (Eds.), *Speech Production: Motor Control, Brain Research, and Fluency Disorders*, pp. 529–546. Elsevier, Amsterdam.

Barlow, S.M., Dusick, A., Finan, D.S., Coltart, S., and Biswas, A. (2001). Mechanically evoked perioral reflexes in premature and term human infants. *Brain Research*, 899, 251–254.

Bosma, J.F. (1970). Summarizing and perspective comments: Part V. Form and function in the infant's mouth and pharynx. In J.F. Bosma (Ed.), *Second Symposium on Oral Sensation and Perception*, pp. 550–555. Charles C. Thomas Publisher, Springfield, Illinois.

Branchereau, P., Morin, D., Bonnot, A., Ballion, B., Chapron, J., and Viala, D. (2000). Development of lumbar rhythmic networks: From embryonic to neonate locomotor-like patterns in the mouse. *Brain Research Bulletin*. 53 (5), 711–718.

Butera, R.J., Rinzel, J., and Smith, J.C. (1999). Models of respiratory rhythm generation in the pre-Bötzinger Complex. I. Bursting pacemaker neurons. *Journal Neurophysiology*, 82, 382–397.

Combes, D., Meyrand, P., and Simmers, J. (1999). Motor pattern specification by dual descending pathways to a lobster rhythm-generating network. *Journal of Neuroscience*, 19 (9), 3610–3619.

Conway, B.A., Hultborn, H., and Kiehn, O. (1987). Proprioceptive input resets central locomotor rhythm in the spinal cat. *Experimental Brain Research*, 68, 643–656.

Delcomyn, F. (1980). Neural basis of rhythmic behavior in animals. *Science,* 210, 492–498.

DeRosier, E.A., Ortega, J.D., Park, S., and **Larson, C.R.** (1987). Effects of PAG Stimulation on Laryngeal EMG and Vocalization in the Awake Monkey, p. 855. Society for *Neuroscience Abstracts,* New Orleans, LA.

DeRosier, E.A., West, R.A., and **Larson, C.R.** (1988). Comparison of Single Unit Discharge Properties in the Periaqueductal Gray and Nucleus Retroambiguus During Vocalization in Monkeys, p. 1237. Society for *Neuroscience Abstracts,* Toronto.

Dubayle, D. and **Viala, D.** (1996). Interactions between medullary and spinal respiratory rhythm generators in the in vitro brainstem spinal cord preparation from newborn rats. *Experimental Brain Research,* 109, 1–8.

Farley, G.R., Barlow, S.M., and **Netsell, R.** (1992a). Factors influencing neural activity in parabrachial regions during cat vocalizations. *Experimental Brain Research,* 89, 341–351.

Farley, G.R., Barlow, S.M., Netsell, R., and **Chmelka, J.V.** (1992b). Vocalizations in the cat: Behavioral methodology and spectrographic analysis. *Experimental Brain Research,* 89, 333–340.

Finan, D.S. (1998). Intrinsic dynamics and phase-dependent mechanosensory modulation of non-nutritive sucking in human infants. Unpublished Doctoral Dissertation, Indiana University.

Finan, D.S. and **Barlow, S.M.** (1996). The actifier and neurophysiological studies of orofacial control in neonates. *Journal of Speech and Hearing Research,* 39, 833–838.

Finan, D.S. and **Barlow, S.M.** (1998). Mechanosensory modulation of non-nutritive sucking in human infants. *Journal of Early Human Development,* 52 (2), 181–197.

Garrett, J.D. and **Luschei, E.S.** (1987). Subglottic pressure modulation during evoked phonation in the anesthetized cat. In T. Baer, C. Sasaki and K. Harris (Eds.), *Laryngeal Function in Phonation and Respiration,* pp. 139–153. College-Hill Press, Boston.

Georgopolous, A.P., Kettner, R.E., and **Schwartz, A.B.** (1988). Primate motor cortex and free arm movements to visual targets in three-dimensional space. II. Coding of the direction of movement by a neuronal population. *Journal of Neuroscience,* 8, 2928–2937.

Glass, L. and **Mackey, M.C.** (1988). *From Clocks to Chaos: The rhythms of Life.* Princeton University Press, Princeton, NJ.

Grillner, S. (1981). Control of locomotion in bipeds, tetrapods and fish. In V.B. Books (Ed.), *Handbook of physiology,* Sec 1, *The nervous system,* Vol II, Part 2, pp. 1179–1236. American Physiological Society, Bethesda.

Grillner, S. (2001). From egg to action. *Brain Research Bulletin,* 53 (5), 473–477.

Hannam, A.G. and **Lund, J.P.** (1981). The effect of intra-oral stimulation on the human masticatory cycle. *Archives Oral Biology,* 26, 865–870.

Ingersoll, E.W. and **Thoman, E.B.** (1994). The breathing bear: Effects on respiration in premature infants. *Physiology and Behavior,* 56 (5), 855–859.

Iriki, A., Nozaki, S., and **Nakamura, Y.** (1988). Feeding behavior in mammals: Corticobulbar projection is reorganized during conversion from sucking to chewing. *Developmental Brain Research,* 44, 189–196.

Kalaska, J.F. and **Crammond, D.J.** (1992). Cerebral cortical mechanisms of reaching movements. *Science,* 255, 1517–1523.

Koshiya, N. and **Smith, J.C.** (1999). Neuronal pacemaker for breathing visualized *in vitro. Nature,* 400, 360–363.

Kriellaars, D.J., Brownstone, R.M., Noga, B.R. and **Jordan, L.M.** (1994). Mechanical entrainment of fictive locomotion in the decerebrate cat. *Journal of Neurophysiology,* 71 (6), 2074–2086.

Larson, C.R. (1985). The midbrain periaqueductal gray: a brainstem structure involved in vocalization. *Journal of Speech and Hearing Research,* 28, 241–249.

Larson, C.R. and **Kistler, M.K.** (1984). Periaqueductal gray neuronal activity associated with laryngeal EMG and vocalization in the awake monkey. *Neuroscience Letters,* 46, 261–266.

Larson, C.R., Wilson, K.E., and **Luschei, E.S.** (1983). Preliminary observations on cortical and brainstem mechanisms of laryngeal control. In D. Bless and J. Abbs (Eds.), *Vocal Fold Physiology: Contemporary Research and Clinical Issues.* College-Hill Press, San Diego.

Lin, L.D., Murray, G.M., and **Sessle, B.J.** (1998). Effects on non-human primate mastication of reversible inactivation by cooling of the face primary somatosensory cortex. *Archives Oral Biology,* 43, 133–141.

Marder, E. and **Bucher, D.** (2001). Central pattern generators and the control of rhythmic movements. *Current Biology,* 11, 986–996.

Nozaki, S., Iriki, A., and **Nakamura, Y.** (1986). Localization of central rhythm generator involved in cortically induced rhythmical masticatory jaw-opening movement in the guinea pig. *Journal of Neurophysiology,* 55 (4), 806–825.

Pavlidis, T. (1973). Entrainment of oscillators by external inputs. In: *Biological Oscillators: Their Mathematical Analysis,* pp. 71–98. Academic Press, London.

Pearson, K.G. (2000). Neural adaptation in the generation of rhythmic behavior. *Annual Review Physiology,* 62, 723–753.

Pearson, K.G. and **Gordon, J.** (2000). Locomotion. In E.R. Kandel, J.H. Schwartz, and T.M. Jessell (Eds.), *Principles of Neural Science,* pp. 737–755. McGraw-Hill, New York.

Pearson, K.G., Ramirez, J.M., and **Jiang, W.** (1992). Entrainment of the locomotor rhythm by group Ib afferents from ankle extensor muscles in spinal cats. *Experimental Brain Research,* 90, 557–566.

Penn, A.A. and **Shatz, C.J.** (1999). Brain waves and brain wiring: the role of endogenous and sensory-driven neural activity in development. *Pediatric Research,* 45 (4), 447–458.

Rossignol, S., Lund, J.P., and **Drew, T.** (1988). The role of sensory inputs in regulating patterns of rhythmical in higher vertebrates. In A. Cohen, S. Rossignol, and S. Grillner (Eds.), *Neural Control of Rhythmic Movements in Vertebrates,* pp. 201–283. John Wiley and Sons, New York.

Sammon, M.P. and **Darnall, R.A.** (1994). Entrainment of respiration to rocking in premature infants: Coherence analysis. *Journal Applied Physiology*, 77 (3), 1548–1554.

Simon, P.M., Zurob, A.S., Wies, W.M., Leiter, J.C., and **Hubmayr, R.D.** (1999). Entrainment of respiration in humans by periodic lung inflations. Effect of state and CO_2. *American Journal of Respiratory Critical Care Medicine*, 160 (3), 950–960.

Simon, P.M., Habel, A.M., Daubenspeck, J.A., and **Leiter, J.C.** (2000). Vagal feedback in the entrainment of respiration to mechanical ventilation in sleeping humans. *Journal Applied Physiology*, 89, 760–769.

Smith, J.C., Ellenberger, H.H., Ballanyi, K., Richter, D.W., and **Feldman, J.L.** (1991). Pre-Bötzinger Complex: A brainstem region that may generate respiratory rhythm in mammals. *Science*, 254, 726–729.

Smith, J.C., Ballanyi, K., and **Richter, D.W.** (1992). Whole-cell patch-clamp recordings from respiratory neurons in neonatal rat brainstem in vitro. *Neuroscience Letters*, 134, 153–156.

Speck, D.F., Karius, D.R., and **Ling, L.** (1993). Respiratory afferents and the inhibition of inspiration. In D.F. Speck, M.S. Dekin, W.R. Revelette, and D.T. Frazier (Eds.), *Respiratory control: Central and Peripheral Mechanisms*, pp. 100–103. University Press of Kentucky, Lexington.

Swensen, A.M. and **Marder, E.** (2001). Modulators with convergent cellular actions elicit distinct circuit outputs. *Journal Neuroscience*, 21, 4050–4058.

Westberg, K.G., Clavelou, P., Sandstrom, G., and **Lund, J.P.** (1998). Evidence that trigeminal brainstem interneurons form subpopulations to produce different forms of mastication in the rabbit. *Journal of Neuroscience*, 18 (16), 6466–6479.

Zacksenhouse, M. (2001). Sensitivity of basic oscillatory mechanisms for pattern generation and detection. *Biological Cybernetics*, 85, 301–311.

PART 4

INTERFACE

INTERACTION OF MOTOR AND LANGUAGE FACTORS IN THE DEVELOPMENT OF SPEECH PRODUCTION

ANNE SMITH AND LISA GOFFMAN

10.1 Introduction

In general, models of language development in childhood (Locke 1993) and language production in adults (Levelt 1989; Levelt *et al.* 1999) do not include explicit accounts of the production process at the level of speech motor control. Models of the control and coordination of speech movements (Barlow and Farley 1989; Smith 1992) are written in the language of motor control theory, for example, of reflexes and centrally generated motor commands, and do not account for the question of how linguistic units act as input to, or emerge from, the production process (one exception to this is the theory of articulatory phonology of Browman and Goldstein 1992, which we discuss below). The growing literature on speech motor development, however, forces our attention on potential language/motor interactions. Clearly, language and speech motor processes co-develop in the child. How does language acquisition affect speech motor development, and how do basic motor processes affect language acquisition? These questions are the central focus of this chapter.

10.2 Language/motor interfaces: theoretical frameworks

Our focus is language/motor interactions, thus we are concerned with theoretical attempts to determine how various levels of linguistic processing, and the units that have been proposed to operate at these levels, are related to speech motor processes. This is a difficult problem, because speech production ultimately depends on the nervous system's control and coordination of the activity of many motoneuron pools. These motoneuron pools innervate muscles of the chest wall, larynx, and supralaryngeal structures. The physiology of the neural control of motor unit recruitment and discharge, muscle forces, and movements is remote from the constructs of linguistic theories.

Many attempts to bridge the gap between language processes and motor aspects of production posit that linguistic units serve as the input to speech motor planning processes. Putative units of production range in size from the phrase (Kozhevnikov and Chistovich 1966), to the syllable (Stetson 1951; Levelt and Wheeldon 1994), to the phoneme (Shattuck-Hufnagel 1987; Guenther *et al.* 1998), to the phonetic feature (Perkell 1980). Much early experimental work in the field of speech production sought evidence for consistent mappings from linguistic units to aspects of the speech acoustic signal and physiological output measures, such as movements and muscle activity (reviewed by MacNeilage 1970). Consistent mappings between linguistic units and output measures were elusive, because the essential nature of speech production involves coproduction across units. The physiological events underlying the production of phrase, syllable, and phoneme units vary as a function of prosody, the surrounding phonemes, word boundaries, and other factors.

The failure to find invariant correlates of linguistic units in acoustic or physiological signals led scientists studying the physiology of speech production to conclude that speech motor output should be studied just as other motor behaviors are studied (Moll *et al.* 1977; Abbs 1986). These authors argued that the explanatory variables of speech motor control models should be the same as those used in the general motor control literature; for example, to account for locomotion or reaching, and experiments should be designed to determine the role of reflexes and central pattern generators in the control and coordination of speech movements. These authors obviously recognized that linguistic units operated as the input to the production process, but they argued that these units were not transparent at the level of analysis of acoustic or physiological signals. Thus, they proposed that experimental questions regarding speech motor processes should not be framed in terms of linguistic constructs. Since the late 1970s, many studies of the physiological bases of speech production focused on speech as a motor behavior without reference to linguistic units. Experiments were designed to examine oral reflexes during speech and to find evidence for the central patterning of speech movements, for example in the sequencing of articulatory movements (reviewed in Smith 1992). The classic perturbation paradigm of the limb motor control literature was applied to speech to determine the role of on-line somatosensory information in the generation of speech movements (Abbs and Gracco 1984; Kelso *et al.* 1984). Modelers of the speech motor control process relegated language processes to a small area of their block diagrams (Barlow and Farley 1989), and experimental results generally were not discussed in relation to linguistic units.

In contrast, the field of psycholinguistics has focused research efforts on linguistic processing components of speech production, with almost no attention to the physiological bases. In these speech production models, linguistic units, generally phonemes (Shattuck-Hufnagel 1987) or syllables (Levelt 1989; Levelt *et al.* 1999) serve as the input to the motor processes that generate speech movements. The complex role of the articulatory system may be acknowledged in psycholinguistic accounts, but movement variables do not contribute to linguistic levels of the speech production hierarchy. As stated by Levelt *et al.* (1999, p. 5), 'the functioning of this [articulatory] system is beyond our present theory. The articulatory system is, of course, not just the muscular machinery that controls lungs, larynx, and vocal tract; it is as much a computational neural system that controls the execution of abstract gestural scores by this highly complex movement system'.

Generally, in psycholinguistic theories (e.g. Levelt 1989; Bock 1995; Levelt *et al.* 1999), multiple levels of a linguistic hierarchy, such as grammatical encoding or metrical and segmental plans, provide input to the motor implementation system, which is simply a downstream executor operating independently from the linguistic levels. Thus, conceptual, syntactic, morphological, and phonological representations are construed as separate from the motor system through which these representations are realized. A primary source of evidence for the separation of processing levels comes from investigations of reaction time during the real time production of words (Levelt *et al.* 1991; Vigliocco *et al.* 2002). Such data support the idea that speech production processes are feed-forward and hierarchical. For example, phonological activation occurs only after lemma selection (Levelt *et al.* 1991). When participants are asked to name a picture (e.g. of a sheep) while listening to auditory primes, semantically (e.g. goat) and phonologically (e.g. sheet), similar words are also activated, as indicated by changes in reaction times. The results were complex and dependent upon stimulus-onset asynchronies; however, there were differential responses to phonological and semantic primes. Such evidence supports that processes related to lemma selection are distinct from those involved in phonological activation. Levelt and his colleagues are quite explicit in proposing that encoding the word as a motor action occurs after selection of the appropriate lemma. Other theorists have interpreted the data from priming experiments to support the interaction of co-activated lemma selection and phonological encoding processes (Dell and O'Seaghdha 1992), but in their model linguistic processing also precedes activation of articulatory planning networks.

Most of the experimental work supporting hierarchical psycholinguistic models has been completed on adult subjects. However, we note that there is some consideration of the relationship between movement and concept in early development. Levelt *et al.* (1999) begin their target article in *Behavioral and Brain Sciences* with a speculation about how, for infants, 'word production emerges from a coupling of two initially independent systems, a conceptual system and an articulatory system' (Levelt *et al.* 1999, p. 1). Early development, under this account, can be conceptualized as a linkage between lexical concepts and 'motor patterns' observed in babbling.

A novel attempt to bridge the gap between the biology of movement and the representation of linguistic units was offered in the dynamical systems theory of articulatory phonology by Browman and Goldstein (1992). This theory posits that gestures, defined as 'abstract characterizations of articulatory events' (Browman and Goldstein 1992, p. 155), are the basic units of phonological contrast. Words are produced by specifying a 'gestural score', an abstract sequence of settings of vocal tract variables, such as lip aperture, tongue tip constriction, velic aperture, etc. (Browman and Goldstein 1991). Further, they argued that the lexicon is composed of dynamically specified gestures. This has implications for both production and perception, 'because the same lexicon is assumed to be accessed whether an individual is speaking or listening, the hypothesis implies that a listener ultimately recovers the set of gestures that are part of a given lexical entry' (Browman and Goldstein 1991, p. 314). This theory is parsimonious in that it strips away levels of representation, and suggests that there is a set of biologically grounded primitives from which complex perceptual and motor behaviors emerge. However, it cannot account for the early acquisition of language. Infants' speech perception abilities precede their production capacity, so that early perception could not take place by recovery of a set of articulatory gestures. Also there is some evidence that phonological contrasts do not emerge from basic gestures in children's speech (see Section 10.4.2 below; Goffman and Smith 1999). Browman and Goldstein (1991, 1992) suggest that gestures are abstractions that are not overtly realized. If the gesture is so abstract as to not be directly measurable, the theory becomes quite difficult to test.

In summary, the literature on the physiology of normal adult speech production has largely abandoned the attempt to relate linguistic units to the motor processes involved in production, and has focused on speech as a motor behavior. Or, under the dynamical view, the relationship of language and motor processes becomes irrelevant, because the units of language are emergent from the production process (Browman and Goldstein 1992). Theories of language production, such as that of Levelt *et al.* (1999), invoke the operation of linguistic units at many levels of a multi-stage process, but do not attempt to account for the potential interleaving of these levels of linguistic processing with motor organization. What we will argue in the sections that follow is that, in the study of the development of speech motor processes in normal and disordered children, the interaction of language and motor processes must be addressed. While we can describe patterns of movement and muscle activity in the language of motor control theories, we find that even these 'low-level' physiological events are shaped in consistent ways by the linguistic goals and capacities of the speaker. At the same time, there is evidence that the physiological characteristics of the effector systems involved in speech production have 'bottom-up' influences on language processes.

10.3 Developmental approaches to language/motor interactions

During early development, it is especially difficult to dissociate cognitive–linguistic from motor processes. Properties of language begin to interact with biological behaviors in canonical babbling, which is viewed as a crucial precursor to speech production (Stark 1980; Oller 2001). Canonical babbling is a movement primitive (Kent 1992; MacNeilage and Davis 2000) that is similar in structure to many other motor behaviors occurring during the same developmental period. It is a rhythmic stereotypy similar to kicking (Thelen 1981) and object banging (Ejiri 1998). In their frame-content model, MacNeilage and Davis (1990, 2000) hypothesize that babbling is comprised of rhythmic oscillations of the jaw that are coordinated with phonation and only later are modified systematically for the production of specified phonetic segments. In this sense, babbling may be viewed initially as a movement primitive for speech. By 'movement primitive' we do not mean to invoke the concept of an abstract gesture, as defined by Browman and Goldstein (1992), rather we would define a movement primitive as a biologically grounded movement pattern that arises initially unrelated to speech, such as an oral open–close sequence. Later in development, these primitives become elaborated and associated with neural networks mediating auditory and linguistic representations (Pulvermuller 1999). However, even during these earliest phases of language learning, experiential factors interact with speech production. Babbling, although an extremely robust phenomenon that occurs across cultures and language groups, may be modified by experience. One striking example of such modification is that infants who are hearing impaired show delayed onset of babbling (Stoel-Gammon and Otomo 1986; Oller and Eilers 1988), indicating that this movement primitive is already linked to auditory experience.

Additional evidence that babbling (and first words, for that matter) is constrained by physiological and anatomic factors (Kent 1984, 1992) is provided by the finding that early phonetic and syllabic inventories are similar regardless of the language being acquired (Locke and Pearson 1992). For example, [h, w, j, p, b, m, t, d, n, k, g] comprise a large proportion of sounds included in first words across multiple languages (Locke 1993; Vihman 1996). At the same time, there are language-specific effects. Adult listeners can discriminate whether an infant at the late babbling phase is acquiring their native language (de Boysson-Bardies *et al.* 1984; de Boysson-Bardies and Vihman 1991). There is a clear interaction between language and motor variables. Already, language learning is an interactive process that incorporates auditory and motor domains. Links between conceptual knowledge and speech production are also emerging during this time period, as children acquire their first communicative intents and words, and relate them to their vocal repertoire (Vihman 1996).

Phrase-level movement primitives, such as speech-like respiratory cycles and falling intonation contours, also begin to interact with language-specific processes toward the end of the first year of life. Respiratory recordings of infant cry show that the speech-like characteristics of brief inspiratory followed by long expiratory phases emerge in the context of this distress behavior (Langlois and Baken 1976; Stark 1989). It is suggested that properties observed during cry are harnessed for the production of speech. However, the relationship between homeostatic and speech functions is complex. In 15-month-old toddlers, speech and quiet breathing show very different patterns of synchrony of rib cage and abdomen movements (Moore *et al.* 2001). Linkages may be observed in specific behaviors, but cannot be generalized to all homeostatic functions.

Falling intonation contours and final lengthening (Snow 1994, 1998) are another example of relatively primitive behaviors that begin to link with utterance level units. Falling intonation contours, for example, are present from the earliest period of language learning. Increasingly complex prosodic contours emerge as linguistic complexity increases. At the word level, strong–weak, or trochaic, syllable sequences are acquired very early in development and, as discussed below, may serve as another example of a physiological bias that is modified for the production of progressively varied linguistic units.

Physiological influences do not simply disappear as development progresses and language contributions become more complex. Although the weighting of physiological factors may be strongest during babbling and first word learning, there is a continued influence into the later childhood years. As an example, Kent (1992) has proposed that segmental development may be described in relation to motor phenomena. Early stop consonants are produced with ballistic movements (Green *et al.* 2002), while later-learned fricatives require fine force regulation. For children acquiring English, the [r] sound is notorious for its difficult acquisition process. These production difficulties cannot be explained on grounds of perceptual salience or frequency of occurrence in the language. Instead, both perceptual (related to the large number of allophonic variations in the language) and movement complexity are likely to explain the protracted developmental course for acquisition of this segment. High movement variability in child versus adult speech production (Kent and Forner 1980; Sharkey and Folkins 1985; Smith and Goffman 1998) also suggests that physiological variables continue to influence development. Our data related to motor variables in later language learning will be elaborated below.

It follows that, if physiological and linguistic mechanisms are co-developing in an interactive manner, both levels would simultaneously influence the sorts of production units that children use. As previously discussed, adult speech production models emphasize the syllable or segment as the organizational unit. Motor control approaches focus on movements as the basic units. The developmental evidence reveals that units change over time, consistent with the claim that both motor and language levels drive production. Perhaps the classic paper of Ferguson and Farwell (1975) was the first to make the claim that the emergence of speech production units needs to be studied carefully in child language. These investigators, relying on detailed transcription evidence, found that word units have primacy, at least during the single-word period. As an example, one of their participants, K, produced the words 'moo' and 'mama' with an initial [b]. Other words that began with the adult target [b] also were produced with [b]. Thus [b] and [m] were not contrastive. Findings such as these suggest that, for young children, contrasts are made at the word, not the segmental, level. Other studies have since replicated this finding (reviewed in Vihman 1996).

As reported above, transcription evidence supports the idea that children's speech-production units may differ from those of adults, and that multiple co-occurring units may operate simultaneously. During the single-word period, the word unit was prominent, but initial segmental contrasts also occurred (Ferguson and Farwell 1975; Vihman 1996). More detailed acoustic studies have reinforced the claim that there is no single or privileged speech production unit. Nittrouer *et al.* (1989, 1996) reported that young children and adults differed in the degree of coarticulation observed across productions of syllable sequences (i.e. [sisi], [susu], [shishi], [shushu]). These investigators found that children produced more coar-ticulated fricatives when compared with adults. These results were interpreted as evidence that children organize their speech movements more broadly than adults, with segmental components emerging later in development. What was not clear from these findings was whether the spreading of an articulatory movement crossed boundaries greater than those associated with a syllable. In sum, many lines of evidence suggest that speech production units change across development, and that such units are influenced in specific ways by changes in motor, auditory, and cognitive–linguistic processes.

10.4 Movement trajectory analysis as a window to language/motor interactions

In recent studies, physiological data have been recorded during speech production in young children and have provided new dimensions to our understanding of the acquisition process. In earlier work from our laboratory, we developed a measure of speech motor control that captured the degree of variability in a set (or class) of time- and amplitude-normalized movement trajectories from one effector produced for a phrase-length utterance (Smith *et al.* 1995). In adults, the motion of a single effector reveals a very consistent spatiotemporal pattern over repeated productions, such that the variability of a set of movement trajectories for a sentence is very low (Smith *et al.* 1995). Smith and Goffman (1998) reported that 4-year-olds and 7-year-olds were much more variable in their movement trajecto-ries for a sentence compared to young adults. Thus, this index of spatiotemporal variability appears to provide one useful window on to the maturation of speech production processes. Analysis of these normalized trajectories is also useful in determining how potential linguistic distinctions are implemented in movement. To this end, we have developed pattern recognition procedures (Smith *et al.* 1995) to apply to normalized movement trajectories, so that we can ask whether speakers produce distinctive movement templates for different linguistic targets. The statistical pattern recognition algorithm we have employed involves creating a template movement pattern for each condition (e.g. for the phrase spoken at different rates in Smith *et al.* 1995, or for a words differing by a single phoneme in Goffman and Smith 1999). This template is computed by averaging the multiple normalized trajectories (usually 10–15 trials) for each subject within each condition. Then each subject's individual trajectories for each condition are compared by cross correlation with the averaged templates for that subject for all conditions. Each single trajectory is then sorted into the condition with which it correlates most highly. We then can compare errors in sorting across groups and conditions. In summary, this algorithm basically sorts movement trajectories into the average group that most closely resembles it in spatiotemporal pattern. Using this approach, it is possible to evaluate changes in movement patterning in relation to changing linguistic goals at multiple levels.

Our overall research strategy is to look for bidirectional influences between language and motor systems. We have used linguistic units of various sizes, from the phrase level to the segment, as an analytic window on speech motor processes. We have designed some studies to determine if there are basic motor system biases that influence the production of speech, especially in younger children. We have also studied speakers with disorders expressed as disturbances in speech motor control (stuttering) and disorders expressed primarily as deficits in language processing (specific language impairment).

10.4.1 Phrase-level analyses

Our work introducing movement analyses for the whole trajectory for a phrase (which includes multiple speech movements) was novel, because earlier speech kinematic studies focused on measures from single movements or from selected points in time (e.g. opening movement duration, displacement, and peak velocity). In the first study from our laboratory reviewed here (Smith *et al.* 1995), a head-mounted strain gauge system was used to collect the oral movement data. In all subsequent studies we have used an optotrak system (small light-emitting diodes are attached to the lips and jaw and their motion is tracked in three-dimensional space with an accuracy of 0.1 mm) to collect the kinematic data. The optotrak system is very easy to use with children as young as 4 years.

In our initial conceptualization of the work on phrase-level trajectory analysis, we were interested in avoiding the traditional assumptions that phonemes or syllables were the basic units of production. Thus, we did not choose to look at single movements or open–close sequences associated with phonemes or syllables (Smith *et al.* 1995, 2000). However, the choice of the length of the segment of movement data to normalize does imply that there is some 'unitness' about that segment (Ward and Arnfield 2001). If not, the data, after normalization, would not converge on to a common template. In all of the studies in which we have normalized phrase-level trajectories, the sets of movement trajectories from multiple repetitions of the phrase do converge on to a common template in both young children and adults (Smith *et al.* 1995; Smith and Goffman 1998). Further, the variability functions across relative time (lower panel Figs 10.1 and 10.2) do not show obvious, marked peaks, which would indicate that the analysis has crossed a boundary in the underlying planning units. These data are strong evidence that phrase-level planning units are used to generate motor commands for speech. It could be suggested that having the speaker repeat a phrase, as we did in our earliest studies, induces a consistent pattern of movement that would not otherwise emerge. However, in later studies we have randomized presentation of the stimuli, such that subjects produce five or more different sentences in an unpredictable order. We find the same level of consistency in the sets of trajectories for a phrase when the sentences are produced in random order. Finally, our earlier work employed analyses of the consistency of movement trajectories for a single articulator, the lower lip. It could be argued that a more relevant parameter in terms of speech production goals is lip aperture, or the distance between the two lips, which involves coordination of the upper lip, lower lip, and jaw. In a recent study (Smith and Zelaznik 2003), we have studied speech motor development using normalization methods to examine consistency of lip aperture trajectories over multiple trials. Similar developmental trends are found using this measure, which reflects a higher-order, coordinative unit.

Although most of our work has employed speech movement analyses, when the same normalization procedure is applied to the lip EMG amplitude envelope, the results are similar (Wohlert and Smith 2002). Children's EMG patterns for speech, like their oral movements, are more variable than those of adults, but after normalization they converge on to a common template. As children and adults compute the neural commands to motorneuron pools to generate 10 repetitions of an utterance, the planning and execution is consistent at the phrase level.

Maner *et al.* (2000) used the phrase-level movement trajectory analysis to examine the effects of length and syntactic complexity on speech motor variability in 5-year-old children and adults. Our hypothesis was that with increased length and complexity of the utterance, phrase-level movement variability would be higher. We compared the movement variability indices for a phrase spoken in isolation and spoken embedded in sentences of varying complexity. Children's sets of movement trajectories for the phrase were more variable when the phrase was spoken in a longer sentence compared to when it was produced in isolation. Adults showed no effect on movement variability of increased length/complexity. Examples of the data from this study are included in Figs 10.1 and 10.2. We included conditions intended to separate the effects of length and syntactic complexity, but this manipulation did not work as expected. Thus, we could not argue that the effects were primarily due to increased syntactic complexity rather than utterance length. Kleinow and Smith (2000) replicated this study with

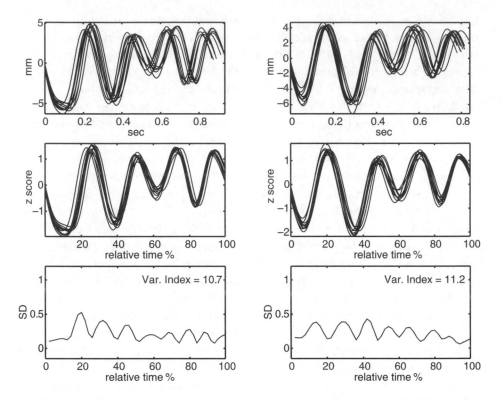

Fig. 10.1 Examples of phrase-level movement trajectory analyses for an adult. The left sets of plots show the lower-lip movement for ten productions of 'buy Bobby a puppy' spoken in isolation. The right set of plots is for the same phrase spoken in the sentence, 'You buy Bobby a puppy now if he wants one.' For both columns of plots, the top traces are the original displacement data. The middle plot shows these movement trajectories after time and amplitude normalization. The bottom plot shows the trajectory variability as a function of normalized time (see Maner *et al.* 2000 for detailed methods). For normal adults, as shown in this example, the movement variability index does not change when the phrase is spoken as part of a longer, more complex sentence.

normally fluent adults and adults who stutter. The adults who stutter, like young children, showed increased phrase-level movement variability when the utterance was longer and more complex. The results of these studies further support the conclusion that phrase-level planning affects speech movement output. In addition, however, we argued that these results support the hypothesis of a closer link between movement planning and execution and premotor linguistic processing in children and disordered speakers. In other words, in a serial ordered model such as that proposed by Levelt *et al.* (1999), one would not predict that increasing processing demands at higher levels would have any effect on movement implementation. The fact that movement output is affected argues that these higher-level processes interact with movement planning and execution. Also, although we did not

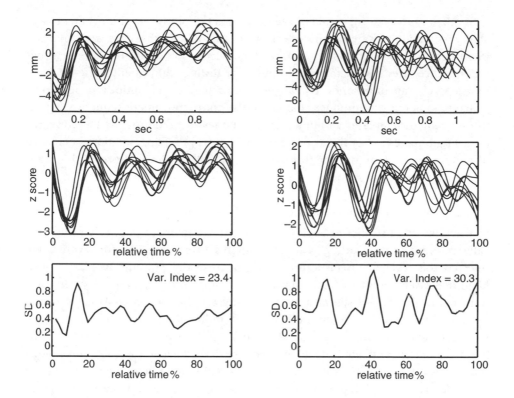

Fig. 10.2 Examples of phrase-level movement trajectory analyses for a 7-year-old child. The left set of plots show the lower-lip movement for ten productions of 'buy Bobby a puppy' spoken in isolation. The right set of plots is for the same phrase spoken in the sentence, 'You buy Bobby a puppy now if he wants one.' For both columns of plots, the top traces are the original displacement data. The middle plot shows these movement trajectories after time and amplitude normalization. The bottom plot shows the trajectory variability as a function of normalized time (see Maner *et al.* 2000 for detailed methods). For young children the movement variability typically increases when the phrase is spoken as part of a longer, more complex sentence.

observe these effects in normal adults, we would posit that there are language/motor interactions in the normal adult, but that our experimental conditions did not place enough linguistic demands on the adults to produce observable effects on their motor output. In an experiment in progress (Kleinow and Smith unpublished), we are testing this hypothesis by using sentence stimuli with higher levels of syntactic complexity. Another important question is whether these effects on kinematic output are attributable specifically to language/motor interactions (as we would argue), or whether the observed increases in kinematic variability reflect the effects of a general increase in central processing demands. Our dependent measures in these experiments do not allow us to make the specificity argument, but some of our observations, outlined below on prosodic targets produced by children, do suggest that the interactions are not simply reflected in increased trajectory variability.

In other study of adult speakers, we have used the phrase-level movement variability analysis to examine the effects of changing speaking rate and intensity (Smith *et al.* 1995; Smith and Kleinow 2000; Kleinow *et al.* 2001). Pattern recognition procedures reveal that adults produce distinct movement patterns for a phrase when rate or loudness is changed. Speaking rate and loudness appear to be global parameters that produce changes in the entire movement sequence. Again, the movement templates within a rate or loudness condition tended to converge on a single pattern after linear normalization, thus providing additional evidence of phrase-level planning and the presence of phrase-level reorganization for changing speech output goals.

10.4.2 Word and phonetic segment level analyses

In the next set of studies to be described, we move to analyses of other linguistically relevant units, starting with experiments examining prosodic words. We selected this level of linguistic processing because the prosodic word has been identified as a differentiable level of processing for children (Gerken 1994). In addition, many theories of speech production suggest that advance planning of the utterance may employ its prosodic structure rather than (or in addition to) its syntactic structure (e.g. Ferreira 1991; Bock 1995). Generally, in these experiments, children and adult speakers produce two-syllable (or four-movement) sequences that are either trochaic (strong–weak) or iambic (weak–strong) in prosodic structure. It has been suggested that, at least for children learning English, the relative ease of acquiring a trochaic prosodic structure reflects an early bias of both perceptual and motor systems. Iambic sequences are more problematic during early language learning (Echols 1993; Gerken 1994; Schwartz and Goffman 1995). A prominent finding from our studies is that the earlier-developing trochaic structure is, perhaps surprisingly, more poorly controlled in oral movement output than the iamb (Goffman 1999; Goffman and Malin 1999). Figure 10.3 shows movement data obtained from a young child producing trochaic and iambic forms of a novel word. As shown in this figure, young children produce lower lip + jaw movement sequences that are unmodulated in the early developing trochaic form. That is, movement patterns associated with strong–weak trochaic sequences are produced with equal amplitude and duration across initial strong and final weak syllables. Although this result is initially counterintuitive, we hypothesize that children are employing a movement primitive of equal-amplitude, sequential oral movements (similar to that observed in earlier canonical babbling) for their production of these 'easier' words. This movement primitive applies to the lip–jaw complex. Acoustic analyses show that fundamental frequency and amplitude are varied as a function of stress (Goffman 1999). Perceptual judgments of stress productions further affirm that children are contrasting iambs and trochees; only productions that are prosodically accurate are included in the analyses. Thus, we hypothesize that the respiratory and laryngeal components of production are developing earlier than

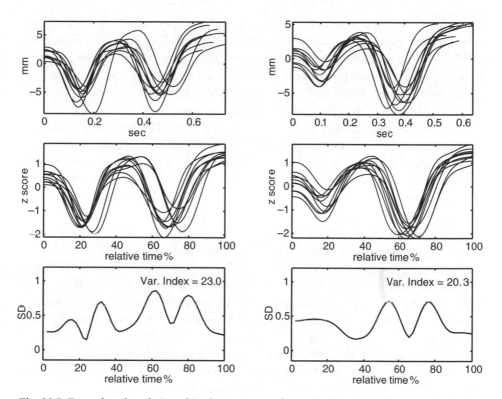

Fig. 10.3 Examples of trochaic and iambic nonce words extracted from the phrase 'It's Bob's [fVfVf]'. These are from a 4-year-old child. The left set of plots shows the lower lip–jaw movement for 10 productions of the novel word trochee ['fʌfəf]. The right set of plots is for the same phonetic sequence, now learned as an iamb [fə'fʌf]. It is important to note that a central vowel was selected for both stressed and unstressed conditions. Since unstressed vowels are typically centralized as a function of stress, this allows for the most possible similarity across stress conditions. For both columns of plots, the top traces are the original displacement data. The middle plot shows these movement trajectories after time and amplitude normalization. The bottom plot shows the trajectory variability as a function of normalized time. Note that, unlike the iamb, the trochaic word is not amplitude modulated (i.e. the two open–close movement sequences for the word are equal in amplitude). Also, as indicated by the trajectory variability index, the trochee is produced with significantly more variability than the iamb. For details of these methods, see Goffman (1999).

articulatory control in relation to the production of this prosodic target. Children rely on an early developing articulatory pattern for the production of the more frequently occurring trochee.

Unlike the earlier developing trochee, also as shown in Fig. 10.3, iambs do show movement amplitude and duration variation with stress, with initial weak syllables produced with substantially smaller and shorter movements than final strong sylla-bles. Apparently, children are deploying more elaborated motor control skills in their production of these more complex forms. Another source of evidence that fewer motor resources are dedicated to the production of trochees is that iambs are produced with a statistically higher degree of spatiotemporal stability (as measured by the trajectory variability index). Overall, it is also important to note that children with specific language impairment (SLI) show less mature movement patterns than their peers who are developing normally.

Our interpretation of these results is that, early in development, children rely on a motor bias, that of rhythmic, unmodulated articulatory movement sequences, to produce trochaic forms. Such a bias is observed initially in canonical babbling and is exploited for the production of true words. Children are required to move away from this physiological bias to achieve increasingly complex communicative goals; new movement categories are built as new linguistic distinctions emerge. As shown in Fig. 10.4, adults produce a larger repertoire of controlled distinctions across different prosodic targets, as indicated by their modulation of trochees as well as their differentiated categories across mono- and multi-morphemic iambs (e.g. 'giraffe' versus 'a dog'; Goffman 2003). Overall, we suggest that the early developing trochaic sequence exploits biases of movement that are already in place from the canonical babbling period, and that increased systematic differentiations of prosodic patterning emerge as communicative demands increase. Although these results are counterintuitive, on reflection it is logical that children initially use the movement primitives they have acquired prelinguistically, and import these into the task of word production. In English, since the majority of content words are trochaic, these primitives are first applied to strong–weak sequences. Weak syllables in iambic sequences are omitted or produced with equal stress during the earliest phases of language production (Gerken 1994; Kehoe et al. 1995). This suggests that the demands for production of iambic sequences are higher. The amplitude-modulated oral sequence is a requirement for the successful production of iambs; to produce perceptually acceptable trochees, children can rely on simpler articulatory movements. As oral motor skills improve and as linguistic task demands increase, the system elaborates until the distinctive adult patterns appear. Thus, overall, these data provide an example of bi-directional influences, with lower-level rhythmic movement primitives influencing the sorts of linguistic distinctions that appear in early speech production.

We have also manipulated the segmental content of an utterance to evaluate the influence of phonetic variation on movement output. In Goffman and Smith (1999), 4-year-old, 7-year-old, and adult speakers produced utterances that varied only in the voicing or nasality of a consonant in an utterance internal word (i.e. Bob saw [man/pan/ban/fan/van] again). One goal was to test a hypothesis of articulatory phonology (Browman and Goldstein 1986, 1992) that phonetic contrasts emerge from differences in the assembly of, for example, close–open articulatory gestures and voicing or velar raising/lowering. Particularly for children, the basic articulatory movement gesture for labial consonants is proposed to consist of a

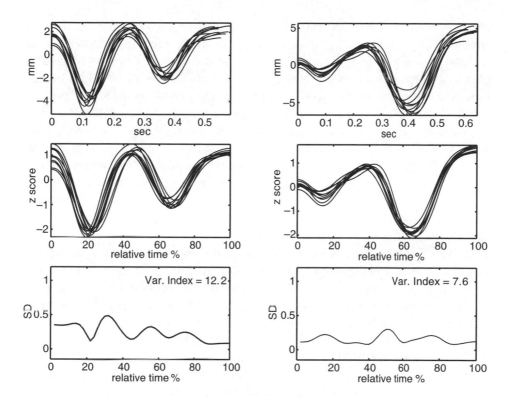

Fig. 10.4 Examples of trochaic and iambic nonce words extracted from the phrase 'It's Bob's [fVfVf]'. These are from an adult speaker. The left set of plots shows the lower lip–jaw movement for 10 productions of the nonce trochee ['fʌfəf]. The right set of plots is for the same phonetic sequence, now learned as an iamb [fə'fʌf]. For both columns of plots, the top traces are the original displacement data. The middle plot shows these movement trajectories after time and amplitude normalization. The bottom plot shows the trajectory variability as a function of normalized time. Note that both the trochee and the iamb are amplitude-modulated for stress. In other words, for the trochee the first open–close movement sequence is larger than the second, while for the iamb the reverse is true. Also, as indicated by the trajectory variability index, the trochee is produced with more variability than the iamb. These individual findings are supported in the larger data set.

generalized movement template. Thus, linguistically relevant contrasts across [m,p,b] and [f,v] would emerge from changes in voice onset time (VOT) or velar raising/lowering. To assess this hypothesis, time- and amplitude-normalized velocity profiles were derived from these simple close–open articulatory movements and subjected to a pattern recognition routine (as described on pp. 233–4). The pattern recognition algorithm reliably sorted the velocity profiles as belonging to specific segments. That is, for example, even for [p] versus [b] or [m] versus [b], aspects of the oral articulatory movements were differentiated, or contained some phoneme specific information. This result was particularly striking, because children were overall more variable than adults and used different movement strategies (e.g. durations and displacements) to attain speech goals. Even in the face of this noisier and less mature speech motor system, the same degree of phonetic differentiation in oral articulatory movements was observed for all age groups. Although multiple explanations (from linguistic to biomechanical) of this result are possible, because of the developmental changes in variability as well as displacement and duration, it is most likely that high-level linguistic units specify aspects of even the most basic articulatory movements. Lower-level motor or biomechanical explanations seem less parsimonious, since the adult and child both achieve the same degree of differentiation. Even a very simple movement trajectory has some constituent structure that is related to different phonetic segments.

In a recent study (Goffman *et al.* 2003), we asked young children and adults to produce two seven-word sentences that varied only in an utterance internal vowel (e.g. 'Mom has the man/moon in the box'). The objective was to evaluate the extent of influence of lip rounding on the entire utterance. Our findings reveal that changing only a single segment influences the movement planning for most or all of the utterance. For both children and adults, the lip rounding gesture had broad influences across a multi-word utterance (far beyond the confines of a syllable or word). Adults showed more organized rounding gestures, but the influence on the entire utterance was similar across age groups.

The account that is beginning to emerge from these data is that biological factors (as in the prosody results) influence the sorts of units that children produce. These young children appear to rely on a basic rhythmic framework for the production of early developing trochaic sequences. However, as communicative demands increase, this bias must be abandoned. The segmental data, in a sense, tell the opposite story. Aspects of higher-level linguistic processing drive even the most basic organization of the close–open movement sequence. The extent of the effects of the various units on movement planning and execution is also quite flexible, as shown by the phrase-level data and the coarticulation results. Also, dependent on the developmental time window, different units and processes may have different weights. In sum, phrase, prosodic word, and segmental level units all converge to systematically influence even the most basic of articulatory movements. It does not seem possible to select either a privileged unit or a privileged direction of influence.

10.5 A parallel multiple unit framework

Many lines of evidence lead to the suggestion that language production involves the activation of many different units during the planning and production of speech. We propose a parallel, multiple unit approach to investigate the development of speech production in children and the characteristics of production in adults. Earlier theoretical accounts have emphasized one level or type of planning unit as the input to the production process. As noted above, linguistic models of adult speech production suggest that either phoneme-sized units or syllables are used to compute the required speech motor sequences (Levelt and Wheeldon 1994; Guenther *et al.* 1998). In some models, for example Levelt *et al.* (1999), other planning units are included, e.g. phrase-level (phonological word-level) syllabification. However, these are assumed to act serially and to have little effect on the actual computation of motor commands. The motor commands are computed from abstract gestural scores for syllables (Levelt and Wheeldon 1994). Levelt and his colleagues have presented compelling evidence for the operation of multiple levels of linguistic processing. Our proposal is that these multiple levels of linguistic representation have direct, detectable effects on motor planning and execution. In other words, at the language–motor interface there are not only phoneme- or syllable-size input units. Rather, these higher levels of representation, for example, syntactic and prosodic levels, must be available to, and used in, shaping the motor planning process. Again, this would not be possible in the model of Levelt and colleagues, because it posits unidirectional flow of information in serially ordered processing modules.

Such a proposal is consistent with evidence from the studies from our laboratory reviewed above, and from many other sources. It is clear that the control processes in speaking must operate over temporal and spatial frames of many different sizes, suggesting that organizational units would likewise operate over multiple levels. Speech breathing cycles last many seconds, while articulatory movements occur over several hundred milliseconds, and control of onset and offset of voicing must occur with tens of milliseconds. In the spatial domain, phonetic contrasts may involve targeted control of local parameters, for example lingual–palatal contact, while other speech parameters, for example, rate or loudness changes, operate globally across respiratory, laryngeal, and orofacial systems (Dromey and Ramig 1998). It is also clear that one level of linguistic processing cannot be assigned to a single subsystem. It might be tempting to argue that the speech breathing control system would only need to integrate information about the syntactic structure of the utterance for control of breathing pauses. However, there is evidence that there are active respiratory adjustments for emphatic stress at the syllable level (Finnegan *et al.* 2000). Further, control of oral articulatory parameters must integrate information from phonetic, syllabic, prosodic, and phrase-level linguistic components, because oral movements change in systematic ways in relation to linguistic goals at these levels (Smith *et al.* 1995; Goffman 1999; Goffman and Malin 1999; Goffman and Smith 1999).

While many developmental studies have focused on the word or syllable level of speech planning and production, some have also emphasized phrase-level processes. Abbeduto (1987) investigated syntactic, semantic, and rhythmic influences on speech motor planning in children and adults. He used syllable duration and consistency of syllable duration as measures of the efficiency of speech motor planning. Children and adults were more efficient at programming multiword utterances when stimuli contain syntactically appropriate structures. Gerard and Clement (1998) employed acoustic analyses of syllable and total phrase duration and fundamental frequency contours to examine the structure and development of prosodic control when phrase-level intonational targets were varied. Their data suggested that phrase-level fundamental frequency contours were pre-planned in children and adults. Children developed prosodic representations gradually, and pitch contours were acquired before durational parameters.

This parallel, multiple unit view of the language/motor interface is also consistent with parallel distributed models of brain organization, such as that of Pulvermuller (1999), which elaborates the Hebbian cell assembly hypothesis to account for language. He suggests that infant babbling is controlled by activity 'in inferior motor, premotor, and prefrontal cortices ... One may well envisage that one specific synfire chain controls the articulation of a given syllable and thus represents its articulatory program' (Pulvermuller 1999, p. 258). He also suggests that the activity of babbling would activate auditory areas and somatosensory areas, so that the infant develops a distributed network that includes motor, auditory, and somatosensory areas for the production of syllables.

In recent work, PET has been employed to examine brain activity prior to speech production in normal adults (Indefrey *et al.* 2001). The left Rolandic operculum, adjacent to Broca's area, shows greater activation for planning utterances with appropriate syntactic structure compared to random words, suggesting a neural correlate of syntactic encoding during pre-speech processing. These areas are also activated when processing syntactic information (Friederici *et al.* 2000). Thus, it seems reasonable to argue that movement planning/production and linguistic encoding processes share some common and co-activated neural mechanisms. Thus we hypothesize that, as syntactic representations of the utterance are formed, as in the model of Levelt *et al.* (1999), associated speech motor planning areas are co-activated, so that the emerging syntactic structure influences the form of the motor sequence that will be generated. We would make the same argument for prosodic representations. These syntactic and prosodic movement frames are also modulated by the specific syllabic and phonetic components that the utterance requires. As noted above, we are not suggesting a progression in the size of the temporal frame for each level of linguistic processing, as a change in a single phoneme can affect the organization of the entire movement sequence for a sentence (Goffman *et al.* 2003). Finally, Diamond (2000), on the basis of studies of children with attention deficit hyperactivity disorder, dyslexia, and SLI, makes a very similar argument about the interaction and co-development of cognitive and motor processes. A parallel argument is also made about children with developmental coordination disorder (Hill and Bishop 1998).

The central question that we posed at the beginning of this chapter was: How can we relate the physiology of muscle activation and movement to the units of language? This remains a difficult question, and our suggestion that there is not a single level of linguistic processing acting at the language–motor interface makes it perhaps even more complex. Ultimately, the question for speech motor control is how the nervous system computes the command sequences to drive all the muscles involved in speech. In a model to generate vowels (DIVA), Guenther *et al.* (1998) assume that the input units are phonemes. They argue that the motor command computation could not be derived from a somatosensory map, but rather these commands must be computed from auditory perceptual space. 'Auditory target regions are hypothesized to arise during development as an emergent property of neural map formation in the auditory system. Furthermore, speech movements are planned as trajectories in auditory perceptual space' (Geunther *et al.* 1998, p. 611). Callan *et al.* (2000) applied the DIVA model to the developing system and demonstrated that it can produce appropriate output in the face of changes due to growth of the vocal tract. These auditory models are in contrast to the gestural model, which assumes an abstract representation of gestures in terms of vocal tract targets (Browman and Goldstein 1992; Levelt and Wheeldon 1994).

Our proposal would be that the infant enters the task of speech production with a set of concepts, a set of auditory representations based on his/her perception of speech (Jusczyk 1997; Kuhl 2000; Werker and Desjardins 2001), and a repertoire of nonspeech oral motor and vocal behaviors (Stark 1980; Oller 2001). We would suggest that, in this beginning set of representations in auditory space, there are already multiple units being formed, including prosodic, word, syllabic, and phonetic units. In other words, there are coexisting, perceptually coherent units at these multiple levels of representation, which, in turn, influence the production process. Language-specific experience modifies how these units cohere as early as the first year of life (Werker and Desjardins 2001). This assertion is also supported by the work showing that infants are sensitive to changes in acoustic input at all of these levels (e.g. Myers *et al.* 1996; Jusczyk 1997).

An essential component of our preliminary framework is the hypothesis that, as speech motor learning occurs over development, the bidirectional influences of language and motor factors are changing. We propose that, as the child matures, the mappings or interactions of language units and movement units change. With the onset of babbling, it seems likely that auditory representations link to movement, and that a sensorimotor–auditory mapping is formed (Pulvermuller 1999). On the production side, during the babbling period, prosodic frames (e.g. fundamental frequency contours) and syllables are most likely the linguistic units with the most weight in shaping the motor command generation process. As the child develops the capacity to produce longer and more complex utterances, word- and phrase-level mappings occur. In this process we would argue that somatosensory and auditory perceptual target space are both essential to compute motor command sequences. Over time, highly stable functional synergies, or collectives of muscles (Bernstein 1967; Saltzman 1978; Sporns and Edelman 1993) acting to achieve peceptual/motor targets, evolve. These functional synergies (e.g. the upper lip, lower lip, and jaw muscles involved in the control of lip aperture) do not map directly on to any single level of linguistic unit, such as the phoneme or syllable. Rather, their activation and sequencing is influenced by the multiple levels of linguistic processing that we have discussed.

As in the learning of any motor behavior, the consistency and accuracy of performance increases over time. Indeed, in the adult, speech is extremely efficient and robust to a variety of perturbations. Data from experiments including older children and adolescents (Walsh and Smith 2002; Smith and Zelaznik 2003) demonstrate that the speech motor learning process is quite protracted. Adult performance is not attained until after 16 years of age. Given that we found no gender differences in articulatory motor control during adolescence, we have argued that these late changes do not predominantly reflect adaptations to peripheral growth. Rather, we suggest that the late maturation of articulatory motor processes is driven primarily by interaction of speech motor systems with co-developing cognitive–linguistic systems, which are also not adult-like until this late period of development (e.g. Holcomb *et al.* 1992). During this long learning process, language–motor linkages become highly stable, and we hypothesize that many highly frequent syllable sequences are stored. It seems reasonable to suggest that we have a mental syllabary (Levelt and Wheeldon 1994), but we would argue further that children and adults would ultimately develop what we would call a multisyllabary. These are stored motor sequences for high-frequency multi-syllable sequences, words, or phrases. We would speculate that ultimately these could be relatively directly accessed and executed.

10.6 Conclusion

Our central argument in this chapter is that links between speech motor processes and linguistic processes are much closer than previous models suggest, and that there are multiple, parallel units operating in preparation of command signals for speech production. During development these mappings between linguistic units and motor output are changing. By studying the emergence and time course of these interactive mappings, we can shed some light on the question of the units of organization of speech production. We have presented a preliminary framework for the investigation of these hypotheses. Models of adult speech production assume the syllable or phoneme as the input unit. However, a single-unit input model cannot account for the characteristics of speech movement organization, nor for the evidence of changing interactions of language and motor processes across developmental periods. Speech motor and psycholinguistic theories are now sufficiently elaborated to begin to fully explicate the entire process of speech production in a coherent framework that integrates linguistic and articulatory components.

Acknowledgements

The work from our laboratories reviewed in this chapter has been supported by the National Institutes of Health, National Institute on Deafness and Other Communicative Disorders, Grants DC00559, DC02527, and DC04826.

References

Abbeduto, L. 1987. Syntactic, semantic, and rhythmic influences on children's and adults' motor programming of speech. *Journal of Psycholinguistic Research, 16,* 201–221.

Abbs, J.H. 1986. Invariance and variability in speech production: a distinction between linguistic intent and its neuromotor implementation. In J. Perkell and D. Klatt (Eds.), *Invariance and variability in speech processes.* Mahwah, NJ: Lawrence Erlbaum, pp. 202–225.

Abbs, J.H. and **Gracco, V.L.** 1984. Control of complex motor gestures: orofacial muscle responses to load perturbations of lip during speech. *Journal of Neurophysiology, 51,* 705–723.

Barlow, S.M. and **Farley, G.R.** 1989. Neurophysiology of speech. In D.P. Kuehn, M.L. Lemme and J.M. Baumgartner (Eds.), *Neural bases of speech, hearing, and language.* Boston: College Hill Press, pp. 146–200.

Bernstein, N.A. 1967. *The coordination and regulation of movements.* Oxford: Pergamon Press.

Bock, K. 1995. Sentence production: from mind to mouth. In J.L. Miller and P.D. Eimas (Eds.), *Speech, language, and communication. Handbook of perception and cognition* (2nd ed.). San Diego, CA: Academic Press, pp. 191–216.

Browman, C.P. and **Goldstein, L.M.** 1986. Towards an articulatory phonology. *Phonology Yearbook, 3,* 219–252.

Browman, C. and **Goldstein, L.,** 1991. Gestural structures: distinctiveness, phonological processes, and historical change. In I.G. Mattingly and M. Studdert-Kennedy (Eds.), *Modularity and the motor theory of speech perception.* Mahwah: Lawrence Erlbaum & Associates, Inc., pp. 313–337.

Browman, C.P. and **Goldstein, L.** 1992. Articulatory phonology: an overview. *Phonetica, 49,* 155–180.

Callen, D.E., Kent, R.D., Guenther, F.H., and **Vorperian, H.K.** 2000. An auditory-feedback-based neural network model of speech production that is robust to developmental changes in the size and shape of the articulatory system. *Journal of Speech, Language, and Hearing Research, 43,* 721–736.

de Boysson-Bardies, B. and **Vihman, M.M.** 1991. Adaptation to language: evidence from babbling and first words in four languages. *Language, 67,* 297–319.

de Boysson-Bardies, B., Sagart, L., and **Durand, C.** 1984. Discernible differences in the babbling of infants according to target language. *Journal of Child Language, 11,* 1–15.

Dell, G.S. and **O'Seaghdha, P. G.** 1992. Stages of lexical access in language production. *Cognition, 42,* 287–314.

Diamond, A. 2000. Close interrelation of motor development and cognitive development and of the cerebellum and prefrontal cortex. *Child Development, 71,* 44–56.

Dromey, C. and **Ramig, L.O.** 1998. Intentional changes in sound pressure level and rate: their impact on measures of respiration, phonation, and articulation. *Journal of Speech, Language, and Hearing Research, 41 (5),* 1003–1018.

Echols, C.H. 1993. A perceptually-based model of children's earliest productions. *Cognition, 46,* 245–296.

Ejiri, K. 1998. Relationship between rhythmic behavior and canonical babbling in infant vocal development. *Phonetica, 55,* 226–237.

Ferguson, C.A. and **Farwell, C.B.** 1975. Words and sounds in early language acquisition: English initial consonants in the first fifty words. *Language, 51,* 419–439.

Ferreira, F. 1991. Effects of length and syntactic complexity on initiation times for prepared utterances. *Journal of Memory and Language, 30,* 210–233.

Finnegan, E.M., Luschei, E.S., and **Hoffman, H.T.** 2000. Modulations in respiratory and laryngeal activity associated with changes in vocal intensity during speech. *Journal of Speech, Language, and Hearing Research, 43(4),* 934–950.

Friederici, A.D., Meyer, M., and **von Cramon, D.Y.** 2000. Auditory language comprehension: an event-related fMRI study on the processing of syntactic and lexical information. *Brain and Language, 75 (3),* 289–300.

Gerard, C. and **Clement, J.** 1998. The structure and development of French prosodic representations. *Journal of Language and Speech, 41 (2),* 117–142.

Gerken, L. 1994. Young children's representation of prosodic phonology: evidence from English-speakers' weak syllable productions. *Journal of Memory and Language, 33,* 19–38.

Goffman, L. 1999. Prosodic influences on speech production in children with specific language impairment: kinematic, acoustic, and transcription evidence. *Journal of Speech, Language, and Hearing Research, 42,* 1499–1517.

Goffman, L. 2003. Rhythmic motor contributions to the acquisition of linguistic stress in content and function words. (Submitted.)

Goffman, L. and **Malin, C.** 1999. Metrical effects on speech movements in children and adults. *Journal of Speech, Language, and Hearing Research, 42,* 1003–1115.

Goffman, L. and **Smith, A.** 1999. Development and phonetic differentiation of speech movement patterns. *Journal of Experimental Psychology: Human Perception and Performance, 25,* 649–660.

Goffman, L., Vink, L., Smith, A., and **Ho, M.** 2003. Effect of segmental motor organization in speech production. (In preparation.)

Green, J.R., Moore, C.A., and **Reilly,** 2002. The sequential development of jaw and lip control for speech. *Journal of Speech, Language, and Hearing Research, 45,* 66–79.

Guenther, F.H., Hamson, M., and Johnson, D. 1998. A theoretical investigation of reference frames for the planning of speech movements. *Psychological Review, 105 (4)*, 611–633.

Hill, E. and Bishop, D.V.M. 1998. A reaching test reveals weak hand preference in specific language impairment and developmental coordination disorder. *Laterality, 3*, 295–310.

Holcomb, P.J., Coffey, S.A., and Neville, H.J. 1992. Visual and auditory sentence processing: a developmental analysis using event-related brain potentials. *Developmental Neuropsychology, 8*, 203–241.

Indefrey, P., Brown, C.M., Hellwig, F., Amunts, K., Herzog, H., Seitz, R.J., and Hagoort, P. 2001. A neural correlate of syntactic encoding during speech production. *Proceedings of the National Academy of Sciences, 98 (10)*, 5933–5936.

Jusczyk, P.W. 1997. *The discovery of spoken language*. Cambridge, MA: MIT Press.

Kehoe, M., Stoel-Gammon, C., and Buder, E. (1995). Acoustic correlates of stress in young children's speech. *Journal of Speech and Hearing Research, 38*, 338–350.

Kelso, J.A.S., Tuller, B., Vatikiotis-Bateson, E., and Fowler, C.A. 1984. Functionally specific articulatory cooperation adaptation to jaw perturbations during speech: evidence for coordinative structures. *Journal of Experimental Psychology: Human Perception and Performance, 10*, 812–832.

Kent, R.D. 1992. The biology of phonological development. In C.A. Ferguson, L. Menn, and C. Stoel-Gammon (Eds.), *Phonological development: Models, research, implications*. Timonium, MD: York Press, pp. 65–90.

Kent, R.D. 1984. Psychobiology of speech development: coemergence of language and a movement system. *American Journal of Physiology, 246*, R888–894.

Kent, R.D. and Forner, L.L. 1980. Speech segment durations in sentence recitations by children and adults. *Journal of Phonetics, 8*, 157–168.

Kleinow, J. and Smith, A. 2000. Influences of length and syntactic complexity on the speech motor stability of the fluent speech of adults who stutter. *Journal of Speech, Language, and Hearing Research, 43*, 548–559.

Kleinow, J., Smith, A., and Ramig, L.O. 2001. Speech motor stability in IPD: effects of rate and loudness manipulations. *Journal of Speech, Language, and Hearing Research, 44*, 1041–1051.

Kozhevnikov, V.A. and Chistovich, L.A. 1966. *Speech: articulation and perception*. United States Department of Commerce, Joint Publications Research Service, 30. Springfield, VA: United States Department of Commerce.

Kuhl, P.K. 2000. Speech, language, and developmental change. In F. Lacerda and C. von Hofsten (Eds.), *Emerging cognitive abilities in early infancy*. Mahwah, NJ: Lawrence Erlbaum Associates, pp. 111–133.

Langlois, A. and Baken, R. 1976. Development of respiratory time-factors in infant cry. *Developmental Medicine and Child Neurology, 18*, 732–737.

Levelt, W.J.M. 1989. *Speaking: From intention to articulation.* Cambridge, MA: MIT Press.

Levelt, W.J.M. and **Wheeldon, L.** 1994. Do speakers have access to a mental syllabary? *Cognition, 50,* 239–269.

Levelt, W.J.M., Schriefers, H., Vorberg, D., and **Meyer, A.S.** 1991. The time course of lexical access in speech production: a study of picture naming. *Psychological Review, 98,* 122–142.

Levelt, W.J.M., Roelofs, A., and **Meyer, A.S.** 1999. A theory of lexical access in speech production. *Behavioral and Brain Sciences, 22,* 1–75.

Locke, J. 1993. *The child's path to spoken language.* Cambridge, MA: Harvard University Press.

Locke, J. and **Pearson, D.M.** 1992. Vocal learning and the emergence of phonological capacity: a neurobiological approach. In C.A. Ferguson, L. Menn, and C. Stoel-Gammon (Eds.), *Phonological development: models, research, implications.* Timonium, MD: York Press, pp. 91–130.

MacNeilage, P. 1970. Motor control of serial ordering of speech. *Psychological Review, 77,* 182–196.

MacNeilage, P.F. and **Davis, B.L.** 1990. Acquisition of speech production: frames then content. In M. Jeannerod (Ed.), *Attention and performance XII: motor representation and control.* Hillsdale, NJ: Lawrence Erlbaum Associates, pp. 453–476.

MacNeilage, P.F. and **Davis, B.L.** 2000. On the origin of internal structure of word forms. *Science, 288,* 527–531.

Maner, K., Smith, A., and **Grayson, L.** 2000. Influences of length and syntactic complexity on speech motor performance of children and adults. *Journal of Speech, Language, and Hearing Research, 43,* 560–573.

Moll, K., Zimmermann, G., and **Smith, A.** 1977. The study of speech production as a human neuromotor system. In M. Sawashima and F.S. Cooper (Eds.), *Dynamic aspects of speech production.* Tokyo: University of Tokyo, pp. 107–127.

Moore, C.A., Caulfield, T.J., and **Green, J.R.** 2001. Relative kinematics of the rib cage and abdomen during speech and nonspeech behaviors of 15-month-old children. *Journal of Speech, Language, and Hearing Research, 44,* 80–94.

Myers, J., Jusczyk, P.W., Kemler Nelson, D.G., Charles-Luce, J., Woodward, A.L., and **Hirsh-Pasek, K.** 1996. Infants' sensitivity to word boundaries in fluent speech. *Journal of Child Language, 23,* 1–30.

Nittrouer, S., Studdert-Kennedy, M. and **McGowen, R.S.** 1989. The emergence of phonetic segments: evidence from the spectral structure of fricative-vowel syllables spoken by children and adults. *Journal of Speech and Hearing Research, 32,* 120–132.

Nittrouer, S., Studdert-Kennedy, M., and **Neely, S.T.** 1996. How children learn to organize their speech gestures: further evidence from fricative-vowel syllables. *Journal of Speech and Hearing Research, 39 (2),* 379–389.

Oller, D.K. 2001. *The emergence of the speech capacity.* Mahwah, NJ: Lawrence Erlbaum Associates.

Oller, D.K. and **Eilers, R.** 1988. The role of audition in infant babbling. *Child Development, 59,* 441–449.

Perkell, J.S. 1980. Phonetic features and the physiology of speech production. In B. Butterworth (Ed.), *Language production,* Vol. 1. New York: Academic Press, pp. 337–372.

Pulvermuller, F. 1999. Words in the brain's language. *Behavioral and Brain Sciences, 22,* 253–336.

Saltzman, E. 1978. Levels of sensorimotor representation. *Journal of Mathematical Biology, 20,* 91–163.

Schwartz, R.G. and **Goffman, L.** 1995. Metrical patterns of words and production accuracy. *Journal of Speech and Hearing Research, 38,* 876–888.

Sharkey, S.G. and **Folkins, J.W.** 1985. Variability of lip and jaw movements in children and adults: implications for the development of speech motor control. *Journal of Speech and Hearing Research, 28,* 8–15.

Shattuck-Hufnagel, S. 1987. The role of word onset consonants in speech production planning: new evidence from speech error patterns. In E. Keller and M. Gopnik (Eds.), *Motor and sensory processing in language.* Hillsdale, NJ: Erlbaum, pp. 17–51.

Smith, A. 1992. The control of orofacial movements in speech. *Critical Reviews in Oral Biology and Medicine, 3,* 233–267.

Smith, A. and **Goffman, L.** 1998. Stability and patterning of speech movement sequences in children and adults. *Journal of Speech, Language, and Hearing Science, 41,* 18–30.

Smith, A. and **Kleinow, J.** 2000. Kinematic correlates of speaking rate changes in stuttering and normally fluent adults. *Journal of Speech, Language, and Hearing Research, 43,* 521–536.

Smith, A. and **Zelaznik, H.** 2003. The development of functional synergies for speech motor coordination in childhood and adolescence. (Submitted.)

Smith, A., Goffman, L., Zelaznik, H., Ying, G. and **McGillem, C.** 1995. Spatiotemporal stability and patterning of speech movement sequences. *Experimental Brain Research, 104,* 493–501.

Smith, A., Johnson, M., McGillem, C. and **Goffman, L.** 2000. On the assessment of stability and patterning of speech movements. *Journal of Speech, Language, and Hearing Research, 43,* 277–286.

Snow, D. 1994. Phrase-final syllable lengthening and intonation in early child speech. *Journal of Speech and Hearing Research, 37,* 831–840.

Snow, D. 1998. Children's imitations of intonation contours: are rising tones more difficult than falling tones? *Journal of Speech, Language, and Hearing Research, 41,* 576–587.

Sporns, O. and **Edelman, G.M.** 1993. Solving Bernstein's problem: A proposal for the development of coordinated movement by selection. *Child Development, 64,* 960–981.

Stark, R.E. 1980. Stages of speech development in the first year of life. In G. Yeni-Komshian, J. Kavanagh, and C. Ferguson (Eds.), *Child Phonology* (Vol. 1). New York: Academic Press, pp. 73–90.

Stark, R.E. 1989. Temporal patterning of cry and non-cry sounds in the first eight months of life. *First Language, 9,* 107–136.

Stetson, R. 1951. *Motor phonetics.* Amsterdam: North-Holland.

Stoel-Gammon, C. and **Otomo, K.** 1986. Babbling development of hearing impaired and normally hearing subjects. *Journal of Speech and Hearing Disorders, 51,* 33–41.

Thelen, E. 1981. Rhythmical behavior in infancy: an ethological perspective. *Developmental Psychology, 17,* 237–257.

Vigliocco, G., Laurer, M., Damian, M.F., and **Levelt, W.J.M.** 2002. Semantic and syntactic forces in noun phrase production. *Journal of Experimental Psychology: Learning, Memory, and Language, 28,* 46–58.

Vihman, M.M. 1996. *Phonological development: the origins of language in the child.* Cambridge, MA: Blackwell.

Walsh, B. and **Smith, A.** 2002. Articulatory movements in adolescents: evidence for protracted development of speech motor control processes. *Journal of Speech, Language, and Hearing Research, 45,* 1119–1133.

Ward, D. and **Arnfield, S.** 2001. Linear and nonlinear analysis of the stability of gestural organization in speech movement sequences. *Journal of Speech, Language, and Hearing Research, 44,* 108–117.

Werker, J.F. and **Desjardins, R.N.** 2001. Listening to speech in the first year of life. In M. Tomasello and E. Bates (Eds.), *Language development: the essential readings.* Malden, MA: Blackwell, pp. 26–33.

Wohlert, A. and **Smith, A.** 2002. Developmental change in variability of lip muscle activity during speech. *Journal of Speech, Language, and Hearing Research, 45,* 1077–1087.

CHAPTER 11

LINGUISTIC PROCESSES AND CHILDHOOD STUTTERING: MANY'S A SLIP BETWEEN INTENTION AND LIP

EDWARD G. CONTURE, COURTNEY T. ZACKHEIM, JULIE D. ANDERSON, AND MARK W. PELLOWSKI

11.1 Introduction

The purpose of this chapter is to present the theoretical base for a programmatic study of linguistic processes in children who stutter (CWS). This theoretical position is based on our own empirical studies of childhood stuttering (e.g. Logan and Conture 1997; Anderson and Conture 2000; Pellowski *et al.* 2001; Pellowski 2002; Zackheim *et al.* 2002; Melnick *et al.* 2003; Zackheim and Conture 2003; Anderson, unpublished) and speculations (e.g. Conture 2001*a*, pp. 27–50) as well as that of others (e.g. Bernstein Ratner 1997; Kolk and Postma 1997; Tetnowski 1998). This chapter, therefore, while attempting to review all pertinent literature, will focus on the rationale for our study of linguistic processes in relationship to childhood stuttering.

11.1.1 Incidence of stuttering

Stuttering has a lifetime incidence (i.e. percentage of adults who report that they stuttered at some point in their lifetime) of nearly 5%, and significantly impacts the academic, emotional, social, and vocational achievements, development, and potential of individuals who stutter (see Bloodstein 1995; Conture 1996; Yairi 1997). Although the incidence of stuttering is generally reported as 5%, 70–80% of those affected discontinue (e.g. Ambrose and Yairi 1999) without significant formal treatment, a phenomenon referred to as 'spontaneous' or 'unassisted' recovery. For the remaining children (i.e. the approximately 1% of children who continue to stutter after 6 years of age), the negative impact of stuttering on their lives and daily activities can be significant, if not devastating. Thus, there is a strong need to determine those variables that may initiate/cause, exacerbate, or perpetuate instances of stuttering, in order to eventually develop more efficient, effective, empirically based approaches to the diagnosis and treatment of the disorder (for a recent overview of lines of evidence contained within empirical studies of stuttering within the past 20 years, see Conture 2001*b*; for recent data-based investigations of onset and development of childhood stuttering, see a series of recent papers by Yairi, Ambrose and colleagues, e.g. Yairi and Ambrose 1992*a, b*; Yairi *et al.* 1996; Yairi and Ambrose 1999; for overview of treatment efficacy research, pertaining to stuttering, see Conture 1996).

11.1.2 Stuttering: behavior versus disorder

As has been described elsewhere (Conture 2001*b*, pp. 19–20), there is some value, from both a theoretical as well as therapeutic perspective, to distinguish between *the behavior* versus *the disorder* described as stuttering. The former, the behavior, comes and goes relatively rapidly, within milliseconds or at least seconds, suggesting that whatever precipitates or causes instances of stuttering must also occur, as well as change, rapidly. The latter, the disorder, comes and goes relatively slowly, across days, weeks, and months, suggesting that less rapid events, for example, temperamental responses to errors, speech–language development, etc. may influence the overall quantity and quality of the disorder of stuttering. Of course, there can be interactions, if not complete overlaps, at times, between variables that create rapid changes in stuttering, the behavior, and those that create slower change in stuttering, the disorder. For purposes of this discussion, it is those variables, in this case linguistic, that rapidly change and hence rapidly influence the *state* of one's speech fluency that are of interest.

   Why do such distinctions matter? Well, it is our basic assumption, as will be mentioned below, that *any* theoretical account of stuttering (or, for that matter, any disorder), must begin by accounting for the behavior or symptoms of the disorder itself. And, in the past, many explanations of stuttering have:

(1) neither explicitly nor specifically accounted for those speech behaviors, for example, sound/syllable repetitions, that comprise the *sine qua non* of stuttering (cf. the theorization of Brutten and Shoemaker 1967, that tried to explain stuttering behaviors from a learning perspective); and/or

(2) posited variables that are either too slow (e.g. conflicts between one's identity as a typical versus atypical speaker) and/or relatively stable or non-changing (e.g. temperamental characteristics) to account for the rapid, second to second changes in speech fluency during conversational speech that are the hallmark of stuttering.

   Of course, while the latter (2) variables may change slowly and/or minimally, they could clearly have an influence on the quality of the behavior. In essence, the present authors suggest that these variables may exacerbate behavior *already* present or occurring; however, it seems less than likely that such slow, minimally changing events could generate the *initial* disruption causing instances of stuttering, behavior that is very rapidly and continuously changing.

What events, therefore, change rapidly and continuously as we communicate? Our first, perhaps obvious, response, is cognition. Our thoughts change very rapidly throughout conversation. The next, of course, is the linguistic plan we develop to express those thoughts. And finally, the means by which the speaker executes the linguistic plan to convey his or her thoughts, intention, or message. Of the three, just the physical work, through time and space, involved with respiratory, phonatory, and articulatory movement, while clearly rapid, generally cannot match the incredibly rapid occurrence of, and change in, thought and linguistic plans. Furthermore, motor behavior is the end-product of the concatenation of cognitive and linguistic events; that is, motor behavior, during communication, typically follows thinking and linguistic planning (or, at best, occur in parallel with aspects of linguistic planning). If these rapidly changing events, that precede motoric planning, control, and/or execution are themselves less efficient, not well integrated, or even slower than typical, is it not possible that they contribute to a person's relative lack of fluent speech? Do we know if they do? No, of course not, but we never will until we look outside the motoric lamplight into the linguistic darkness for the keys to stuttering

11.1.3 Change in the Zeitgeist

While *motoric* variables (e.g. speech motor control of articulation, phonation, and respiration) have received considerable attention during the past 20 years (e.g. for review, see Conture 1991a; van Lieshout 1995; Ingham 1998; Caruso *et al.* 1999), developing lines of evidence suggest that *linguistic* variables such as phonology, semantics, and syntax may contribute just as much as motoric processes to childhood stuttering (Louko *et al.* 1999). For example, adults who stutter, when compared to adults who do not stutter, retrieve semantic information more slowly (Bosshardt and Fransen 1996) and/or require more processing capacity for sentence generation (Bosshardt *et al.* 2002).

Likewise, of particular salience to the present paper, developing lines of evidence indicate that linguistic variables impact the fluency of CWS. In specific, CWS, when compared to children who do not stutter (CWNS), exhibit:

(1) semantic development that appears to lag behind that of their syntactic development (Anderson and Conture 2000);

(2) increased stuttering frequency as utterance length and complexity increase (e.g. Logan and Conture 1995, 1997), a relationship that appears to also hold for stutterings that occur in clusters (Logan and LaSalle 1999) as well as singletons (e.g. Melnick and Conture 2000);

(3) most of their stutterings occurring in utterances that are longer than their mean length of utterance (Zackheim and Conture, 2003); and

(4) lower receptive vocabulary scores on standardized tests (Williams *et al.* 1969; Westby 1974; Murray and Reed 1977; Anderson and Conture 2000).

Similarly, Weber-Fox (2001) has shown that adults who stutter may exhibit 'alterations in processing ... related to neural functions that are common to word classes and perhaps involve shared, underlying processes for lexical access' (p. 814; cf. Packman *et al.* 2001; Onslow and Packman 2002, regarding stuttering and lexical retrieval).

Of course, exceptions to the above trends can be noted, for example, Ryan's (1992) finding that CWS scored lower than CWNS on a test of receptive vocabulary, but not significantly so [although subsequent follow-up (Ryan 2001), with many of these same subjects, indicated that scores on standardized tests of articulation and language at initial testing were major predictors of stuttering for children whose stuttering persisted approximately 2 years later]. An additional exception to the aforementioned trends is Logan's (2001) finding that utterance length and complexity seem to have less influence on the stutterings of older individuals who stutter. Whatever the case, in terms of CWS, it seems difficult to account for the preceding general trends *solely* by means of motoric explanations of stuttering (e.g. the notion that instances of stuttering are primarily or solely caused by planning, initiation, and execution of speech motor acts). In other words, while changes in speech motor behaviors are clearly involved with the 'speech acts' listeners perceive as stuttering, the current authors believe that linguistic behaviors are also highly likely to be involved with the disturbances in planning and production that contribute to stuttering.

11.1.4 Gone but not forgotten hypothesis

In fact, the above-noted exceptions, in older children and adults, may actually be telling us something about the rule during childhood. Perhaps, differences in the relationship between linguistic variables and stuttering between children and adults who stutter suggest that events that earlier were contributory to stuttering (e.g. difficulties retrieving and encoding words) but resolve with development, may have 'influence beyond the grave'. That is, during the time period when the initiating event existed (i.e. impairment), the child may learn various adaptations to that event, for example, repetitions of sounds, syllables, and words that occur while the child is 'waiting' for the 'word to emerge'. If such learning takes place, such adaptation may persist long after the initiating event has been resolved or at least minimized. This might be similar to the situation where a child whose tonsils were inflamed, swollen, and painful for an extended time may learn compensatory chewing and swallowing behaviors that persist long after the tonsils are surgically removed. Thus, events that initiate stuttering in childhood may be gone, but not forgotten, in adulthood, in the form of learned, compensatory, but maladaptive behaviors. What is attractive about this hypothesis is that rather than expecting to find more differences in speech–language planning between people who do and do not stutter, as people grow older, one would expect, for the group, fewer differences. That is not to say that the quality and/or quantity of instances of stuttering doesn't change with development, far from it, but that the presence or strength of originating sources may diminish and/or become less apparent as people who stutter grow older. Thus, originating difficulties may be gone but not forgotten in the form of compensatory, learned adaptations to a less apparent, if not marginalized, earlier problem [note that van Lieshout (1995) makes a similar argument regarding a motor (learning) problem in stuttering].

Such possibilities, of course, seemingly call out for developmental studies of the aforementioned linguistic variables, from the time of onset of stuttering (i.e. 30–36 months of age) through adulthood, to assess whether the 'gone but not forgotten' speculation has any empirical support. Such notions are similar to the study by Howell *et al.* (1999) of how changes in stuttering loci from function to content words occur from preschool children to adults who stutter, and Peters and Starkweather's (1989) earlier attempt to show how three domains—motor, language, and psycho-social—impact stuttering across five stages of development, from children to adults. And while empirical study of speech motor control in adults, which comprises the vast majority of the work in this area during the past 20 years, has definite value in terms of describing the nature of stuttering in adults, it cannot *by itself* completely address the foregoing suggestions, especially those relating to developing linguistic variables and childhood stuttering. To do that, children and events involving their cognitive and linguistic planning, in addition to adults and speech motor control, must also be studied [e.g. the study by Maner *et al.* (2000) of the bi-directional influence of utterance length/complexity and speech motor performance].

What appears to be needed, therefore, as a starting point, is a theoretical account for those linguistic processes (e.g. semantics, syntax, and phonology) involved with the planning for speech–language production, processes these authors believe appreciably influence instances of stuttering. Increasing our understanding of these processes and their relationship to childhood stuttering should broaden our perspective on stuttering and provide meaningful insights into the role that linguistic processes play in the initiation and/or cause of instances of stuttering in children.

11.2 Theoretical background: general

In attempts to develop a theoretical account for how disruptions in linguistic processes may contribute to instances of stuttering, we have employed the theoretical and empirical work of Levelt and his colleagues regarding normal speech and language production (e.g. Levelt and Wheeldon 1994; Levelt *et al.* 1999; Roelofs 2003), as well as constructs from a Levelt-influenced model of stuttering, the covert repair hypothesis (e.g. Postma and Kolk 1993; Kolk and Postma 1997). Greatly simplifying Levelt *et al.*'s elegant speculation, the process of speech–language production is partitioned into three components:

(1) the *conceptualizer*, where the speaker's 'intention' is created;
(2) the *formulator*, where the speaker's 'intent' is converted into a 'linguistic plan'; and
(3) the *articulator*, where the speaker realizes or executes the linguistic plan in the form of overt communication.

[For views contrary to such modular distinctions between grammar and the lexicon, see, for example, Bates and Goodman (1997) for a more unified lexicalist or anti-modularist account of speech–language development and production, as well as Plunket *et al.* (1997) for a more dynamical neural network oriented model.]

Although each of these three components has relevance to speech–language production, in this paper we will focus on the formulator component (whose sub-components consist of such processes as syntactic, semantic, and phonological encoding). Such focus is based on results of our own studies (e.g. Yaruss and Conture 1996; Anderson and Conture 2000; Pellowski *et al.* 2001; Zackheim *et al.* 2002; Melnick *et al.* 2003; Zackheim and Conture 2003) as well as that of others (e.g. Bernstein and Sih 1987; Kadi-Hanifi and Howell 1992). Interestingly, imbalances between semantic and syntactic development have also been reported for developmentally language-disordered children who frequently exhibit speech disfluencies (Hall *et al.* 1993; Hall 1996; Boscolo *et al.* 2002). Whether these imbalances will be similar to any observed in CWS is, of course, presently unclear. However, the possibility remains, and needs to be empirically assessed, that differing levels of mastery and/or differential development among sub-components of formulative processes (i.e. semantics, syntax, and phonology) may contribute to the difficulties CWS have establishing reasonably fluent speech–language production.

11.2.1 Planning for speech–language production and stuttering

Our basic assumption, that the cause and/or initiation of instances of stuttering is as much related to the process of *planning for* as it is the *execution of* speech and language, has led us to suggest that the most common instances of childhood stuttering (e.g. sound/syllable repetitions, sound prolongations, and single-syllable whole-word repetitions) reflect relatively *slow, inefficient* (when compared to normal) *planning* (formulation) for speech–language production. We believe this is especially true for those processes that must interface rapidly, smoothly, and accurately with one another to communicate the speaker's intent. This does not mean that people who stutter cannot, or do not, exhibit slow-to-initiate phonation, difficulties with temporal organization of speech movement control, or differences in complex movement tasks (for a review, see Caruso *et al.* 1999). However, to date, very few, if any, such concerns with speech motor control have been shown to be either necessary or sufficient for the occurrence of instances of stuttering (for earlier, critical discussions of these issues, see Conture 1991*c*; Ingham 1998). And, of course, the same could be said about linguistic variables, but at present, far less is known regarding the contributions that linguistic variables may make to stuttering. Whatever the case, what one perceives in terms of disfluency is likely to depend on the timing and location of the system involved, and perhaps even the task itself (e.g. van Lieshout *et al.* 1997). Thus, only through a combination of different perspectives/methodologies will we eventually be able to circumscribe the entirety of events associated with the onset and development of stuttering.

On the contrary, linguistic variables, for example, length and grammatical complexity, have been shown repeatedly to be associated with instances of stuttering (for review, see Bernstein-Ratner 1997; Tetnowski 1998; Conture 2001*b*). Of course, correlations between two variables does not mean that one variable causes the other; however, neither do they suggest that linguistic variables are not relevant to stuttering. Furthermore, certain types of speech disfluency (i.e. monosyllabic whole-word repetitions) may be related to greater disparities between semantic and syntactic development (Anderson and Conture 2000). This latter finding is consistent with the finding of Hall and colleagues that such disparities are apparent for highly disfluent language-impaired children (e.g. Hall *et al.* 1993), but is in need of further empirical study [see Pellowski and Conture (2002) for a detailed assessment of different disfluency types in relationship to salient measures/variables associated with childhood stuttering]. Similarly, Wolk *et al.* (1993) reported that CWS, with disordered phonology, when compared to those without disordered phonology, exhibited significantly more sound prolongations. Again, such observations can not be easily or solely explained, it would seem, on the basis of speech motor control accounts of stuttering.

11.2.3 Possible problematic 'sites' within speech–language planning

Many aspects of semantic, syntactic, and phonological planning/formulation may be problematic and potentially related to childhood stuttering. However, our theoretical, as well as observational, work to date (e.g. Anderson and Conture 2000; Pellowski 2002; Melnick *et al.* 2003) leads us to suggest that slowness and/or inefficiencies during four linguistic 'processes' or interactions appear particularly salient:

(1) morphological–syntactic construction of surface structure;
(2) retrieving the lemma (i.e. syntactic/meaning aspects of word) from the mental lexicon; and/or
(3) mapping the lemma onto the lexeme (see Levelt *et al.* 1999 for a more general description of mapping lemma to lexeme); and/or
(4) phonological 'spell-out' of the lemma or the creation of the lexeme (i.e. phonological aspects of the word).

Others (e.g. Perkins *et al.* 1991) have suggested that the integration of suprasegmental with segmental information may be problematic for people who stutter;

however, our research to date has concentrated on the above three processes. Most importantly, difficulties with these and/or other linguistic processes need not necessarily result in clinically significant 'language, vocabulary or phonology problems'. That is, subtle inefficiencies in selection, encoding, or organization of various linguistic variables, while not necessarily becoming manifest as 'clinically significant' grammar, vocabulary, or phonological problems, may none the less appreciably contribute to and/or precipitate instances of stuttering in children.

Slowness and inefficiencies in any or all of these processes, separately or in combination, it would seem, have potential to increase delays and/or errors in speech planning. Such difficulties should result in various infelicities in speech–language production that may be reacted to by the speaker and lead to instances of stuttering. Whether the above speculation is ultimately shown to be tenable, in whole or in part, one point needs to be made: this line of investigation is *not* trying to determine whether these possible difficulties result from genetic, environmental, or combined genetic–environmental factors. Rather, our study of linguistic processes relative to childhood stuttering attempts to determine whether *slow, relatively inefficient functioning* of any one, two or more *formulative (linguistic planning) processes* are exhibited by CWS, and whether these difficulties have potential to contribute to the onset, development, and maintenance of childhood stuttering.

11.2.4 Psycholinguistic theory of stuttering

It seems reasonable to suggest that Wingate (1988) set the stage for modern psycholinguistic approaches to stuttering by suggesting that 'There is ample evidence to indicate that the defect is not simply one of motor control or coordination, but that it involves more central functions of the language production system' (p. 238). Since that time, Postma and Kolk's covert-repair hypothesis (CRH) (e.g. Kolk 1991; Postma and Kolk 1993; Kolk and Postma 1997) has become one of the more comprehensive, psycholinguistically driven explanations of stuttering [see Bernstein Ratner (1995, 1997), Conture (2001a) and Tetnowski (1998) for review of applied as well as theoretical linguistic/psycholinguistic accounts of stuttering]. This theory explicitly attempts to account for the occurrence of sound/syllable repetitions and sound prolongations (i.e. instances of stuttering) and is grounded in the aforementioned Levelt model of speech–language production (e.g. Levelt 1989; Levelt *et al.* 1999; Indefrey and Levelt 2000) as well as empirical studies of speech disfluencies and errors (e.g. Levelt 1983; Blackmer and Mitton 1991; Bredart 1991; Dell and Juliano 1991; Clark and Wasow 1998).

The basic premise of the CRH is that the speech sound units of young CWS are *slow to activate*, a fact that means their intended speech units are more apt to remain in competition (for being selected) with unintended speech units for a longer period of time (for an overview of this and related speculation, see Conture 2001a, pp. 33–45). It is hypothesized that if CWS experience a lengthened period of competition—due to the slowness of their speech target activation—there will be increased chances for misselection during the process of phonological encoding, particularly if these children attempt to initiate speech and/or make speech sound selections at an inappropriately fast rate. If they do, they are thought to be more apt to produce speech sound selection errors because the child's rate of selection has exceeded his/her rate of speech unit activation (an 'automatic' process). With an increased number of such misselections, these children are thought to be more apt to revise their 'phonological plan', a revision that often entails tracing back to the beginning of the sound, syllable, or word. That is, as the speaker self-repairs an 'unintended message' or speech error having (1) just occurred, (2) been in the process of occurring, or (3) been about to occur, an instance of stuttering (e.g. sound/syllable repetition) is thought to result as a by-product of these repairs.

One caveat to the above speculation is that the precise nature of 'normal' (and abnormal) speech errors is still uncertain (Mowrey and MacKay 1990). Thus, instances of stuttering may not necessarily occur where we perceive them, nor involve a phoneme or larger 'unit' as a whole, even though that is how the stuttering is perceived. To paraphrase our title, perhaps, there also may be a slip between perception and lip! Of course, the covert repair hypothesis (CRH), like any theory, is not without concern (see van Lieshout 1995). However, it has clearly generated empirical attempts to assess its basic tenets (e.g. Yaruss and Conture 1996; Logan and Conture 1997; Hartsuiker *et al.* 2003; Melnick *et al.* 2003), something that has not always been true with regard to theories of stuttering.

The CRH, essentially an impairment-adaptation theory (see Kolk 1991), suggests that many speech events, assumed to be self-repairs, exhibited by people who stutter, reflect their attempts to accommodate for, or adapt to, an impaired (i.e. slower-than-normal) ability to 'phonologically encode'. And, while psycholinguists appear divided about the *nature* of linguistic planning problems that may create speech disfluencies such as repetitions (cf. Clark and Wasow 1998 versus Postma and Kolk 1993), more than a few researchers appear to believe that speech disfluencies are reactions to problems that occur *during* the planning for speech–language production. In other words, due to 'impairment', more errors 'wind up' in the phonological plan of people who stutter. And, due to a person's 'adaptation' to difficulties, whether speech or other issues (e.g. difficulties with balance, walking, or writing), people who stutter may attempt to correct/repair such errors with the by-product of such attempts being the overt speech disfluencies that are the *sine qua non* of stuttering [see Conture (1991*b*) and Yairi (1997) for overview of speech disfluencies and related issues associated with childhood stuttering].

11.2.5 Rationale for studying linguistic processes of CWS

Extending the aforementioned speculation (i.e. slow encoding → increased misselections/errors → increased self-repairs → increased stuttering), we hypothesize that CWS have slow or impaired abilities in one or more of their linguistic processes for speech–language production, not only phonological. While the possibility of phonological slowness, or lack of organization is supported by some empirical evidence (e.g. Wijnen and Boers 1994; cf. Burger and Wijnen 1999; Melnick *et al.* 2003), there is mounting evidence to suggest that more than just phonological encoding may be involved with childhood stuttering (e.g. Logan and Conture 1997; Howell *et al.* 1999; Yaruss 1999; Anderson and Conture 2000; Watkins *et al.* 2000; Pellowski 2002; Zackheim *et al.* 2002; Anderson, unpublished).

In specific, some CWS may also exhibit *slowness, inefficiencies* in their ability to retrieve the lemma from the mental lexicon and/or map the word's lemma on to its lexeme. Still other children, it is speculated, may exhibit slowness in morphological–syntactic construction of surface structure (i.e. grammatical form) or clausal constituents of an utterance. And some, of course, may exhibit concerns with two or more of these variables (e.g. phonology, semantics, or syntax). Again, it should be pointed out that it is quite possible that individuals who stutter can exhibit differences in linguistic processing of speech and language even when their articulatory, lexical, and grammatical abilities are shown, through standardized paper-and-pencil testing, to be non-significantly different from that of their normally fluent peers (e.g. Weber-Fox 2001; Pellowski 2002; Anderson, unpublished). As mentioned before, people who stutter do not need to exhibit a clinically significant problem in grammar, vocabulary, or phonology to exhibit apparent, if at times subtle, slowness, inefficiency, or less than well-organized linguistic processing.

As with our speculation regarding slowness in phonological encoding, slowness in semantic and/or syntactic encoding would not be a problem as long as the child makes his or her lexical and/or syntactic selections at a rate commensurate with his or her system's rate of activation for these variables (see Conture 2001*a*, Figures 1.3 and 1.4 for related analogies). If, however, for whatever reason, the child initiates or selects too soon (e.g. the child's internal or external environment encourages him or her to rush the planning of speech–language production), chances increase that inappropriate sounds, words and/or surface structure elements will get placed into the phonetic *plan*. We are, in essence, suggesting that CWS may exhibit *slowness* and *inefficiencies*, not only in phonological spell-out, but *lexical (lemma) retrieval* and/or *morpho-syntactic construction of surface structure* as well. Again, it is entirely possible for a child to exhibit such difficulties in only one, or two or more of these processes, a possibility we are currently attempting to assess. Further, it is also possible for these children to also exhibit motor control difficulties (see the reviews of Denny and Smith 1997; Ingham 1998; Caruso *et al.* 1999) and/or 'relatively unadaptive' temperamental characteristics (see Guitar 1998; Conture 2001*a*; Anderson *et al.* 2002). We believe, however, that for most CWS, these latter events—speech motor control and temperamental characteristics—are more of an influence on the *quality* (e.g. duration, associated physical tension) than on the quantity (e.g. frequency) of instances of stuttering. Of course, while such a dialectic could tide back and forth, suffice it to say that, at this point, one could argue the reverse. That is, linguistic variables influence the quality, whereas temperament and motoric variables influence the quantity of stuttering.

11.3 Different types of speech disfluency may reflect different underlying processes

Some of our preliminary data (e.g. Wolk *et al*. 1993; Anderson and Conture 2000) suggests that the child's different types of speech disfluency may provide clues as to what linguistic processes are involved. The notion that different processes relate to different disfluencies is consistent with Levelt's (1989) speculation that different speech errors and/or disfluency types have different origins. It is also consistent with our previously stated assumption that one prerequisite for a viable theoretical account of stuttering is that it first attempt to explain the essential speech–language characteristics of stuttering, that is, sound/syllable repetitions, sound prolongations, etc. We hasten to point out that the 'definition' of stuttering is, at this point, and for the foreseeable future, based on listener perception, and that some of the variance or differences in disfluency type is based on perception rather than production [see Ingham and colleagues' attempts to develop a time-interval means to improve the reliability of measuring stuttering; e.g. Cordes *et al*. (1992); Ingham *et al*. (1993)]. For example, Zebrowski and Conture (1989) empirically demonstrated how mothers of CWS and mothers of CWNS are similar, as well as different, in their percepts of exactly the same duration and type of speech disfluencies.

However, our speculations in this area would be seriously flawed if it were shown that the most common speech disfluency exhibited by CWS was randomly distributed throughout the population, from one study to the next. However, just the opposite is indicated by the findings of Yaruss *et al*. (1998), based on a clinical sample of 100 CWS, as well as those of Pellowski and Conture (2002), involving a more controlled, randomized research study of 36 CWS and 36 age- and gender-matched normally fluent peers. Results of these two studies indicate that there are a finite, non-randomly distributed number of speech disfluencies that characterize the most common disfluency type of CWS, with sound/syllable repetitions being the most common disfluency types for 47–50% of subjects, sound prolongations as the most common disfluency type for 25–26% of subjects, monosyllabic whole-word repetitions for 13–25%, and about 10–12% exhibiting either revisions, interjections, or phrase repetitions as their most common type of disfluency. In essence, the most common disfluency types of CWS do not appear to be randomly distributed within or between samples of CWS. Thus, if there is anything to the notion that different disfluency types reflect different underlying concerns, perhaps there are also a finite number of non-randomly distributed problems that underlie the occurrence of instances of speech disfluencies/stuttering in children.

11.3.1 Rationale for chronometric measures of linguistic processes

Much of the above speculation, regarding the basic impairment causing stuttering, (in)directly implicates *time* (e.g. slowness of lemma retrieval). As Kent (1984) suggests, the very definition of stuttering (i.e. a disruption in the rhythm or fluency of speech) suggests that *stuttering is a disruption in temporal processes* [see similar reasoning by Caruso *et al.* (1999), from a motor perspective]. To date, however, empirical studies of time or temporal variables (i.e. chronometric measures) in stuttering have focused on description of speech behaviors and/or perceptions of people who stutter (e.g. Barrasch *et al.* 2000) as well as experimental manipulation of their motor execution (e.g. Cross and Luper 1983), rather than linguistic planning for speech–language production [although exceptions, e.g. Bosshardt (1994), van Lieshout *et al.* (1995) can be found where the interaction between linguistic and motor has been discussed/studied relative to speech fluency].

To be sure, measures of 'time' cannot be made in a vacuum, without reference to 'space' or 'spatial movement of a structure'; however, the same goes for measures of 'space', they must be referenced to time for the most complete description of events being studied. Be that as it may, it is a given that structures are moving through space when we are talking about how fast that structure is moving or the 'time' elapsed during that movement. This is similar to how we would assume that a car is moving from point A to point B when we talk about 'how fast it went'. Thus, we are not suggesting, when we focus on time, that spatial considerations are immaterial. Rather, it is merely to suggest that disturbances in the temporal domain—whether in planning or execution of speech–language production—seem highly likely, in some shape or form, to contribute to disruptions in the initiation and/or continuation of fluent, conversational speech. (Some recent findings suggest that spatial aspects, in particular movement amplitude, may be one underlying source of instability relative to stuttering; see Chapters 3 and 13, this volume).

More specifically, in recent years, some (e.g. Perkins *et al.* 1991; Postma and Kolk 1993; Conture 2001*a*) have begun to suggest that slowness, inefficiencies, or dyssynchronies within the *linguistic planning* component of speech–language production are as central to stuttering as disturbances at the level of speech–language execution. However, to investigate behaviors or events associated with linguistic planning, one must examine speech–language production in an online, dynamic (e.g. during actual speech–language production) versus offline, static fashion (e.g. comparing the performance of CWS and CWNS on standardized tests).

One interesting approach to this issue was recently reported by Weber-Fox (2001) in a study of adults who do and do not stutter (mean age of both groups = 23 years). Weber-Fox studied event-related potentials associated with yes/no linguistic decisions (indicated by subjects' button-pushing responses) regarding whether sentence stimuli made sense. She reported differences between these talker groups in functional brain activity; for example, reduced negative amplitudes in select evoked response potentials (ERPs) for adults who stutter. Therefore, even during linguistic decisions that do not involve overt speech–language production, adults who stutter exhibit differences in cortical activities associated with language processing. And, in passing, it bears pointing out that cortical events are not only involved with linguistic and motoric activity. Emotional activities also manifest themselves in cortical events, for example, right hemispheric activity (in ventromedial prefrontal cortex) is strongly correlated with negative affect (Zald *et al.* 2002). This is not a trivial consideration for a problem like stuttering, which many (e.g. Guitar 1998) believe to be, at the least, exacerbated by emotional factors.

However, despite the intriguing nature of Weber-Fox's findings, they do not involve activity associated with overt speech–language production, the 'communicative site' during which stuttering occurs. Probably more salient, for present purposes, ERP methodology are quite problematic to employ with preschool, 'pre-cooperative' CWS (who typically neither read nor write), the age during which stuttering is most apt to begin. Thus, to systematically study the aforementioned psycholinguistic variables in these preschool children, the present authors have turned to another methodology widely used by psycholinguists, that is, picture–word interference tasks. This procedure, while often used with older children and adults, is one that has merit, as our preliminary studies will suggest, for the study of psycholinguistic variables associated with childhood stuttering.

As reviewed by Bloodstein (1995, Table 15, pp. 189–194) and Conture (2001*a*, Appendix A, p. 26), there have been numerous studies of phonatory, oral, and manual reactions of people who do and do not stutter. To date, most such studies have focused on motoric aspects or interpretations of speech reaction time. However, there are some studies of speech reaction time with children (Maske-Cash and Curlee 1995) and adults (Dembrowski and Watson 1991; Peters *et al.* 1989), where the influence of length and complexity of utterances on speech reaction time, of people who do and do not stutter, have been considered. In essence, these findings indicate that both people who do and do not stutter are slower to respond when producing longer, more complex utterances, with some indication (Maske-Cash and Curlee 1995) that the time needed to plan as well as execute speech–language may differ between CWS with concomitant versus those without concomitant problems (cf. van Lieshout 1996).

One difficulty with most of the aforementioned studies of speech reaction time is that the final measure, speech reaction time, is the end-product or result of a complex melding of cognitive, planning, and execution events. While perhaps obvious, no temporal measure of speech–language output can ever be truly divorced from the cognitive, planning, etc. processes that precede it (perhaps like the old song said, 'the hip bone is connected to the leg bone and the leg bone is connected to the shin bone'). However, there do appear to be ways to manipulate linguistic cognitive planning while leaving motoric responses fairly constant, to study the relationship the former have to stuttering. For example, phonological priming (e.g. Brooks and MacWhinney 2000) or structural or grammatical priming (e.g. Smith and Wheeldon 2001) paradigms permit the investigator to manipulate aspects of semantic, syntactic, and phonological planning and then compare reaction times between no-primed and primed conditions through use of what is described as a picture–word interference task.

Of course, one cannot absolutely, categorically, or definitely disambiguate linguistic from motor contributions (or vice versa) with any known paradigm requiring participants to overtly produce speech and language. However, one does not need to achieve such absolute distinctions to come to some relative understanding of the role that linguistic and motor variables may play during a particular paradigm. For example, studies such as Smith and Wheeldon (2001) that involve a priming paradigm, typically establish a 'priming effect' based on subtracting speech reaction time in a control from speech reaction time in the experimental condition. Often, with such studies, the only apparent difference between control and experimental conditions is a cognitive/linguistic manipulation (e.g. participant hears 'duh' milliseconds before seeing picture of 'dog' to be named) while the speaking tasks remain the same for all conditions. Given that the speaking task remains the same for all conditions, one can make the reasonable assumption that concomitant motor difficulties should affect both conditions equally and, therefore, leave the priming effect essentially intact. In other words, one reasonably straightforward way to interpret a priming effect that occurs in association with experimental manipulation of a linguistic variable is that the linguistic variable, in all likelihood, makes some, if not a significant, contribution to the priming effect.

11.3.2 Picture–word interference tasks

As mentioned above, one-well established means for studying temporal aspects of linguistic processes is a picture–word interference task (e.g. Levelt *et al.* 1991; Meyer and Schriefers 1991; Glasner 1992; Levelt 1999; Brooks and MacWhinney 2000; Smith and Wheeldon 2001). Such a task permits one to study dependent variables (e.g. speech reaction time) that appear to provide insight into the time course of semantic (for a review, see Neeley 1991), syntactic (for a review, see Pickering and Branigan 2000), as well as phonological, encoding (for a review, see Meyer and Schriefers 1991). [For a general overview of chronometric measures and human information processes, the interested reader is referred to Coles *et al.* (1995)]. Such insight is important given the aforementioned speculation that the *speed* and/or *time course* of such linguistic events is importantly related to instances of stuttering. And while this methodology, like all methodologies, is not without analytical (e.g. Ratcliff 1993) as well as procedural (e.g. Snodgrass and Vanderwart

1980; Cycowicz *et al.* 1997; Barrow *et al.* 2000) challenges, picture-naming inter- ference tasks have shown themselves to be quite useful in the study of human information processes (e.g. Coles *et al.* 1995; Levelt 1999).

Briefly, the aforementioned picture–word interference task (Glasner 1992) typically involves the use of an interfering stimulus (IS) consisting of a sound, syllable, word, or utterance that is similar to, or different (along various dimen- sions) from, a picture (target) to be named (from this point on, the acronym IS will be used interchangeably with the word 'prime'). With this paradigm, one assumes that presentation of the IS or 'prime' just before, during, or after a picture (hereafter 'target') to be named, leads to activation of the IS's represen- tation within the mental lexicon. If the target and prime are *related* (e.g. phono- logically, semantically, etc.), this may *facilitate* the encoding of the target so that a shorter/faster naming latency occurs. When IS and target are *unrelated*, however, this may *inhibit* encoding of the target, leading to a longer or slower naming latency. [Our generalizations regarding the effects of related versus unre- lated 'primes' do not describe *all* possible outcomes of priming experiments, a fact that is related to present space limitations as well as the general, rather than exhaustive, nature of this brief overview.] It is thought that this paradigm permits the experimenter to manipulate/investigate the time course or speed of the covert processes that influence subjects' overt speech–language responses. For, as Coles *et al.* (1995, p. 87) suggest, one may use '… measures of reaction time … to make inferences about the dynamics of information processing and the architecture of the processing system … [to] answer … questions about the structure and function of a covert system from measures of overt behavior'. Specifically, for our studies of linguistic processes of CWS, we have (e.g. Melnick *et al.* 2003) and are presently using (e.g. Pellowski 2002; Anderson, unpublished; Zackheim, *et al.* 2003) this paradigm to investigate temporal aspects of phono- logical, semantic, and syntactic encoding that we speculate are related to instances of speech disfluency in CWS.

11.3.3 Implicit retrieval

Methodologically, it should be noted that some studies of syntactic priming (also called *structural priming* or *syntactic persistence*, see Pickering and Branigan 2000) with adults (e.g. Bock *et al.* 1992; Branigan *et al.* 1995; Bock and Griffin 2000) and children (e.g. Brooks and Tomasello 1999; Leonard *et al.* 2000) require the subject to name the prime (a procedure used, among various reasons, to conceal the true purpose of the study). However, this procedure, based on our preliminary study of phonological, lexical, and syntactic priming with young children (e.g. Pellowski, 2002; Melnick *et al.* 2003; Anderson, unpublished), appears problematic for young (3- and 4-year-old) children, in that it requires them to produce, in relatively rapid order, two different utterances. That is, they first must repeat the prime and then, shortly thereafter, name the picture. Based on our experience with young children, this two-utterance task is likely to confuse more than a few of them, given that most of them find it a challenge to rapidly name or describe the picture once, let alone twice!

Thus, during our syntactic, semantic, and phonological priming studies, we have auditorily presented the prime to the child and, shortly thereafter, followed it with a picture for the child to describe. In other words, our priming tasks involve, we believe, *implicit retrieval* or relatively automatic syntactic, semantic, or phonological retrieval. Such retrieval is thought to involve little or no awareness on the subject's part that their memory and/or retrieval skills are being assessed. This approach seems reasonable, given our desire to assess whether the *automatic* process of syntactic, semantic, and phonological encoding of CWS is slower, perhaps less efficient, than that of their normally fluent peers.

11.3.4 Semantic, phonological, and syntactic priming of young CWS: overview of preliminary findings

To date, most of our work in this area has been, in essence, developing methodology that would reliably permit us to manipulate experimentally the speech reaction time of 3- to 5-year-old CWS (and their age- and gender-matched peers who do not stutter) during picture-naming or picture-description tasks. Simply employing methodologies in this area, developed with older children and/or adults, is not feasible with pre-reading, pre-writing, and, in more than a few cases, pre-cooperative, young children. Thus, we do not have large amounts of data to share, but will have in the next few years. What follows, therefore, are preliminary findings pertaining to these studies.

11.3.4.1 Phonological priming

After establishing a corpus of pictures that 3- to 5-year-old children could name reasonably quickly, accurately and fluently, Melnick *et al.* (2003) have been able to successfully prime phonologically eighteen 3- to 5-year-old children who do and do not stutter. In this study, and all the ones to be reported below, 'experimental' or priming conditions will be compared to a 'no prime' condition as well as, when appropriate, each other. While many interesting methodological as well as theoretical findings result from this preliminary work, for the present space, two seem particularly relevant. First, findings make apparent that, with appropriate adjustments for age and development, it is possible to prime phonologically 3- to 5-year-old children, who, much like adults, exhibit a tendency to produce faster speech reaction times when sounds related to the word-initial sound of the picture to be named are preactivated by an auditorily presented prime (i.e. consonant–vowel). Secondly, it was also found that CWNS, in both no-prime and experimental conditions, exhibit a strong negative correlation between their speech reaction time and their score on a standardized test of articulatory mastery (i.e. faster [shorter] speech reaction time correlated with higher score on standardized test); however, CWS exhibit no such relationship. The take-away from this, albeit preliminary, work is that the articulatory/ phonological systems of CWS, as a group, seems less well organized, even for those whose articulation and phonology was screened to be within normal limits. While these are, of course, group findings, and any one individual, in either talker group, may differ from the central tendency, findings do suggest, at the least, the need for continued study of the articulatory/phonological systems of CWS in attempts to better understand how these systems may contribute to stuttering (e.g. Zackheim *et al.* 2002).

11.3.4.2 Semantic priming

Another of our studies, conducted in parallel with Melnick *et al.* (2003), involved semantic priming (Pellowski 2002), using different, but similar ages and type of participants (i.e. children who do versus do not stutter). In this study, after a series of pilot studies, it was shown to be possible to semantically prime 3- to 5-year-old children who do and do not stutter [approximately 20 in each talker group, at this writing; see McNamara and Holbrook (2002) and Neeley (1991) for review of semantic priming]. This was done, for example, by having the child hear 'cat' just before (i.e. 700 ms before) he or she sees a picture of 'dog' to name (related prime condition), and, in another condition, hearing 'car' just before seeing a picture of 'dog' to name (unrelated prime condition). This is a rather long (i.e. 700 ms) stimulus–onset asynchrony (SOA)—time from onset of prime to onset of target/picture—when compared to studies with adults in this area. Our relatively long SOA was necessitated by the fact that 3- to 5-year-old children do not read. Thus, the 'primes' had to be presented auditorily, not as visually presented orthographic words. Use of visual primes (e.g. an orthographic word) would have permitted the use of much shorter SOAs. In essence, our auditory presentation of primes to pre-reading children necessitated longer SOAs to insure that the auditorily presented prime onset and offset occurred *before* the onset of the visually presented picture. That is, like the Melnick *et al.* (2003) study, there was no apparent temporal overlap between auditorily presented prime and visually presented picture to name. Pellowski (2002) reported several methodological, as well as theoretically interesting, findings, but the seemingly most salient finding is that CWNS, as to be expected, speed-up (shorten) their speech reaction time during a related semantic prime condition. Conversely, children who do stutter actually get slower! Whether this means that lexical priming facilitates (i.e. speeds up) CWNS but inhibits (i.e. slows down) CWS is unclear, given the need to replicate these findings with more participants, refined methodologies, etc. However, it does seem, even more so than with phonological behavior, that the lexical retrieval and/or encoding systems of CWS appears different from typical; again, results based on preliminary findings. These subtle but perhaps important differences in lexical processes may significantly contribute to the inability to establish reasonably fluent speech oftentimes exhibited by preschool CWS.

11.3.4.3 Syntactic priming

Another member of our group, Anderson (unpublished), conducted a study that attempted to syntactically or structurally prime 3- to 5-year-old children who do and do not stutter (for a review of syntactic priming, see Bock 1986; Pickering and Branigan 2000). This study was conducted in parallel with Pellowski (2002), using, in many cases, the same participants; however, for various performance variables (e.g. fatigue, attention difficulties, etc.), some children could perform and provide reliable data for one task but not the other. Again, after a series of pilot studies, Anderson has shown that it is possible to syntactically prime 3- to 5-year-old children successfully who do ($N = 16$) and do not stutter ($N = 16$), matched for age and gender. The experimental pictures used in this study consisted of pictures that children could readily describe using a simple active affirmative declarative (SAAD) structure (e.g. the boy is hugging the dog), an active transitive construction. Typical actions, for example, included hugging, sitting, and petting, performed in the context of events such as a boy hugging a dog, a girl sitting in a chair, and a girl petting a cat. In the syntactic prime condition, children were shown the same pictures as in the no prime condition (i.e. the 17 experimental pictures and 5 'filler' pictures, the latter depicting actions that could be described with non-SAAD structures). However, in the syntactic priming condition, 2000 ms prior to the onset of presentation of the picture, the child was presented with an auditory priming sentence, composed of a simple active affirmative declarative (SAAD) structure (e.g. 'the boy is walking the dog') that in all obvious respects appeared dissimilar to the picture (e.g. a picture of a girl throwing a stick). Results essentially suggest that the syntactic priming makes the CWS perform more like the CWNS, in terms of speech reaction time. This suggests that while their morpho-syntactic construction may be a somewhat slow and/or inefficient, it is somewhat malleable to external stimulation, something their phonological as well as semantic systems seem less prone to be. Again, the above is preliminary and in need of continued study, with more participants, using refined methodology; however, these findings do suggest that differences in linguistic encoding are associated with childhood stuttering, differences that may ultimately be shown to contribute to their stuttering.

11.3.4.4 Holistic versus incremental processing

Finally, in a further study of the phonological system of CWS, Zackheim *et al.* (2002), following a series of pilot studies, evaluated holistic versus incremental processing (see Charles-Luce and Luce 1990; Walley 1988). Holistic processing refers to the processing of a word as a whole, whereas incremental processing refers to the processing of a word in a segmental or sound by sound fashion. As children increase the size of their mental lexicon, they are thought to decrease their use of holistic phonological representations. To investigate this developmental shift from holistic to incremental processing, this study involved phonological priming in picture naming of young CWNS, findings that will be compared later to those obtained for children who do stutter. Results indicated that, for 3-year-olds, speech reaction time is fastest when presented with a 'holistic' prime (e.g. primes containing the nucleus and coda of the word), whereas for 5-year-olds speech reaction time is fastest when presented with an 'incremental' prime (e.g. primes containing only the initial consonant of the word). Findings appear to lend support to the theory that young children begin to process phonological representations holistically and then, with development, process such representations incrementally. Perhaps, future empirical studies employing this priming paradigm with CWS will indicate that they are delayed in their ability to shift from holistic to incremental processing, a delay that may contribute to the difficulties CWS are thought to have with phonological encoding.

For the present, however, we will continue to assess syntactic, semantic, and phonological aspects of speech–language planning and production in the hope of circumscribing the contributions, if any, these variables have to the onset, development, and maintenance of stuttering. As an example of one such study, and speculation associated with it, the following describes our theorizations regarding linguistic variables that may be associated with sound/syllable repetitions in young CWS.

11.4 Future studies: for example, CWS who have difficulties with phonological encoding

We predict that some CWS may have difficulties in appropriately selecting speech units at a rate commensurate with their phonological encoder's ability to activate speech units, with resulting repairs, as mentioned above, leading to sound/syllable repetitions. The slowness of the 'segmental spell-out' within their phonological encoding system would also mean that these children might experience difficulties in rapidly mapping the syntactic/meaning aspect of a word (i.e. lemma) on to the phonological form of a word (i.e. lexeme), the latter experience perhaps leading to the oft-mentioned remark of people who stutter: 'I know what I want to say, I just can't say it ...' [See Levelt et al. (1999) for discussion of difficulties with lemma/lexeme interactions; cf. van Lieshout in this reference for the notion, hereby paraphrased, 'I know what I want to say, I can even say it, if (part of) my motor system did not block during the (otherwise correct) movements', a blocking effect that van Lieshout attempts to explain in the context of neuro-sensorimotor entrainment.]

11.4.1 Expected findings: difficulties with phonological encoding

We expect some CWS, particularly those who perform poorer on standardized, norm-based tests of phonology and articulation, to be *less influenced by phonological priming* than their non-stuttering peers and/or CWS, and to exhibit phonological abilities in the upper ends of normal limits. We would expect that these children would be most apt to exhibit, as their most common disfluency type, sound/syllable repetitions, a type of disfluency speculated to reflect their attempts to correct an error in their phonetic plan. If sound/syllable repetitions are the most common disfluency type for approximately 50% of CWS (Pellowski 2002), and if such repetitions are associated with articulatory/ phonological processes, as we hypothesize, perhaps most of these CWS may also exhibit articulatory abilities within the lower end of normal limits. In other words, if such disfluencies are the most common disfluency types (which our data suggest they are), then the number of CWS in the lower ends of normal limits articulatorily should also be considerable.

11.5 Conclusion

In closing, none of the above should be taken to suggest that other variables, in particular temperamental characteristics (for review, see Conture 1991*a*, 2001*a*; Embrechts *et al.* 1998; Guitar 1998; Strelau 1998; Zebrowski and Conture 1998) and speech motor control (for review, see van Lieshout 1995; Denny and Smith 1997; Ingham 1998; Caruso *et al.* 1999), might not, at the least, exacerbate, perhaps perpetuate, instances of stuttering. Furthermore, while slowness and inefficiencies in speech–language planning may contribute to the occurrences of instances of stuttering in children, they may do so in conjunction with other variables, such as speech motor control and temperamentally related emotional reactivity and regulation (see Conture and Zackheim 2002). For example, with regard to temperamental characteristics, for instances of stuttering to be overtly manifest, exacerbated, or perpetuated, the child may need to be highly reactive to environmental changes, in particular mistakes or errors in speech–language planning/production. This might mean that the child quickly or readily notices and strongly reacts to changes, differences, or mistakes in his or others' behavior, especially mistakes that occur during actual speech–language planning and/or production. If the child tends to react *intensely* as well as *continuously* (for a review of temperamental variables, see Strelau 1998) to the mistake or change, long after the 'mistake' has been detected, such emotional reactivity could conceivably contribute to the occurrence, if not exacerbation, of instances of childhood stuttering. Likewise, a child could exhibit a history of subtly to clinically significant chewing and swallowing problems with or without difficulties articulating certain speech sounds (i.e. /r,l,w/) and/or subtle to very apparent (non)speech movement control issues that make it difficult to produce fluent speech and language quickly and accurately. However, as said at the outset of this paper, while emotional reactivity, temperamental, and/or speech motor control variables may be of issue for people who stutter, they are, more than likely, a part rather than the whole of the mosaic of variables that contribute to childhood stuttering.

Therefore, we are suggesting that the rapidity of changes, as well as possible disruptions in planning for speech–language production [see van Turennout *et al.* (1998) for a data-based description of the high-speed nature of linguistic planning] is very consistent with the rapidity of changes in instances of stuttering during conversational speech. While stuttering, almost by definition, involves disruptions in motoric execution of speech, it is somewhat difficult to understand how such disruptions can be both a symptom as well as a cause of stuttering! Of course, this is not to deny, if speech motor control is contributory to instances of stuttering, that the motoric symptoms of stuttering could be different than those motoric events that created or led to the motoric symptoms of stuttering. Whether the origin of the difficulties that lead to instances of stuttering is to be found in the speech motor control system, in the linguistic system, or in some complex melange of the two (see Chapter 10, this volume), is an open, perhaps empirical question. All that these present authors are suggesting is that the link between symptoms of childhood stuttering and the linguistic system warrants serious consideration and further empirical study.

Of course, it is entirely possible that speech motor variables may still be shown to co-vary with, and/or precipitate, instances of stuttering. While this is possible, it does not seem extremely probable, given the fact that after nearly 20 years of empirical study of the speech motor control abilities of people who stutter, no such co-variation or precipitation has been uncovered empirically and reported. This does not mean there is no motoric evidence to be found, but, at the least, we may not have been looking in the right direction, with the right methodology to find it. Perhaps, therefore, it is time to mine other shafts of information as well, in attempts to uncover nuggets of information seemingly directly related to the occurrence of instances of childhood stuttering. And to that end, our study of linguistic processes and childhood stuttering has been directed.

Acknowledgement

We would like to acknowledge the many contributors to this work of Drs. Kenneth S. Melnick and Ralph N. Ohde. We would also like to acknowledge Dr. Herman Kolk for his initial inspiration, guidance, and support that helped us conduct this line of inquiry into the possible causes of developmental stuttering.

References

Ambrose, N. and **Yairi, E.** (1999). Normative disfluency data for early childhood stuttering. *Journal of Speech, Language, and Hearing Research, 42*, 895–909.

Anderson, J. and **Conture, E.** (2000). Language abilities of CWS: a preliminary study. *Journal of Fluency Disorders, 25,* 283–304.

Anderson, J., Pellowski, M., Conture, E., and **Kelly, E.** (2003). Temperamental characteristics of young children who stutter, *Journal of Speech, Language and Hearing Research, 46*(5), 1221–1233

Barrasch, C., Guitar, B., McCauley, R., Absher, R. (2000). Disfluency and time perception. *Journal of Speech Language and Hearing Research, 43,* 1429–1439.

Barrow, I. M., Holbert, D., and **Rastatter, M. P.** (2000). Effect of color on developmental picture-vocabulary naming of 4-, 6-, and 8-year old children. *American Journal of Speech-Language Pathology, 9*(4), 310–318.

Bates, E. and **Goodman, J.** (1997). On the inseparability of grammar and the lexicon: evidence from acquisition, aphasia and real-time processing. *Language and Cognitive Processes, 12*(5/6), 507–584.

Bernstein Ratner, N. (1995). Language complexity and stuttering in children. *Topics in Language Disorders, 15*(3), 32–47.

Bernstein Ratner, N. (1997). Stuttering: a psycholinguistic perspective. In R. Curlee and G. Siegel (Eds), *Nature and treatment of stuttering: new directions* (2nd edn) (pp. 99–127). Boston, MA: Allyn & Bacon.

Bernstein Ratner, N. and **Sih, C.** (1987). Effects of gradual increases in sentence length and complexity on children's disfluency. *Journal of Speech and Hearing Disorders, 52,* 278–287.

Blackmer, E. and **Mitton, J.** (1991). Theories of monitoring and the timing of repairs in spontaneous speech. *Cognition, 39,* 173–194.

Bloodstein, O. (1995). *A handbook on stuttering* (5th edn). San Diego, CA: Singular Publishing Group, Inc.

Bock, K. (1986). Syntactic persistence in language production. *Cognitive Psychology, 18,* 355–387.

Bock, K. and **Griffin, Z.** (2000). The persistence of structural priming: transient activation or implicit learning. *Journal of Experimental Psychology: General, 129*(2), 177–192.

Bock, K., Loebell, H., and **Morey, R.** (1992). From conceptual roles to structural relations: bridging the syntactic cleft. *Psychological Review, 99,* 150–171.

Boscolo, B., Bernstein Ratner, N., and **Rescorla, L.** (2002). Fluency of school-aged children with a history of specific expressive language impairment: an exploratory study. *American Journal of Speech-Language Pathology, 11,* 41–49.

Bosshardt, H-G. (1994). Temporal coordination between pre-motor and motor processes in speech production. In C. W. Starkweather and H. F. M. Peters (eds). *Stuttering: proceedings of the first world congress on fluency disorders* (Vol. 1) (pp. 107–112). Nijmegen, The Netherlands: University Press Nijmegen.

Bosshardt, H-G. and **Fransen, H.** (1996). Online sentence processing in adults who stutter and adults who do not stutter. *Journal of Speech and Hearing Research, 39,* 785–797.

Bosshardt, H-G., Ballmer, W., and **de Nil, L.F.** (2002). Effects of category and rhyme decisions on sentence production. *Journal of Speech, Language, and Hearing Research,* 45, 844–857.

Branigan, H., Pickering, M., Liversedge, S., Stewart, A. and **Urbach, T.** (1995). Syntactic priming: investigating the mental representation of language. *Journal of Psycholinguistic Research,* 24, 489–502.

Bredart, S. (1991). Word interruption in self-repairing. *Journal of Psycholinguistic Research,* 20, 123–138.

Brooks, P. and **MacWhinney** (2000). Phonological priming in children's picture naming. *Journal of Child Language,* 27, 335–366.

Brooks, P. and **Tomasello, M.** (1999). Young children learn to produce passives with nonsense verbs. *Developmental Psychology,* 25(1), 29–44.

Brutten, G. and **Shoemaker, D.** (1967). *The modification of stuttering.* Englewood Cliffs, NJ: Prentice-Hall.

Burger, R. and **Wijnen, F.** (1999). Phonological encoding and word stress in stuttering and nonstuttering subjects. *Journal of Fluency Disorders,* 24, 91–106.

Caruso, A., Max, L., and **McClowry, M.** (1999). Perspectives on stuttering as a motor speech disorder. In A. Caruso and E. Strand (eds). *Clinical management of motor speech disorders in children.* New York: Thieme.

Charles-Luce and **Luce, P.A.** (1990). Similarity neighborhoods of words in young children's lexicon. *Journal of Child Language,* 17, 205–215.

Clark, H. and **Wasow, T.** (1998). Repeating words in spontaneous speech. *Cognitive Psychology,* 37, 201–242.

Coles, M., Smid., H., Scheffers, M., and **Otten, L.** (1995). Mental chronometry and the study of human information processing. In M. Rugg and M. Coles (eds). *Electrophysiology of mind: event-related brain potentials and cognition* (pp. 86–131). Oxford, UK: Oxford University Press.

Conture, E. (1991*a*). Young stutterers' speech production: a critical review. In H.F.M. Peters, W. Hulstijn, and C.W. Starkweather (eds). *Speech motor control and stuttering* (pp. 365–384). Amsterdam: Elsevier/ Excerpta Medica.

Conture, E. (1991*b*). Childhood stuttering: what is it and who does it? *ASHA Reports,* 18, 2–14.

Conture, E. (1991*c*). Young stutterers' speech production: a critical review. In H.F.M. Peters, W. Hulstijn, and C.W. Starkweather (eds). *Speech motor control and stuttering* (pp. 365–384). Amsterdam: Elsevier/Excerpta Medica.

Conture, E. (1996). Treatment efficacy: stuttering. *Journal of Speech and Hearing Research,* 39, S18–S26.

Conture, E. (2001*a*). *Stuttering: its nature, diagnosis and treatment* (3rd edn). Needham Heights, MA: Allyn & Bacon.

Conture, E. (2001*b*). Dreams of our theoretical nights meet the realities of our empirical days: stuttering theory and research. In H.-G. Bosshardt, J. Yaruss, and H. Peters (eds). *Stuttering: research, therapy and self-help* (pp. 3–30). Nijmegen, The Netherlands: University of Nijmegen Press.

Conture, E. and **Zackheim, C.** (2002). The long and winding road of developmental stuttering: from the womb to the tomb. Keynote scholarly address presented to The Sixth Oxford Disfluency Conference, Oxford, UK.

Cordes, A., Ingham, R., Frank, P., and **Ingham, J.** (1992). Time-interval analysis of interjudge and intrajudge agreement for stuttering event judgements. *Journal of Speech and Hearing Research, 38,* 382–386.

Cross, D. and **Luper, H.** (1983). Relation between finger reaction time and voice reaction time in stuttering and nonstuttering children and adults. *Journal of Speech and Hearing Research, 26,* 356–361.

Cycowicz, Y., Friedman, D., and **Rothstein, M.** (1997). Picture naming by young children: norms for naming agreement, familiarity and visual complexity. *Journal of Experimental Child Psychology, 65,* 171–237.

Dell, G. and **Juliano, C.** (1991). Connectionist approaches to the production of words. In H.F.M. Peters, W. Hulstijn, and C.W. Starkweather (eds). *Speech Motor Control and Stuttering* (pp. 11–36). Amsterdam, The Netherlands: Elsevier Science Publishers B.V.

Dembrowski, J. and **Watson, B.** (1991). Preparation time and response complexity effects on stutterers' and nonstutterers' acoustic LRT. *Journal of Speech and Hearing Research, 34,* 49–59.

Denny, M. and **Smith, A.** (1997). Respiratory and laryngeal control in stuttering. In R. Curlee and G. Siegel (eds). *Nature and Treatment of Stuttering: New Directions* (2nd edn) (pp. 128–142). Needham Heights, MA: Allyn & Bacon.

Embrechts, M., Ebben, H., Franke, P., and **van de Poel, C.** (1998). Temperament: A comparison between CWS and CWNS. In E.C. Healey and H.F.M. Peters (eds), *Stuttering: Proceedings of the Second World Congress on Fluency Disorders* (Vol. 2). Nijmegen, The Netherlands: University Press Nijmegen.

Glasner, W. (1992). Picture naming. In W.J.M Levelt (ed.). *Lexical Access in Speech Production* (pp. 61–105). Cambridge, MA: Blackwell Publishers.

Guitar, B. (1998). *Stuttering: An Integrated Approach to its Nature and Treatment* (2nd edn). Baltimore, MD: Williams and Wilkins.

Hall, N. (1996). Language and fluency in child language disorders: changes over time. *Journal of Fluency Disorders, 21,* 1–32.

Hall, N., Yamashita, T., and **Aram, D.** (1993). Relationship between language and fluency in children with developmental language disorders. *Journal of Speech and Hearing Research, 36,* 568–579.

Hartsuiker, R., Kolk, H., and **Lickley, R.** (2003). Stuttering on function words and content words: a computational test of the Covert Repair Hypothesis. In R. Harsuiker, R. Bastiaanse, A. Postma, and F. Wijnen (eds). *Phonological Encoding and Monitoring in Normal and Pathological Speech.* Hove, UK: Psychology Press, in press.

Howell, Au-Yeung, J., and Sakin, S. (1999). Exchange of stuttering from function words to content words with age. *Journal of Speech, Language and Hearing Research, 42*, 345–354.

Indefrey, P. and Levelt, W. (2000). The neural correlates of language production. In M. Gazzaniga (ed.), *The New Cognitive Neurosciences* (2nd edn). Cambridge, MA: MIT Press.

Ingham, R. (1998). On learning from speech-motor control research on stuttering. In A. Cordes and R. Ingham (eds). *Treatment Efficacy for Stuttering: A Search for Empirical Bases* (pp. 67–102). San Diego, CA: Singular Publishing Group.

Ingham, R., Cordes, A., and Finn, P. (1993). Time-interval measurement of stuttering: systematic replication of Ingham, Cordes, & Gow (1993). *Journal of Speech and Hearing Research, 36*, 1168–1176.

Kadi-Hanifi, K. and Howell, P. (1992). Syntactic analysis of the spontaneous speech of normally fluent and stuttering children. *Journal of Fluency Disorders, 17*, 151–170.

Kent, R. (1984). Stuttering as a temporal programming disorder. In R. Curlee and W. Perkins (eds), *Nature and Treatment of Stuttering: New Directions* (pp. 283–302). Boston: College-Hill.

Kolk, H. (1991). Is stuttering a symptom of adaptation or of impairment? In H.F.M. Peters, W. Hulstijn, and C.W. Starkweather (eds), *Speech Motor Control and Stuttering* (pp. 131–140). Amsterdam: Elsevier/Excerpta Medica.

Kolk, H. and Postma, A. (1997). Stuttering as a covert repair phenomenon. In R. Curlee and G. Siegel (eds.), *Nature and Treatment of Stuttering: New Directions* (2nd edn) (pp. 182–203). Boston, MA: Allyn & Bacon.

Leonard, L., Miller, C., Grela, B., Holland, A., Gerber, E., and Petucci, M. (2000). Production operations contribute to the grammatical morpheme limitations of children with specific language impairment. *Journal of Memory and Language, 43*, 362–378.

Levelt, W. (1983). Monitoring and self-repair in speech. *Cognition, 14*, 41–104.

Levelt, W. (1989). *Speaking: From Intention to Articulation*. Cambridge, MA: Bradford Books/The MIT Press.

Levelt, W. (1999). Models of word production. *Trends in Cognitive Sciences, 3*(6), 223–232.

Levelt, W. and Wheeldon, L. (1994). Do speakers have access to a mental syllabary? *Cognition, 50*, 239–269.

Levelt, W., Schriefers, H., Vorberg, D., Meyer, A., Pechman, T., and Havinga, J. (1991). The time course of lexical access in speech production: a study of picture naming. *Psychological Review, 98*, 122–142.

Levelt, W., Roelofs, A., and Meyer, A. (1999). A theory of lexical access in speech production. *Behavioral and Brain Sciences, 22*, 1–75.

Logan, K. (2001). The effect of syntactic complexity upon the speech fluency of adolescents and adults who stutter. *Journal of Fluency Disorders, 26*, 85–106.

Logan, K. and Conture, E. (1995). Relationships between length, grammatical complexity, rate and fluency of conversational utterances in CWS. *Journal of Fluency Disorders, 20,* 35–61.

Logan, K. and Conture, E. (1997). Selected temporal, grammatical and phonological characteristics of conversational utterances produced by CWS. *Journal of Speech, Language, and Hearing Research, 40,* 107–120.

Logan, K. and LaSalle, L. (1999). Grammatical characteristics of children's conversational utterances that contain disfluency clusters. *Journal of Speech, Language, and Hearing Research, 42,* 80–91.

Louko, L., Conture, E., and Edwards, E. (1999). Treating children who exhibit co-occurring stuttering and disordered phonology. In R. Curlee (ed.), *Stuttering and Related Disorders of Fluency* (2nd edn) (pp. 124–138). New York: Thieme Medical Publishers, Inc.

McNamara, T.P. and Holbrook, J.B. (2002). Semantic memory and priming. In I.B. Weiner (Series ed.), A.F. Healy and R. Proctor (Vol. eds), *Comprehensive Handbook of Psychology (Vol. 4).* Experimental Psychology. John Wiley & Sons.

Maner, K., Smith, A., and Grayson, L. (2000). Influences of utterance length and complexity on speech motor performance in children and adults. *Journal of Speech, Language, and Hearing Research, 43,* 560–573.

Maske-Cash, W. and Curlee, R. (1995). Effect of utterance length and meaningfulness on the speech initiation times of CWS and CWNS. *Journal of Speech and Hearing Research, 38,* 18–25.

Melnick, K. and Conture, E. (2000). Relationship of length and grammatical complexity to the systematic and onsystematic speech errors and stuttering of CWS. *Journal of Fluency Disorders, 25,* 21–45.

Melnick, K., Conture, E., and Ohde, R. (2003). *Phonological priming in picture naming of young CWS, Journal of Speech, Language and Hearing Research.*

Meyer, A. and Schriefers, H. (1991). Phonological facilitation in picture-word interference experiments: effects of stimulus onset asynchrony and types of interfering stimuli. *Journal of Experimental Psychology: Learning, Memory, and Cognition, 17,* 1146–1160.

Mowrey, R.A. and MacKay, I.R. (1990). Phonological primitives: electromyographic speech error evidence. *Journal of Acoustical Society of America, 88,* 1299–1312.

Murray, H. and Reed, C. (1977). Language abilities of preschool stuttering children. *Journal of Fluency Disorders, 2,* 171–176.

Neeley, J. (1991). Semantic priming effects in visual word recognition: a selective review of current findings and theories. In D. Besner and G. Humphreys (eds), *Basic Processes in Reading: Visual Word Recognition* (pp. 264–336). Hillsdale, NJ: Erlbaum.

Onslow, M. and Packman, A. (2002). Stuttering and lexical retrieval: inconsistencies between theory and data. *Clinical Linguistics and Phonetics, 16,* 295–298.

Packman, A., Onslow, M. Coombes, T., and Goodwin, A. (2001). Stuttering and lexical retrieval. *Clinical Linguistics and Phonetics, 15,* 487–498.

Pellowski, M. (2002). *Lexical priming in picture naming of children who do and do not stutter*, submitted.

Peters, H.F.M., Hulstijn, W., and **Starkweather, C.** (1989). Acoustic and physiological reaction times of stutterers and nonstutterers. *Journal of Speech and Hearing Research, 32,* 668–680.

Pickering, M. and **Branigan, H.** (2000). Syntactic priming in language production. *Trends in Cognitive Sciences, 3*(4), 136–141.

Plunkett, K., Karmiloff-Smith, A., Bates, E., Elman, J.L., and **Johnson, M.H.** (1997). Connectionism and development psychology. *Journal of Child Psychology and Psychiatry, 38,* 53–80.

Postma, A. and **Kolk, H.** (1993). The covert repair hypothesis: prearticulatory repair processes in normal and stuttered disfluencies. *Journal of Speech and Hearing Research, 36,* 472–487.

Ratcliff, R. (1993). Methods for dealing with reaction time outliers. *Psychological Bulletin, 114*(3), 510–532.

Roelofs, A. (2003). Spoken word planning, comprehending, and self-monitoring: Evaluation of WEAVER++. In R. Harsuiker, R. Bastiaanse, A. Postma, and F. Wijnen (eds), *Phonological Encoding and Monitoring in Normal and Pathological Speech*. Hove, UK: Psychology Press, in press.

Ryan, B. (1992). Articulation, language, rate and fluency characteristics of stuttering and nonstuttering preschool children. *Journal of Speech and Hearing Research, 35,* 333–342.

Ryan, B. (2001). A longitudinal study of articulation, language, rate and fluency of 22 preschool CWS. *Journal of Fluency Disorders, 26,* 107–128.

Smith, M. and **Wheeldon, L.** (2001). Syntactic priming in spoken sentence production—an online study. *Cognition, 78,* 123–164.

Snodgrass, J. and **Vanderwart, M.** (1980). A standardized set of 260 pictures: norms for name agreement, image agreement, familiarity, and visual complexity. *Journal of Experimental Psychology: Human Learning and Memory, 6,* 174–215.

Strelau, J. (1998). *Temperament: A Psychological Perspective*. New York: Plenum Press

Tetnowski, J. (1998). Linguistic effects on disfluency. In R. Paul (ed.), *Exploring the Speech–language Connection* (Vol. 8), (pp. 227–251), Baltimore, MD: Paul R. Brookes Publishing Co.

van Lieshout, P. (1995). Motor planning and articulation in fluent speech of stutterers and nonstutterers. Doctoral dissertation, University of Nijmegen, Nijmegen, The Netherlands.

van Lieshout, P. (1996). From planning to articulation in speech production: what differentiates a person who stutters from a person who does not stutter? *Journal of Speech and Hearing Research, 39,* 546–564.

van Lieshout, P., Starkweather, C., Hulstijn, W., and **Peters, H.** (1995). Effects of linguistic correlates of stuttering on emg activity in nonstuttering speakers. *Journal of Speech and Hearing Research, 38,* 360–372.

van Lieshout, P., Hulstijn, W., Peters, H. (1996). Speech production in people who stutter: testing the motor plan assembly hypothesis. *Journal of Speech and Hearing Research, 39,* 76–92.

van Lieshout, P., Peters, H., and **Bakker, K.** (1997). En route to a speech motor test: a first halt. In W. Hulstijn, H.F. M. Peters, & P.H.H.M. van Lieshout (eds). *Speech Production: Motor Control, Brain Research and Fluency Disorders.* Amsterdam: Elsevier.

van Turennout, M., Hagoort, P., and **Brown, C.** (1998). Brain activity during speaking: from syntax to phonology in 40 milliseconds. *Science, 280,* 572–574.

Walley, A.C. (1988). Spoken word recognition by young children and adults. *Cognitive Development, 3,* 137–165.

Watkins, R., Yairi, E., Ambrose, N., DeThorne, L., Johnson, B., Mullen, C., and **Berg, J.** (2000). *Grammatical influences on stuttering in young children.* Paper presented to Annual Conference of American Speech Language Hearing Association, Washington, DC.

Weber-Fox, C. (2001). Neural systems for sentence processing in stuttering. *Journal of Speech, Language, and Hearing Research, 44,* 814–825.

Westby, C. (1974). Language performance of stuttering and nonstuttering children. *Journal of Communication Disorders, 12,* 133–145.

Wijnen, F. and **Boers, I.** (1994). Phonological priming effects in stutterers. *Journal of Fluency Disorders, 19,* 1–20.

Williams, D., Melrose, B., and **Woods, C.** (1969). The relationship between stuttering and academic achievement in children. *Journal of Communication Disorders, 2,* 87–98.

Wingate, M. (1988). *The Structure of Stuttering.* New York: Springer Verlag.

Wolk, L., Edwards, M.L., and **Conture, E.G.** (1993). Coexistence of stuttering and disordered phonology in young children. *Journal of Speech and Hearing Research, 36,* 906–917.

Yairi, E. (1997). Disfluency characteristics of childhood stuttering. In R.F. Curlee and G.M. Siegel (eds) *Nature and Treatment of Stuttering* (2nd edn) (pp. 49–78). Needham Heights, MA: Allyn & Bacon.

Yairi, E. and **Ambrose, N.** (1992*a*). A longitudinal study of stuttering in children: a preliminary report. *Journal of Speech and Hearing Research, 35,* 755–760.

Yairi, E. and **Ambrose, N.** (1992*b*). Onset of stuttering in preschool children: selected factors. *Journal of Speech and Hearing Research, 35,* 782–788.

Yairi, E. and **Ambrose, N.** (1999). Early childhood stuttering I: persistence and recovery rates. *Journal of Speech Language Hearing Research, 42,* 1097–1112.

Yairi, E., Ambrose, N., Paden, E. and **Throneburg, R.** (1996). Predictive factors of persistence and recovery: pathways of childhood stuttering. *Journal of Communication Disorders, 29,* 51–77.

Yaruss, J.S. (1999). Utterance length, syntactic complexity, and childhood stuttering. *Journal of Speech and Hearing Research, 42,* 329–344.

Yaruss, J. and **Conture, E.** (1996). Stuttering and phonological disorders in children: examination of the covert repair hypothesis. *Journal of Speech and Hearing Research, 39,* 349–364.

Yaruss, J., LaSalle, L. and **Conture, E.** (1998). Evaluating stuttering in young children: diagnostic data. *American Journal of Speech-Language Pathology, 7,* 62–76.

Zackheim, C. and **Conture, E.** (2003). Childhood stuttering in relation to mean length of utterance, *Journal of fluency disorders,* 28, 115–143.

Zackheim, C., Conture, E., and **Ohde, R.** (2002). *Phonological priming in children: holistic versus incremental processing.* Poster presentation to the Annual Conference of American Speech Language Hearing Association, Atlanta, GA.

Zald, D. H., Mattson, D., and **Pardo, J.V.** (2002). Brain activity in ventromedial prefrontal correlates with individual differences in negative affect. *Proceedings of the National Academy of Science USA 99*(4), 2450–2454.

Zebrowski, P. and **Conture, E.** (1989). Judgements of disfluency by mothers of stuttering and normally fluent children. *Journal of Speech and Hearing Research, 32,* 625–634.

Zebrowski, P. and **Conture, E.** (1998). Influence of non-treatment variables on treatment effectiveness for school-age CWS. In A. Cordes and R. Ingham (eds), *Treatment Efficacy for Stuttering: A Search for Empirical Bases* (pp. 293–310). San Diego, CA: Singular Publishing Group.

PART 5

MOTOR CONTROL IN DISORDERS

CHAPTER 12

MOTOR CONTROL PERSPECTIVES ON MOTOR SPEECH DISORDERS

RAY D. KENT AND KRISTIN ROSEN

12.1 Introduction

Like Janus, the study of dysarthria has had two faces. One of these is the description of speech abnormalities, typically by perceptual means (although acoustic analysis is increasingly used). The other is physiological analysis, whether by inference or by direct observation. The two faces are explicit in the classic work by Darley *et al.* (1969*a*, *b*). Their data took the form of auditory–perceptual ratings of speech disturbances, but they inferred the physiologic basis of these disturbances by reference to classic neurologic pathophysiology. That is, one face of dysarthria was perceptually described, the other inferred.

The heart of the perceptual method was a multidimensional perceptual description that assumed the independence of the 38 component dimensions used in their analysis. This was a good start, and one that remains influential, but we know today that perceptual dimensions such as the ones used by Darley and associates are not psychophysically uniform, and are not independent (Kent 1996). Rather, the dimensions are different in kind, are often interdependent, and are sometimes hierarchical. Which is to say, dysarthria assessment is not really a process of answering 38 sequential questions. Indeed, it is not the common clinical practice to assess dysarthria in this way. Instead, the clinician listens for the most salient perceptual dimensions and may disregard entirely the dimensions that do not apply (Duffy and Kent 2001).

Darley *et al.* (1969*b*) wrote that a major achievement of their research was the opportunity to define the neuromuscular basis for deviant clusters. They concluded from their observations that 'speech follows neurology', that is, speech disturbances can be understood within classical neurology. If this is true, then the understanding of motor speech disorders should be a straightforward interpretation of general neurology to the particular case of speech. The extreme version of this perspective would be that we do not have to study speech movements at all, because all we need to do is to make appropriate translations of the movement data from more accessible motor systems, such as the limbs, to the muscles of the respiratory, laryngeal, pharyngeal, and orofacial systems. But there are reasons to doubt that motor speech disorders can be understood so easily, and these reasons may point to motor control interpretations that are unique to speech.

Darley *et al.* (1969*a, b*) welcomed research to test their hypotheses on the presumed pathophysiologic foundations of dysarthria. Several subsequent studies attempted to determine these foundations. These efforts were important because they measured, rather than assumed, physiologic abnormalities. Interestingly, these studies did not bring about a widely accepted alternative classification. Some early studies were consistent with the predictions of classic neurology (Leanderson *et al.*1972; Hunker *et al.* 1982; Hirose 1986; Moore and Scudder 1989), but others were not (Neilson *et al.* 1979; Neilson and O'Dwyer 1981; O'Dwyer *et al.* 1983). Put together, these studies give at best a clouded view of how speech disorder relates to movement abnormality. As Netsell (1986) remarked, 'Collectively, the motor control studies of the past decade have pointed out that the perceptual–physiologic relationships are much more complex than suggested by the initial hypotheses (Darley *et al.*, 1969a, 1969b)' (p. 46). Netsell went on to assert that causal relationships remain to be established between auditory–perceptual features or neurologic signs and the associated motor control abnormalities. The same challenge remains in effect today.

A long term goal of research on motor speech disorders has been to document, rather than simply infer, the sensorimotor impairments. This remains an important, and largely unrealized, goal. This information is needed for the basic understanding of motor speech disorders and also to plan clinical interventions. The immediate problem is to identify the types of sensorimotor impairments. If we wish to develop measurable correlates of dysarthria at the level of motor performance, then we need to select sensitive and feasible measures. In definitions of dysarthria, the most frequently noted sensorimotor correlates are slowness, paralysis, weakness, and incoordination. However, these are not uniform with respect to potential quantification. Slowness and weakness can be directly (albeit perhaps imperfectly) measured, but paralysis and incoordination are not always measured so readily. The neuromuscular bases of dysarthria proposed by Darley *et al.* were the following.

(1) tone (*balanced hypertonus*, in which agonist and antagonist muscle groups have a nearly equal state of increased tone; *biased hypertonus*, in which one muscle group has a dominant level of increased tone; and *hypotonus*, in which muscles have decreased tone);
(2) control of phasic movements (rate of speed, range of movements, force of movements, direction of movements);
(3) rate and rhythm;
(4) diadochokinesis; and
(5) coordination.

Not all of these potential neuromuscular or motor variables have been studied carefully or extensively in acoustic or physiologic studies of speech. The ones that have been examined most extensively are rate of movement, force or strength, rate and rhythm, diadochokinesis, and coordination. Accordingly, this paper will address these variables in particular. In fact, these are not necessarily independent factors. For example, abnormal diadochokinesis may be rooted in hypertonus, slow rate of movement, or poorly coordinated movement. There are other complications. First, there may be co-impairments, or the co-existence of two or more abnormalities. Secondly, compensations to the neurologic disorder may be difficult to distinguish from the motor disorder itself. Thirdly, motor abnormalities increase with age, even in individuals who are considered neurologically normal, meaning that normal aging processes must be taken into account to identify the pathophysiologic bases of dysarthria. The same comment applies to motor speech disorders in children, in which case the problem is to distinguish abnormalities in motor control from developmental changes. That is, the effects of neurological disorders must be considered against maturational status in children and aging phenomena in older adults. Several examples of these factors are mentioned in this paper, but it should be emphasized that we are only beginning to understand the interactions of disease with development and aging.

This chapter emphasizes the dysarthrias but comments are included on apraxia of speech, which is a challenging disorder because it has been explained as an impairment of linguistic phonological processing, motor control, or both of these. A consideration of motor control issues in apraxia of speech is timely because of recent arguments that the motor control impairment in this disorder reached beyond speech and can affect nonspeech movements of the orofacial motor system (Ballard *et al.* 2000).

12.2 Rate of movement, rate of speech

Altered rate is one of the most frequently observed features of dysarthria, across several perceptual types of dysarthria (Duffy 1995). According to Darley *et al.* (1969*a*, *b*), slow rate and/or prolonged intervals were particularly notable in ataxic, hyperkinetic (chorea), spastic, and spastic–flaccid types of dysarthria. However, on a more general scale, dysarthric speech is typically slow, although hastening phenomena occasionally occur, especially in Parkinson's disease. There are two major ways of measuring rate in discrete motor tasks such as speaking, typing, or tapping. One way is to measure *events per unit time*, as in the classic task of diadochokinesis (also termed alternating motion rate, AMR, when the task is confined to simple reciprocal movements such as repetition of the syllable /ta/) or as in the determination of speaking rate for more complex speech samples, typically passage reading or conversation. Speech has special status in this respect, as it may be the fastest discrete motor performance that humans can perform. The other way of measuring rate is to determine the speed of an individual structure, such as tongue or lip. Such measures are often termed *articulatory velocities* and are expressed in units such as mm/s. Because this kind of measurement requires special apparatus, it is not commonly used in clinical assessment. It may seem logical, even inevitable, that an increase in events per unit time is achieved through an increased velocity of individual effectors that perform the discrete motor task. However, at least in speech, an increase in events per unit time (e.g. syllables/s) is often achieved in part—and sometimes exclusively—by reducing the distance moved by the effector and not by increasing velocity (Kent *et al.* 1974; Westbury and Dembowski 1993; McClean 2000). The reduction in distance can be large enough that an increase in events per unit time is actually achieved with *slower* velocities of the effector. This point is important because the bulk of evidence that dysarthria is slow is in the form of events-per-unit-time measures, not velocities. It should be emphasized that both ways of measuring rate are valid and useful. But they should not be confused with one another, and it should not even be assumed that they are corre-lated in all speakers. The safest assumption is that the two types of measures are complementary in the analysis of rate of movement.

The common strategy of achieving rate increases through reductions of articula-tory displacement raises questions about whether individuals with motor speech impairments can deploy the same means of speaking rate adjustment. For some individuals with dysarthria, the displacement envelope of articulatory movement may be severely constrained so that adjustments within this envelope are not made easily. One example is amyotrophic lateral sclerosis (ALS), in which articulatory movements become increasingly limited in both displacement and rate. In an acoustic study, Turner *et al.* (1995) assessed vowel production at three different speaking rates (habitual, fast, slow) in nine ALS patients and nine control subjects. One of the acoustic indexes determined was the F1–F2 planar area for the tradi-tional vowel quadilateral. As shown in Fig. 12.1, the ALS subjects had smaller vowel plane areas than the neurologically normal controls. In addition, the subjects with ALS had more variable relations between vowel plane area and speaking rate. Although the subjects with ALS made some adjustments of vowel area in relation to speaking rate, these adjustments are quite small compared to the adjustments made by the control subjects.

The literature is replete with AMR data showing slow rates in dysarthria (Duffy 1995; Kent *et al.* 1998*a*). However, relatively few of the AMR studies have reported a finer analysis of the durations of component segments, such as syllables and intersyllable pauses. Recent work demonstrates the value of such microanalyses, including the ability to distinguish among dysarthria types. Ozawa *et al.* (2001) concluded that slow AMRs observed in spastic and ataxic dysarthria had different temporal mechanisms, with lengthening of syllable duration in the former and lengthening of pause (gap) duration in the latter. These differences may reflect different motor control deficiencies underlying the two forms of dysarthria. Nishio

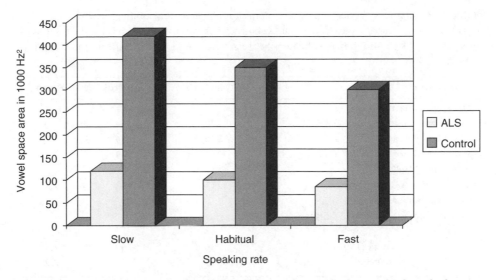

Fig. 12.1 Areas of the F1–F2 vowel quadrilateral for speakers with amyotrophic lateral sclerosis (ALS) and neurologically normal controls producing speech at three rates (habitual, fast, slow). (Adapted with permission from Turner *et al.* 1995.)

and Niimi (2001) concluded that speaking rate is a sensitive measure of abnormal speech motor control in several types of dysarthria in Japanese speakers, including flaccid, spastic, ataxic, hypokinetic, hyperkinetic, and UUMN. However, slow speaking rate is not linked to the same phenomena across types of dysarthria. Nishio and Niimi concluded that articulation rate accounts for the slow rate in spastic, ataxic, and UUMN dysarthria, but that pause time is needed to account for the slow rate in flaccid and hypokinetic dysarthria. If this result pertains to languages other than Japanese, then we must consider another complication of speaking rate analysis, one that invites microanalysis. It also has been shown that speakers with ataxic dysarthria differ from neurologically normal speakers in the adjustment of syllable and inter-syllable pause durations as speaking rate is varied (Kent *et al.* 1997).

Stevens (1998) summarized articulatory kinematics as measures of unidirectional movement from one configuration to another (e.g. abducted to adducted vocal folds) and cyclic movement from one configuration to another and return to the original configuration (e.g. abducted to adducted to abducted vocal folds). The typical AMR task can be used to derive estimates of movement time for both unidirectional (consonant to vowel) and cyclic movement (consonant to vowel to consonant). Table 12.1 shows data for cyclic movement times obtained from AMR data for dysarthric and control subjects. For each study represented in the table, the speakers with dysarthria have extended cycle durations compared to the controls.

Table 12.1 Durations of cyclic movements derived from alternating motion rate (AMR) tasks in dysarthric versus normal speech. The values shown are means in milliseconds for the three syllables /p^/, /t^/, /k^/. Also shown is the ratio between the values for the dysarthric and control subjects

Comparison	Dysarthria	Control	Ratio
Ataxia versus normal			
(a) Portnoy and Aronson (1982)	270	164	1.6
(b) Kent *et al.* (2000)	256	154	1.7
Spastic versus normal speech (Portnoy and Aronson 1982)	244	164	1.5
Parkinson disease versus normal speech (Canter 1965)	217	152	1.4
Traumatic brain injury versus normal speech			
(a) Blumberger *et al.* (1995)	236	169	1.4
(b) Wang *et al.* (2003)	341	153	2.2

With respect to evidence of reduced articulatory velocities, relatively few sources of data are available, but studies have shown that articulatory velocities are reduced in at least some subjects with cerebellar ataxia, Parkinson's disease (PD), and amyotrophic lateral sclerosis (ALS). Figure 12.2 shows velocity data for closing movements of the lower lip from three different studies involving a comparison of neurologically normal controls with individuals with dysarthria. Across these studies, articulatory velocities were reduced in the individuals with dysarthria compared to the neurologically normal talkers.

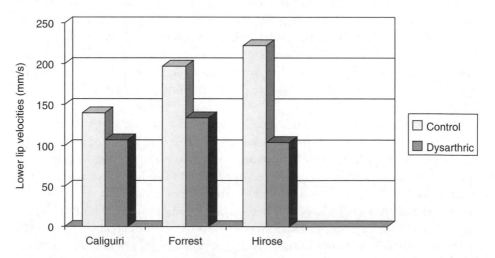

Fig. 12.2 Velocities of lower lip movement in three studies that compared dysarthric and neurologically normal speakers: Caligiuri (1987), Forrest *et al.* (1989), and Hirose (1986).

However it is measured, speaking rate is one factor in dysdiadochokinesis, or abnormal performance on a maximal-rate syllable repetition. At the minimum, dysdiadochokinesis can be quanitified by measures of syllable rate, mean durations of subcomponents (e.g. syllable and pause segments), and the variability in the durations of the subcomponents. Consideration of the syllable-to-syllable energy profile adds another dimension that may distinguish patterns of dysdiadochokinesis (Kent *et al.* 1999). These refinements in analysis have the potential to enhance the clinical value of the task, especially in view of progress in other research domains, including:

(1) neuroimaging to reveal areas of cortical activation associated with syllable repetition (Lotze *et al.* 2000; Riecker *et al.* 2000; Wildgruber *et al.* 2001); and
(2) the interaction between speaking task performance and the type of motor speech disorder (Kent and Kent 2000; Ziegler 2002).

12.2.1 Conclusion

Published data converge on the principle that slow rate is a nearly universal characteristic of dysarthria. However, finer levels of analysis are needed to determine if slow rate is a consequence of reduced articulatory velocities, longer steady-state durations, longer pause durations, or some combination of these. Moreover, the cause of slow rate is generally not known. A slow rate may reflect weakness, rigidity, inefficient temporal processing, or even compensation. Accordingly, slow rate is properly viewed as a global description of a speech disorder and is not easily interpreted in terms of hypotheses concerning underlying pathophysiologies, motor control abnormalities, or behavioral adjustments. This issue is not unique to dysarthria. It has been suggested that bradykinesia in Parkinson's disease is not fully explained by weakness, tremor, and rigidity but also involves sensory and motor scaling and sensorimotor integration (Berardelli *et al.* 2001). An understanding of slow speaking rate in relation to neurological disease will require a consideration of both event rates and articulatory velocities in different speaking tasks performed with different rates. A further consideration, considered more fully later in this chapter, is the possibility that a slow speaking rate is at least partly a compensation for neurologic lesion.

12.3 Strength and endurance

Weakness often is implicated as an underlying factor in dysarthria. But, as Luschei (1991) observed, 'There are many reasons why a muscle may be weak' (p. 9). Different neurologic diseases have different points of attack—on muscle contraction directly, on the myoneural junction, on the peripheral nerves, and on motoneurons. Weakness can be detected on a single assessment but it also can arise from repeated use of a muscle system, in which case the term fatigue may be used. The relevant published studies typically assess strength (often in the form of a maximum force) and endurance (maintenance of a specified force over time).

Strength and endurance of the orofacial muscles have been quantitatively examined primarily for stroke, Parkinson's disease, myasthenia gravis, and traumatic brain injury, each of which is considered briefly below.

12.3.1 Stroke

Thompson *et al.* (1995) included measures of tongue strength and endurance in their study of 16 subjects who had upper motor neuron lesions and dysarthria. This study also included measures of articulation, intelligibility, and rate of repetitive movements. Although tongue strength, tongue endurance, and rates of tongue movement were reduced in the clinical group compared to a matched control group, Thompson *et al.* did not observe systematic relationships between the instrumental data and perceptual data.

12.3.2 Parkinson's disease

A similar lack of congruity between physiologic and perceptual measures was reported by Solomon *et al.* (2000) for Parkinson's disease. Individuals with Parkinson's disease and dysarthria had reduced tongue strength and endurance, but no significant correlations were found between these measures and perceptual measures of speech production. Gentil *et al.* (1998), in a comparison of the effects of levodopa on finger and orofacial movements, concluded that the treatment had favorable effects on finger movements in the form of improved motor scores and force production, but that the treatment had negligible, or even negative, effects on force production in the orofacial system. In a related study, Gentil *et al.* (1999) examined isometric force production in the lips, tongue, and forefinger of individuals with Parkinson's disease. Force production impairments included a slower rate of force development, difficulties in maintaining a given contraction, and variability in force generation. It was also noted that force control was dissimilar between the orofacial and finger muscles, and even between the lips and tongue.

12.3.3 Myasthenia gravis

Weijnen *et al.* (2000) investigated tongue force in patients with bulbar myasthenia gravis, patients with ocular myasthenia gravis, and patients in clinical remission who had previously had bulbar myasthenia gravis. Healthy subjects were included as controls. It was determined that patients with bulbar myasthenia gravis had significantly reduced tongue force in the lateral direction. It was further observed that patients in the remission group had only incomplete recovery of lateral tongue force.

12.3.4 Traumatic brain injury

Control of orofacial force by individuals with traumatic brain injury (TBI) has been the focus of several studies (McHenry *et al.* 1994*a*, *b*; Theodoros *et al.* 1995; Goozee *et al.* 2001). McHenry *et al.* (1994*b*) compared two groups of individuals who differed in speech intelligibility. Dynamic and static force generation was assessed for the upper lip, lower lip, tongue, and jaw. The only difference between these two groups was in the ability to sustain a 2 N force level with the tongue. Theodoros *et al.* reported that their subjects with traumatic brain injury differed from control subjects on lip and tongue function on strength, endurance, and rate of repetition of movements. Goozee *et al.* concluded that their subjects with TBI differed from normal control subjects in tongue endurance (sustained force) and rate of repetitive movement, but not in tongue strength or fine pressure control. It was also noted that there were only weak correlations between the physiological nonspeech tongue parameters and deviant perceptual articulatory features of the subjects with TBI.

12.3.5 Interpretation

These disparate results are not easily placed in a common perspective on the value of force measures in assessing motor speech disorders. Furthermore, the search for effects of fatigue on speech and voice functions in healthy individuals has led to mixed results. For example, Beukers (1998) concluded that voice fatigue could not be demonstrated with the Voice Interval Test, but Stemple *et al.* (1995) reported significant changes in certain phonatory behaviors following prolonged voice use. The changes included shifts in fundamental frequency and the appearance of anterior glottal chinks.

There are several reasons why fatigue may be difficult to observe in the muscles of speech and phonation, including the possibility that the muscle fibers are fatigue resistant. Resistance to fatigue has been observed in laryngeal, tongue, and mandibular muscles. Han *et al.* (1999) reported that the vocalis muscle compartment of the thyroarytenoid muscle contains a large number of slow tonic muscle fibers (STF). Unlike most muscle fibers, STF do not exhibit a twitch contraction but rather show contractions that are prolonged, stable, precisely controlled, and fatigue resistant. Because STF have not been observed in the vocal folds of other mammals, Han *et al.* proposed that STF 'may be a unique human specialization for speech' (p. 146). Research on the rat tongue also has identified motor units that are fatigue resistant (Sokoloff 2000). Human masticatory muscle fibers are distinctive in that they contain at least four different isoforms of myosin heavy chain, exhibit a continuous range of contraction speeds, and have a high oxidative capacity and are therefore highly fatigue resistant (Weijs 1997).

It is a reasonable hypothesis that many muscles used in speech are fatigue resistant, which would limit the generalization of fatigue-related processes from skeletal muscle to the orofacial and laryngeal muscles. Another possible reason for the limited success in relating measures of strength to ratings of speech is that the forces typical of speech are quite modest compared to the maximal forces that can be developed (Kent *et al.* 1987). Therefore, reduction of the maximal force capacity does not necessarily produce a limitation on speech. What may be more important in speech is the rate of force development, especially because speech requires the relatively rapid generation of forces to execute the successive movements of a complex serial behavior. There are indications that slowness to develop force may be as important as limitations in maximum force, especially for the performance of movements that demand rapid generation of forces (Canning *et al.* 1999).

The limited progress in the quantification of weakness does not mean that weakness is unimportant in speech motor assessment. Perhaps some of the most compelling evidence for the role of weakness in explaining dysarthria comes from obvious clinical signs such as tongue deviation. Umapathi *et al.* (2000) reported that in a study of 300 patients with acute unilateral ischemic motor strokes, tongue deviation was observed in 29% of the patients, and 90% of these had dysarthria. This report accords with the suggestion of Urban *et al.* (1996, 1997) that the pathogenesis of dysarthria in stroke is the disruption of corticolingual fibers.

Because many dysarthrias are associated with neurodegenerative diseases that occur especially in older individuals, one of the challenges in clinical assessment is to distinguish weakness as a pathophysiologic sign from the weakness that tends to occur with age, as discussed later in this chapter.

12.3.6 Conclusion

Although weakness is often assumed as a contributing factor in the pathogenesis of dysarthria, limited progress has been made toward the confirmation of weakness by instrumental methods and explaining the role of weakness in contributing to speech and voice disorders. A particular problem has been to show that measures of weakness are correlated with perceptual measures of speech adequacy (intelligibility, communicative adequacy, quality).

12.4 Coordination

It is usually assumed that speech is a highly coordinated motor behavior and, further, that the coordination of movements in speech would be highly susceptible to disruption by neurologic disease or damage. In fact, the coordination of movements in speech remains an active research question. As a working definition, coordination 'is a repeatable spatiotemporal pattern of movement in relation to a behavioral act or goal' (Kent and Adams 1989). This definition emphasizes that coordinated movements are reliably observable as a subject performs a particular motor response. Speech is remarkable for its temporal and spatial precision. Lackner and Levine (1975) commented on the resolution of the articulatory system, noting that it 'appears to be the most precisely controlled movement system of the human body' (p. 107). It would not be surprising if neurologic damage would disrupt this precision. But what, then, is dyscoordination, and how can it measured in the laboratory or clinic? Dyscoordination may be defined in terms of instability, that is, as a poorly repeatable spatiotemporal pattern of movement. But could it also could be a highly repeatable, albeit maladaptive or inefficient, movement sequence? Can errors of coordination be detected from a single, non-repeated motor performance? These questions are considered in the following.

12.4.1 Repeatability of speech motor sequences

Although it might seem logical that speakers with neurologic speech disorders would have excessive variability in the repeated performance of speech tasks, the evidence is not completely clear on this point. Neilson and O'Dwyer (1984) concluded that the variability of speech muscle activity in speakers with athetoid cerebral palsy was not greater than in healthy control speakers. Study of this issue is clouded by a number of factors, such as the confound with speaking rate. Generally, slow speakers have greater variability in their temporal speech patterns than do fast speakers. Because dysarthric speakers, as a rule, are slower than neurologically normal speakers, the former would be expected to have greater variability just because of their slow rates.

The idea of repeatability is central to a composite measure of spatial and temporal variability, termed the spatiotemporal index (STI; Smith *et al.* 1995). The 'STI reflects the degree to which a set of movement trajectories produced for multiple repetitions of a motor behavior converge onto a single movement template after linear normalization' (Kleinow *et al.* 2001, p. 1042). High STI values may be evidence of a disordered state. Kleinow *et al.* compared STI values in the speech of individuals with Parkinson's disease for the conditions of altered rate and loudness. STI values increased with slowed rate but were stable with loudness changes. It was concluded that changes in vocal effort did not alter the stability associated with preferred production modes. But it is also possible that resistance training can lead to improved coordination (Carroll *et al.* 2001). The STI is a promising quantitative index for the study of dysarthria, but its suitability to disrupted movement patterns needs to be explored. In addition, Ward and Arnfield (2001) have recommended that a nonlinearly normalized analysis of the movement data may be preferable to the linear normalization used in the studies to date.

Calculation of an index such as STI for repeated tokens of an utterances is one valuable approach for the study of dysarthria or other motor speech disorders. However, the clinical assessment of dysarthria rarely requires the clinician to listen to multiple repetitions of an utterance. To the contrary, judgments regarding dyscoordination are rendered on the basis of single tokens of several different utterances, as though the lack of coordination can be identified from only one production of an articulatory sequence. If dyscoordination can be identified from single tokens, then indexes based on multiple tokens of an utterance may not entirely capture the errant pattern.

12.4.2 Coarticulation

Another approach is to use coarticulation as an index of coordination. To the extent that dysarthria is the result of dyscoordination, then coarticulation should be different from that seen in neurologically normal speech. Coarticulation has been studied especially in cerebellar disease (Hertrich and Ackermann 1999) and Parkinson's disease (Tjaden 2000). It appears that coarticulatory disturbances, when present at all, are relatively minor, especially if appropriate controls are exercised over speaking rate. Except in very severe dysarthria, coarticulatory patterns do not readily disintegrate. Studies of coarticulation in patients with apraxia of speech also has produced discrepant results, with some reports of delayed or deficient coarticulation (Ziegler and von Cramon 1985, 1986*a*, *b*; Tuller and Story 1987; Southwood *et al.* 1997) and others indicating normal patterns (Katz 1987, 1988).

Furthermore, because the mechanism of coarticulation is not completely clear, interpretation of coarticulatory abnormalities as evidence of coordination problems carries much uncertainty. In both the window model of coarticulation (Keating 1990) and the DIVA model of speech production (Guenther 1994, 1995), coarticulation arises primarily because of variability in the allowable range of articulatory positions. This is illustrated in Fig. 12.3, which shows a hypothetical target zone (a window in Keating's model and a convex target in Guenther's model) for a normal speaker (black cube) and a motorically impaired speaker (gray cube). Each cube represents a three-dimensional target defined by the articulatory positions of lip, tongue, and jaw. Variability in articulatory positioning may result in a larger target for the impaired than for the normal speaker. The larger the target, the greater the allowable coarticulation with surrounding sounds. Consider, for example, a child with developmental apraxia of speech who lacks articulatory precision. Because of this variability, the child's target is abnormally large, which permits extensive coarticulation and also provides highly variable feedback concerning articulation. In this reasoning, coarticulation as a temporal phenomenon is explained on the basis of permissible articulatory error for the articulatory positions specified for individual segments. This is not to say that coarticulatory abnormalities could not arise for other reasons, but only to indicate one possible explanation for unusual coarticulation in individuals with neurologic impairments.

12.4.3 Coordination: other aspects

Another problem is that coordination occasionally takes unexpected forms, one example being the coordination of movements in the face of tremor. Tremor is involuntary rhythmic oscillation occurring about an equilibrium position of either the whole body or some part of the body (Rondot *et al.* 1978). Of all movement disorders, essential tremor is the most common (Britton 1995). Frequencies

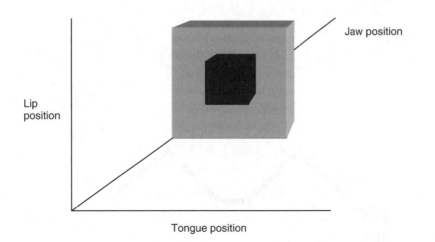

Fig. 12.3 Illustration of an articulatory target for a hypothetical speech sound, as produced by a neurologically impaired speaker (gray cube) and a neurologically normal speaker (black cube). The impaired speaker has a larger target zone, which presumably allows a greater coarticulation with surrounding sounds (the cube essentially defines the limits of coarticulation).

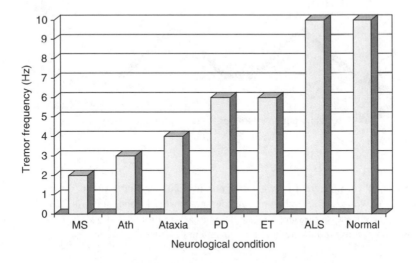

Fig. 12.4 Typical tremor frequencies for selected neurological conditions: multiple sclerosis (MS), athetosis (Ath), ataxia, Parkinson's disease (PD), essential tremor (ET), amyotrophic lateral sclerosis (ALS), and normal physiologic tremor.

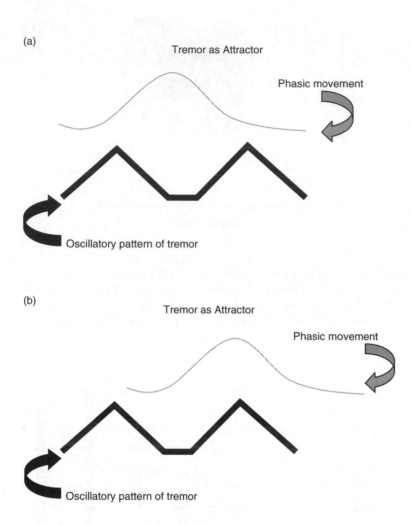

Fig. 12.5 Hypothetical diagram showing how phasic (voluntary) movements can be timed with a severe tremor. With timing as shown in A, the tremor would essentially cancel much of the phasic movement because they are opposite in phase. With timing as shown in B, the tremor and phasic movement would combine in a movement of larger amplitude.

observed in normal and pathologic tremor vary from 1 or 2 Hz up to about 16 Hz (Fig. 12.4). One way of contending with tremor is to use it as the rhythm for voluntary phasic movement, as illustrated in Fig. 12.5. That is, tremor can be an attractor for phasic voluntary movements. The individual with a severe tremor may find it advantageous to time a phasic movement with the tremor cycle so as to minimize interference with the intended movement (compare lines A and B in Fig. 12.5). Evidence for this phenomenon has been presented for Parkinson's disease (Hertrich *et al.*1993; Staude *et al.* 1995), essential vocal–oromandibular tremor (Kent *et al.* 1998*b*), and cerebellar ataxia (Kent *et al.* 2000). The role of tremor as an internal pacemaker for the coordination of movement is abnormal, perhaps, but it is a good example of motoric adaptation to a chronic abnormality. If coordination is defined as movements specified within a low-dimensional space of order parameters (Jeka and Kelso 1989), then tremor-based speech is co-ordinated speech.

12.4.4 Conclusion

The coordination of speech is not readily measured in ways that reflect neurologic disorder. Coordination remains a rather abstract concept, at least in relation to observable events that might be used to identify and grade dyscoordination in the speech motor disorders. There is no simple index of dyscoordination that is widely used clinically, but recent research points to promising methods, such as the STI.

12.5 Evidence of speech-specific pathophysiology

Effects of medical interventions and the physiology of craniofacial muscles provide evidence that neuropathology of the speech system motor system is not completely congruent with that for the limbs. Therefore, disturbances in motor control are not entirely generalizable from nonspeech to speech motor systems.

12.5.1 Effects of medical interventions: speech vs. nonspeech motor systems

One factor to be considered in defining the pathophysiologic correlates of dysarthria is that various interventions that quite consistently lead to improvements in nonspeech motor control (especially limb movements) sometimes have neutral or even negative outcomes for speech. This pattern of results has been reported for levodopa therapy (Gentil *et al.* 1998; Poluha *et al.* 1998; Louis *et al.* 2001); unilateral or bilateral posteroventral pallidotomy (Scott *et al.* 1998; Ghika *et al.* 1999; Schrag *et al.* 1999); fetal dopamine transplants (Bakker *et al.* 1997); and pallidal or thalamic stimulation (Gross *et al.* 1997; Pahwa *et al.* 1999; Taha *et al.* 1999). Indeed, some studies have shown a benefit for speech from these interventions (Leanderson *et al.* 1972; Robertson and Hammerstad 1996; Jiang *et al.* 1999), but the essential point is that these positive outcomes for speech have not been readily or consistently demonstrated to accompany improvements in nonspeech functions. If the speech disorder is to be understood within the classical foundations of neuropathology, then it is puzzling that treatments with positive outcome for nonspeech motor behavior often have neutral or negative outcomes for speech.

In Parkinson's disease, it appears that the neural control for facial expression and limb movements is accomplished primarily through dopaminergic systems, whereas the neural control for speech is achieved largely through nondopaminergic systems (Levy *et al.* 2000).

12.5.2 Distinctive properties of craniofacial muscles in developmental biology

The clinical differentiation between speech and nonspeech effects of neurologic disease is consistent with genetic and developmental studies. Recent evidence indicates that craniofacial and lingual muscles differ from skeletal muscles in their developmental patterns, functional properties, and molecular phenotypes (Noden *et al.* 1999; Shuler and Dalrymple 2001; Mootoosamy and Dietrich 2002). The distinctive properties of craniofacial and lingual muscles are important considerations in understanding the effects of neurologic disease, and may help to explain why a given disease may not have the same consequences on speech and nonspeech muscles. Although current knowledge is limited, the further exploration of contractile, metabolic, and genetic differences in muscle groups may open the door to a better interpretation of clinical manifestations of neurologic disease.

12.6 Challenges to the study of pathophysiologic correlates of dysarthria

This section considers several additional obstacles to the specification of pathophysiologic abnormalities in dysarthria, namely, the effects of compensation, aging, and gender.

12.6.1 Compensatory mechanisms and strategies

One of the greatest challenges in the analysis of dysarthria is the identification of compensatory mechanisms and strategies that a speaker may have adopted in response to a motor speech disorder. Although compensation and adaptation are frequently mentioned in the general clinical literature, it is quite difficult to distinguish compensations from the direct effects of a neurologic disorder. It is possible that some compensations may result in an apparent pathophysiology. Table 12.2 lists some examples of sensorimotor deficits, their kinematic or kinesthetic manifestations, and possible compensatory strategies. It should be emphasized that the intent of the table is not to claim that the responses described are necessarily and always compensatory, but, rather, to suggest ways in which compensations may arise. Confirmation that compensatory mechanisms are at work remains a challenge to investigators and clinicians alike. In a study of dysarthria following TBI, Goozee *et al.* (2001) speculated that the lack of clear relationships between physiological and perceptual data may reflect individual differences in the compensations for physiological impairments.

Table 12.2 Relationships between sensorimotor deficit, kinematic or kinesthetic manifestations of a neurologic disorder, and possible compensatory strategies

Sensorimotor deficit	Kinematic/kinesthetic manifestations	Compensatory strategy
Dyscoordination	Inconsistent unit lengths	Equalize units (scanning speech) (Kent *et al.* 1979) 'Freeze' structures to reduce degrees of freedom
	Difficulty scaling movement	Increase muscular force to produce contrasting durations (Ackermann *et al.* 1995)
	Difficulty initiating and terminating movements	Continuous voicing and subtle velopharyngeal incompetence to simplify sequential adjustments (Kent and Netsell 1978)
Weakness		
Articulators	Difficulty achieving articulatory positions	Recruitment of other muscle fibers, groups, or structures Modify movement target (e.g. substitute phonemes) (Duffy 1995) Exaggerate movements (e.g. increased movements of jaw to compensate for weak lip muscles (Duffy 1995)
Laryngeal	Difficulty producing audible voice	Increase respiratory effort (Netsell 2001)
Respiratory	Difficulty producing long phrases on a single breath; decreased loudness	Use larger lung volumes or terminate phrases on larger lung volumes (Hixon 1990) Hyper-adduction of vocal folds, resulting in strained–strangled voice quality
Rigidity, bradykinesia	Difficulty producing long phrases on a single breath	Produce fewer syllables on a single breath (Solomon and Hixon 1993)
Spasticity (hypertonus)	Laryngeal hyperfunction	Hypofunctional laryngeal adjustments (Murdoch *et al.* 1994)
Hyperkinesia	Interference with reaching or maintaining targets and producing smooth movements	
Tremor	Rhythmic disruption	Timing of phasic movement to coincide with tremor, resulting in delayed movement or tremor-paced sequences (see references in text)
Chorea	Nonrhythmic disruption	Attempts to suppress unwanted movements may increase intensity of extraneous movements

12.6.2 Considerations of aging

Research on aging has made it clear that a variety of changes are noted in individuals who are regarded as healthy. With aging, (1) simple reaction time increases at a rate of 0.5–1.6 ms/year, starting at the age of 20 years; (2) muscle power in the arms and legs decreases by 21–45% between 20 and 80 years; (3) various coordination tasks show a loss of 14–27% between 20 and 80 years; (4) simulated activities of daily living tasks show an average loss of 30% between 20 and 80 years of age; and (5) motor stability reduces during the performance of dual tasks, indicating that attention requirements change with age (Mahant and Stacy 2001; Woolacott and Shumway-Cook 2002). Furthermore, studies of aging show that apparently healthy individuals present with a variety of abnormal neurological signs. Bennett *et al.* (1999) reported a study of the frequency of abnormal neurological signs in a sample of 467 normal elderly residents over 65 years of age. In this sample, (1) bradykinesia was noted in 30% of individuals over the age of 85 years; (2) lower extremity rigidity was seen in more than 40% of individuals over the age of 85; and (3) gait disturbance (shuffling gait) occurred in 6% of individuals in the age group of 65–74 years, and 30% of those in the age group of 75–84 years. In addition, evidence of age-related weakness in healthy subjects is compelling (Booth *et al.* 1994; Roos *et al.* 1997; Ranganathan *et al.* 2001; Kodama *et al.* 2002). The use of age-matched controls is therefore essential to identify useful clinical measures of strength and endurance.

More specifically for the purposes of this chapter, age-related changes in the speech production system are manifold. A complete discussion goes beyond the scope of the current chapter, but it is notable that healthy older individuals have been reported to show slower vocal reaction times, reduced perioral strength, diminished orosensory discrimination, and a greater variability in articulatory kinematics (Martin *et al.* 1994; Wohlert 1996; Fozo and Watson 1998; Wolhert and Smith 1998). These changes are part of the background on which disease-related sensorimotor changes will take their full effect.

12.6.3 Gender differences in neurologic disease

The early studies of dysarthria rarely considered the possibility of gender differences in either the perceptual features of dysarthria or the underlying pathophysiology. More recent studies have been identified sex differences in the dysarthria associated with Parkinson's disease, cerebellar disease, and amyotrophic lateral sclerosis (Hertrich *et al.* 1998; Luschei *et al.* 1999; Stelzig *et al.* 1999; Holmes *et al.* 2000; Kent *et al.* 1992, 2000). In some respects, sex-related differences are not surprising given the sexual dimorphism of the speech production system and sex-related differences in the effects of aging on speech and voice. But the gender differences may extend to motor control strategies. Koenig (2000) concluded that 'differences in laryngeal structure and aerodynamic quantities may require men and women to adopt somewhat different strategies for achieving distinctive consonantal voicing contrasts' (p. 1211). It is interesting to note that voicing contrasts are differentially affected in men and women by certain neurologic diseases (Kent *et al.* 1992). However, these differences have not been carefully examined across different neurologic disorders, and many questions remain as to the distribution of these differences over the various tissues and functions of the speech production system.

Gender differences in neurologic disease are not restricted to speech. Scott *et al.* (2000) concluded from a questionnaire study of 948 individuals with Parkinson's disease that males reported a higher frequency of writing difficulties, fumblingness, gait problems, speech problems, increased flow of saliva, and lack of initiative. A study of 630 patients with Parkinson's disease (Lyons *et al.* 1998) revealed that gender differences emerge with disease progression. Men had more severe parkinsonian motor features, while women experienced more levodopa-induced dyskinesia.

12.7 Overall conclusion

Darley *et al.* (1969*a*, *b*) followed a reasonable and parsimonious line of thought in explaining the neuromuscular substrates of motor speech disorders in terms of classic neuropathology. This line of thought should not be abandoned casually, but there are reasons to revise the simple maxim that 'speech follows neurology'. Speech has its own neurology, distinct in some respects from the neurology of skeletal movements. This 'speech neurology' is informed by:

(1) speech motor dysfunction associated with neurologic disease;
(2) response of speech and nonspeech motor systems to surgical and pharmacological interventions;
(3) genetic, molecular, and functional studies of craniofacial and laryngeal muscles;
(4) gender differences in speech motor control;
(5) the effects of aging on speech; and
(6) capabilities for compensation to disorder.

Acknowledgement

This work was supported in part by research grant No. 5 R01 DC00319 from the National Institute on Deafness and Other Communicative Disorders (NIDCD-NIH).

References

Ackermann, H., Hertrich, I., and **Scharf, G.** (1995). Kinematic analysis of lower lip movements in ataxic dysarthria. *Journal of Speech and Hearing Research, 38,* 1252–1259.

Bakker, K. K., Ramig, L. O., Johnson, A. B., and **Freed, C. R.** (1997). Preliminary voice and speech analysis following fetal dopamine transplants in 5 individuals with Parkinson disease. *Journal of Speech, Language, and Hearing Research, 40,* 615–626.

Ballard, K. J., Granier, J. P., and **Robin, D. A.** (2000). Understanding the nature of apraxia of speech: theory, analysis, and treatment. *Aphasiology, 14,* 969–995.

Bennett, D. A., Shannon, K. M., Beckett, L. A., and **Wilson, R. S.** (1999). Dimensionality of parkinsonian signs in aging and Alzheimer's disease. *Journal of Gerontology Series A-Biological Sciences & Medical Sciences, 54,* M191–M196.

Berardelli, S., Rothwell, J. C., Thompson, P. D., and **Hallet, M.** (2001). Pathophysiology of bradykinesia in Parkinson's disease. *Brain, 124,* 2131–2146.

Beukers, R. (1998). Are voice endurance tests able to assess vocal fatigue? *Clinical Otolaryngology and Allied Sciences, 23,* 533–538.

Blumberger, J., Sullivan, S. J., and **Clement, N.** (1995). Diadochokinetic rate in persons with traumatic brain injury. *Brain Injury, 9,* 797–804.

Booth, F. W., Weeden, S. H., and **Tseng, B. S.** (1994). Effect of aging on human skeletal muscle and motor function. *Medicine and Science in Sportsand& Exercise, 26,* 556–560.

Britton, T. C. (1995). Essential tremor and its variants. *Current Opinion in Neurology, 8,* 314–319.

Caligiuri, M.P. (1987). Labial kinematics during speech in patients with Parkinsonian rigidity. *Brain, 110,* 1033–1044.

Canning, C. G., Ada, L., and **O'Dwyer, N.** (1999). Slowness to develop force contributes to weakness after stroke. *Archives of Physical Medicine and Rehabilitation, 80,* 66–70.

Canter, G. J. (1965). Speech characteristics of patients with Parkinson's disease: III. Articulation, diadochokinesis, and over-all speech adequacy. *Journal of Speech and Hearing Disorders, 30,* 217–224.

Carroll, T. J., Barry, B., Riek, S., and **Carson, R. G.** (2001). Resistance training enhances the stability of sensorimotor coordination. *Proceedings of the Royal Society of London—Series B: Biological Sciences, 268,* 221–227.

Darley, F. L., Aronson, A. E., and **Brown, J. R.** (1969a). Differential diagnostic patterns of dysarthria. *Journal of Speech and Hearing Research, 12,* 249–269.

Darley, F. L., Aronson, A. E., and **Brown, J. R.** (1969b). Clusters of deviant speech dimensions in the dysarthrias. *Journal of Speech and Hearing Research, 12,* 462–496.

Duffy, J. R. (1995). *Motor speech disorders: Substrates, differential diagnosis, and management.* St. Louis: Mosby Year-Book.

Duffy, J. R. and **Kent, R. D.** (2001). Darley's contributions to the understanding, differential diagnosis, and scientific study of the dysarthrias. *Aphasiology, 15,* 275–289.

Forrest, K., Weismer, G., and **Turner, G. S.** (1989). Kinematic, acoustic, and perceptual analyses of connected speech produced by Parkinsonian and normal geriatric adults. *Journal of the Acoustical Society of America, 85,* 2608–2622.

Fozo, M. S. and **Watson, B. C.** (1998). Task complexity effect on vocal reaction time in aged speakers. *Journal of Voice, 12,* 404–414.

Gentil, M., Tournier, C. L., Perrin, S., and **Pollak, P.** (1998). Effects of levodopa on finger and orofacial movements in Parkinson's disease. *Progress in Neuro-Psychopharmacology and Biological Psychiatry, 22,* 1261–1274.

Gentil, M., Perrin, S., Tournier, C. L., and **Pollak, P.** (1999). Lip, tongue and forefinger force control in Parkinson's disease. *Clinical Linguistics and Phonetics, 13,* 45–54.

Ghika, J., Ghika-Schmitd, F., Fankhauser, H., Assal, G., Vingerhoets, F., Albanese, A., Bougousslavsky, J., and **Favre, J.** (1999). Bilateral contemporaneous posteroventral pallidotomy for the treatment of Parkinson's disease: neuropsychological and neurological side effects – Report of four cases and review of the literature. *Journal of Neurosurgery, 91,* 313–321.

Goozee, J. V., Murdoch, B. E., and **Theordoros, D. G.** (2001). Physiological assessment of tongue function in dysarthria following traumatic brain injury. *Logopedics, Phoniatrics, Vocology, 26,* 51–65.

Gross, C., Rougier, A., Guehl, D., Boraud, T., Julien, M. and **Bioulac, C.** (1997). High-frequency stimulation of the globus pallidus internalis in Parkinson's disease: a study of seven cases. *Journal of Neurosurgery, 87,* 491–498.

Guenther, F. H. (1994). A neural network model of speech acquisition and motor equivalent speech production. *Biological Cybernetics, 72,* 43–53.

Guenther, F. H. (1995). Speech sound acquisition, coarticulation, and rate effects in a neural network model of speech production. *Psychological Review, 102,* 594–621.

Han, Y. S., Wang, J., Fischman, D. A., Biller, H. F., and **Sanders, I.** (1999). Slow tonic muscle fibers in the thyroarytenoid muscles of human vocal folds: a possible specialization for speech. *Anatomical Record, 256,* 146–157.

Hertrich, I. and **Ackermann, H.** (1999). Temporal and spectral aspects of coarticulation in ataxic dysarthria: an acoustic analysis. *Journal of Speech, Language, and Hearing Research, 42,* 367–381.

Hertrich, I., Ackermann, H., Ziegler, W., and **Kaschel. R.** (1993). Speech iterations in parkinsonism—a case study. *Aphasiology, 7,* 395–406.

Hertrich, I., Spieker, S., and **Ackermann, H.** (1998). Gender-specific phonatory dysfunctions in disorders of the basal ganglia and the cerebellum: acoustic and perceptual characteristics. In W. Ziegler and K. Deger (eds.), *Clinical phonetics and linguistics* (pp. 448–457). London: Whurr.

Hirose, H. (1986). Pathophysiology of motor speech disorders (dysarthria). *Folia Phoniatrica, 38,* 61–88.

Holmes, R. J., Oates, J. M., Phyland, D. J., and **Hughes, A. J.** (2000). Voice characteristics in the progression of Parkinson's disease. *International Journal of Language and Communication Disorders, 35,* 407–418.

Hunker, C. J., Abbs, J. H., and **Barlow, S. M.** (1982). The relationship between parkinsonian rigidity and hypokinesia in the orofacial system: a quantitative analysis. *Neurology, 32,* 749–754.

Jeka, J. J. and **Kelso, J. A. S.** (1989). The dynamic pattern approach to coordinated behavior: a tutorial review. In S. W. Wallace (ed.), *Perspectives on the coordination of movement* (pp. 3–45). Amsterdam: North-Holland.

Jiang, J., Lin, E., Wang, J., and **Hanson, D. G.** (1999). Glottographic measures before and after levodopa treatment in Parkinson's disease. *Laryngoscope, 109,* 1287–1294.

Katz, W. F. (1987). Anticipatory labial and lingual coarticulation in aphasia. In J. H. Ryalls (ed.), *Phonetic approaches to speech production in aphasia and related disorders* (pp. 221–242). Boston, MA: College-Hill Press.

Katz, W. F. (1988). Anticipatory coarticulation in aphasia: acoustic and perceptual data. *Brain and Language, 35,* 340–368.

Keating, P. A. (1990). The window model of coarticulation: articulatory evidence. In J. Kingston and M. E. Beckman (eds), *Papers in laboratory phonology I. Between the grammar and physics of speech* (pp. 451–470). Cambridge, England: Cambridge University Press.

Kent, R. D. (1996). Hearing and believing: some limits to the auditory–perceptual assessment of speech and voice disorders. *American Journal of Speech–Language Pathology, 7,* 7–23.

Kent, R. D. and **Adams, S. G.** (1989). The concept and measurement of coordination in speech disorders. In S. A. Wallace (ed.), *Perspectives on the coordination of movement* (pp. 415–450). Amsterdam: North Holland.

Kent, R. D. and **Kent, J. F.** (2000). Task-based profiles of the dysarthrias. *Folia Phoniatrica et Logopaedica, 52,* 48–53.

Kent, R. D. and **Netsell, R.** (1978). Articulatory abnormalities in athetoid cerebral palsy. *Journal of Speech and Hearing Disorders, 43,* 353–373.

Kent, R. D., Carney, P. J., and **Severeid, L.** (1974). Velar movement and timing: evaluation of a model for binary control. *Journal of Speech and Hearing Research, 17,* 470–488.

Kent, R. D., Netsell, R., and **Abbs, J.** (1979). Acoustic characteristics of dysarthria associated with cerebellar disease. *Journal of Speech and Hearing Research, 22,* 627–648.

Kent, R. D., Kent, J. F., and **Rosenbek, J. C.** (1987). Maximum performance tests of speech production. *Journal of Speech and Hearing Disorders, 52,* 367–387.

Kent, J. F., Kent, R. D., Rosenbek, J. C., Weismer, G., Martin, R. E., Sufit, R. L. and **Brooks, B. R.** (1992). Quantitative description of the dysarthria in women with amyotrophic lateral sclerosis. *Journal of Speech and Hearing Research, 35,* 723–733.

Kent, R. D., Kent, J. F., Rosenbek, J. C., Vorperian, H. K., and **Weismer, G.** (1997). A speaking task analysis of the dysarthria in cerebellar disease. *Folia Phoniatrica et Logopaedica, 49,* 63–82.

Kent, R. D., Kent, J. F., Duffy, J. R., and **Weismer, G.** (1998a). The dysarthrias: speech–voice profiles, related dysfunctions, and neuropathologies. *Journal of Medical Speech–Language Pathology, 6,* 165–211.

Kent, R. D., Duffy, J. R., Vorperian, H. K., and **Thomas, J. E.** (1998b). Severe essential vocal and oromandibular tremor: a case report. *Phonoscope, 4,* 237–253.

Kent, R. D., Duffy, J., Kent, J. F., and **Vorperian, H. K.** (1999). Quantification of motor speech abilities in stroke: time-energy analyses of syllable and word repetition. *Journal of Medical Speech–Language Pathology, 7,* 83–90.

Kent, R. D., Kent, J. F., Duffy, J. R., Thomas, J. E., Weismer, G., and **Stuntebeck, S.** (2000). Ataxic dysarthria. *Journal of Speech, Language, and Hearing Research, 43,* 1275–1289.

Kleinow, J., Smith, A., and **Ramig, L.** (2001). Speech motor stability in IPD: effects of rate and loudness manipulations. *Journal of Speech, Language, and Hearing Research, 44,* 1041–1051.

Kodama, T., Nakagawa, M., Arimura, K., Koriyama, C., Akiba, S., and **Osame, M.** (2002). Cross-sectional analysis of neurological findings among healthy elderly: study in a remote island in Kagoshima, Japan. *Neuroepidemiology, 21,* 36–43.

Koenig, L. L. (2000). Laryngeal factors in voiceless consonant production in men, women, and 5-year-olds. *Journal of Speech, Language, and Hearing Research, 43,* 1211–1228.

Lackner, J. R. and **Levine, K. B.** (1975). Speech production: evidence for syntactically and phonologically determined units. *Perception and Psychophysics, 17,* 107–113.

Leanderson, R., Meyerson, B., and **Persson, A.** (1972). Lip muscle function in parkinsonian dysarthria. *Acta Otolaryngologica, 73,* 1–8.

Levy, G., Tang, M. X., Cote, L. J., Louis, E. D., Alfaro, B., Mejia, H., Stern, Y., and **Marder, K.** (2000). Motor impairment in PD-Relationship to incident dementia and age. *Neurology, 55,* 539–544.

Lotze, M., Seggawies, G., Erb, M., Grodd, W., and **Birbaumer, N.** (2000). The representation of articulation in the primary sensorimotor cortex. *Neuroreport, 11,* 2985–2989.

Louis, E. D., Winfield, L., Fahn, S., and **Ford, B.** (2001). Speech dysfluency exacerbated by levodopa in Parkinson's disease. *Movement Disorders, 16,* 562–565.

Luschei, E. S. (1991). Development of objective standards of nonspeech oral strength and performance: an advocate's views. In C. A. Moore, K. M. Yorkston, and D. R. Beukelman (eds), *Dysarthria and apraxia of speech: perspectives on management* (pp. 3–14). Baltimore: Paul H. Brookes.

Luschei, E. S., Ramig, L. O., Baker, K. L., and **Smith, M. E.** (1999). Discharge characteristics of laryngeal single motor units during phonation in young and older adults and in persons with parkinson disease. *Journal of Neurophysiology, 81,* 2131–2139.

Lyons, K. E., Hubble, J. P., Troster, A. I., Pahwa, R., and **Koller, W. C.** (1998). Gender differences in Parkinson's disease. *Clinical Neuropharmacology, 21,* 118–121.

Mahant, P. R. and **Stacy, M. A.** (2001). Movement disorders and normal aging. *Neurologic Clinics, 19,* 543–563.

Martin, J. H., Diamond, B., Aviv, J. E., Jones, M., E., Keen, M. S., and **Wee, T. A.** (1994). Age-related changes in pharyngeal and supraglottic sensation. *Annals of Otology, Rhinology, and Laryngology, 103,* 749–752.

McClean, M. D. (2000). Patterns of orofacial movement velocity across variations in speech rate. *Journal of Speech, Language, and Hearing Research, 43,* 205–216.

McHenry, M. A., Minton, J. T., and **Wilson, R. L.** (1994*a*). Increasing the efficiency of articulatory force testing of adults with traumatic brain injury. In J. A. Till, K. M. Yorkston, and D. R. Beukelman (eds), *Motor speech disorders: advances in assessment and treatment* (pp. 135–146). Baltimore: Paul H. Brookes.

McHenry, M. A., Minton, J. T., Wilson, R. L., and **Post, Y. V.** (1994*b*). Intelligibility and nonspeech orofacial strength and force control following traumatic brain injury. *Journal of Speech and Hearing Research, 37,* 1271–1283.

Moore, C. A. and **Scudder R. R.** (1989). Coordination of jaw muscle activity in parkinsonian movement: description and response to traditional treatment. In K. M. Yorkston and D. R. Beukelman (eds), *Recent advances in clinical dysarthria.* Boston: College-Hill.

Mootoosamy, R. C. and **Dietrich, S.** (2002). Distinct regulatory cascades for head and trunk myogenesis. *Development, 129,* 573–583.

Murdoch, B. E., Thompson, E. C., and **Stokes, P. D.** (1994). Phonatory and laryngeal dysfunction following upper motor neuron vascular lesions. *Journal of Medical Speech-Language Pathology, 2,* 177–189.

Neilson, P. D. and **O'Dwyer, N. J.** (1981). Pathophysiology of dysarthria in cerebral palsy. *Journal of Neurology, Neurosurgery and Psychiatry, 44,* 1013–1019.

Neilson, P. D. and **O'Dwyer, N. J.** (1984). Reproducibility and variability of speech muscle activity in athetoid dysarthria of cerebral palsy. *Journal of Speech and Hearing Research, 27,* 502–519.

Neilson, P. D., Andrews, G., Guitar, B. E., and **Quinn, P. T.** (1979). Tonic stretch reflexes in lip, tongue and jaw muscles. *Brain Research, 178,* 311–327.

Netsell, R. (1986). *A neurobiologic view of speech production and the dysarthrias.* San Diego: College-Hill Press.

Netsell, R. (2001). Speech aeromechanics and the dysarthrias: implications for children with traumatic brain injury. *Journal of Head Trauma Rehabilitation, 16,* 415–425.

Nishio, M. and **Niimi, S.** (2001). Speaking rate and its components in dysarthric speakers. *Clinical Linguistics and Phonetics, 15,* 309–317.

Noden, D. M., Marchcio, R., Borycki, A.-G., and **Emerson, C. P., Jr** (1999). Differentiation of avian craniofacial muscles: I. Patterns of early regulatory gene expression and myosin heavy chain synthesis. *Developmental Dynamics, 216,* 96–112.

O'Dwyer, N. J., Neilson, P. D., Guitar, B. E., Quinn, P. T., and **Andrews, G.** (1983). Control of upper airway structures during nonspeech tasks in normal and cerebral palsied subjects: EMG findings. *Journal of Speech and Hearing Research, 31,* 162–170.

Ozawa, Y., Shiromoto, O., Ishizaki, F., and **Watamori, T.** (2001). Symptomatic differences in decreasing alternating motion rates between individuals with spastic and with ataxic dysarthria: an acoustic analysis. *Folia Phoniatrica et Logopedica, 53,* 67–72.

Pahwa, R., Lyons, K. L., Wilkinson, S. B., Carpenter, M. A., Troster, A. I., Searl, J. P., Overman, J., Pickering, S., and Koller, W. C. (1999). Bilateral thalamic stimulation for the treatment of essential tremor. *Neurology, 53,* 1447–1450.

Poluha, P. C., Teulings, H. L., and Brookshire, R. H. (1998). Handwriting and speech changes across the levodopa cycle in Parkinson's disease. *Acta Psychologica, 100,* 71–84.

Portnoy, R. A. and Aronson, A. E. (1982). Diadochokinetic syllable rate and regularity in normal and in spastic and ataxic dysarthric subjects. *Journal of Speech and Hearing Disorders, 47,* 324–328.

Ranganathan, V. K., Siemionow, V., Sahgal, V., and Yue, G. H. (2001). Effects of aging on hand function. *Journal of the American Geriatrics Society, 49,* 1478–1484.

Riecker, A., Ackermann, H., Wildgruber, D., Meyer, J., Dogil, G., Haider, H., and Grodd, W. (2000). Articulatory/phonetic sequencing at the level of the anterior perisylvian cortex: a functional magnetic resonance imaging (fMRI) study. *Brain and Language, 75,* 259–276.

Robertson, L. T. and Hammerstad, J. P. (1996). Jaw movement dysfunction related to Parkinson's disease and partially modified by levodopa. *Journal of Neurology, Neurosurgery, and Psychiatry, 60,* 41–50.

Rondot, P., Jedynak, C. P. and Ferrey, G. (1978). Pathologic tremors: nosological correlates. In J. F. Desmedt (ed.), *Physiological tremor, pathological tremors and clonus. Progress in Clinical Neurophysiology. Vol. 5* (pp. 95–113). Basel: Karger.

Roos, M. R., Rice, C. L., and Vandervoort, A. A. (1997). Age-related changes in motor unit function. *Muscle and Nerve, 20,* 679–690.

Schrag, A., Samuel, M., Caputo, E., Scaravilli, T., Troyer, M., Marsden, C. D., Thomas, D. G. T., Lees, A. J., Brooks, D. J., and Quinn, N. P. (1999). Unilateral pallidotomy for Parkinson's disease: results after more than 1 year. *Journal of Neurology, Neurosurgery and Psychiatry, 67,* 511–517.

Scott, R., Gregory, R., Hines, N., Carroll, C., Hyman, N., Papanasstasiou, V., Leather, C., Rowe, J., Silburn, P., and Aziz, T. (1998). Neuropsychological, neurological and functional outcome following pallidotomy for Parkinson's disease—a consecutive series of eight simultaneous bilateral and twelve unilateral procedures. *Brain, 121,* 659–675.

Scott, B., Borgman, A., Engler, H., Johnels, B., and Aquilonius, S. M. (2000). Gender differences in Parkinson's disease symptom profile. *Acta Neurologica Scandinavica, 102,* 37–43.

Shuler, C. F. and Dalrymple, K. R. (2001). Molecular regulation of tongue and craniofacial muscle differentiation. *Critical Reviews in Oral Biology and Medicine, 12,* 3–17.

Smith, A., Goffman, L., Zelaznik, H., Ying, G., and McGillem, C. (1995). Spatiotemporal stability and patterning of speech movement sequences. *Experimental Brain Research, 104,* 493–501.

Sokoloff, A. J. (2000). Localization and contractile properties of intrinsic longitudinal motor units of the rate tongue. *Journal of Neurophysiology, 84,* 827–835.

Solomon, N. P. and **Hixon, T. J.** (1993). Speech breathing in Parkinson's disease. *Journal of Speech and Hearing Research, 36,* 294–310.

Solomon, N. P., Robin, D. A., and **Luschei, E. S.** (2000). Strength, endurance, and stability of the tongue and hand in Parkinson disease. *Journal of Speech, Language, and Hearing Research, 43,* 256–267.

Southwood, M. H., Dagenais, P. A., Sutphin, S. M., and **Garcia, J. M.** (1997). Coarticulation in apraxia of speech: a perceptual, acoustic, and electropalatographic study. *Clinical Linguisticsand⅋ Phonetics, 11,* 179–203.

Staude, G., Wolf, W., Ott, M., Oertel, W. H., and **Dengler, R.** (1995). Tremor as a factor in prolonged reaction times of Parkinsonian patients. *Movement Disorders, 10,* 153–162.

Stelzig, Y., Hochhaus, W., Gall, V., and **Henneberg, A.** (1999). Laryngeal findings of patients with Parkinson's disease. *Laryngo-Rhino-Otologie, 78,* 544–551[in German].

Stemple, J. C., Stanley, J., and **Lee, L.** (1995). Objective measures of voice production in normal subjects following prolonged voice use. *Journal of Voice, 9,* 127–133.

Stevens, K. N. (1998). *Acoustic phonetics.* Cambridge, MA: MIT Press.

Taha, J. M., Janszen, M. A., and **Favre, J.** (1999). Thalamic deep brain stimulation for the treatment of head, voice, and bilateral limb tremor. *Journal of Neurosurgery, 91,* 68–72.

Theodoros, D. G., Murdoch, B. E., and **Stokes, P.** (1995). A physiological analysis of articulatory dysfunction in dysarthric speakers following severe closed-head injury. *Brain Injury, 9,* 237–254.

Thompson, E. C., Murdoch, B. E., and **Stokes, P. D.** (1995). Lip function in subjects with upper motor neuron type dysarthria following cerebrovascular accidents. *European Journal of Disorders of Communication, 30,* 451–466.

Tjaden, K. (2000). An acoustic study of coarticulation in dysarthric speakers with Parkinson disease. *Journal of Speech, Language, and Hearing Research, 43,* 1466–1480.

Tuller, B. and **Story, R. S.** (1987). Anticipatory coarticulation in aphasia. In J. H. Ryalls (ed.), *Phonetic approaches to speech production in aphasia and related disorders.* Boston: College-Hill Press.

Turner, G. S., Tjaden, K., and **Weismer, G.** (1995). The influence of speaking rate on vowel space and speech intelligibility for individuals with amyotrophic lateral sclerosis. *Journal of Speech and Hearing Research, 38,* 1001–1013.

Umapathi, T., Venketasubramanian, N., Leck, K. J., Tan, C. B., Lee, W. L., and **Tjia, H.** (2000). Tongue deviation in acute ischaemic stroke: a study of supranuclear twelfth cranial nerve palsy in 300 stroke patients. *Cerebrovascular Diseases, 10,* 462–465.

Urban, P. P., Hopf, H. C., Zorowka, P. G., Fleischer, S., and **Andreas, J.** (1996). Dysarthria and lucunar stroke—Pathophysiologic aspects. *Neurology, 47,* 1135–1141.

Urban, P. P., Hopf, H. C., Fleischer, X., Zorowka, P. G., and **Mullerforell, W.** (1997). Impaired cortico-bulbar tract function in dysarthria due to hemispheric stroke—Functional testing using transcranial magnetic stimulation. *Brain, 120,* 1077–1084.

Wang, Y.-T., Kent, R. D., Duffy, J. R., Thomas, J. E., and **Weismer, G.** (2004). Syllable alternating motion rates as an index of motor speech abilities in traumatic brain injury, submitted.

Ward, D. and **Arnfield, S.** (2001). Linear and nonlinear analysis of the stability of gestural organization in speech movement sequences. *Journal of Speech, Language, and Hearing Research, 44,* 108–117.

Weijnen, F. G., Kuks, J. B. M., van der Bilt, A., van der Glas, H. W., Wassenberg, M. W. M., and **Bosman, F.** (2000). Tongue force in patients with myasthenia gravis. *Acta Neurologica Scandinavica, 102,* 303–308.

Weijs, W. A. (1997). [Masticatory muscles Part II. Functional properties of the masticatory muscle fibers]. *Nederlands Tijdschrift voor Tandheelkunde, 104,* 210–213 [in Dutch].

Westbury, J. and **Dembowski, J.** (1993). Articulatory kinematics of normal diadochokinetic performance. *Annual Bulletin, Research Institute of Logopedics and Phoniatrics, University of Tokyo,* No. 27, 13–36.

Wildgruber, D., Ackermann, H., and **Grodd, W.** (2001). Differential contributions of motor cortex, basal ganglia, and cerebellum to speech motor control: effects of syllable repetition rate evaluated by fMRI. *Neuroimage, 13,* 101–109.

Wohlert, A. B. (1996). Tactile perception of spatial stimulation on the lip surface by young and older adults. *Journal of Speech and Hearing Research, 39,* 1191–1198.

Wohlert, A. B. and **Smith, A.** (1998). Spatiotemporal stability of lip movements in older adult speakers. *Journal of Speech, Language, and Hearing Research, 41,* 41–50.

Woollacott, M. and **Shumway-Cook, A.** (2002). Attention and the control of posture and gait: a review of an emerging area of research. *Gaitand& Posture, 16,* 1–14.

Ziegler, W. (2002). Task-related factors in oral motor control: speech and oral diadochokinesis in dysarthria and apraxia of speech. *Brain and Language, 80,* 556–575.

Ziegler, W. and **von Cramon, D.** (1985). Anticipatory coarticulation in a speaker with apraxia of speech. *Brain and Language, 26,* 117–130.

Ziegler, W. and **von Cramon, D.** (1986a). Disturbed coarticulation in apraxia of speech: acoustic evidence. *Brain and Language, 29,* 34–47.

Ziegler, W. and **von Cramon, D.** (1986b). Timing deficits in apraxia of speech. *European Archives of Psychiatry and Neurological Sciences, 236,* 44–49.

CHAPTER 13

SEARCHING FOR THE WEAK LINK IN THE SPEECH PRODUCTION CHAIN OF PEOPLE WHO STUTTER: A MOTOR SKILL APPROACH

PASCAL H. H. M. VAN LIESHOUT, WOUTER HULSTIJN, AND HERMAN F. M. PETERS

13.1 Introduction

> Stuttering is essentially a neuromuscular disorder whose core consists of tiny lags and disruptions in the timing of the complicated movements required for speech
>
> (Van Riper 1990, p. 317)

This statement from Charles van Riper reflects on the nature of stuttering and casts little doubt about the involvement of the speech motor system in stuttering. In this chapter, we will provide arguments and empirical evidence that stuttering can be linked to the speech motor system, but not necessarily in terms of a 'speech motor disorder'. Rather, the central theme of our chapter will be that, for people who stutter (PWS), the speech motor control system is the weak link in the chain of events that lead to the production of speech. A weak link in terms of limited skill or ability to prepare and perform the motor actions that are required to implement the various demands imposed by cognitive, linguistic, emotional, and motor aspects of speech (Hulstijn and van Lieshout 1998). In this, we take the position that speech is similar to other motor tasks that involve a certain amount of accuracy and speed, and where humans demonstrate large individual differences in skill, even when amount and extent of practice is taken into account. We will use the term 'speech clumsiness' to label our view on stuttering by analogy with the term 'clumsiness' used for children who 'puzzle scientists because there is no very obvious reason for their difficulties. These children have no biochemical, anatomical or sensory deficiency, show no hard signs of neurological impairment and are intellectually able. Nevertheless, they find it extraordinarily difficult to acquire the movement skills they need, in order to function adequately in every day life' (Barnett *et al.* 1998, p. 436). We do not claim that stuttering children should be classified as a subgroup of children with developmental coordination disorder (DCD), but we do notice that in the traditional diagnosis of (fine) motor problems in clumsy children, speech production has always been left out (Henderson and Barnett 1998), mostly because speech is not the focus for the traditional disciplines involved in DCD (occupational therapy, psychiatry, and neurology). [Developmental Coordination Disorder (DSM IV) is the official term adopted by the American Psychiatric Association for 'clumsy' children (Henderson and Barnett 1998)]. None the less, there are striking parallels between stuttering and DCD in terms of the questionable reliability of assessment of symptoms and the lack of valid standardized tests; the absence of clear evidence for specific neurological lesions; the potential relevance of feedback (more on this later in this chapter); the issue of spontaneous recovery versus perseverance of symptoms at later ages; the ambiguity regarding pathology or maturity (delay); the variability of symptoms across and within tasks; the potential overlap with other types of disorders (including language and attention functions); and the emotional and social problems that accompany both (for a recent overview, see Henderson and Barnett 1998). The overlap with other (developmental) disorders has inspired some to suggest that the notion of separate developmental disorders (which may include stuttering) could actually be misguided by the way we tend to categorize symptoms into syndromes, and that, in fact, all these problems can be related and often co-occur as part of a more general problem based on an atypical brain development due to subtle lesions in the cerebrum/cerebellum (Kaplan *et al.* 1998). This is not the place to discuss these issues further, although they clearly deserve more attention, certainly in light of popular views on stuttering that embrace the concept of multi-causality (Adams 1995; Smith and Kelly 1997). In this chapter, if we use the term 'speech clumsiness' it denotes our view on stuttering as a limitation in speech motor skill, without claiming further direct associations with DCD. We do not exclude that possibility, but there is simply not enough research in this area to corroborate such an association. In the next section, we will briefly elaborate on the concept of speech motor skill, and what aspects of speech production relate to it. Then in Section 13.3, we will summarize early research attempts (before 1995) that tried to address the notion of speech motor skill in people who stutter. This will be followed with a critical review of current research in this area in Section 13.4. Section 13.5 will discuss possible future directions of research that may allow us to test our notion of 'speech clumsiness' in stuttering in more detail. Finally, Section 13.6 will provide a summary and our main conclusions.

13.2 Speech motor skill: can we define it?

To submit the claim that people who stutter have limited speech motor skills has no value if we cannot define the concept of 'motor skill' more precisely. The literature in motor control provides various definitions to choose from: 'Skill consists in the ability to bring about some end result with maximum certainty and minimum outlay of energy, or of time and energy' (Guthrie 1952, p. 136); 'Skills: movements that are dependent on practice and experience for their execution, as opposed to being genetically defined' (Schmidt 1988, p. 17); and 'A skilled response is … highly organized, both spatially and temporally. The central problem for skill learning is how such organization or patterning comes about' (Paul Fitts as cited in Kelso 1995).

The common notion reflected in all three descriptions (rather than real definitions) is that motor skill requires practice, a high spatial and temporal organization, and effectiveness (in terms of energy and time costs). Only the first description by Guthrie also alludes to the fact that skilful actions require a purpose or perhaps, in broader terms, a context. We also want to add another component that we think is necessary to describe skilful actions, namely adaptability (van Lieshout *et al.* 1997*a*). Performing a task in a simple, rigid way, regardless of changes in context or purpose, would not classify as a skilful action in our perspective. The capability to adapt to ongoing and often unexpected changes in task requirements allows us to distinguish between true motor skill and purely automated performance.

Does speech fit these descriptions? Obviously, speech movements are not innate and require practice for an extended period of time (into adolescence) before they reach a certain level of skill (Smith and Goffman 1998; Green *et al.* 2000, 2002). Speech movements are without doubt characterized by a high spatial and temporal organization (e.g. Smith 1992; Gracco 1997). They are also very effective as they accomplish their goals with a minimum of effort if possible (Lindblom 1990; MacNeilage *et al.* 2000), as typically demonstrated in the phenomenon of motor equivalence (e.g. Guenther 1994). The latter aspect also indicates their natural flexibility to change, even when perturbed at a subconscious level (e.g. Folkins and Zimmermann 1982; Abbs and Gracco 1984; Saltzman *et al.* 1998). Finally, they have a clear context, namely to generate acoustic information that will communicate the speaker's intentions to a listener. In short, producing speech is indeed a motor skill. This may seem a trivial conclusion, but it is not, or better, we wish it were. The concept of a motor skill entails the concept of learning and practice (see above), but clearly, that is not sufficient. If learning and practice were not only necessary but also sufficient to determine skill, we could all potentially become stars in sports and music if only we would practice enough. We know this is not true, and that for each 'star', there are plenty of individuals who are more committed to practice than the stars themselves, but never reach the same level of skill. Motor skill (for a given task) comes in various levels across a normal population. Apart from motor processes, a variety of other factors (cognition, emotion, motivation, social environment, etc.) play a role in this skill continuum. We all seem to accept this concept of a continuum readily when it concerns sports, art, or professional motor skills, as in surgery, but somehow seem reluctant to apply it to speech. Most studies in this area assume that all adults are speech motor 'stars' and use this as a reference to indicate if and when children have reached a mature motor skill level, namely, when they become similar to adults in terms of (mostly) a limited number of movement parameters (e.g. Smith *et al.* 1998; Green *et al.* 2000, 2002). However, even in assuming that these parameters actually reflect speech motor skill, adults do show a lot of variability between subjects, and even within a subject when sampled at different times (e.g. Alfonso and van Lieshout 1997). Such individual differences are easily masked if we focus on group data only, but this approach is not very fruitful if we want to take the concept of motor skill seriously. Our knowledge of normal variation in speech motor skill is limited, and this means that defining cut-points to determine different levels of skill is rather arbitrary. In fact, it is even fairly arbitrary to define a cut-point between normal and so-called pathological motor skill levels. Sure, the extreme cases at either end of a continuum can be identified with relative ease. However, it is the individual somewhere in between that creates the challenge. A decision on normal versus abnormal is often based on an a priori knowledge or assumption regarding a lesion somewhere in the speech-production system. For example, if someone is labelled a 'stutterer', then his or her motor behaviour must be pathological if it is different. Only recently, we have become aware of the circular nature of this approach, and have started to question the validity of this assumption (e.g. van Lieshout *et al.* 1993, 1996*b*). What aspects should we consider in assessing individual differences in speech motor skill?

First, we need to define our domain of inquiry. Traditionally, speech motor skill is not considered to be involved in the conceptualization and formulation of a language code. There is certainly some evidence to suggest an evolutionary relationship between motor factors and language development (Allott 1989; MacNeilage *et al.* 2000) as well as between the emergence of hand and speech gestures in infants (Locke *et al.* 1995), suggesting close ties between motor aspects of speech production and language development. Recent studies also suggest that phonetic (motor) aspects arising in babbling during the acquisition of speech movements may also play a role in the future language development of an individual child (Jakielski 1998). In addition, the preponderance of co-occurring (speech) motor and language delays in children (e.g. Kaplan *et al.* 1998) does suggest that during development these functions share neural resources. This seems in line with recent arguments that a strict separation between language and motor functions in terms of neural networks is an oversimplification (Lieberman 1995; Aboitiz and Garcia 1997; Bates and Dick 2002). Still, for ease of interpretation and discussion, we will assume in the context of this chapter that, at least at a superficial level, we can make a clear difference between speech motor and linguistic functions. (Obviously, to make this a more valid comparison we would also need to incorporate other functions such as cognition, emotion, and attention, but this would be beyond the scope of this chapter.) Whereas linguistic functions are concerned with the semantic and structural properties of the message, the speech motor functions deal with the implementation of this message in terms of enabling, initiating, and executing the required motor tasks. There are different models one could adhere to in order to make a cut-point between these two main functions. In more traditional linguistic models, the cut-point would be at the phonetic encoding stage (cf. Levelt *et al.* 1999). We prefer a somewhat different view in which the speech motor system starts at the level where motor tasks are defined as coordinated actions or gestures (Browman and Goldstein 1997). The gestural specifications determine the location and amount of constriction that needs to take place in order to generate specific changes in the vocal tract that will generate the appropriate aerodynamic conditions for acoustic transmission. In subsequent stages, these specifications are mapped on to specific articulator movements as part of a series of conversion stages, the details of which can be found elsewhere (Saltzman and Kelso 1987; see also Chapter 3, this volume). Linguistic contrasts for sound production arc incorporated at the level of the coordinated actions and, therefore, gestures are phonological in nature (Browman and Goldstein 1991). We also adhere to the notion that inner speech is a subliminal articulation and a product of the speech motor system (e.g. Ackermann *et al.* 1998; Shergill *et al.*, 2001). Inner speech immediately precedes the actual execution of movements and is influenced by the same processes that would influence overt articulation, except for those that are an immediate consequence of biomechanical interactions, which obviously do not happen during inner speech. In practical terms then, any type of experimental task that would involve the covert or overt generation of articulation taps into aspects that relate to speech motor skill. (Obviously, other motor systems as related to phonation and respiration are involved as well, but for practical reasons we will not discuss this aspect here.) This is confirmed by some recent findings which suggest that imagery motor training can be as effective as actual motor training, suggesting a clear link between mental and real manifestations of motor actions (Wilson *et al.* 2002).

In creating this somewhat artificial, but for the purpose of this paper practical, distinction between linguistic and motor functions in speech, we do not claim that both operate independently from each other. Linguistic contrasts will have immediate consequences for the ongoing demands on speech motor skill; for example, in requiring the speaker to change rate or amplitude of movements. Obviously, the challenge will be to define demands on speech motor skill as presented by changes in linguistic contrasts or structure. We think that some of the more recent studies in this area provide some clues as how to tackle this challenge (see Section 13.4).

13.3 Earlier research on speech motor control in people who stutter

In the past 30 years, a number of studies on movement control have shown significant group differences between people who stutter (PWS) and matched control speakers (for reviews, see Alfonso 1991, 1995; van Lieshout 1995; Hulstijn and van Lieshout 1998; Ingham 1998; Peters *et al.* 2000). In studies where group differences were found, the problems concentrate on the timing and coordination of motor events and/or the appropriate scaling of muscle output for a given speech task. Appropriate coordination and scaling of motor actions are an intrinsic part of what we earlier defined as speech motor skill (see Section 13.2). Traditionally, these findings have been interpreted in the perspective of a motor control deficit (e.g. Zimmermann *et al.* 1981). However, the fact that not all stuttering individuals show these differences to the same extent, or at all, has generated some criticism about the tenability of this claim (e.g. Ingham 1998). The basic claim of this type of criticism is that if a motor deficit exists, there should be a common pattern of motor issues for all people who stutter. This, somewhat simplistic notion, ignores the fact that, for many clinically known speech motor disorders, speech motor problems are not identical for every subject for a given disorder, or on all conditions significantly different from matched control subjects (e.g. Forrest and Weismer 1995; Ackermann *et al.* 1997; Adams 1997). The effect of lesions in (sub)cortical brain centres related to motor control on speech movements is a combination of impairment caused by dysfunction and the individual's capability to deal with it under various demands imposed by task and environment. Separating causal effects from compensatory ones is not easy, as we will discuss in more detail in Section 13.4.5.3. Take, for example, the very common finding of a slower motor performance in people who stutter (compared to normal speakers), as demonstrated in a number of studies (for reviews, see van Lieshout 1995; Peters *et al.* 2000). Generally, this is taken as direct evidence for some sort of lesion in the brain. However, as subsequent studies have shown, delays in the timing and executing of movements can also be interpreted as part of a complex compensatory strategy to reduce the demands on the motor task at hand (e.g. van Lieshout *et al.* 1993, 1994, 1996a; Hulstijn and van Lieshout 1998). The latter interpretation is given some weight in light of the fact that slower motor performance is a fairly common characteristic in many patients with a variety of different causes, as observed in speech (e.g. Ackermann *et al.* 1997) and non-speech motor tasks (e.g. Dingwell *et al.* 2000). The latter study highlights the potential strategic component of slowing down in order to provide stability in motor control. For stuttering, the reduced speed has been linked to a less mature control system, with a stronger reliance on the processing of sensory information (van Lieshout *et al.* 1996a; Neilson and Neilson 1987). In other words, to potential differences in speech motor skill.

Earlier studies differed considerably in task requirements, methodology, and subject selection, which makes it hard to compare the results and their impact on identifying motor control problems in PWS (Alfonso 1991). Furthermore, most of these studies have focused on perceptually fluent speech, where the differentiation between limitation or compensation is often hard to make (see Section 13.4.5.3).

It is also important to realize that the motor skill approach entails the concept of individual variability along a continuum for *all* speakers, not just people who stutter. This was confirmed in a recent study by Alfonso and van Lieshout (1997). In the mid-zone of this motor skill continuum people who stutter and so-called normal speakers could be very close, differing only in extremely subtle ways of coping with demands on their speech motor system. For simple tasks, such differences will not occur and they will seem indistinguishable. For more demanding tasks, the differences will show up, provided the task requirements exceed the range of flexibility allowed for by potential compensatory strategies that would otherwise mask them. Similar individual differences can also be observed for children with developmental coordination disorder (e.g. Kaplan *et al.* 1998; Volman and Geuze 1998).

In the next section, we will review a selection of mainly recent studies (published after 1995) that tried to investigate in more detail the nature of the motor response and/or the demands on the motor system in order to clear up some of the ambiguities related to changes in linguistic (and other higher-order) variables. The discussion of these studies will focus on how they can provide support for our 'speech clumsiness' hypothesis in stuttering, regardless of whether they were set up with this purpose in mind.

13.4 What do recent studies tell us about speech motor skills in people who stutter?

13.4.1 General issues

As described in the previous sections, one of the main challenges facing researchers in speech motor control is to expose and identify potential differences in speech motor skill that may exist between PWS and people who do not stutter (PNS). In this chapter, we will focus on the potential motor control limitations that in our view define 'speech clumsiness'. To this end, researchers have focused on conditions that are known to change the severity of an individual's stuttering, in the assumption that whatever makes them stutter more is also putting a greater demand on their speech motor system. The latter obviously has to be demonstrated beyond measuring simply stuttering frequency, to avoid circularity in this type of reasoning. Greater demands on motor skills have to be translated in terms of how changes in task requirements affect the various components that comprise motor skill (see Section 13.2). We have already stated that speech motor skill requires practice and is evident in highly organized (temporal and spatial) movement sequences, performed in an adaptive, cost-effective, and purposeful way. If people who stutter have limited (speech) motor skills, this could show up in the extent and time of practice for a given task, the robustness of the organization/

coordination of movements, the effectiveness to compensate for ongoing changes in demands, and the appropriateness of movements for a given context.

Often, a limitation in motor skill translates as a reduced ability to stabilize motor behaviours for a given task (for an example with children with DCD, see Volman and Geuze 1998). The most likely option then, to find problems in verbal motor skill for PWS, is in identifying factors that (de)stabilize speech motor behaviours. In the past 5–6 years, three main factors have emerged as being critical in this respect. The *first factor* deals with rate of speech (Section 13.4.1), starting from the intuitively simply notion that faster rates make it more difficult for a speaker to maintain stability, especially when he or she has motor skill limitations (cf. Volman and Geuze 1998). The opposite is also thought to be true, namely, that if rate of speech slows down, it becomes easier to maintain or induce stability (cf. Dingwell *et al.* 2000 for a non-speech example). A *second factor* deals with the potential inter-action between higher-order processes related to cognition, language formulation, and speech motor control (Section 13.4.2). The general idea is that an increase in the processing demands for language formulation or other cognitive tasks will tax the capacity for someone with limited speech motor skills to maintain stability (for a discussion of this topic, see also van Lieshout 1998). Finally, as a *third factor*, the role of various forms of feedback in speech production has regained new interest as a potential influence in (de)stabilizing motor control (Section 13.4.3). Each of these three factors will be reviewed in the following subsections, in light of their success in revealing differences in motor skill between inviduals who stutter and matched normal speaking peers. In subsection 13.4.4, we will more specifically address the notion of variability in movement control in PWS. We will review some of the recent studies that have looked into this issue and address the poten-tial and limitations of the concept of movement variability. Subsection 13.4.5 will present a summary and some preliminary conclusions regarding support for our claim on limitations in (speech) motor skills or speech clumsiness in PWS.

13.4.2 Speech rate

13.4.2.1 The effects of increasing rate

The basic idea behind manipulations in speech rate is that faster rates are assumed to make it more difficult for PWS to maintain stability in motor control, and thus precipitate stuttering. A recent study by Ward (1997) indeed showed that for his group of stuttering individuals, faster rates induced more variability in movement coordination in fluent speech production. Extrapolating his results to stuttering, one would then expect more stuttering for faster rates as well. Vanryckeghem and colleagues (Vanryckeghem *et al.* 1999) showed that for their severe PWS subjects, faster rates induced more disfluency. However, for milder PWS, the rate effect was not apparent, suggesting that their speech motor systems are more stable. The latter interpretation would be in line with the motor skill interpretation of stuttering discussed in Section 13.2. Unfortunately, the simple connection between rate and stuttering seems less tenable when we look at the findings of some other studies. For example, a number of studies by Kalinowski and colleagues (e.g. Kalinowski *et al.* 1995; Kalinowski and Stuart 1996) failed to show a clear relationship between rate manipulations and the number of disfluencies for their stuttering subjects. Similarly, a study on lower lip movements did not find support for the claim that PWS as a group are less stable at faster rates than a matched group of control speakers (Smith and Kleinow 2000). Clearly, just making a PWS speak faster does not necessarily lead to an increase in stuttering. In itself, this is not as surprising as it might sound. Faster speaking rates can be realized in many different ways. One can simply reduce pauses between lexical items, make faster movements while reducing the amplitude, increase the overlap between articulatory gestures and thus reduce movement accuracy, or do all these things in some combined fashion (cf. van Lieshout *et al.* 1995; Smith and Kleinow 2000). It is possible that some of these strategies facilitate (rather than impede) movement control. As argued in Hulstijn and van Lieshout (1998), the key issue may not be rate, but rather movement accuracy, or to be more precise, in the way speed and accuracy are balanced in terms of Fitt's law of movement control (Fitts 1954). Support for our claim that a mere increase in movement rate could actually facilitate movement control was found in preliminary data from a study by Namasivayam and Van Lieshout (2001). In this study, the effects of speech rate clearly showed that individual speakers (PWS and controls) became more alike in terms of movement symmetry and movement speed when requested to simply speak faster. One way to interpret this finding is in terms of coordination dynamics (Kelso 1995). According to this theory, the coupling strength between coordinated elements becomes less at faster rates of movement, and the system initially regresses to the most stable and basic pattern of coordination. If pushed further by increasing rate even more, the coupling will eventually become unstable, unless other degrees of freedom can be invoked to re-stabilize the system (cf. Buchanan and Kelso 1999). A tell-tale sign of a system that is on the edge of either switching to a different coupling state or becoming unstable is an increase in the variability of relative phase, a measure of movement coupling (cf. Kelso *et al.* 1986; van Lieshout and Moussa 2000). The data reported by Ward (1997) on higher variability in relative phase at faster speech rates for his group of PWS could indicate such a sign. Speech motor skill very likely relates to the capability to postpone the occurrence of instability as induced by increases in rate. For example, if our experimental designs encourage or permit subjects to 'regress' to use more basic and stable movement patterns or manipulate the degrees of freedom for a given task (e.g. either in terms of different movement directions or reduced contributions for a particular articulator), a prescribed rate increase may not lead to disfluencies. However, if rate is increased beyond the capabilities of a subject to maintain a stable performance, or if additional requirements for accuracy prevent the use of more basic patterns, instability, and most likely disfluency, will occur. Thus, speaking fast and at the same time complying with certain accuracy demands during speech production (in terms of intelligibility) is extremely difficult, and would provide the most demanding context at which different levels of speech motor skill could be differentiated (cf. Hulstijn and van Lieshout 1998). In this respect, it is interesting to look at the results of a study by Kloth *et al.* (1995). They investigated a group of young children (between 23 and 58 months) with a parental history of stuttering, who at their first assessment did not stutter. The only difference they found between those children of this group who did develop stuttering problems as compared to those who did not, was in their rate of articulation, with the former group speaking faster then their peers (for similar results, see also Hall *et al.* 1999). If, indeed, faster speaking rates in these young children restrict the amount of flexibility that is available to the control system—as suggested above—this could be a limiting factor in developing adequate speech control strategies to maintain fluency under increasingly more complex linguistic demands.

A study by Howell *et al.* (1999) adds another interesting dimension to this discussion. They found that local (as opposed to global) rate variations, related to the size of a prosodic unit, correlated well with stuttering frequency. That is, lexical items in longer prosodic units were produced at a relatively faster rate and this paralleled an increase in the number of disfluent items. Their results seem to suggest that it is not so much an overall rate increase, but rather local variations in rate that could be problematic for PWS. Speaking at a normal habitual rate and being forced to make local rate adjustments to accommodate the size of a specific unit of coordination might demand a flexibility in rate control that is not readily available to PWS, if indeed, as we claim, their speech motor skills are more limited. In contrast, global increases in speaking rate might reduce local rate differences and, thus, the associated demands on coordination flexibility (see also subsection 13.4.4). Further evidence suggesting that flexibility in rate control might be an issue for PWS is found in another recent study (McClean and Runyan 2000), in which severely stuttering subjects showed greater speed differences between jaw and other articulators than mildly stuttering subjects and controls for a given speech task. Speed differences between articulators are a potential source for instability in motor control (see, for example, Amazeen *et al.* 1995; Treffner and Turvey 1996; and Chapter 3, this volume).

13.4.2.2 The effects of decreasing rate

What about performing speech tasks at a slower pace? In general, it is expected that this will help PWS to speak more fluently. However, the study by Vanryckeghem *et al.* (1999) did not find a significant reduction in stuttering at slow rates as compared to normal rate. In addition, perceptually fluent speech can be achieved without actually slowing down (e.g. Kalinowski and Stuart 1996; Onslow *et al.* 1996; Natke *et al.*

2001). This is also clear from a study on the physiological effects of different fluency-enhancing conditions (Stager *et al.* 1997). These authors found that the strongest improvements in fluency occurred under conditions in which peak airflow and peak pressure values had decreased. However, speech rate did not vary consistently with changes in fluency. The relevance of controlling air pressure is emphasized in the results from a recent study (Boucher and Lamontagne 2001), where it was found that normal speakers can influence vocal fold vibration via changes in intraoral pressure as they occur during normal and fast rates. In the discussion of their data, the authors state that 'if one considers the negative effects of excessive intraoral pressure on the vocal folds, modifying the behaviour of pressure-building maneuvres may be a more essential goal of therapy than a modification of speaking rate per se' (Boucher and Lamontagne 2001, p. 1012). The reduction in peak pressure values found for the most beneficial fluency-enhancing conditions (Stager *et al.* 1997), speaks to this assumption. It also concurs with the following statement that 'slowing speaking rate may be sufficient to enhance fluency, [but] it does not seem to be a necessary condition' (Story *et al.* 1996, p. 1003). The relationship between rate and intraoral pressures is an important aspect that deserves further study, especially in light of other findings that show deviant patterns of sub-glottal pressure patterns in PWS for both fluent and non-fluent speech (Peters and Boves 1988; Peters *et al.* 1995).

13.4.2.3 Summary

To summarize the data on the effects of speech rate on motor control and fluency, it can be concluded that the two simple assumptions stated at the beginning of the subsection (i.e. faster means less fluent, slower means more fluent) are in need of refinement. Changing global speech rates in either direction may have little direct consequence for fluency and, by implication, for motor control, as long as people have the motor skills to find alternative solutions to maintain stability. If, however, demands for flexibility in speech motor control are increased (in terms of accuracy or local rate variations), possible limitations in motor control skills will surface. The findings on intraoral pressure issues in people who stutter suggest a direct connection between motor control skills and aerodynamic consequences. For example, an increase in rate could lead to a limited flexibility in motor control (as argued in Section 13.4.2.1) and thus reduce the possibility for a speaker to modify peak intraoral pressures, leading to negative consequences for maintaining voicing during speech. Slowing down will only have a beneficial effect on fluency if it allows for a more effective (= flexible) control of aerodynamic processes (cf. Boucher and Lamontagne 2001). This link between rate and aerodynamics also provides a motor skill alternative to the assumption that the assumed effects of speech rate on fluency are related to linguistic planning (cf. Howell *et al.* 1999; Oomen and Postma 2001*b*). In the next subsection, the potential influence of higher-order processes on speech motor control will be discussed in more detail.

13.4.3 Linguistic and cognitive demands

13.4.3.1 Linguistic demands

Although it is well known that PWS may have problems with certain linguistic features of the verbal material they produce (e.g. size of a word or sentence, position of a word in a sentence, frequency of a word) (for reviews, see Karniol 1995; van Lieshout *et al.* 1995), a good explanation of how such linguistic features interfere with motor control is still lacking (van Lieshout 1998). A recent study showed that longer words and words at the beginning of a sentence were associated with higher muscular activity compared with short words and words in other sentence positions (van Lieshout *et al.* 1995). These EMG findings were accompanied by local reductions in vowel durations and interpreted as an increase in articulatory effort. A more recent study reported similar changes in local durations as a function of the size of the linguistic (tone) unit (Howell *et al.* 1999). However, a simple increase in sentence length does not necessarily lead to more effort (van Lieshout *et al.* 1995) or movement instability (Kleinow and Smith 2000). Interestingly, the latter study did show more movement variability for syntactically more complex utterances. Apparently, simply adding (filler) words to a sentence without increasing syntactic complexity may allow a subject to maintain, or even simplify, his coordination patterns by speaking faster but with less accuracy, as discussed in the previous subsection (see also van Lieshout *et al.* 1995). A recent study by Yaruss (1999) investigated the influence of syntactic complexity and sentence length in more detail with stuttering boys aged between 3.3 and 5.5 years. His data suggested that although utterance length was a better predictor for the occurrence of stuttering than syntactic complexity, neither factor could adequately account for the presence of dysfluency. These findings seem to contradict the findings from Kleinow and Smith's study in which movement variability for syntactically more complex utterances was stronger for PWS compared to control speakers (Kleinow and Smith 2000). Obviously, the two studies are hard to compare, as Yaruss reports on children younger than 6 years (Yaruss 1999) and Kleinow and Smith on older subjects. What seems clear is that linguistically more complex sentences require more flexibility in motor control, as indicated by greater movement variability for all speakers (Kleinow and Smith 2000; see also van Lieshout *et al.* 2002). For PWS, these demands on motor skill might form a challenge and thus lead to a more variable performance compared to normal speakers if compensatory strategies are ineffective. It would be interesting to know whether the type of variability shown in both groups of speakers is actually the same, as variability based on flexibility is different than variability based on instability (see Chapter 3, this volume; and Section 13.5.2).

13.4.3.2 Cognitive demands

Current explanations for linguistic effects on motor control are mostly stated in terms of increased motor complexity (linguistically more difficult is motorically more difficult) or, alternatively, in referring to competing demands for shared central processing resources (Oomen and Postma 2001*a*; see also van Lieshout 1998). An interpretation based on shared resource competition would entail that limited speech motor skills require a more controlled mode of movement initiation and execution (van Lieshout 1995). Any task that competes with resources needed to control the speech motor system would potentially interfere with movement stability. Experimentally, this claim can be tested using a dual-task paradigm, based on the assumption that the allocation of processing resources might underlie the disruptive effects of performing two different tasks at the same time (for example, see Brown and Marsden 1991; Dalen 1993).

Recent neuroimaging work shows that activity in brain areas involved in motor control [in particular supplementary motor area (SMA), cingulate cortex, insula, and post-central gyrus] is reduced in the context of a dual-task performance in which attention is shifted away from the primary motor task (Johansen-Berg and Matthews 2002). Others argue for a more direct influence in the way two tasks both involve the same motor areas and thus interfere with each other (Herath *et al.* 2001). The latter interpretation seems plausible in the light of recent findings that PWS show an increase in stuttering frequency in the context of dual-task situations that involve a silent and overt speech task (Bosshardt 1997, 2002). The assumption would be that mental calculation involves silent articulation which recruits the same motor areas as used for the overt speech task. There is indeed support for the assumption that mental calculation includes articulatory loop components (Cowell *et al.* 2000) and that such components show activity in areas that are also involved in overt articulatory motor control (McGuire *et al.* 1996; Ryding *et al.* 1996; Desmond *et al.* 1997; Shergill *et al.* 2001).

How does this all relate to motor skill? Recent studies indicate that the effect of dual-task situations and its potential to distract from the main task at hand, will have different consequences for those with higher or lower levels of motor skill. People with lower skills benefit from attention and thus may show a performance degradation in dual-task paradigms, whereas skilled people under such circumstances may actually do better because their performance is more automated (Beilock *et al.* 2002). If the same situation applies to speech motor skill, the increase in stuttering under dual-task situations could indeed suggest a lower skill level for PWS, whereas normal speakers are not affected in terms of speech disfluency (Bosshardt 2002), suggesting higher speech motor skill levels.

Obviously, the effects of dual-task situations on speech requires further study. Alternative explanations need to be investigated. For example, a dual-task situation requiring simultaneous speaking and mental calculation may involve some kind of supervisory or executive type of control (cf. Schumacher *et al.* 2001), suggesting a cognitive-based source for interference. Others have suggested that a very specific type of dual-task situation (Stroop Color Word task) induces cognitive stress that underlies the increase in stuttering frequency (Caruso *et al.* 1994). Interestingly, from recent studies in motor control, cognitive stress is associated with increased attention or consciousness in control, leading to reduced flexibility and affecting skilled performers negatively (Higuchi 2000). However, as argued above, increased attention should benefit unskilled performers, and if this applied to PWS for speech motor tasks, they should stutter less, not more, under cognitive stress. Some support for the latter assumption was found in a study by Peters and colleagues (Peters *et al.* 1989), who found that PWS stuttered less under high time-stress as compared to lower time-stress conditions. Obviously, time-stress does not equal cognitive stress, but it seems reasonable to assume that forcing people to respond very quickly using feedback and frequent reminders does introduce a certain level of cognitive stress.

13.4.3.3 Summary

This global review of some recent findings on linguistic and cognitive factors in stuttering emphasizes that we need to be able to identify the mechanisms by which these higher-order influences actually impact on motor control (see also Chapter 10, this volume). Based on the recent findings in this area, there is some evidence to support our assumption that if PWS have limitations in speech motor skill, linguistic features that require flexibility in motor control and cognitive demands that draw away attention from motor control might destabilize movement patterns in these individuals. It is also clear that the relationship between (types of) stress, attention, and motor skill in speech production needs more study, as some recent studies on the effects of cognitive stress on limb control provides an interesting challenge to the traditional assumption that (like the situation for normal speakers) stress causes people who stutter to become more disfluent.

13.4.4 Feedback

The potential role of feedback in speech production is a complex issue (for general reviews of the role of different sources of feedback, see Hood, 1998; Barlow *et al.* 1999; Postma, 2000). For PWS, feedback (or problems in the use of it) as a factor in explaining their speech problems focuses on two types: auditory and kinaesthetic feedback (for a review of earlier studies, see van Lieshout 1995). These and other factors will be discussed in more detail in the following subsections.

13.4.4.1 Auditory feedback

With respect to auditory feedback, it has been known for a long time that changing its temporal characteristics may have a beneficial effect on stuttering (e.g. Van Riper 1970; Webster *et al.* 1970). Inspired by the pioneering work of Peter Howell and colleagues in this area (e.g. Howell 1983, 1990), others have looked in more detail at the effects of delayed auditory feedback (DAF) and frequency altered feedback (FAF) on stuttering. The findings suggest that the general fluency-enhancing effect of DAF/FAF occurs regardless of speech rate (e.g. Kalinowski *et al.*

1993; Hargrave *et al.* 1994; Kalinowski and Stuart 1996; Stuart *et al.* 1997), although the effect appears to be task and subject specific (Armson and Stuart 1998; Ingham *et al.* 1997). A recent study found the clinical effects for DAF stronger compared to those of FAF (Natke 2000).

What can explain the influence of a change in auditory feedback on the fluency of speech (both for normal speakers and PWS, but in opposite directions)? Findings reported by Stager *et al.* (1997) indicated that fluency enhancement for delayed auditory feedback (and other fluency enhancement techniques) might relate to changes in peak respiratory flow and pressures. However, the authors could not clarify why peak flow and pressure changed under these conditions. One possible explanation is offered in a recent study by Jones and Munhall (2000), who found that (subconscious) changes in auditory feedback were closely followed by (equally subconscious) compensations in voice production. In other words, changes in auditory feedback affect motor production in an almost online fashion. The air pressure and flow changes observed by Stager and colleagues (Stager *et al.* 1997) under DAF might results from such motor adaptations. The potential relationship between auditory feedback and phonation (and its relevance for stuttering) is detailed in the 'audio-phonatory coupling' theory by Kalveram (1993). This theory claims that auditory feedback modulates phonation duration in a reflex-like manner. This coupling is high for stressed syllables, but for unstressed syllables children have to learn to inhibit this coupling, making the control of phonation in non-stressed syllables more feedforward. For PWS, the theory assumes that the inhibition phase for non-stressed syllables is 'misguided' (in terms of the authors) during development, which basically refers to a motor skill learning issue. This means that the auditory-phonatory coupling remains strong for all syllables, which leads to temporal inaccuracies in the control of phonation and, by assumption, to disfluencies (Kalveram and Natke 1997). Problems in the processing of auditory feedback have been mentioned before as a possible source for stuttering (e.g. Stromsta 1972; Timmons and Boudreau 1972; Harrington 1988; but see Postma and Kolk 1992). It finds a close analogue in the assumption of feedback processing problems in children with developmental coordination disorder or clumsiness (Laszlo and Sainsbury 1993; see Section 13.1).

13.4.4.2 Visual feedback

Is fluency enhancement restricted to changes in auditory feedback only? Not necessarily. A recent study showed that visual gestures of speech, which mimic a situation of unison speaking, also induced fluency (Kalinowski *et al.* 2000). This could suggest a common basis to the type of information that is conveyed to the receiver in both visual speech gestures and acoustic signals. For example, both visual and auditory information is structured by the motor actions that generate it (Dekle *et al.* 1992; Fowler 1996; Hogden *et al.* 1996) and, especially the latter, could underlie the capability to shadow speech at very short latencies (Porter and Lubker

1980). More recently, this issue was raised in a paper by Pihan and colleagues (Pihan *et al.* 2000), who stated that 'shadowing studies suggest that perceived speech is rapidly represented by neural networks, which provide an interpretation of the acoustic structure in terms of a motor program' (p. 2348). If such information is available to PWS, this might provide them with temporal and/or spatial cues regarding their own articulation and thus explain the fluency enhancement effect of shadowing speech (e.g. Healey and Howe 1987).

13.4.4.3 Kinaesthetic feedback and proprioception

The other type of feedback that has received some attention with respect to speech motor control in normal speakers and PWS is movement related and includes kinaesthesia and proprioception (De Nil and Abbs 1991*a*, *b*; Loucks and De Nil 2001). Although both terms have been used as if interchangeable, it seems appropriate to maintain a distinction. Proprioception encompasses various sensory systems that encode movement information which is relayed to specific neural networks, whereas kinaesthesia has to do with how that basis sensory information is perceived and used in motor control (for a detailed discussion of concepts of sensation, specification, and perception, see Stoffregen and Bardy 2001). The idea that PWS may have problems with the processing of sensory information is not new (e.g. Zimmermann *et al.* 1981; Neilson and Neilson 1991). Recent work that addresses this issue shows that when PWS are asked to make a minimal movement under visual and non-visual conditions, PWS make larger minimal movements than their normally speaking counterparts under a non-visual feedback condition (De Nil *et al.* 1991*a*; Howell *et al.* 1995; Archibald and De Nil 1999; Loucks and De Nil 2001). It remains unclear whether this reflects a limited sensory–motor integration process or a reduced signal-to-noise ratio in their neural pathways. Support for the latter interpretation was found in the spectral analysis of force data in a study that compared PWS and matched control speakers in visual and non-visual conditions while they tried to maintain specified force levels (Grosjean *et al.* 1997). Problems in the use of kinaesthetic feedback has also been suggested to characterize children with developmental coordination disorder (Laszlo and Sainsbury 1993), emphasizing the intimate relationship between motor control and sensory information during development. Recent studies on adult speakers have provided some evidence that people who stutter may show a stronger reliance on kinaesthetic feedback compared to normal speakers (van Lieshout *et al.* 1993, 1996*a*, *b*). The latter would suggest that feedback processing is not necessarily disturbed, but that PWS are showing immature (as in less skilful) motor control strategies.

13.4.4.4 Probing the use of feedback

One powerful way to study the use of feedback in speech is to employ perturbation paradigms. In this set-up, an articulator is either immobilized using a biteblock (e.g. Folkins and Zimmermann 1981; Fowler and Turvey 1981; Baum *et al.* 1996) or perturbed by applying a temporary subconscious mechanical load during ongoing movements (e.g. Folkins and Zimmermann 1982; Kelso *et al.* 1984; Shaiman and Gracco 2002). The latter type of perturbation is also known as dynamic perturbation, whereas the first paradigm can be referred to as static perturbation. What is known about PWS under such conditions?

One early study on the effects of dynamic perturbation in PWS showed that compared to matched controls they had longer latencies and reduced upper lip EMG amplitudes, suggesting a less than adequate compensation (Caruso *et al.* 1987). However, a more recent study failed to replicate significant group findings in compensation responses to mechanical loads applied to the jaw (Bauer *et al.* 1997). Regarding static perturbations, preliminary data from the lab of the first author (Namasivayam and van Lieshout 2001) showed that PWS are able to compensate for the biteblock effect, but their response patterns showed a greater global physiological effort in both lips, compared to a more specific dominant response in the lower lip only for control speakers. This tendency for a global, less refined, response to the perturbation seems similar to the more primitive movement patterns found in young children for lip closing during early stages of speech motor development (see Chapter 10, this volume) and, in our view, are indicative for what we call 'speech clumsiness' (see also Hulstijn and van Lieshout 1998).

13.4.4.5 *Summary*

This general overview of some recent studies on the use of various forms of feedback in speech production does suggest that PWS are different from controls. The data do not seem to point to a clinically significant disorder, but rather to a differential task performance that seems indicative of a difference in motor skill, as reflected in less refined and more basic movement patterns for PWS (even for non-speech fine-motor tasks). Another dimension that needs to be added in this respect is variability in movement control. If PWS have indeed a limited speech motor skill, we could expect to see more variability in movement patterns under more demanding conditions, similar to that shown for young children during early stages of speech motor development (for a review, see Chapter 10, this volume). This issue will be addressed next.

13.4.5 Variability

13.4.5.1 *General issues*

Variability in speech motor performance has always been a hot topic in research with PWS (for a discussion see, for example, Alfonso 1991). Some recent studies suggest that with respect to movement coordination (Ward 1997) and syllable timing (Boutsen *et al.* 2000) PWS are more variable than matched controls. One could assume that such variability underlies the presence of stuttering, but the findings of a study by Wieneke and colleagues (Wieneke *et al.* 2001) showed no difference in segment durational variability in fluent and non-fluent utterances of their group of PWS. More in line with our speech clumsiness perspective are the findings from recent studies by Anne Smith and colleagues. They showed that greater movement variability might not be a general characteristic of PWS (Smith and Kleinow 2000), *unless* specific demands on the motor system are increased, such as using syntactically more complex utterances (Kleinow and Smith 2000; for other studies in this area see Chapter 10, this volume).

One of the issues with respect to variability is the notion that it is something that should be avoided, and in a 'normal' system is minimal or even absent. So, when Caruso *et al.* (1988) reported a consistent sequencing of lips and jaw for their control subjects and much more variability in their group of PWS, this was taken as evidence for an impairment in movement sequencing. However, as later studies have shown, articulatory sequencing is not as consistent in control speakers as originally thought (e.g. De Nil 1995) and is closely related to the absolute relative timing between lips and jaw: the closer events are in time, the less critical the actual sequence seems to be (van Lieshout *et al.* 1994; Alfonso and van Lieshout 1997).

13.4.5.2 Variability versus flexibility

In evaluating variability in movement patterns, one needs to address the critical balance between sufficient flexibility to perform a difficult task versus avoiding too much variability that would impede achieving the task's goals. Variability in lower lip movement patterns seems the norm in younger children while performing speech tasks, and this variability gradually improves with age, which is generally interpreted as an index of motor skill maturation (Chapter 10, this volume). Of course, variability in one articulator does not mean that it would impede normal speech. For example, a recent study on children with a repaired upper cleft lip showed that although the upper lip showed smaller and more variable movements than the lower lip for this group of speakers compared to controls, coordination of lips was not affected (van Lieshout *et al.* 2002). These children achieved their speech goals despite the physical limitations in their upper lip movements, emphasizing the fact that speech is about coordination and not about single articulator movements. The same study also showed that for linguistically more complex utterances, variability in movement patterns increased for all speakers, similar to the findings reported by Smith and colleagues (see Chapter 10, this volume, for a review of their findings). That is, variability as such can be part of a normal speech motor system displaying an element of flexibility to accommodate fast-changing demands on the speed and accuracy of individual movements and their couplings (van Lieshout *et al.* 1997*a*; Hulstijn and van Lieshout 1998). An overly stable (= rigid) movement pattern would rather impede than facilitate speech motor control under such conditions. On the other hand, in performing highly automatic simple movement patterns, for example repeating the word 'apa' continuously at the same rate, would not require much movement flexibility and might actually benefit from a absolute stable pattern. The importance of differentiating between absolute (or rigid) coordination and relative (or flexible) coordination is addressed most notably in the work by Scott Kelso and his colleagues, who were inspired by the work of Nikolai Aleksandrovitsj Bernstein (1896–1966) and Eric von Holst (1908–1962), among others (see Kelso 1995 for an excellent discussion of this topic and Chapter 3, this volume).

13.4.5.3 Adaptation versus limitation

So, where does this leave us regarding variability in PWS? As mentioned in Section 13.4.5.1, variability in the behaviours of PWS has always been pushed as a hall-mark characteristic of the disorder. The problem is that the link between variabil-ity or the lack of variability has not been demonstrated to relate directly to the occurrence of disfluency. We know that non-fluent passages or word productions can be associated with movement or acoustic variability, but this only demon-strates that if the speech motor system of PWS is in a non-fluent mode, things do not happen as regularly as they (seem to) do normally (cf. Wieneke *et al.* 2001). That is not surprising. What we need to address is the issue of how to differentiate between adaptation effects and direct manifestations of underlying mechanisms related to stuttering.

So, how can we distinguish between adaptation effects and direct manifestations of potential motor skill limitations? Adaptation and plasticity are frequently used concepts, but a good methodology to differentiate their effects from the direct unmediated effects of the limitation itself is still lacking. A *first solution* would be to prevent the adaptation, either by instruction or certain experimental methods, and observe if the disorder, for instance the amount of stuttering, will manifest itself more clearly. One suggested method to achieve this is to push the subjects near to, or even over, their limits (van Lieshout 1995; Hulstijn and Peters 2001). However, this strat-egy poses two major obstacles. One is that the adaptation might have been trained and used for such a long period of time that it has become a habit that cannot easily be eliminated by simple instruction or experimental manipulation. Secondly, not all acquired adaptations might be beneficial. Superstitious learning might lead to adap-tations that are non-beneficial or even lead to a decrement in performance. The sole aim of many therapies is to remove these extra unwanted negative or non-beneficial behaviours, while the core of the disorder is left untouched.

A *second solution* to assess whether a motor phenomenon is the result of adapta-tion would be to investigate its relation with the movement errors under study. In the case of stuttering, one option is to study its relation with the amount of dysfluency. Most of the speech motor research on stuttering is performed on perceptually fluent speech. What would happen if we study our motor phenom-enon, i.e. the amount and direction of articulatory sequencing difference, in non-fluent speech? We could get three types of results. First, we might observe exactly the same timing pattern in both fluent and in non-fluent utterances. If that were the case, we could conclude that this timing event might be a secondary symptom that accompanies stuttering but is not instrumental in the production of the symptoms of stuttering. On the other hand, if we observe a timing pattern in dysfluent speech that is more like that of the control speakers, we could infer that the person who stuttered has not been able to use his 'normal' adaptation procedure which usually prevents him or her from stuttering, which, in turn, would imply that our motor phenomenon signals adaptation rather than disorder. If, by contrast, we observe that in non-fluent utterances the difference between stutterers and control speakers becomes larger, then we can conclude that our phenomenon is not an adaptation mechanism, but that it bears a direct relation with speech motor skill limitations. This simple research strategy has seldom been pursued, and we think it warrants serious reconsideration. It can also be refined by studying individual moment-by-moment changes in movement or coordination parameters before, during, and after a stutter event. Thus, we would gain more insight in the dynamic nature of control mechanisms underlying fluent and dysfluent speech production. An example of this can be seen in Fig. 13.1, which displays tongue body and lip closing gestures for a person who stutters while saying the non-word /tipa/. These data were collected with an electro-magnetic midsagittal articulograph or EMMA system (AG100, van Lieshout and Moussa 2000).

Figure 13.1 shows the acoustic signal (Audio; top graph displays its wideband spectrogram), the movements of tongue tip (TT; actually, the coil is positioned 1 cm behind the tongue tip and, anatomically, this position refers to tongue blade movements, but functionally it parallels movements of the tongue tip), tongue body (TB) and bilabial closure (BC = lips + jaw), with arrows indicating the specific movement targets for a fluent token of /tipa/. During the interval demarcated '1' the speaker experiences a short block, followed by an almost normal realization of the target item. Subsequent, in interval 2 a sustained block occurred, followed by a release and a transition into interval 3 where fluent speech execution is no longer achieved. Notice the clear increase in movement cycle durations during interval 3, which could be either an attempt to regain fluency or a consequence of a series of interruptions similar to those shown in interval 1. Both for the short block at interval 1 and the long block at interval 2, the interruption occurs right at the end of the closing movement for the tongue tip (i.e. past and not at the phoneme boundary). The interesting other issue that can be observed is that the TB target position for the /i/ vowel, relative to the TT target position for /t/ closure, is reached much earlier in both cases, compared to the fluent tokens. Further comparisons with fluent speech tokens from normal speakers would allow us to differentiate these phenomena in terms of adaptation versus limitation signs, as discussed above. For the fluent portion (< interval 1) of this trial, both gestures showed two spectral components in their movement signals, referred to as motion primitives (see Chapter 3, this volume for more details on the concept of motion primitives). The stronger or dominant motion

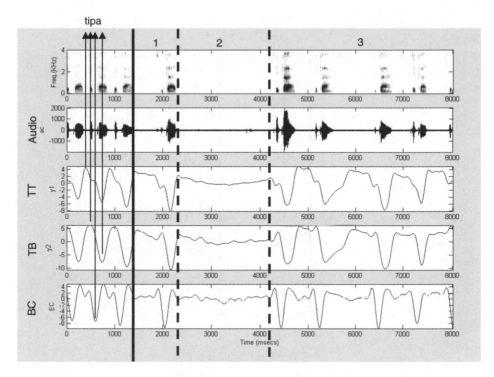

Fig. 13.1 Example of EMMA speech movement data for a person who stutters while repeating the non-word /tipa/: the actual movements for tongue tip (TT), tongue body (TB), and bilabial closing gestures, as well as the acoustic signal (Audio) and spectrogram.

primitive was at 2 Hz (Figure 13.2(A)) and the second primitive was at 4 Hz (Figure 13.2(B)). In Figure 13.2, Panels (A) and (B) show the coupling (expressed in relative phase, labelled 'Phi' in both panels) between both gestures for each primitive and their amplitudes (see 'Amp'). The amplitude for the dominant primitive (A) decreases just before the onset of the block in interval 1 and remains low after that. The second primitive shows a more varied pattern with alterations in amplitude at various moments during the trial. Fluctuations in the coupling (see Phi in (B)) between both gestures are clearly evident for the second primitive in interval 1. Low-amplitude values are associated with instabilities in relative phase for the long block (interval 2) as is evident for both primitives. Notice how, in interval 3, the second primitive sometimes regains stability at points of larger amplitude, which is not seen for the dominant primitive (it should be noted that for the calculation of relative phase, signals are amplitude normalized and changes in relative phase are not a measurement artefact caused by amplitude variations of the signals as displayed in (A) and (B)). Hence, both primitives clearly behave independently from

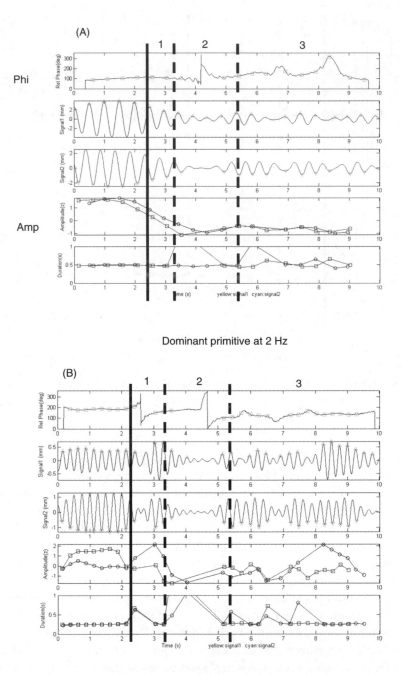

Dominant primitive at 2 Hz

Second primitive at 4 Hz

Fig. 13.2 Panels A and B show the relative phase (Phi) and amplitude (Amp) data for the extracted motion primitives at 2 and 4 Hz. See text for more details.

each other in both nature and stability of their coupling throughout the trial. Given the preliminary nature of these data, we do not want to speculate about possible distal causal relationships, but it is clear that an immediate proximal cause for the stuttering events is a destabilization of the coupling between the two gestures, which, in turn, seems to be related to a reduction in amplitude for the underlying motion primitives. Only when both primitives appear to be strong in amplitude, are stability in coupling present and speech fluent (see events before interval 1, Figure 13.1).

This example shows that factors that might induce a destabilizing influence, may act in a very non-linear way. When amplitude decreases to a certain (likely idio-syncratic) threshold, the system responds with a clear, dramatic change in behaviour. The mechanisms behind these changes in stability are not entirely clear, but it is claimed that kinaesthetic signals are coupled to a neural oscillator in order to stabilize the output signals for a given effector system, and smaller movement amplitudes reduce the feedback gain and thus the coupling strength between the neural oscillator and effector (cf. Peper and Beek 1998; Fink *et al.* 2000a; Kelso *et al.* 2001; van Lieshout *et al.* 2002). This type of coupling has been implemented in robotics, where, indeed, a reduction in feedback below a certain threshold destabi-lized the coupling between the robot arm and its controller network. Interestingly, the destabilization resulted in a sudden block of the arm movement during an ongoing task (Williamson 1998). Surely, the sudden block of a robot arm and the sudden block of an ongoing tongue gesture in a PWS is not the same thing, but the similarity in underlying mechanism (amplitude drop) and resulting behaviour is compelling. This example stresses the importance of feedback in motor coordination from a non-linear dynamical systems point of view (see Chapter 3, this volume) and in our view provides a potential source for the motor skill limitations in PWS.

A *third solution* to potentially differentiate between adaptation and limitation is to assess the effect of fluency enhancing or reducing methods on the motor phenom-enon under study (e.g. Stager *et al.* 1997). For example, if we believe that some measure of variability, like spatiotemporal index (STI) (Chapter 10, this volume) or the standard deviation of the continuous measurement of relative phase (Hulstijn and van Lieshout 1998; van Lieshout and Moussa 2000; Chapter 3, this volume), is a direct reflection of a coordination disorder, then this can be tested by investigat-ing changes in these measures under a stuttering reducing condition (e.g. see Zmarich *et al.* 2001).

13.4.6 Summary

This global review of recent studies on speech motor control in speakers who do and no not stutter illustrates that PWS do have limitations in their speech motor skills. In particular, there is evidence from various sources discussed in this section that they lack a certain ability to optimize the use of proprioceptive information in specific task conditions, and that local variations in speech rate and increased demands on linguistic/cognitive processing may interfere with smooth movement execution. We think these findings mirror a combination of limited (speech) motor skills and related compensatory strategies (see also van Lieshout 1995; Hulstijn and van Lieshout 1998). What is currently lacking is a better understanding of the mechanisms involved in stabilizing or destabilizing a speech motor system and whether these could explain how fluent speech actually becomes disfluent, as illustrated in our example (Section 13.4.5.3). In the final part of this chapter, we will briefly discuss other issues that need to be addressed in future research in this area.

13.5. Where do we go from here?

This question is not an easy one to answer. Depending on one's perspective on the nature and cause(s) of stuttering, different answers will come up. Obviously, stuttering as a clinical manifestation is more than just a (potential) problem in speech motor skills. Many other factors come into play as a result of being faced with limitations in expressing oneself in a fluent and (for outsiders) acceptable manner. Just imagine the frustration of a child who lacks the skills to play tennis (or any other motor task), but none the less is forced (due to circumstances and/or environment) to be on the tennis court every day and perform under high demands for years and years. This is an unlikely scenario for this child playing tennis (at least we hope so), but it is reality for someone who stutters. No doubt, for many of these children mental concepts and behavioural patterns will emerge that potentially can create all sorts of problems in self-esteem, emotional and physical well-being (Stein *et al.* 1996; Blood *et al.* 1997; Mahr and Torosian, 1999). These are the kind of problems clinicians often face in addition to the speech issues (Menzies *et al.* 1999), and this is very similar for other developmental problems, including developmental coordination disorder (e.g. Cantell *et al.* 1994). We also recognize that other factors, such as potential weaknesses in linguistic processing, may play a role in childhood stuttering (see Chapter 11, this volume), as they do in many developmental 'disorders' (Bishop 1990; see Section 13.1). However, our focus will be on speech motor control and the potential issues that accompany people who stutter in dealing with speaking (and other motor) tasks, because we believe this research has not met its final destination (cf. Ingham 1998). So, what do we think needs to be done?

13.5.1 Key variables in motor control

First of all, we need to define the key variables that will allow us to probe into mechanisms of motor control and how they relate to activities in the central and peripheral nervous system. One example of a potential key variable, namely movement amplitude in motion primitives, was mentioned in our example above. If we can identify these key variables and the mechanisms by which they lead the oral motor control system through different optimal (flexible yet stable) and non-optimal (rigid or highly variable) solutions, we can address the issues of potential causation and remediation in stuttering, and, possibly, other speech disorders (e.g. van Lieshout *et al.* 2002; Chapter 3, this volume). To access the normal extent of flexibility in these behaviours, it is important to measure them at different points in time for the same subject (Alfonso and van Lieshout 1997; van Lieshout and Moussa 2000), and to identify such behaviours at an individual basis as opposed to comparing group data (Vicente and Torenvliet 2001). Although the mechanisms are very likely to be of a general nature, individuals may differ in the thresholds that determine ranges of flexibility and stability, with PWS being at the lower end of this continuum. For speech, this aspect has hardly been addressed, and we need studies in which such key variables are systematically varied along a continuum, while controlling for other factors such as linguistic context. The latter aspect can also be exploited to study the interactions between linguistic and motor processing in more detail (see Chapter 10, this volume; van Lieshout *et al.* 1999).

Another important issue that needs to be addressed is how subjects can recruit additional degrees of freedom to stabilize the execution of motor patterns in the context of new or increasing demands (e.g. Buchanan *et al.* 1997; Fink *et al.* 2000*b*). In speech, research data on this issue do not exist and it is entirely possible that speech motor skills in PWS are characterized by a lack of flexibility to recruit additional degrees of freedom to stabilize the coordination between articulatory structures during speech production.

13.5.2 What kind of behaviours do we need to study?

What sort of behaviours do we need to measure in order to be able to identify these key variables? Preferably, they should be as close as possible to the actual control system, in this case, the oral motor system. Although *stuttering counts* do serve a meaningful purpose, certainly in clinical settings, they carry little specific information about the underlying motor control mechanisms (van Lieshout 1995). *Reaction time* studies have a similar problem. They can help to identify certain conditions that require extra processing (or execution) time, but the source of these variations can be difficult to pinpoint and may differ from one model to another (van Lieshout *et al.* 1996*b*). Although some believe that speech research should focus primarily on *acoustic measures* (Weismer and Liss 1991), these only indirectly relate to the motor events that gave rise to them in the first place. Besides, there can be a lot of relevant articulation going on even if there is no sound. For example, prolonged vowel durations could be based on longer movement durations, larger movements, segregated movements (multiple peaks in velocity profile), or a simple prolonged static position in the oral tract. The same acoustic signature could relate to different tongue positions, and different acoustic signatures might relate to the same tongue position (Maurer *et al.* 1993). Finally, in the acoustic but especially *perceptual analysis* of speech errors and disfluencies, meaningful motor events are often hard (if not impossible) to identify, leading to misguided conclusions about their nature and origin (e.g. Mowrey and MacKay 1990; Kent 1996).

Aerodynamic measures (pressure, flow, airway resistance) also have an indirect relationship to the actual motor events that generated them, but with some clever experimental design, and in particular in combining these measures with motor events in respiration, phonation, and articulation, they potentially could provide insight in some of the underlying mechanisms that may be involved in stuttering (e.g. Peters and Boves 1988; Stager *et al.*, 1997; Boucher and Lamontagne 2001). *Multi-dimensional measurements* will, more than ever, be of great importance to quantify and qualify the relationships between motor events happening at the various levels of speech production (Ludlow 1991; Peters *et al.* 2000; van Lieshout *et al.* 1997*b*) in order to detect relationships between these events and the way they interact with the communicative environment. A very nice example of the latter issue was demonstrated in a recent study (McFarland 2001), showing that the kinematic respiratory signals of conversational partners were strongly coupled, which bears a close resemblance to distant couplings in limb control studies (e.g. Schmidt *et al.* 1990; Treffner 1999) and dyadic conversation (e.g. Buder 1996).

If we focus on actual *motor behaviours* (kinematics, muscle activity), one of the first challenges to tackle is the issue of passive versus active control. Some of the motor events we measure may have less to do with actual nervous system involvement, and reflect the biomechanical interactions between coupled systems. For example, recent studies by Ostry and colleagues have provided evidence that biomechanical influences on jaw movements underlie changes in movement parameters that are traditionally attributed to co-articulation planning strategies (Ostry *et al.* 1996). Interactions between control signals and structural dynamics need to be taken into account in modelling the behaviours of tongue, jaw, and other structures involved in speech and other oral tasks (e.g. Laboissiere *et al.* 1996; Sanguineti *et al.* 1998). Such models will help us to understand how the nervous system is able to exploit these dynamics in maximizing the chances of achieving the task's goal and, at the same time, minimizing the physical effort needed to accomplish this.

13.5.3 Stuttering in a broader context

Developmental stuttering, as already indicated in Section 13.1, has interesting parallels to developmental coordination disorder or DCD. However, this is not the only interesting comparison that can be made, and we think that broadening the scope towards other speech 'disorders' is an important and necessary step for motor control research in stuttering (e.g. Molt 1999).

In the literature to date, some have speculated that stuttering is a form of focal action *dystonia* (Kiziltan and Akalin 1996). Action dystonia is associated with abnormal cortical motor excitability (Ikoma *et al.* 1996), which could be related to abnormal outputs from the extrapyramidal motor system, in particular the basal ganglia and thalamic structures (e.g. Berardelli *et al.* 1998; Artieda *et al.* 2001) and affect speech functions, in particular respiration and phonation (e.g. Braun *et al.* 1995; Lagueny *et al.* 1995). The role of the basal ganglia in dystonia, in particular as related to dopaminergic dysfunction (e.g. Madhusudanan 1999), is interesting in the light of recent claims that stuttering involves an overactive dopamine system in brain regions that are involved in speech production (Wu *et al.* 1997). In terms of treatment, abnormal motor activity in focal dystonia is often suppressed with botulinum toxin (e.g. Giladi 1997). Similarly, in comparing stuttering to spasmodic dysphonia (a form of local dystonia), some have tried to treat stuttering with laryngeal injections of botulinum toxin (Brin *et al.* 1994; see also Ludlow 1990 for an overview of the use of botulinum toxin in the treatment of speech and voice disorders). However, as indicated by Smith *et al.* (1996), excessive laryngeal EMG activity might not be a major or consistent problem for PWS, thus questioning the benefit of botulinum toxin treatment for stuttering.

Following the idea that stuttering might involve a disturbed functioning of the extrapyramidal system, it has been claimed that, in terms of its pathogenesis, it is related to Tourette's syndrome (Abwender *et al.* 1998). However, a recent study suggests that in terms of speech problems, Tourette's syndrome may be more similar to cluttering than to stuttering (Van Borsel and Vanryckeghem 2000). Others have claimed that stuttering is definitely not a variant form of Tourette's syndrome (Pauls *et al.* 1993) and a recent (yet unpublished) study indicated that for a relatively large group of patients with Tourette's syndrome, stuttering (when appropriately defined) was not a major issue (De Nil *et al.* unpublished).

A very different type of speech disorder that has been compared to stuttering is verbal apraxia (Rosenbek 1980; Byrd and Cooper 1989). It is interesting to notice that some authors have labelled developmental coordination disorder with the term apraxia or dyspraxia (for a review of this topic, see Henderson and Barnett 1998). In light of claims that stuttering involves a speech motor planning deficit (e.g. Peters *et al.* 1989; Salmelin *et al.* 2000; but see van Lieshout *et al.* 1996*b*, *c*), one would expect a clear relationship between stuttering and verbal apraxia, since the latter disorder is also assumed to be related to verbal motor planning difficulties (e.g. Clark and Robin 1998; McNeil *et al.* 1997). However, studies in this area are scarce and, although it has been reported that stuttering children were very similar on all subtests of the Blakely Screening Test for Developmental Apraxia of Speech (STDAS) to children with developmental apraxia (Byrd *et al.* 1989), this does not provide evidence that there is a underlying connection in terms of some shared (patho)neurophysiology. In fact, the kind of errors that dominate the speech of children with verbal apraxia—speech errors, in particular with respect to place of articulation (e.g. Maassen *et al.* 1997)—are not found to be a major distinguishing factor in children who stutter (e.g. Wolk *et al.* 1993; Melnick and Conture 2000) or adults (Postma and Kolk 1990). It is possible that there may be some complex relationship between phonological errors and stuttering (Postma and Kolk 1993;

LaSalle and Conture 1995, 1997; Wolk *et al.* 2000) or that phonological disturb-ances co-occur with stuttering (Wolk *et al.* 1993; Louko 1995; Yaruss and Conture 1996), but the evidence for limited phonological abilities as a direct source for disfluency is not yet compelling (Paden and Yairi 1996; Burger and Wijnen 1999; but see Chapter 11, this volume for a different view). The whole issue is further complicated by a potential confounding between perceptually/acoustically catego-rized phonological speech errors and (more differentiated) speech motor-based disfluencies (Mowrey and MacKay 1990), as already indicated in the previous subsection and illustrated in the example data shown in Fig. 13.1.

In sum, at this point, comparing stuttering to other speech problems with similar or different involvement of certain brain areas requires further study, as the topic is barely scratched in the current literature. We do see parallels, but there are also clear differences that need to be accounted for. Studying and comparing the behav-ioural aspects of these individuals and the influence of the key variables on stabil-ity in motor control (Section 13.5.1) will tell us more about the possible idiosyn-cratic relationships between causal mechanisms (shared or not) and behavioural consequences, both in terms of limitations and adaptations (see Section 13.4.5.3).

13.6 Summary and some conclusions

This chapter focused intentionally and specifically on speech motor skills in people who stutter. Other factors are important and need to be considered (see various chapters in this volume), but first and foremost we believe that stuttering needs to be approached from the point of view that a person who stutters knows what to say, could even say it, if (part of) the motor system did not block during the (other-wise correct) movements (see Chapter 11, this volume, for a linguistic take on this). The evidence provided in this chapter is not yet conclusive or complete, but we do think that it supports our claim that the weaker link in individuals who stutter is to deal with (oral) fine-motor tasks, in particular speech, in the skilful manner as defined in the first section of this chapter. Their motor behaviours tend to be less effective, more variable, and more basic, perhaps even 'immature', in their handling of the complex coordination between individual articulators. Speech motor skill is not a dichotomy but a continuum, and individuals can be traced along the entire continuum, there being some extremely good and bad speakers, as well a 'grey zone' where 'normal' and stuttering individuals could be fairly close in their performance and responses to demands. In this sense, we hesi-tate to call stuttering (yet) a disorder, since the label 'disorder' implies we have a good and complete understanding of what is normal in speech production. We do not. Similar problems exist for other areas, for example in the diagnosis of devel-opmental coordination disorder (Henderson and Barnett 1998). For now, we prefer the term 'speech clumsiness' to indicate their limitation in speech motor skills, as this is less absolute and does not need to imply a structural deficit. It is even possible that for adult PWS the actual 'cause' for their problems has dissipated, but the remaining behaviours are inefficient in promoting fluent speech as part of early compensatory strategies that were created in response to an early problem during development (van Lieshout 1995; see Chapter 11, this volume for a similar line of reasoning but regarding linguistic variables). Speech motor research in stuttering and in general will have to be informed by other approaches, some of which are presented in this volume, in order to keep an open perspective and to recognize the fact that for a truly complex system such as the human brain, nothing happens in isolation (Freeman *et al.* 2001). We started this chapter with a quote from Van Riper, and we will end it with a paraphrase of his statement to reflect our current understanding of stuttering:

> Stuttering is a complex communication problem whose core consists of idiosyncratic limitations in speech motor skill as evidenced in more vari- able, less effective and more basic movement patterns in dealing with high demands for movement accurary and speed required for speech.

References

Abbs, J. H. and **Gracco, V. L.** (1984). Control of complex motor gestures: orofacial muscle responses to load perturbations of lip during speech. *Journal of Neurophysiology*, 51, 705–723.

Aboitiz, F. and **Garcia, R.** (1997). The evolutionary origin of the language areas in the human brain. A neuroanatomical perspective. *Brain Research Reviews*, 25, 381–396.

Abwender, D. A., Trinidad, K. S., Jones, K. R., Como, P. G., Hymes, E., and **Kurlan, R.** (1998). Features resembling Tourette's syndrome in developmental stutterers. *Brain and Language*, 62, 455–464.

Ackermann, H., Hertrich, I., Daum, I., Scharf, G., and **Spieker, S.** (1997). Kinematic analysis of articulatory movements in central motor disorders. *Movement Disorders*, 12, 1019–1027.

Ackermann, H., Wildgruber, D., Daum, I., and **Grodd, W.** (1998). Does the cere- bellum contribute to cognitive aspects of speech production? A functional magnetic resonance imaging (fMRI) study in humans. *Neuroscience Letters*, 247, 187–190.

Adams, M. R. (1995). The demands and capacities model I: theoretical Elaborations. *Journal of Fluency Disorders*, 15, 135–141.

Adams, S. G. (1997). Hypokinetic dysarthria in Parkinson's disease. In M. R. McNeil (Ed.), *Clinical management of sensorimotor speech disorders* (pp. 261–285). New York: Thieme.

Alfonso, P. J. (1991). Implications of the concepts underlying task-dynamic modeling on kinematic studies of stuttering. In H. F. Peters, W. Hulstijn, and C. W.

Starkweather (Eds), *Speech motor control and stuttering* (pp. 79–100). Amsterdam: Elseviers Publishers.

Alfonso, P. J. (1995). Respiratory function in stutterers. In F. Bell-Berti and L. J. Raphael (Eds), *Producing speech: contemporary issues* (pp. 199–213). New York: AIP Press.

Alfonso, P. J. and **van Lieshout, P.** (1997). Spatial and temporal variability in obstru-ent gestural specification by stutterers and controls: Comparisons across sessions. In W. Hulstijn, H. F. Peters, and P. H. H. M. van Lieshout (Eds), *Speech production: motor control, brain research and fluency disorders* (pp. 151–160). Amsterdam: Elsevier Publishers.

Allott, R. (1989). *Motor theory of language origin.* Lewes, UK: Book Guild.

Amazeen, P. G., Schmidt, R. C., and **Turvey, M. T.** (1995). Frequency detuning of the phase entrainment dynamics of visually coupled rhythmic movements. *Biological Cybernetics,* 72, 511–518.

Archibald, L. and **De Nil, L. F.** (1999). The relationship between stuttering severity and kinesthetic acuity for jaw and lip movements in adults stutterers. *Journal of Fluency Disorders,* 24, 25–42.

Armson, J. and **Stuart, A.** (1998). Effect of extended exposure to frequency-altered feedback on stuttering during reading and monologue. *Journal of Speech Language and Hearing Research,* 41, 479–490.

Artieda, J., Garcia De Casasola, M. C., Pastor, M. A., Alegre, M., and **Urriza, J.** (2001). [The pathophysiological basis of dystonia]. *Revista de Neurologia* 32, 549–558.

Barlow, S. M., Farley, G. R., and **Andreatta, R. D.** (1999). Neural systems in speech physiology. In S. M. Barlow (Ed.), *Handbook of clinical speech physiology* (pp. 101–163). San Diego, CA: Singular Publishing Group, Inc.

Barnett, A. L., Kooistra, L., and **Henderson, S. E.** (1998). 'Clumsiness' as syndrome and symptom. *Human Movement Science,* 17, 435–444.

Bates, E. and **Dick, F.** (2002). Language, gesture, and the developing brain. *Developmental Psychobiology,* 40, 293–310.

Bauer, A., Jaencke, L., and **Kalveram, K. T.** (1997). Mechanical perturbation of the jaw during speech in stutterers and nonstutterers. In W.Hulstijn, H. F. M. Peters, and P. H. H. M. van Lieshout (Eds), *Speech production: motor control, brain research and fluency disorders* (pp. 191–196). Amsterdam: Elsevier Science Publishers.

Baum, S. R., McFarland, D. H., and **Diab, M.** (1996). Compensation to articulatory perturbation: perceptual data. *Journal of the Acoustical Society of America,* 99, 3791–3794.

Beilock, S. L., Carr, T. H., MacMahon, C., and **Starkes, J. L.** (2002). When paying attention becomes counterproductive: impact of divided versus skill-focused atten-tion on novice and experienced performance of sensorimotor skills. *Journal of Experimental Psychology: Applied,* 8, 6–16.

Berardelli, A., Rothwell, J. C., Hallett, M., Thompson, P. D., Manfredi, M., and **Marsden, C. D.** (1998). The pathophysiology of primary dystonia. *Brain,* 121 (Pt 7), 1195–1212.

Bishop, D. V. M. (1990). Handedness, clumsiness and developmental language disorders. *Neuropsychologia*, 28, 681–690.

Blood, I. M., Wertz, H., Blood, G. W., Bennett, S., and **Simpson, K. C.** (1997). The effects of life stressors and daily stressors on stuttering. *Journal of Speech Language and Hearing Research*, 40, 134–143.

Bosshardt, H. G. (1997). Speech fluency under dual-task conditions. *Journal of Fluency Disorders*, 22, 113.

Bosshardt, H. G. (2002). Effects of concurrent cognitive processing on the fluency of word repetition: comparison between persons who do and do not stutter. *Journal of Fluency Disorders*, 27, 93–114.

Boucher, V. and **Lamontagne, M.** (2001). Effects of speaking rate on the control of vocal fold vibration: clinical implications of active and passive aspects of devoicing. *Journal of Speech Language and Hearing Research*, 44, 1005–1014.

Boutsen, F. R., Brutten, G. J., and **Watts, C. R.** (2000). Timing and intensity variability in the metronomic speech of stuttering and nonstuttering speakers. *Journal of Speech Language and Hearing Research*, 43, 513–520.

Braun, N., Abd, A., Baer, J., Blitzer, A., Stewart, C., and **Brin, M.** (1995). Dyspnea in dystonia. A functional evaluation. *Chest*, 107, 1309–1316.

Brin, M. F., Stewart, C., Blitzer, A., and **Diamond, B.** (1994). Laryngeal botulinum toxin injections for disabling stuttering in adults. *Neurology*, 44, 2262–2266.

Browman, C. P. and **Goldstein, L.** (1991). Gestural structures: distinctiveness, phonological processes, and historical change. In I. G. Mattingly and M. Studdert-Kennedy (Eds), *Modularity and the motor theory of speech perception* (pp. 313–338). Hillsdale: Lawrence Erlbaum Associates.

Browman, C. P. and **Goldstein, L. M.** (1997). The Gestural Phonology Model. In W.Hulstijn, H. F. M. Peters, and P. H. H. M. van Lieshout (Eds), *Speech production: motor control, brain research, and fluency disorders* (pp. 57–71). Amsterdam: Elsevier Science Publishers.

Brown, R. G. and **Marsden, C. D.** (1991). Dual task performance and processing resources in normal subjects and patients with Parkinson's disease. *Brain*, 114 (Pt 1A), 215–231.

Buchanan, J. J. and **Kelso, J. A.** (1999). To switch or not to switch: recruitment of degrees of freedom stabilizes biological coordination. *Journal of Motor Behavior*, 31, 126–144.

Buchanan, J. J., Kelso, J. A. S., deGuzman, G. C., and **Ding, M.** (1997). The spontaneous recruitment and suppression of degrees of freedom in rhythmic hand movements. *Human Movement Science*, 16, 1–32.

Buder, E. H. (1996). Dynamics of speech processes in dyadic interaction. In J.H.Watt and C. A. Vanlear (Eds), *Dynamic patterns in communication processes* (pp. 301–325). Thousand Oaks, CA: Sage.

Burger, R. and **Wijnen, F.** (1999). Phonological encoding and word stress in stuttering and nonstuttering subjects. *Journal of Fluency Disorders*, 24, 91–106.

Byrd, K. and **Cooper, E. B.** (1989). Apraxic speech characteristics in stuttering, developmentally apraxic, and normal speaking children. *Journal of Fluency Disorders*, 14, 215–229.

Cantell, M. H., Smyth, M. M., and **Ahonen, T. P.** (1994). Clumsiness in adolescence—educational, motor, and social outcomes of motor delay detected at 5-years. *Adapted Physical Activity Quarterly*, 11, 115–129.

Caruso, A. J., Gracco, V. L., and **Abbs, J. H.** (1987). A speech motor control perspective on stuttering: preliminary observations. In H. F. M.Peters and W. Hulstijn (Eds), *Speech motor dynamics in stuttering* (pp. 245–258). Vienna: Springer-Verlag.

Caruso, A. J., Abbs, J. H., and **Gracco, V. L.** (1988). Kinematic analysis of multiple movement coordination during speech in stutterers. *Brain*, 111 (Pt 2), 439–456.

Caruso, A. J., Chodzko-Zajko, W. J., Bidinger, D. A., and **Sommers, R. K.** (1994). Adults who stutter: responses to cognitive stress. *Journal of Speech Language and Hearing Research*, 37, 746–754.

Clark, H. M. and **Robin, D. A.** (1998). Generalized motor programme and parameterization accuracy in apraxia of speech and conduction aphasia. *Aphasiology*, 12, 699–713.

Cowell, S. F., Egan, G. F., Code, C., Harasty, J., and **Watson, J. D.** (2000). The functional neuroanatomy of simple calculation and number repetition: a parametric PET activation study. *Neuroimage*, 12, 565–573.

Dalen, K. (1993). Hemispheric asymmetry and dual-task performance in children: a finger-tapping study. *International Journal of Neuroscience*, 69, 85–95.

Dekle, D. J., Fowler, C. A., and **Funnell, M. G.** (1992). Audiovisual integration in perception of real words. *Perceptual Psychophysiology*, 51, 355–362.

De Nil, L. F. (1995). The influence of phonetic context on temporal sequencing of upper lip, lower lip and jaw peak velocity and movement onset during bilabial consonants in stuttering and nonstuttering adults. *Journal of Fluency Disorders*, 20, 127–144.

De Nil, L. F. and **Abbs, J. H.** (1991a). Kinaesthetic acuity of stutterers and non-stutterers for oral and non-oral movements. *Brain*, 114 (Pt 5), 2145–2158.

De Nil, L. F. and **Abbs, J. H.** (1991b). Oral and finger kinesthetic thresholds in stutterers. In H. F. M. Peters, W. Hulstijn, and C. W. Starkweather (Eds), *Speech motor control and stuttering* (pp. 123–130). Amsterdam: Elsevier Science Publishers.

Desmond, J. E., Gabrieli, J. D., Wagner, A. D., Ginier, B. L., and **Glover, G. H.** (1997). Lobular patterns of cerebellar activation in verbal working-memory and finger-tapping tasks as revealed by functional MRI. *Journal of Neuroscience*, 17, 9675–9685.

Dingwell, J. B., Cusumano, J. P., Sternad, D., and **Cavanagh, P. R.** (2000). Slower speeds in patients with diabetic neuropathy lead to improved local dynamic stability of continuous overground walking. *Journal of Biomechanics*, 33, 1269–1277.

Fink, P. W., Foo, P., Jirsa, V. K., and **Kelso, J. A.** (2000a). Local and global stabilization of coordination by sensory information. *Experimental Brain Research* 134, 9–20.

Fink, P. W., Kelso, J. A. S., Jirsa, V. K., and **de Guzman, G. C.** (2000*b*). Recruitment of degrees of freedom stabilizes coordination. *Journal of Experimental Psychology: Human Perception and Performance*, 26, 671–692.

Fitts, P. M. (1954). The information capacity of the human motor system in controlling the amplitude of movement. *Journal of Experimental Psychology*, 47, 381–391.

Folkins, J. W. and **Zimmermann, G. N.** (1981). Jaw-muscle activity during speech with the mandible fixed. *Journal of the Acoustical Society of America*, 69, 1441–1445.

Folkins, J. W. and **Zimmermann, G. N.** (1982). Lip and jaw interaction during speech: responses to perturbation of lower-lip movement prior to bilabial closure. *Journal of the Acoustical Society of America*, 71, 1225–1233.

Forrest, K. and **Weismer, G.** (1995). Dynamic aspects of lower lip movement in parkinsonian and neurologically normal geriatric speakers' production of stress. *Journal of Speech and Hearing Research*, 38, 260–272.

Fowler, C. A. (1996). Listeners do hear sounds, not tongues. *Journal of the Acoustical Society of America*, 99, 1730–1741.

Fowler, C. A. and **Turvey, M. T.** (1981). Immediate compensation in bite-block speech. *Phonetica*, 37, 306–326.

Freeman, W. J., Kozma, R., and **Werbos, P. J.** (2001). Biocomplexity: adaptive behavior in complex stochastic dynamical systems. *Biosystems*, 59, 109–123.

Giladi, N. (1997). The mechanism of action of botulinum toxin type A in focal dystonia is most probably through its dual effect on efferent (motor) and afferent pathways at the injected site. *Journal of Neurological Science*, 152, 132–135.

Goffman, L. and **Smith, A.** (1999). Development and phonetic differentiation of speech movement patterns. *Journal of Experimental Psychology: Human Perception and Performance*, 25, 649–660.

Gracco, V. L. (1997). A neuromotor perspective on speech production. In W.Hulstijn, H. F. M. Peters, and P. H. H. M. van Lieshout (Eds), *Speech production: motor control, brain research and fluency disorders* (pp. 37–56). Amsterdam: Elsevier Science Publishers.

Green, J. R., Moore, C. A., Higashikawa, M., and **Steeve, R. W.** (2000). The physiologic development of speech motor control: Lip and jaw coordination. *Journal of Speech Language and Hearing Research*, 43, 239–255.

Green, J. R., Moore, C. A., and **Reilly, K. J.** (2002). The sequential development of jaw and lip control for speech. *Journal of Speech Language and Hearing Research*, 45, 66–79.

Grosjean, M., Van Galen, G. P., de Jong, W. P., van Lieshout, P. H. H. M., and **Hulstijn, W.** (1997). Is stuttering caused by failing neuromuscular force control? In W. Hulstijn, H. F. M. Peters, and P. H. H. M. van Lieshout (Eds), *Speech production: motor control, brain research and fluency disorders* (pp. 197–204). Amsterdam, The Netherlands: Elsevier Science Publishers.

Guenther, F. H. (1994). A neural network model of speech acquisition and motor equivalent speech production. *Biological Cybernetics*, 72, 43–53.

Guthrie, E. R. (1952). *The psychology of learning*. New York: Harper and Row.

Hall, K. D., Amir, O., and **Yairi, E.** (1999). A longitudinal investigation of speaking rate in preschool children who stutter. *Journal of Speech Language and Hearing Research*, 42, 1367–1377.

Hargrave, S., Kalinowski, J., Stuart, A., Armson, J., and **Jones, K.** (1994). Effect of frequency-altered feedback on stuttering frequency at normal and fast speech rates. *Journal of Speech and Hearing Research*, 37, 1313–1319.

Harrington, J. (1988). Stuttering, delayed auditory feedback, and linguistic rhythm. *Journal of Speech and Hearing Research*, 31, 36–47.

Healey, E. C. and **Howe, S. W.** (1987). Speech shadowing characteristics of stutterers under diotic and dichotic conditions. *Journal of Communication Disorders*, 20, 493–506.

Henderson, S. E. and **Barnett, A. L.** (1998). The classification of specific motor coordination disorders in children: some problems to be solved (Reprinted from Perspectives on the classification of specific developmental disorders). *Human Movement Science*, 17, 449–469.

Herath, P., Klingberg, T., Young, J., Amunts, K., and **Roland, P.** (2001). Neural correlates of dual task interference can be dissociated from those of divided attention: an fMRI study. *Cerebral Cortex*, 11, 796–805.

Higuchi, T. (2000). Disruption of kinematic coordination in throwing under stress. *Japanese Psychological Research*, 42, 168–177.

Hogden, J., Lofqvist, A., Gracco, V., Zlokarnik, I., Rubin, P., and **Saltzman, E.** (1996). Accurate recovery of articulator positions from acoustics: new conclusions based on human data. *Journal of the Acoustical Society of America*, 100, 1819–1834.

Hood, L. J. (1998). An overview of neural function and feedback control in human communication. *Journal of Communication Disorders*, 31, 461–469.

Howell, P. (1983). The effect of delaying auditory feedback of selected components of the speech signal. *Perceptual Psychophysiology*, 34, 387–396.

Howell, P. (1990). Changes in voice level caused by several forms of altered feedback in fluent speakers and stutterers. *Language and Speech*, 33 (Pt 4), 325–338.

Howell, P., Sackin, S., and **Rustin, L.** (1995). Comparison of speech motor development in stutterers and fluent speakers between 7 and 12 years old. *Journal of Fluency Disorders*, 20(3), 243–255.

Howell, P., Au-Yeung, J., and **Pilgrim, L.** (1999). Utterance rate and linguistic properties as determinants of lexical dysfluencies in children who stutter. *Journal of the Acoustical Society of America*, 105, 481–490.

Hulstijn, W. and **Peters, H. F. M.** (2001). Stuttering: A disorder of motor control? In B. A. M. Maassen, W. Hulstijn, R. D. Kent, H. F. M. Peters, and P. H. H. M. van Lieshout (Eds), *Speech motor control in normal and disordered speech* (pp. 316–321). Nijmegen: Vantilt.

Hulstijn, W. and van Lieshout, P. H. H. M. (1998). A motor skill approach to stuttering. In W.Ziegler and K. Deger (Eds), *Clinical phonetics and linguistics* (pp. 391–404). London, UK: Whurr Publishers.

Ikoma, K., Samii, A., Mercuri, B., Wassermann, E. M., and Hallett, M. (1996). Abnormal cortical motor excitability in dystonia. *Neurology*, 46, 1371–1376.

Ingham, R. J. (1998). On learning from speech-motor control research on stuttering. In A. K.Cordes and R. J. Ingham (Eds), *Treatment efficacy for stuttering: a search for empirical bases* (pp. 67–101). San Diego: Singular Publishing Group.

Ingham, R. J., Moglia, R. A., Frank, P., Ingham, J. C., and Cordes, A. K. (1997). Experimental investigation of the effects of frequency-altered auditory feedback on the speech of adults who stutter. *Journal of Speech Language and Hearing Research*, 40, 361–372.

Jakielski, K. (1998). *Motor organization in the acquisition of consonant clusters*. Ph.D thesis, Ann Arbor, MI.

Johansen-Berg, H. and Matthews, M. (2002). Attention to movement modulates activity in sensori-motor areas, including primary motor cortex. *Experimental Brain Research*, 142, 13–24.

Jones, J. A. and Munhall, K. G. (2000). Perceptual calibration of F0 production: evidence from feedback perturbation. *Journal of the Acoustical Society of America*, 108, 1246–1251.

Kalinowski, J. and Stuart, A. (1996). Stuttering amelioration at various auditory feedback delays and speech rates. *European Journal of Disorders of Communication*, 31, 259–269.

Kalinowski, J., Armson, J., Roland-Mieszkowski, M., Stuart, A., and Gracco, V. L. (1993). Effects of alterations in auditory feedback and speech rate on stuttering frequency. *Language and Speech*, 36 (Pt 1), 1–16.

Kalinowski, J., Armson, J., and Stuart, A. (1995). Effect of normal and fast articulatory rates on stuttering frequency. *Journal of Fluency Disorders*, 20, 293–302.

Kalinowski, J., Stuart, A., Rastatter, M. P., Snyder, G., and Dayalu, V. (2000). Inducement of fluent speech in persons who stutter via visual choral speech. *Neuroscience Letters*, 281, 198–200.

Kalveram, K. T. (1993). A neural-network model enabling sensorimotor learning: application to the control of arm movements and some implications for speech-motor control and stuttering. *Psychological Research* 55, 299–314.

Kalveram, K. T. and Natke, U. (1997). Stuttering and misguided learning of articulation and phonation, or why it is extremely difficult to measure the physical properties of limbs. In W. Hulstijn, H. F. M. Peters, and P. H. H. M. van Lieshout (Eds), *Speech production: motor control, brain research and fluency disorders* (pp. 89–98). Amsterdam: Elsevier Science Publishers.

Kaplan, B. J., Wilson, B. N., Dewey, D., and Crawford, S. G. (1998). DCD may not be a discrete disorder. *Human Movement Science*, 17, 471–490.

Karniol, R. (1995). Stuttering, language, and cognition: a review and a model of stuttering as suprasegmental sentence plan alignment (SPA). *Psychological Bulletin*, 117, 104–124.

Kelso, J. A. S. (1995). *Dynamic patterns. The self-organization of brain and behavior.* Cambridge, MA: A Bradford Book (MIT Press).

Kelso, J. A., Tuller, B., Vatikiotis-Bateson, E., and **Fowler, C. A.** (1984). Functionally specific articulatory cooperation following jaw perturbations during speech: evidence for coordinative structures. *Journal of Experimental Psychology: Human Perception and Performance*, 10, 812–832.

Kelso, J. A. S., Saltzman, E., and **Tuller, B.** (1986). The dynamical theory in speech production: Data and theory. *Journal of Phonetics*, 14, 29–60.

Kelso, J. A., Fink, P. W., DeLaplain, C. R., and **Carson, R. G.** (2001). Haptic information stabilizes and destabilizes coordination dynamics. *Proceedings of the Royal Society of London B, Biological Sciences*, 268, 1207–1213.

Kent, R. D. (1996). Hearing and believing: some limits to the auditory–perceptual assessment of speech and voice disorders. *American Journal of Speech–Language Pathology*, 5, 7–23.

Kiziltan, G. and **Akalin, M. A.** (1996). Stuttering may be a type of action dystonia. *Movement Disorders*, 11, 278–282.

Kleinow, J. and **Smith, A.** (2000). Influences of length and syntactic complexity on the speech motor stability of the fluent speech of adults who stutter. *Journal of Speech Language and Hearing Research*, 43, 548–559.

Kloth, S. A. M., Janssen, P., Kraaimaat, F. W., and **Brutten, G. J.** (1995). Speech-motor and linguistic skills of young stutterers prior to onset. *Journal of Fluency Disorders. Special Issue: Festschrift to Gene J. Brutten*, 20(2), 157–170.

Laboissiere, R., Ostry, D. J., and **Feldman, A. G.** (1996). The control of multi-muscle systems: human jaw and hyoid movements. *Biological Cybernetics*, 74, 373–384.

Lagueny, A., Burbaud, P., Le Masson, G., Bergouignan, F. X., Ferrer, X., and **Julien, J.** (1995). Involvement of respiratory muscles in adult-onset dystonia: a clinical and electrophysiological study. *Movement Disorders*, 10, 708–713.

LaSalle, L. R. and **Conture, E. G.** (1995). Disfluency clusters of children who stutter—relation of stutterings to self-repairs. *Science*, 38, 965–977.

Laszlo, J. I. and **Sainsbury, K. M.** (1993). Perceptual–motor development and prevention of clumsiness. *Psychological Research–Psychologische Forschung*, 55, 167–174.

Levelt, W. J., Roelofs, A., and **Meyer, A. S.** (1999). A theory of lexical access in speech production. Behavioral and Brain Sciences, 22, 1–38.

Lieberman, P. (1995). Manual versus speech motor control and the evolution of language. *Behavioral and Brain Sciences*, 18, 197–198.

Lindblom, B. (1990). Explaining phonetic variation: a sketch of the H&H theory. In W. Hardcastle and A. Marchal (Eds), *Speech production and speech modelling* (pp. 403–439). Amsterdam: Kluwer Academic Publishers.

Locke, J. L., Bekken, K. E., McMinn-Larson, L., and **Wein, D.** (1995). Emergent control of manual and vocal-motor activity in relation to the development of speech. *Brain and Language*, 51, 498–508.

Logan, K. J. and **Conture, E. G.** (1997). Selected temporal, grammatical, and phonological characteristics of conversational utterances produced by children who stutter. *Journal of Speech Language and Hearing Research*, 40, 107–120.

Loucks, T. M. and **De Nil, L. F.** (2001). Oral kinesthetic deficit in stuttering evaluated by movement accuracy and tendon vibration. In B. Maassen, W. Hulstijn, R. D. Kent, H. F. M. Peters, and P. H. H. M. van Lieshout (Eds.), *Speech motor control in normal and disordered speech* (pp. 307–310). Nijmegen, The Netherlands: Uitgeverij Vantilt.

Louko, L. J. (1995). Phonological characteristics of young-children who stutter. *Topics in Language Disorders*, 15, 48–59.

Ludlow, C. L. (1990). Treatment of speech and voice disorders with botulinum toxin. *Journal of the American Medical Association*, 264, 2671–2675.

Ludlow, C. L. (1991). Measurement of speech motor control processes in stuttering. In H. F. M Peters, W. Hulstijn, and C. W. Starkweather (Eds), *Speech motor control and stuttering* (pp. 479–491). Amsterdam, The Netherlands: Elsevier Science Publishers.

Maassen, B., Thoonen, G., and **Boers, I.** (1997). Quantitative assessment of dysarthria and developmental apraxia of speech. In W. Hulstijn, H. F. M. Peters, and P. H. H. M. van Lieshout (Eds), *Speech production: motor control, brain research and fluency disorders* (pp. 611–619). Amsterdam: Elsevier Science Publishers.

MacNeilage, P. F., Davis, B. L., Kinney, A., and **Matyear, C. L.** (2000). The motor core of speech: a comparison of serial organization patterns in infants and languages. *Child Development*, 71, 153–163.

Madhusudanan, M. (1999). Dystonia : emerging concepts in pathophysiology. *Neurology India*, 47, 263–267.

Mahr, G. C. and **Torosian, T.** (1999). Anxiety and social phobia in stuttering. *Journal of Fluency Disorders*, 24, 119–126.

Maner, K. J., Smith, A., and **Grayson, L.** (2000). Influences of utterance length and complexity on speech motor performance in children and adults. *Journal of Speech Language and Hearing Research*, 43, 560–573.

Maurer, D., Grone, B. F., Landis, T., Hoch, G., and **Schonle, P. W.** (1993). Re-examination of the relation between the vocal tract and the vowel sound with electromagnetic articulography (EMA) in vocalization. *Clinical Linguistics and Phonetics*, 7, 129–143.

McClean, M. D. and **Runyan, C. M.** (2000). Variations in the relative speeds of orofacial structures with stuttering severity. *Journal of Speech Language and Hearing Research*, 43, 1524–1531.

McFarland, D. H. (2001). Respiratory markers of conversational interaction. *Journal of Speech Language and Hearing Research*, 44, 128–143.

McGuire, P. K., Silbersweig, D. A., Murray, R. M., David, A. S., Frackowiak, R. S. J., and Frith, C. D. (1996). Functional anatomy of inner speech and auditory verbal imagery. *Psychological Medicine*, 26, 29–38.

McNeil, M. R., Robin, D. A., and Schmidt, R. A. (1997). Apraxia of speech: Definition, differentiation, and treatment. In M. R. McNeil (Ed.), *Clinical management of sensorimotor speech disorders* (pp. 311–344). New York, USA: Thieme.

Melnick, K. S. and Conture, K. G. (2000). Relationship of length and grammatical complexity to the systematic and nonsystematic speech errors and stuttering of children who stutter. *Journal of Fluency Disorders*, 25, 21–45.

Menzies, R. G., Onslow, M., and Packman, A. (1999). Anxiety and stuttering: exploring a complex relationship. *American Journal of Speech–Language Pathology*, 8, 3–10.

Molt, L. (1999). *The Basal Ganglia's possible role in stuttering: an examination of similarities between stuttering, Tourette Syndrome, Dystonia, and other neurological-based disorders of movement*. International Stuttering Awareness Day Internet Conference, 1–22 October 1999 .

Mowrey, R. A. and MacKay, I. R. (1990). Phonological primitives: electromyographic speech error evidence. *Journal of the Acoustical Society of America*, 88, 1299–1312.

Namasivayam, A. K. & van Lieshout, P. H. H. M. (2001). Compensation and adaptation to static perturbations in people who stutter. In B. Maassen, W. Hulstijn, R. D. Kent, H. F. M. Peters, and P. H. H. M. van Lieshout (Eds), *Speech motor control in normal and disordered speech* (pp. 253–257). Nijmegen, The Netherlands: Uitgeverij Vantilt.

Natke, U. (2000). [Reduction of stuttering frequency using frequency-shifted and delayed auditory feedback]. *Folia Phoniatrica Logopedica*, 52, 151–159.

Natke, U., Grosser, J., and Kalveram, K. T. (2001). Fluency, fundamental frequency, and speech rate under frequency-shifted auditory feedback in stuttering and nonstuttering persons. *Journal of Fluency Disorders*, 26, 227–241.

Neilson, M. D. and Neilson, P. D. (1987). Speech Motor Control and Stuttering— A Computational Model of Adaptive Sensory–Motor Processing. *Speech Communication*, 6, 325–333.

Neilson, M. D. and Neilson, P. D. (1991). Adaptive model theory of speech motor control and stuttering. In H. F. M. Peters, W. Hulstijn, and C. W. Starkweather (Eds), *Speech motor control and stuttering* (pp. 149–156). Amsterdam: Elsevier Science Publishers.

Onslow, M., Costa, L., Andrews, C., Harrison, E., and Packman, A. (1996). Speech outcomes of a prolonged-speech treatment for stuttering. *Science*, 39, 734–749.

Oomen, C. C. E. and Postma, A. (2001a). Effects of divided attention on the production of filled pauses and repetitions. *Journal of Speech Language and Hearing Research*, 44, 997–1004.

Oomen, C. C. E. and Postma, A. (2001b). Effects of time pressure on mechanisms of speech production and self-monitoring. *Journal of Psycholinguistic Research*, 30, 163–184.

Ostry, D. J., Gribble, P. L., and Gracco, V. L. (1996). Coarticulation of jaw movements in speech production: is context sensitivity in speech kinematics centrally planned? *Journal of Neuroscience*, 16, 1570–1579.

Paden, E. P. and Yairi, E. (1996). Phonological characteristics of children whose stuttering persisted or recovered. *Science*, 39, 981–990.

Pauls, D. L., Leckman, J. F., and Cohen, D. J. (1993). Familial relationship between Gilles de la Tourette's syndrome, attention deficit disorder, learning disabilities, speech disorders, and stuttering. *Journal of the American Academy of Child and Adolescent Psychiatry*, 32, 1044–1050.

Peper, C. E. and Beek, P. J. (1998). Distinguishing between the effects of frequency and amplitude on interlimb coupling in tapping a 2:3 polyrhythm. *Experimental Brain Research*, 118, 78–92.

Peters, H. F. M. and Boves, L. (1988). Coordination of aerodynamic and phonatory processes in fluent speech utterances of stutterers. *Science*, 31, 352–361.

Peters, H. F., Hulstijn, W., and Starkweather, C. W. (1989). Acoustic and physiological reaction times of stutterers and nonstutterers. *Journal of Speech and Hearing Research*, 32, 668–680.

Peters, H. F. M., Hietkamp, R., and Boves, L. (1995). Aerodynamic and phonatory processes in disfluent speech utterances in stutterers. In C. W. Starkweather and H. F. M. Peters (Eds), (pp. 76–81). Nijmegen, The Netherlands: The International Fluency Association, University Press Nijmegen.

Peters, H. F., Hulstijn, W., and van Lieshout, P. H. (2000). Recent developments in speech motor research into stuttering. *Folia Phoniatrica et Logopedica*, 52, 103–119.

Pihan, H., Altenmuller, E., Hertrich, I., and Ackermann, H. (2000). Cortical activation patterns of affective speech processing depend on concurrent demands on the subvocal rehearsal system. A DC-potential study. *Brain*, 123 (Pt 11), 2338–2349.

Porter, R. J. Jr and Lubker, J. F. (1980). Rapid reproduction of vowel-vowel sequences: evidence for a fast and direct acoustic–motoric linkage in speech. *Journal of Speech and Hearing Research*, 23, 593–602.

Postma, A. (2000). Detection of errors during speech production: a review of speech monitoring models. *Cognition*, 77, 97–132.

Postma, A. and Kolk, H. (1990). Speech errors, disfluencies, and self-repairs of stutterers in two accuracy conditions. *Journal of Fluency Disorders*, 15, 291–303.

Postma, A. and Kolk, H. (1992). Error monitoring in people who stutter: evidence against auditory feedback defect theories. *Journal of Speech and Hearing Research*, 35, 1024–1032.

Postma, A. and Kolk, H. (1993). The covert repair hypothesis: prearticulatory repair processes in normal and stuttered disfluencies. *Journal of Speech and Hearing Research*, 36, 472–487.

Rosenbek, J. (1980). Apraxia of speech–relationship to stuttering. *Journal of Fluency Disorders*, 5, 233–253.

Ryding, E., Bradvik, B., and **Ingvar, D. H.** (1996). Silent speech activates prefrontal cortical regions asymmetrically, as well as speech-related areas in the dominant hemisphere. *Brain and Language*, 52, 435–451.

Salmelin, R., Schnitzler, A., Schmitz, F., and **Freund, H. J.** (2000). Single word reading in developmental stutterers and fluent speakers. *Brain*, 123 (Pt 6), 1184–1202.

Saltzman, E. and **Kelso, J. A.** (1987). Skilled actions: a task-dynamic approach. *Psychological Review*, 94, 84–106.

Saltzman, E., Lofqvist, A., Kay, B., Kinsella-Shaw, J., and **Rubin, P.** (1998). Dynamics of intergestural timing: a perturbation study of lip–larynx coordination. *Experimental Brain Research*, 123, 412–424.

Sanguineti, V., Laboissiere, R., and **Ostry, D. J.** (1998). A dynamic biomechanical model for neural control of speech production. *Journal of the Acoustical Society of America*, 103, 1615–1627.

Schmidt, R. A. (1988). *Motor control and learning: a behavioral emphasis*. Champaign, IL: Human Kinetics.

Schmidt, R. C., Carello, C., and **Turvey, M. T.** (1990). Phase transitions and critical fluctuations in the visual coordination of rhythmic movements between people. *Journal of Experimental Psychology: Human Perception and Performance*, 16, 227–247.

Schumacher, E. H., Seymour, T. L., Glass, J. M., Fencsik, D. E., Lauber, E. J., Kieras, D. E. *et al.* (2001). Virtually perfect time sharing in dual-task performance: uncorking the central cognitive bottleneck. *Psychological Science*, 12, 101–108.

Shaiman, S. and **Gracco, V. L.** (2002). Task-specific sensorimotor interactions in speech production. *Experimental Brain Research*, 146, 411–418.

Shergill, S. S., Bullmore, E. T., Brammer, M. J., Williams, S. C., Murray, R. M., and **McGuire, P. K.** (2001). A functional study of auditory verbal imagery. *Psychological Medicine*, 31, 241–253.

Smith, A. (1992). The control of orofacial movements in speech. *Critical Reviews in Oral Biology and Medicine*, 3, 233–267.

Smith, A. and **Goffman, L.** (1998). Stability and patterning of speech movement sequences in children and adults. *Journal of Speech Language and Hearing Research*, 41, 18–30.

Smith, A. and **Kelly, E. M.** (1997). Stuttering: a dynamic, multifactorial model. In R. F. Curlee and G. M. Siegel (Eds), *Nature and treatment of stuttering: new directions* (pp. 204–217). Boston, MA: Allyn and Bacon.

Smith, A. and **Kleinow, J.** (2000). Kinematic correlates of speaking rate changes in stuttering and normally fluent adults. *Journal of Speech Language and Hearing Research*, 43, 521–536.

Smith, A., Denny, M., Shaffer, L. A., Kelly, E. M., and **Hirano, M.** (1996). Activity of intrinsic laryngeal muscles in fluent and disfluent speech. *Science*, 39, 329–348.

Stager, S. V., Denman, D. W., and **Ludlow, C. L.** (1997). Modifications in aerodynamic variables by persons who stutter under fluency-evoking conditions. *Journal of Speech Language and Hearing Research*, 40, 832–847.

Stein, M. B., Baird, A., and **Walker, J. R.** (1996). Social phobia in adults with stuttering. *American Journal of Psychiatry*, 153, 278–280.

Stoffregen, T. A. and **Bardy, B. G.** (2001). On specification and the senses. *Behavioural Brain Science*, 24, 195–213.

Story, R. S., Alfonso, P. J., and **Harris, K. S.** (1996). Pre- and posttreatment comparison of the kinematics of the fluent speech of persons who stutter. *Journal of Speech and Hearing Research*, 39, 991–1005.

Stromsta, C. (1972). Interaural phase disparity of stutterers and nonstutterers. *Journal of Speech and Hearing Research*, 15, 771–780.

Stuart, A., Kalinowski, J., and **Rastatter, M. P.** (1997). Effect of monaural and binaural altered auditory feedback on stuttering frequency. *Journal of the Acoustical Society of America*, 101, 3806–3809.

Timmons, B. A. and **Boudreau, J. P.** (1972). Auditory feedback as a major factor in stuttering. *Journal of Speech and Hearing Disorders*, 37, 476–484.

Treffner, P. J. (1999). Resonance contraints on between-person polyrhythms. In M. A. Grealy and J. A. Thomson (Eds), *Studies in perception and action V* (pp. 165–169). Mahwah, NJ: Erlbaum.

Treffner, P. J. and **Turvey, M. T.** (1996). Symmetry, broken symmetry, and handedness in bimanual coordination dynamics. *Experimental Brain Research*, 107, 463–478.

Van Borsel, J. and **Vanryckeghem, M.** (2000). Dysfluency and phonic tics in Tourette syndrome: a case report. *Journal of Communication Disorders*, 33, 227–239.

van Lieshout, P. H. H. M. (1995). *Motor planning and articulation in fluent speech of stutterers and nonstutterers*. University of Nijmegen, The Netherlands.

van Lieshout, P. H. H. M. (1998). Linguistic and motor determinants: how well can they be separated? In E. C. Healey and H. F. M. Peters (Eds), *Proceedings of the Second World Congress on Fluency Disorders, San Francisco, August 18–22, 1997* (pp. 15–23). Nijmegen, The Netherlands: IFA.

van Lieshout, P. and **Moussa, W.** (2000). The assessment of speech motor behaviors using electromagnetic articulography. *The Phonetician*, 81, 9–22.

van Lieshout, P. H., Peters, H. F., Starkweather, C. W., and **Hulstijn, W.** (1993). Physiological differences between stutterers and nonstutterers in perceptually fluent speech: EMG amplitude and duration. *Journal of Speech and Hearing Research*, 36, 55–63.

van Lieshout, P., Alfonso, P. J., Hulstijn, W., and **Peters, H. F.** (1994). Electromagnetic midsagittal articulography (EMMA). In F. J. Maarse, A. E. Akkerman, A. N. Brand, L. J. M. Mulder, and M. J. Van der Stelt (Eds), *Computers in Psychology: Applications, Methods, and Instrumentation* (pp. 62–76). Lisse: Swets and Zeitlinger.

van Lieshout, P. H., Starkweather, C. W., Hulstijn, W., and Peters, H. F. (1995). Effects of linguistic correlates of stuttering on EMG activity in nonstuttering speakers. *Journal of Speech and Hearing Research*, 38, 360–372.

van Lieshout, P. H., Hulstijn, W., and Peters, H. F. (1996a). From planning to articulation in speech production: what differentiates a person who stutters from a person who does not stutter? *Journal of Speech and Hearing Research*, 39, 546–564.

van Lieshout, P. H., Hulstijn, W., and Peters, H. F. (1996b). Speech production in people who stutter: testing the motor plan assembly hypothesis. *Journal of Speech and Hearing Research*, 39, 76–92.

van Lieshout, P., Hulstijn, W., Alfonso, P. J., and Peters, H. F. (1997a). Higher and lower order influences on the stability of the dynamic coupling between articulators. In W. Hulstijn, H. F. Peters, and P. van Lieshout (Eds), *Speech production: motor control, brain research and fluency disorders* (pp. 161–170). Amsterdam: Elsevier Science Publishers.

van Lieshout, P. H. H. M., Peters, H. F. M., and Bakker, A. J. (1997b). En route to a speech motor test: a first halt. In W. Hulstijn, H. F. M. Peters, and P. H. H. M. van Lieshout (Eds), *Speech production: motor control, brain research and fluency disorders* (pp. 463–471). Amsterdam: Elsevier.

van Lieshout, P. H. H. M., Hijl, M., and Hulstijn, W. (1999). Flexibility and stability in bilabial gestures: 2) evidence from continuous syllable production. In J. J. Ohala, J. J. Hasegawa, M. Ohala, D. Granville, and A. C. Bailey (Eds), (pp. 45–48). San Francisco: American Institute of Physics.

van Lieshout, P. H. H. M., Rutjens, C. A. W., and Spauwen, P. H. M. (2002). The dynamics of interlip coupling in speakers with a repaired unilateral cleft-lip history. *Journal of Speech Language and Hearing Research*, 45, 5–19.

Van Riper, C. (1970). The use of DAF in stuttering therapy. *British Journal of Disorders of Communication*, 5, 40–45.

Van Riper, C. (1990). Final thoughts about stuttering. *Journal of Fluency Disorders*, 15, 317–318.

Vanryckeghem, M., Glessing, J. J., Brutten, G. J., and McAlindon, P. (1999). The main and interactive effect of oral reading rate on the frequency of stuttering. *American Journal of Speech–Language Pathology*, 8, 164–170.

Vicente, K. J. and Torenvliet, G. L. (2001). The Earth is spherical (p < 0.05): alternative methods of statistical inference. *Theoretical Issues in Ergonomics Science*, 1, 248–271.

Volman, M. C. J. R. and Geuze, R. H. (1998). Relative phase stability of bimanual and visuomanual rhythmic coordination patterns in children with a Developmental Coordination Disorder. *Human Movement Science*, 17, 541–572.

Ward, D. (1997). Intrinsic and extrinsic timing in stutterers' speech: Data and implications. *Language and Speech*, 40, 289–310.

Webster, R. L., Schumacher, S. J., and **Lubker, B. B.** (1970). Changes in stuttering frequency as a function of various intervals of delayed auditory feedback. *Journal of Abnormal Psychology* 75, 45–49.

Weismer, G. and **Liss, J. M.** (1991). Reductionism is a dead-end in speech research: perspectives on a new direction. In C. A. Moore, K. M. Yorkston, and D. R. Beukelman (Eds), *Dysarthria and apraxia of speech: perspectives on management* (pp. 15–27). Baltimore, MA: Paul H. Brookes Publishing Co.

Wieneke, G. H., Eijken, E., Janssen, P., and **Brutten, G. J.** (2001). Durational Variability in the Fluent Speech of Stutterers and Nonstutterers. *Journal of Fluency Disorders*, 26, 13–53.

Williamson, M. M. (1998). Neural control of rhythmic arm movements. *Neural Networks*, 11, 1379–1394.

Wilson, P. H., Thomas, P. R., and **Maruff, P.** (2002). Motor imagery training ameliorates motor clumsiness in children. *Journal of Child Neurology*, 17, 491–498.

Wolk, L., Edwards, M. L., and **Conture, E. G.** (1993). Coexistence of stuttering and disordered phonology in young children. *Journal of Speech and Hearing Research*, 36, 906–917.

Wolk, L., Blomgren, B., and **Smith, A. B.** (2000). The frequency of simultaneous disfluency and phonological errors in children: a preliminary investigation. *Journal of Fluency Disorders*, 25, 269–281.

Wu, J. C., Maguire, G., Riley, G., Lee, A., Keator, D., Tang, C. *et al.* (1997). Increased dopamine activity associated with stuttering. *Neuroreport*, 8, 767–770.

Yaruss, J. S. (1999). Utterance length, syntactic complexity, and childhood stuttering. *Journal of Speech Language and Hearing Research*, 42, 329–344.

Yaruss, J. S. and **Conture, E. G.** (1996). Stuttering and phonological disorders in children: examination of the Covert Repair Hypothesis. *Journal of Speech and Hearing Research*, 39, 349–364.

Zimmermann, G. N., Smith, A., and **Hanley, J. M.** (1981). Stuttering: in need of a unifying conceptual framework. *Journal of Speech and Hearing Research*, 24, 25–31.

Zmarich, C., Hulstijn, W., Bernardini, S., and **Nijland, L.** (2001). *Bilabial and labiodental movement patterns in stuttering and nonstuttering children during speech*. 4th International Speech Motor Conference, June 13–16, Nijmegen, The Netherlands.

CHAPTER 14

STUTTERING AND INTERNAL MODELS FOR SENSORIMOTOR CONTROL: A THEORETICAL PERSPECTIVE TO GENERATE TESTABLE HYPOTHESES

LUDO MAX

14.1 Introduction

Stuttering is characterized by disruptions in speech motor behavior (repeated or prolonged articulatory and phonatory actions) that result in sound and syllable repetitions, audible and inaudible sound prolongations, and broken words. The importance of this fact, that moments of stuttering are associated with disruptions in motor behavior, cannot be overemphasized. Clearly, the association itself does not warrant the conclusion that stuttering is a speech motor disorder, because the process may have broken down at a pre-motor level. Nevertheless, it does indicate that any role played by cognitive–linguistic or psychological–emotional processes in either the distal (related to etiology) or proximal (related to individual moments of stuttering) causes of stuttering requires an explanation of how disruptions in those processes would result in the articulatory and phonatory repetitive movements and fixed postures observed during stuttering.

I will propose in this chapter a specific version of the perspective that stuttering is in fact a disorder affecting the control and organization of movements. Doing so is consistent with previous suggestions by others, but the details of the hypothesis proposed here—heavily based on recent insights in the areas of neuroscience and motor control—differ considerably from most previous proposals. Specifically, I will suggest that the onset of stuttering during childhood may be related to the use of inaccurate, or incorrectly updated, internal models of the dynamics of the effector system to evaluate generated motor commands prior to execution, and that the resulting mismatch between predicted and actual sensory consequences may lead to repetitive attempts at completing the planned movements or re-setting the system. This proposal borrows from work by others (Neilson and Neilson 1987, 1991), but expands it considerably, by (1) integrating concepts from the most recent movement neuroscience literature, and (2) explaining how this perspective could account for the basic characteristics of the disorder, as well as a large number of associated phenomena (age of onset, fluency-enhancing conditions, treatment outcomes, etc.). Although largely speculative at this time, the primary value of the proposed perspective lies in the fact that it offers a comprehensive theoretical framework that can generate several testable hypotheses. Indeed, progress in unraveling the intricate mechanisms underlying stuttering may be significantly enhanced by focusing our research efforts on the empirical testing of *theoretically motivated* hypotheses.

To develop this theoretical framework, I will review in Section 14.2 relevant data from other research groups as well as from my own laboratory. The review will emphasize work showing that stuttering and nonstuttering individuals differ in the central control of movements, that these differences do not provide strong support for the common interpretation of a specific timing disorder, that they are not restricted to the speech motor system, and that they are often associated with difficulties in sensory processing or sensorimotor integration and learning. To place these findings in a more global perspective on the central control of movements, Section 14.3 will present recent theoretical notions and empirical data that have led to important new insights in the area of nonspeech motor control and neuroscience, and that may prove to be valuable pieces in the scientific puzzle of stuttering. Emphasis will be placed on new information regarding the acquisition/updating of internal models for motor control and the neural activation patterns associated with sensorimotor processing in speech and nonspeech motor systems. Based on that information, I will describe in Section 14.4 the sensorimotor perspective on stuttering that is the focus of this chapter.

It should be noted that the ideas developed here are not meant to imply that linguistic, environmental, and psychological–emotional variables are unimportant in the development of stuttering, for the loci of stuttering, in the experiences of individuals who stutter, or in their treatment. On the contrary, there is no doubt that both normal and disordered speech and nonspeech motor systems are influenced by nonmotor variables. An excellent illustration for disordered motor systems is easily found in Parkinson's disease. Generally accepted to be a neuropathology of the nigrostriatal dopaminergic pathways, the motor symptoms of this disease are influenced by environmental–perceptual variables, such as the presence of visual patterns. Similarly, other variables, such as environmental stressors, are also known to exacerbate motor symptoms in Parkinson's disease. Hence, it is clear that disorders that are appropriately considered motor disorders can be *influenced* by several nonmotor variables.

14.2 Research on stuttering as a neuromotor problem

I will first summarize selected speech and nonspeech motor control and brain activation studies by others and then discuss in more detail recent findings from our own ongoing programs of stuttering research at the University of Connecticut and Haskins Laboratories.

14.2.1 Other research laboratories

14.2.1.1 Speech movements

Numerous investigators have used reaction-time paradigms to investigate the speech motor capacities of stuttering individuals. With very few exceptions, these studies have demonstrated that, as a group, stuttering individuals are slower than nonstuttering individuals in initiating both phonation and articulation (Bloodstein 1995).

Another extensive line of research consists of acoustic studies examining temporal aspects of the perceptually fluent speech of individuals who stutter (Bloodstein 1995). Briefly, findings can be summarized as follows. Several studies have shown longer voice onset times (VOT) in stuttering versus nonstuttering speakers, although such differences were sometimes limited to only a few phonetic contexts or levels of complexity. More consistent are data indicating that, for adults, stuttering individuals show longer vowel durations than nonstuttering individuals. Two additional acoustic measures, consonant–vowel (CV) transition duration and stop gap duration, have also been shown to be longer for stuttering than for nonstuttering individuals, although, again, inconsistent findings have been reported.

Recognizing the benefits of analyzing speech movements in ways similar to those used for nonspeech motor behavior, several investigators have analyzed kinematic aspects of stuttering individuals' speech movements. Zimmermann (1980) found that stuttering subjects, as compared with nonstuttering subjects, showed longer movement durations and longer latencies between various kinematic and phonatory events during bilabial opening movements in consonant–vowel–consonant (CVC) sequences. Caruso et al. (1988a) observed similar kinematic between-group differences during bilabial closing movements. McClean et al. (1990), on the other hand, reported that such differences may be limited to stuttering speakers who recently participated in stuttering treatment.

One aspect of speech movement organization that has been discussed extensively in relation to stuttering is the sequencing of kinematic events across different articulators. It has been shown repeatedly that normally fluent speakers typically organize the movement onsets and peak velocities associated with bilabial closing for the first /p/ in *sapapple* in the order upper lip–lower lip–jaw (UL–LL–J; Caruso et al. 1988a; Gracco 1994; De Nil 1995). In the study by Caruso et al. (1988a), however, five of six stuttering individuals predominantly used sequencing patterns that were different from those most commonly seen in the nonstuttering individuals. Similar differences in articulatory sequencing were reported by Alfonso (1991) for tongue and jaw closing movements during alveolar stops and fricatives.

Although these differences initially appeared very promising, their interpretation remained unclear. Some reasons for this problem can be found in contradictory results regarding the effects of speech rate (McClean *et al.* 1990; De Nil and Abbs 1991), therapy history (McClean *et al.* 1990; Story and Alfonso cited in Alfonso 1991), and phonetic context and speech task (Gracco 1994; De Nil 1995). Interestingly, the only replication study (De Nil 1995) with the same task and target word as in Caruso *et al.* (1988a) did reveal a between-group difference in articulatory sequencing, whereas other tasks and other target words have failed to reveal a difference (De Nil 1995; Jäncke *et al.* 1995a, b).

A different approach to studying speech movement timing can be found in work using a spatiotemporal index (STI) that reflects variability of lower lip movement across repeated productions of an utterance. Kleinow and Smith (2000) found that adults who stutter showed overall higher STI values (i.e. more variability) than adults who do not stutter, and that the stuttering adults' STI values increased even more with increasing complexity of the produced utterances. However, in a different study, Smith and Kleinow (2000) found no statistically significant STI difference between stuttering and nonstuttering adults.

Another important aspect of speech motor control pertains to the coordination of oral and laryngeal movements. In a study by Peters and Hulstijn (1987), stuttering individuals produced the target utterances with labial EMG activity preceding laryngeal EMG activity, whereas the nonstuttering individuals initiated labial and laryngeal EMG activity at approximately the same time. Yoshioka and Löfqvist (1981) and Hutchinson and Watkin (1976) suggested that stuttering moments are associated with laryngeal movements that are improperly timed relative to the oral or respiratory movements. Borden and Armson (1987), on the other hand, concluded that oral–laryngeal coordination could be appropriate even during moments of stuttering. Caruso *et al.* (1988b) reached the same conclusion, based on comparisons of both the duration and sequencing of physiological events within and across the articulatory and phonatory subsystems in dysfluent productions by stuttering children versus fluent productions by nonstuttering children.

Most investigators have used perceptually fluent speech to study the coordination of oral and laryngeal movements. Jäncke *et al.* (1995b) reported that stuttering adults showed a tendency toward increased intra-individual variability in oral–laryngeal coordination as compared with nonstuttering adults. For children, Conture *et al.* (1988) found no between-group differences in physiological indices of the coordination of articulation and phonation during perceptually fluent speech.

Based on acoustic analyses, Boutsen (1995) and Zebrowski *et al.* (1985) reported that nonstuttering adults and children, respectively, showed a negative correlation between stop gap (SG) duration and aspiration duration or VOT, whereas stuttering individuals showed no correlation or only a very small one. These correlation analyses were based on data points defined by coordinates corresponding to each participant's mean SG duration and VOT. However, within-subject data reflecting adjustments in the same variables across multiple productions of target consonants were reported by Borden *et al.* (1987), who found no negative correlation between SG duration and VOT for either nonstuttering or stuttering speakers.

The possible role of a *sensory* problem in stuttering has been recognized primarily in suggestions focusing on auditory feedback disruptions (Bloodstein 1995). Less attention has been paid to the possibility that stuttering may involve a proprioceptive dysfunction. Caruso *et al.* (1987) applied inferiorly directed perturbations to the lower lip of three stuttering and three nonstuttering adults during bilabial closing gestures (load direction opposite movement direction). Stuttering individuals' compensatory movements showed longer latencies and smaller displacements than those of nonstuttering individuals. Furthermore, McClean (1996) found that, immediately preceding fluently produced monosyllabic words, only 4 of 14 adults who stutter showed the same attenuation of mechanically elicited reflexes in the upper and lower lips that was shown by 11 of 14 adults who do not stutter. Thus, results from the perturbation and the evoked reflex paradigms suggest that stuttering may be associated with an aberrant afferent information system, with difficulties in the central processing of the afferent information, or in the use of afferent information for updating efferent commands.

Overall, it can be concluded from these acoustic and physiological speech data that, compared with nonstuttering individuals, stuttering individuals typically take longer to initiate and complete articulatory as well as phonatory movements; that, despite numerous studies, the evidence for a specific timing/sequencing or coordination disorder remains very limited; and that there is at least some initial evidence that warrants a more in-depth exploration of the possibility that at least some observed between-group differences have a sensory basis.

14.2.1.2 Nonspeech movements

Unfortunately, the results from studies of nonspeech movements in individuals who stutter are difficult to integrate with the data obtained for articulatory movements, because of the absence of comparable measurements across the motor systems. Nevertheless, the results generally suggest that nonspeech motor differences between stuttering and nonstuttering individuals may be task-dependent. On the one hand, differences have been observed in the ability to make very small or accurate orofacial and finger movements (De Nil and Abbs 1991; Howell *et al.* 1995; Loucks and De Nil 2001), behavioral measures of finger movement sequencing accuracy, initiation time and execution time (Webster 1997), manual reaction times (Bishop *et al.* 1991; Webster and Ryan 1991), and bimanual coordination (Zelaznik *et al.* 1997; Forster and Webster 2001). On the other hand, no differences were found for manual rhythmic timing (for a review see Max and Yudman 2003) or isometric force generation tasks (Zelaznik *et al.* 1994), although one study with a nonspeech lip force production task (Grosjean *et al.* 1997) found stuttering subjects to have less accurate isometric force control than nonstuttering subjects when visual feedback was added.

It is interesting that, similar to the situation for speech movements, there is evidence suggesting that the nonspeech motor difficulties of stuttering individuals are, at least in part, based on sensory deficiencies. Studying kinesthetic acuity for oral and non-oral movements, De Nil and Abbs (1991) asked stuttering and control subjects to make the smallest possible movements with the jaw, lower lip, tongue, or finger. In the absence of visual feedback, the stuttering group produced oral movements that were larger than those produced by the nonstuttering group. When visual feedback was provided, performance of the two groups was similar. Howell *et al.* (1995) obtained comparable results for lip movements in stuttering versus nonstuttering children. Loucks and De Nil (2001) later found that stuttering adults also performed more poorly than control subjects in making accurate jaw opening movements to visually presented spatial targets. Stuttering subjects again differed from nonstuttering subjects when only kinesthetic feedback was available whereas performance of the two groups was similar when visual feedback was provided. Moreover, a bimanual coordination task used by Forster and Webster (2001) yielded identical results with regard to the presence versus absence of visual feedback.

The most appropriate conclusion to draw from these nonspeech data appears to be that differences between stuttering and nonstuttering individuals are indeed not limited to speech movements. Rather, the two groups also differ with regard to certain movement parameters when using the orofacial structures for nonspeech purposes or when using an unrelated effector system such as the fingers or hands. In addition, there is preliminary evidence that these nonspeech motor difficulties in stuttering individuals are based on difficulties with the processing of sensory information or with the integration of sensory and motor signals.

14.2.1.3 Brain activation patterns

Brain imaging data obtained during speech production have consistently revealed differences between stuttering and nonstuttering subjects. These differences— although not always localized in the same cortical, subcortical or cerebellar areas— typically reflect either reduced left hemisphere or increased right hemisphere activation in the stuttering group (Wu *et al.* 1995; Braun *et al.* 1997; De Nil *et al.* 2000, 2001; Fox *et al.* 1996, 2000; Ingham 2001). However, the finding of reduced left hemisphere lateralization may be of limited importance. First, data from some studies suggest that, among normal speakers, women show less left hemisphere lateralization when compared with men (Shaywitz *et al.* 1995; Medland *et al.* 2002). The paradoxical situation is that the prevalence of stuttering is lower, rather than higher, among women than among men. Secondly, increased right-hemisphere lateralization across a variety of tasks has been demonstrated in subject samples in which the altered lateralization is most likely a result of neural plasticity due to previous motor experiences—for example, judo wrestlers (Mikheev *et al.* 2002).

In a positron emission tomography (PET) study with four stuttering subjects, Wu *et al.* (1995) observed left caudate nucleus hypometabolism. Later, they reported increased presynaptic dopaminergic (i.e. inhibiting) activity in cortical and subcortical areas of three stuttering adults (Wu *et al.* 1997). Furthermore, pharmaceutical studies with dopamine receptor antagonists have shown both increased striatal activation (Riley *et al.* 2001) and reductions in stuttering frequency (Maguire *et al.* 2000). In light of the above-discussed speech and nonspeech sensorimotor difficulties in stuttering individuals, the most critical implications of these findings may be related to the now well-known role of the basal ganglia dopaminergic system in motor coordination and planning (Fattapposta *et al.* 2002; Mattay *et al.* 2002) as well as sensorimotor integration and learning (Huda *et al.* 2001; Fattapposta *et al.* 2002).

Regarding sensorimotor integration, it is intriguing that Fox *et al.* (1996, 2000) found that, during solo reading, stuttering subjects not only showed increased activation of cerebral and cerebellar motor areas, but also failed to activate, or sometimes even deactivated (relative to rest), auditory cortical areas. During fluent speech induced by chorus reading, both the hyperactivity of the motor areas and the lack of activation or deactivation of auditory areas were reduced or eliminated. In a later study, 4 of the 10 subjects were re-scanned during overt stuttered speech, imagining reading with stuttering, fluent chorus reading, and imagining reading without stuttering (Ingham *et al.* 2000). Brain areas associated with both overt and imagined stuttering, as compared with actual and imagined fluency, essentially matched those from the previous investigation in which speech had been actually produced. It is important to note, however, that this finding does not indicate that stuttering must be a problem of nonmotor, higher-level linguistic processes. It is well known now that imagery of movement actually results in activation of motor, premotor, supplementary motor, anterior cingulate, parietal, sensorimotor, and cerebellar areas (Lotze *et al.* 1999; Binkofski *et al.* 2000; Buccino *et al.* 2001) and even the activation of peripheral muscles (Lotze *et al.* 1999; Jeannerod 2001).

The finding that stuttering is associated with reduced or reversed left hemisphere lateralization, hyperactivation of premotor and motor areas, and a failure to activate or a deactivation of auditory (as well as somatosensory) areas was replicated in a study by Braun *et al.* (1997), who compared stuttered versus fluent speech, as well stuttering versus nonstuttering speakers. In fact, in a review paper, Ingham (2001) concluded that the most critical findings across studies may be the atypical activation of premotor systems in combination with the lack of activation or deactivation of auditory areas, thus implicating movement preparation and sensory monitoring or sensorimotor integration as potentially deficient processes in stuttering. Along the same lines, De Nil *et al.* (2001) interpreted their own findings on cerebellar activation as indicating an increased need for sensory or motor monitoring in stuttering subjects. With regard to the level at which breakdowns in speech production occur in individuals who stutter (i.e. cognitive–linguistic versus motor), it is noteworthy that Braun *et al.* (1997) found that differences between stuttering and nonstuttering individuals in the activation of motor and sensory cortical areas were present even during nonspeech oral movement tasks.

Summarizing the brain-imaging studies with stuttering subjects is difficult, given the use of different imaging technologies, different experimental tasks, and often different results. Nevertheless, the most consistent findings across studies appear to be that, during speech production, stuttering individuals show hyperactivation of cerebral and cerebellar motor areas, reduced or reversed hemispheric lateralization of those motor areas, and absent or reduced activation of the cortical auditory areas.

14.2.2 Studies from our own program of research

14.2.2.1 Kinematics of speech, orofacial nonspeech, and finger movements

We investigated the hypothesis that neuromotor differences between stuttering and nonstuttering adults are not limited to the movements involved in speech production (Max *et al.* 2003*a*). Kinematic data were obtained for perceptually fluent speech movements (UL, LL, J) as well as for orofacial nonspeech movements (UL, LL, J) and finger movements [metacarpophalangeal (MCP) and proximal interphalangeal (PIP) joint of the index finger, and interphalangeal joint of the thumb (IP)]. The work revealed several interesting findings. First, differences were found between the stuttering and nonstuttering individuals in several measures of lip and jaw closing, but not opening, movements for bilabial stop consonants. Secondly, the magnitude of these differences varied across different levels of utterance length (larger differences for shorter utterances) and across different locations of the target movement within an utterance (larger differences close to the beginning). Thirdly, not only the speech task, but also the finger movement task, revealed differences between the stuttering and nonstuttering groups. Analogous to the speech data, the finger movement data showed such differences in finger flexion but not finger extension. The kinematic variables that most consistently differentiated the two groups in both the speech task and the finger movement task were total movement duration and duration from movement onset to peak velocity. Hence, findings indicated that the groups of stuttering and nonstuttering subjects showed generalized differences in certain goal-directed movements across unrelated motor systems.

14.2.2.2 Sequencing of speech, orofacial nonspeech, and finger movements

To specifically address aspects of motor timing, data from the speech, orofacial nonspeech, and finger movement tasks described above were also analyzed to compare stuttering and nonstuttering individuals with regard to the sequencing of the moments of movement onset or peak velocity for the effectors contributing to a single gesture such as a bilabial closing or index finger–thumb opposition movement. The results showed more similarities than differences between the stuttering and nonstuttering individuals. In fact, sequencing patterns of the two groups were most similar during the speech task. Consistent across the four conditions of this task, both groups performed most closing gestures with an UL–J–LL sequence and most opening gestures with a J–LL–UL sequence. For all four conditions of the orofacial nonspeech task, both groups again showed a preference for UL-lead sequences during closing movements and J-lead sequences during opening movements. For all four conditions of the finger movement task, both groups showed a preference for PIP-lead sequences during the closing movements. No clear trends were observed in the finger opening movement data.

14.2.2.3 Isochronous rhythmic timing of speech, orofacial nonspeech, and finger movements

Different aspects of motor timing were investigated in a study during which the same groups of stuttering and nonstuttering subjects performed isochronous (i.e. equal interresponse intervals) rhythmic timing tasks in a synchronization–continuation paradigm (Max and Yudman 2003). Auditory stimuli with 450 ms, 650 ms, or 850 ms inter-stimulus onset intervals were presented through headphones, and subjects started performing the target response in synchrony with the auditory stimuli whenever they felt ready to do so. After 10 responses, the auditory stimuli ceased, and the subject's task was to maintain the exact same movement rhythm. Responses consisted of bilabial contact in the syllable 'pa' during a speech task, bilabial contact in a 'lip popping' orofacial nonspeech task, and thumb–index finger contact in a finger movement task. Based on the relevant kinematic events, multiple analyses of timing accuracy and variability were completed for both the synchronization and continuation phases, including decomposition of total timing variance into central clock and motor implementation variance, according to the Wing–Kristofferson model (Wing and Kristofferson 1973). The combined results from descriptive comparisons, statistical significance testing, and effect size computations indicated that the stuttering and nonstuttering participants showed highly similar levels of both timing accuracy and timing variability. This was true (1) for all three motor tasks, (2) at all movement rates, and (3) for synchronization as well as continuation movements.

14.2.2.4 Relative timing of oral and laryngeal events

We first examined oral–laryngeal coordination in a preliminary study (Max and Glass 2001) and subsequently in a more in-depth study (Max and Gracco 2003). The latter work included both acoustic and physiological data [electroglottography

(EGG) and articulatory kinematics] obtained for productions of /p/ in perceptually fluent speech (all data were collected in the paradigm described above for Max *et al.* 2003*a*). Dependent variables included the duration of various intervals defined by either acoustic events or events within and across the EGG and kinematic traces, as well as a number of proportional measures specifically reflecting oral–laryngeal relative timing [e.g. acoustic and physiological devoicing symmetry, a measure that reflects the percentage of the devoicing interval (DI) occurring prior to the articulatory release for the stop consonant].

Results revealed similar within-subject correlations between acoustic measures of SG and VOT for the stuttering versus nonstuttering individuals. The acoustic data further indicated that the stuttering individuals showed longer DIs and VOTs than the nonstuttering individuals. However, no between-group difference in either central tendency or variability was observed for a relative measure of oral–laryngeal relative timing. Similarly, the physiological data (lip aperture kinematics and laryngeal EGG) revealed differences in the absolute duration of intervals defined within and across the kinematic and EGG data, but not in the *relative timing* of the involved articulatory and phonatory events.

Thus, findings appear to reflect a general slowness in the stuttering group, rather than a difference specifically in oral–laryngeal relative timing. Of course, all analyses were completed on perceptually fluent utterances and, therefore, do not provide information regarding the possibility that individuals who stutter may experience intermittent oral–laryngeal coordination difficulties that occur only during moments of stuttering.

14.2.2.5 Adaptation and the role of motor learning

In a series of publications, we have shown that stuttering adaptation occurs as a result of repeated reading rather than repeated stuttering, and that some of the changes observable in the acoustic speech signal during the repeated readings are consistent with changes known to occur during nonspeech motor practice (Max *et al.* 1997; Max and Caruso 1998). We have suggested that the improvements in speech fluency during an adaptation paradigm may represent a form of motor learning, albeit with rather short-term benefits due to very limited amount of practice.

Recently, we have also examined the phenomenon of adaptation in an individual with acquired neurogenic stuttering. If, as has been suggested by others, individuals with acquired neurogenic stuttering do indeed fail to show a capability to reduce their stuttering with repeated readings, then the fact that individuals with developmental stuttering do benefit from motor practice may provide an important piece of information in our attempts to understand the mechanisms underlying developmental stuttering. It is therefore interesting that our case study of a 57-year-old male who started stuttering after ischemic lesion to the orbital surface of the right frontal lobe and the pons did not show an improvement in fluency during an adaptation paradigm (Balasubramanian *et al.* 2003).

14.2.3 Conclusions based on the reviewed empirical data

The finding that is, by far, most consistent across the reviewed studies is that stuttering individuals perform both speech and nonspeech movements with longer durations than do nonstuttering individuals. Evidence to support the much more specific hypothesis that stuttering is a disorder of speech timing remains very limited. Indeed, it appears that the timing hypothesis has been motivated merely by the myriad of studies revealing differences in temporal parameters of speech. A critical point, however, is that one cannot simply assume that longer movement durations (or even dysfluent speech) *must* indicate a timing problem. This point is easily illustrated as there are a number of neurological disorders that are associated with aberrant movements (including repetitive movements and sustained postures) and movement slowness, but that are not considered to be specifically disorders of movement timing; for example, Parkinson's disease (Hallett and Khoshbin 1980), Huntington's disease (Thompson *et al.* 1988), Wilson's disease (Hefter *et al.* 1993), and idiopathic dystonia (Jahanshahi *et al.* 2001). Although each of these disorders is associated with movements characterized by aberrant temporal patterns (in each case longer movement durations), the underlying mechanisms are likely to be very different. For example, some slow movements in Parkinson's disease are performed with appropriate sequencing of agonist and antagonist activity but with repeated cycles of electromyographic bursts, even though each burst by itself may be of normal duration (Hallett and Khoshbin 1980). It has been suggested that such multiple cycles of activation may be used to compensate for an inadequate scaling of the magnitude of the agonist activity (Berardelli *et al.* 1996). For patients with Huntington's disease, on the other hand, slowness may be accompanied by prolonged contraction of the agonist and antagonist muscles (Thompson *et al.* 1988). This situation is more similar to that seen in idiopathic dystonia, a motor disorder characterized by excessive and prolonged co-contraction of antagonistic muscle groups due to failure of reciprocal inhibition via inhibitory interneurons or, possibly, abnormal central commands (Jahanshahi *et al.* 2001).

These examples of other motor disorders are offered only to make the point that one should be careful before concluding that movements that do not have the normal temporal characteristics are necessarily a result of mistiming. If, on the other hand, one wants to use the terminology *timing disorder* in a descriptive manner for any disorder in which movements do not enfold over time as expected, regardless of what caused this abnormality, then the term also applies to several speech disorders besides stuttering. For this reason, I believe that it is important to continue investigating whether it is specifically the timing versus other aspects of movement control that are affected in stuttering. In the next section, I will discuss selected topics from the contemporary movement neuroscience literature that will then form the foundation for a theoretical perspective on stuttering that does not assume a timing disorder. In particular, I will describe new insights that contribute directly to the proposed neuromotor perspective on stuttering, or that may account for some of the phenomena known to be associated with the disorder.

14.3 New insights from the neuroscience of motor control

14.3.1 Forward and inverse internal models

A critical question regarding the mechanisms underlying adaptive control of both speech and nonspeech movements relates to the ability of the central nervous system (CNS) to generate accurate motor commands to effector systems characterized by intricate dynamics. Indeed, the transformation from central commands to movements is very complex, due to multiple conversions (e.g. from shoulder, elbow, and wrist joint angles to hand position) and the time-varying influence of several variables that depend on neural and muscular physiological factors (e.g. neural discharge pattern, structural–chemical processes causing the sliding of myosin and actin filaments), the current state of the system (e.g. length–force and velocity–force relationships of the neuromuscular system), and biomechanics (e.g. inertia, gravity-related forces).

One potential solution that is currently widely accepted in the nonspeech motor control literature proposes that, for precision control in the presence of these intricate transformations, the CNS maintains internal representations of the properties of the motor systems and environment (Kawato and Wolpert 1998; Thoroughman and Shadmehr 1999). These internal representations consist of forward or inverse models, or a combination of both forward and inverse models (Shadmehr and Mussa-Ivaldi 1994; Wolpert *et al.* 1998*a*; Bhushan and Shadmehr 1999). A forward model is a 'map' from motor commands to sensory consequences; in other words, a forward model allows a prediction of the sensory consequences of a given set of motor commands by evaluating an efference copy of the generated motor commands with the internal model. This prediction can then be used to further refine the motor commands and to generate compensatory responses, in parallel with the changing task conditions, as the actions enfold (e.g. due to interaction torques, load forces, etc). An inverse model is a 'map' from the desired sensory consequences to the central commands necessary to achieve those consequences. If the actual motor output differs from the desired output, the internal model requires updating as a new mapping needs to be learned so that different commands are generated for future attempts.

It is important to note that these internal models:

(1) are fundamentally different from, and indeed bear no direct relationship to, either traditional or generalized motor programs, given that the internal models represent information regarding the forward or inverse *transformations* between motor commands and movement consequences rather than instructions for the muscle contractions that generate those movements;

(2) describe such transformations for effector systems and the environment/objects that the effector system interacts with, rather than for specific movements or movement sequences;

(3) are compatible with various theoretical perspectives on motor control as they do not impose any restrictions on the nature of the motor commands; and

(4) also integrate sensory information with ongoing central commands to respond online to afferent error signals during the movements (Wang *et al.* 2001).

Experimental studies based on the notion of internal models have already uncovered many important aspects of how movements are adjusted based on their predicted or actual sensory consequences. The two most widely used paradigms have investigated (1) how much and which information is taken into account by the motor system when anticipating the sensory consequences of movements; and (2) how, and to what extent, movements are adjusted in the presence of sensory perturbations.

Studies investigating the anticipation of movement consequences have examined, among other things, the suppression of self generated versus externally generated tactile stimuli (Blakemore *et al.* 1998*b*) and adjustments in the force with which an object is held in relation to the self-generated forces that are used to move the object (Blakemore *et al.* 1998*a*). These phenomena strongly support the notion that the CNS uses internal models to predict the sensory consequences of movements and show appropriate anticipatory responses. Anticipatory adjustments in grip force that are appropriately scaled in relation to the generated load forces, for example, can be accomplished only if internal models of the limb and object dynamics are used to evaluate a copy of the motor commands and accurately predict the object's motion and associated forces.

A particularly interesting question is whether the motor system develops internal models that contain only a coarse approximation or a very detailed and accurate representation of the dynamic transformations. Flanagan and Lolley (2001) were able to show that highly specific aspects of limb dynamics, such as the inertial anisotropy of the arm (differences in inertial resistance for movements in different directions), are correctly predicted by the motor system. When sliding an object with the tip of their index finger, subjects precisely scaled the amount of vertical force on the object in relation to direction-dependent variations in hand acceleration. In other words, subjects' internal models were sufficiently detailed and precise to make the motor system generate a larger vertical force on the object for movement directions that are associated with lower inertial resistance and thus higher acceleration. It is believed that such internal models are acquired early in life and then continually updated to accommodate gradual changes in system biomechanics and improved neural control.

Evidence in support of the idea that, after their initial acquisition, internal models are continuously updated, comes from studies investigating movement adjustments in the presence of sensory perturbations. If movements and/or their sensory consequences are experimentally manipulated, the central commands normally generated for the task will result in sensory feedback that differs from the predicted and desired feedback, and the internal model needs to be updated such that a different set of central commands is generated to achieve the desired outcome on future trials. Such adjustments, known as sensorimotor adaptation, have indeed been observed in various motor systems and tasks. Examples are studies investigating arm movements to visual targets in the presence of either visual perturbation conditions or in velocity-dependent force fields.

For example, when subjects wear prism glasses while performing a reaching task, the glasses introduce a lateral displacement of the visual field. Under these conditions, subjects adapt to the altered sensory information, and they learn to successfully reach for the target. When the prism glasses are removed after a relatively large number of trials, errors (known as aftereffects) are observed in the direction opposite the previously imposed displacement of the visual field. Similar sensorimotor adaptation and aftereffects have been observed for arm movements in force fields (Shadmehr and Mussa-Ivaldi 1994; Bhushan and Shadmehr 1999; Thoroughman and Shadmehr 1999). In these tasks, subjects move a robotic manipulandum towards visual targets while the robot motor generates forces that perturb the hand movements. As a result of the manipulation, subjects initially show curved rather than relatively straight movement trajectories. However, after some experience with the force field, sensorimotor adaptation occurs and the hand movement trajectories return to the relatively straight path seen in a null field. Such sensorimotor adaptation and subsequent aftereffects indicate that subjects can re-learn, and have access to, representations of the mapping between afferent information and the motor commands requisite for successful completion of the task.

Recently, initial data have become available regarding sensorimotor adapation in speech articulation. For whispered and normally voiced speech, respectively, Houde and Jordan (1998) and Max *et al.* (2003c) have demonstrated that normal speakers show adaptation and aftereffects as a result of auditory perturbations. These researchers showed that when the formant frequencies in the auditory feedback signal are experimentally shifted up or down, subjects compensate by adjusting their own formant frequencies in the opposite direction of the applied shifts.

A last issue regarding the acquisition and updating of internal models that deserves a brief discussion here because of its potential application to stuttering research, is related to the underlying neural processes. Current theoretical models and empirical data suggest particularly the cerebellum (Miall *et al.* 1993; Wolpert *et al.* 1998a; Imamizu *et al.* 2000; Blakemore *et al.* 2001) and posterior parietal cortex (Wolpert *et al.* 1998b) as the primary locations for the formation of internal models. Interestingly, it appears that newly acquired internal models may gradually become more resistant to interference (Brashers-Krug *et al.* 1996, Shadmehr and

Brashers-Krug 1997), and brain imaging studies have revealed continued changes in neural activation during this stage of motor memory consolidation even when motor performance remains unchanged. Specifically, these studies have shown an initial increase in cerebellar blood flow at the early learning stages, followed by a gradual decrease as learning proceeds, or an activation shift from prefrontal to premotor, posterior parietal, and cerebellar regions (Grafton *et al.* 1994; Seitz *et al.* 1994; Flament *et al.* 1996; van Mier *et al.* 1998). Others have suggested that widespread changes in cerebellar activation reflect learning processes, whereas local changes in an area near the posterior superior fissure (which continued to show activation even after learning was complete) may reflect the actual formation of an internal model (Imamizu *et al.* 2000).

The important difference between movement acquisition and consolidation or internal model formation is further demonstrated by a study in which a monkey reached for visual targets while wearing prism glasses (Yin and Kitazawa 2001). Even when the monkey practiced for 250 trials and movement error had been eliminated by that time, practice had only transient effects, as no aftereffects could be observed after 24 hours. However, when the monkey practiced for an additional 250 trials, aftereffects could be observed for at least 3 days. Thus, additional repetition with minimal errors was necessary to achieve consolidation. This study emphasizes not only the importance of differentiating between skill acquisition and consolidation for brain imaging research, but also the fact that consolidation of an improved motor skill may require extensive practice and repetition of movements that show the desired characteristics and outcomes.

14.3.2 Cortical activation patterns during speech and nonspeech tasks

Using magnetoencephalography (MEG), it has been demonstrated that the auditory cortex M100 response (which has a latency of approximately 100 ms) is reduced in amplitude during vowel production as opposed to hearing a tape-recording of one's own vowel productions (Houde *et al.* 2002). The M100 response to short tones is also reduced in amplitude during reading aloud as compared with reading silently (Numminen *et al.* 1999) or with hearing a recording of one's own speech (Curio *et al.* 2000; Houde *et al.* 2002). In the study by Curio *et al.* (2000), self-uttered syllables also delayed the peak response in both hemispheres, although the effect was larger on the left. Furthermore, auditory cortex did not react with an additional response to a rare syllable during a self-uttered sequence, although it did do so for a rare syllable in a replayed sequence. Thus, these MEG data convincingly demonstrate short-latency inhibiting or delaying effects on auditory cortex that are specific to actually producing speech.

Moreover, studies using PET technology (which has a lower temporal resolution), and thus investigating cortical activation on a slower time scale, have shown overall activation of auditory cortical areas during speech production (Fox *et al.* 1996, 2000; Braun *et al.* 1997). In fact, fMRI data have shown that even while subjects subvocally named visually presented objects, the dorsal portion of the left posterior superior temporal gyrus was activated (Hickok *et al.* 2000). When speech was whispered but auditory feedback was blocked by masking, activation of secondary auditory cortex was still observed (Paus *et al.* 1996).

It should be noted that these MEG and PET data indicating speech-related modulation of auditory cortex activity are consistent with aforementioned differences in the perception of self-generated versus externally generated tactile stimuli and compensatory motor responses to self-generated versus externally generated loads. That is, the speech findings also reveal motor-to-sensory priming for self-generated utterances, consistent with the view that a copy of the central commands is forwarded and evaluated by an internal model, such that the involved sensory systems are activated and anticipate the subsequent afferent signals.

Another interesting fact that has become increasingly clear, and that I will also use later to account for some of the data with regard to stuttering, is that even brain areas that were previously thought to be involved only in one specific task may be recruited by seemingly unrelated tasks. One relevant example here is the finding that auditory cortex and neighboring areas, such as middle and superior temporal gyrus and superior temporal sulcus, are activated bilaterally in response to *visual* perception of a speaker's silent speech movements, or even nonspeech movements that can be interpreted as speech movements (Calvert *et al.* 1997; Campbell *et al.* 2001). A second example is the activation of premotor, supplementary motor, Broca's, anterior cingulate, and parietal areas while *observing* or *imagining* movements (Lotze *et al.* 1999; Binkofski *et al.* 2000; Buccino *et al.* 2001). For Broca's region, this was also true, under certain presentation conditions, for visually observing silent speech movements (Campbell *et al.* 2001).

14.4 A sensorimotor perspective on stuttering

14.4.1 Stuttering as a result of incorrect or unstable internal models for sensorimotor control

It would seem appropriate to summarize the stuttering research discussed in Sections 14.2.1 and 14.2.2 in the following five points. First, when individuals who stutter experience actual moments of stuttering, the involved muscle systems show oscillatory or prolonged contractions that give rise to sound- or syllable repetitions, sound prolongations, and broken words. Unless stuttering individuals differ from nonstuttering individuals in peripheral neuromuscular or biochemical characteristics—and there currently seems to be no evidence that they do—it can be assumed that the neural drive to the musculature is aberrant during moments of stuttering. Neural drive is the result of an interaction among central commands for phasic activation, central commands for antagonist co-activation, muscle length-dependent afferent inputs facilitating both phasic and tonic reflexes, and other continuous proprioceptive and tactile afferent inputs that are integrated online for adaptive motor responses. Therefore, the neural drive resulting in articulatory and/or phonatory oscillations or fixations could reflect a wide variety of underlying mechanisms, including, but not limited to, an incorrect specification of phasic central commands to the involved muscle systems, an incorrect specification of co-activation commands, inappropriate excitatory or inhibitory responses triggered by incorrect or incorrectly integrated afferent inputs, or attempts to correct real or perceived errors in the planned commands.

Second, with regard to stuttering individuals' perceptually fluent speech, it seems that one of the few conclusions that can be drawn with a reasonable degree of certainty is that stuttering individuals typically move more slowly than nonstuttering individuals. Interestingly, the longer movement durations seem to be found not only in the speech motor system but also in nonspeech motor systems, such as that controlling finger movements. Again, several suggestions could be consistent with these observations. For example, movement slowness could be a result of, among other things, a deficiency in the fast generation of agonist muscle activity or in precisely scaling the magnitude of this activity (Wlld *et al.* 1996), abnormally high levels of co-activation of antagonist muscle groups (Mink and Thach 1991), or a strategy to cope with the complexity of, or difficulty with, a motor task (Grosjean *et al.* 1997; Swinnen *et al.* 1997).

Thirdly, the available evidence suggests that stuttering individuals have problems with the processing of certain modalities of sensory information, or possibly with the integration of sensory and motor signals. Similar to the aforementioned movement slowness, these problems with the use of sensory information seem to be generalized rather than limited to the speech system (Forster and Webster 2001). Interestingly, the performance of stuttering individuals on tasks that rely heavily on an efficient and accurate use of sensory information (e.g. kinesthetic) typically improves when an additional source of sensory information (e.g. visual) is provided (De Nil and Abbs 1991; Howell *et al.* 1995; Forster and Webster 2001).

Fourthly, it is well documented now that stuttering adults differ from nonstuttering adults in the extent and localization of brain activity during stuttered as well as fluent speech. Such areas showing different activation are widely distributed throughout the brain, but it has been suggested that, overall, they point at an involvement of motor areas involved in the central preparation of muscle commands, as well as areas involved in sensory detection and processing, including the auditory system. An initial increase and then gradual decrease in brain activation after intensive stuttering treatment have been shown to occur in the cerebellum (De Nil *et al.* 2001).

Fifthly, behavioral data from stuttering adaptation paradigms indicate that individuals with developmental stuttering, but not those with stuttering acquired as a result of a brain lesion, typically become more fluent when repeatedly producing the same utterances. There is evidence from both behavioral and acoustic analyses suggesting that this decrease in stuttering frequency across repeated productions may be a form of motor learning.

Based on the reviewed information in general and these five summary statements in particular, I suggest here the possibility that individuals who stutter may have, or at least may have had during childhood, problems with the acquisition and/or refinement of the multiple internal models that allow adaptive sensorimotor control in the presence of varying conditions and task demands (see also Neilson and Neilson 1987, 1991). In other words, the essence of the disorder may lie in an inability to learn stable or correct mappings between motor and sensory signals and to update these mappings in the presence of rapid neural and craniofacial maturation during speech development. In addition to the complexity of the transformations already described above, speech production requires one or more additional transformations as the CNS also needs accurate forward and inverse representations of the conversion from articulatory movements to acoustic output.

After their initial acquisition during babbling and early speech, these internal models require continuous updating, due to the rapid developmental changes in neural, anatomical, and biomechanical characteristics during childhood. The developmental changes require that the internal representations of the commands-to-output transformations be updated in parallel. Indeed, rather dramatic anatomical changes that take place in the vocal tract during development have been well documented (Kent and Vorperian 1995). Consequently, children's motor systems face the challenging task of acquiring and updating multiple internal models for a continually changing neuromotor system. If, for some reason, the CNS would fail to accurately update the internal models to match the currently applicable transformations, it would become unable to predict with great precision the sensory consequences of planned movements and to derive the necessary commands for a desired sensory outcome.

If, then, the CNS determines that unexpected sensory consequences are encountered, or that incorrect commands were generated (i.e. there is a mismatch between expected and actual feedback), a possible result could be that it responds by re-attempting the movement and re-issuing the central commands, sustaining the already ongoing commands, generating modified commands, or applying a more general re-setting strategy—with each of these attempted 'repairs' resulting in prolonged or repeated muscle contractions until the sensory consequences are interpreted as matching the expected consequences or the motor commands are interpreted as correct. Interpreting the sensory consequences as different from the expected ones could happen when evaluating an efference copy of the motor commands with incorrect or unstable (e.g. inappropriately changing in response to time-varying features of feedback) internal models or, alternatively, when there is an actual error in the sensory transmission or processing. Judging the motor commands to be incorrect could also happen when evaluating a copy of those commands with unstable or incorrect internal models or, alternatively, when there is an actual error in movement preparation or execution. In either case, central commands to the muscles could be sustained (resulting in an audible or inaudible sound prolongation) or repeated (resulting in a sound or syllable repetition) until a correct prediction is made with a forward model and the sensory consequences are no longer unexpected, until a different set of commands is derived with an inverse model, or until the conflict is resolved or avoided by relying on online moment-to-moment feedback and related movement corrections.

In order to minimize the frequency of occurrence of the described maladaptive responses to motor–sensory mismatches—and thus to increase the likelihood that speech is produced fluently—the CNS of stuttering individuals may prefer a motor control strategy that involves longer movement durations, because longer durations allow more time for the processing and integration of sensory information. This feedback could be used for subtle adjustments during completion of the movement, and, therefore, to compensate for the reduced efficiency of the typical control scheme that relies heavily on internal models. Hence, the slower movements observed in stuttering speakers may represent a preferred motor strategy rather than a physiological limitation in movement speed. This suggestion has also been made by others, and it is in keeping with our own finding that individuals who stutter slow down much more, relative to individuals who do no stutter, on bilabial closing movements than on bilabial opening movements (Max *et al.* 2003*a*)—the relevance of this finding follows from the fact that both our own and others' studies have made it clear that closing movements are performed with shorter durations and, for most speakers, greater velocities than opening movements (Gracco 1994). In addition, the perspective is also consistent with the cerebellar imaging data of De Nil *et al.* (2001), which suggested that stuttering speakers' movements may be less automatized and more dependent on sensory or motor monitoring than those of nonstuttering speakers. Similarly, the brain imaging data from Wu and colleagues (Wu *et al.* 1995, 1997; Riley *et al.* 2001), implicating basal ganglia involvement in stuttering, are highly compatible with the proposed model, given that recent data have suggested a major role of dopaminergic systems in sensorimotor integration and learning (Huda *et al.* 2001; Suri *et al.* 2001; Fattapposta *et al.* 2002).

Clearly, these speculative ideas represent only the core elements of a broad framework that, if shown to be potentially useful, needs considerable further development. Indeed, for a number of key features associated with stuttering, it may be unclear at this point whether or not a satisfactory explanation can be formulated. Moreover, one could formulate a related, but alternative, proposal by suggesting that the internal models of stuttering individuals are as accurate and stable as those of nonstuttering individuals, but that the former group typically relies on a movement strategy that is inappropriately based toward afferent feedback control (Max *et al.* 2003*b*). At any rate, many critical features and research findings do seem to be compatible with the described perspective, and, in the following section, I will discuss how this perspective could possibly account for various phenomena known to be associated with stuttering.

14.4.2 Can the theoretical perspective account for the phenomena associated with stuttering?

I already mentioned earlier how the proposed internal model perspective on stuttering was derived from, and is compatible with, a large body of research that was reviewed and summarized above. Probably the greatest challenge for any perspective on stuttering, however, is to demonstrate how it can also account for numerous well-documented phenomena that are known to be associated with the disorder. I discuss here briefly how some of these phenomena could be interpreted in light of the proposed internal model perspective.

14.4.2.1 The peak years for onset of stuttering and spontaneous recovery during childhood

The perspective is highly compatible with an onset that occurs during early childhood—with the peak years between 2 and 4 years of age—but that shows relatively large variability across children. It is specifically proposed that stuttering may be related to an insufficient or incorrect learning or updating of the various dynamic, kinematic, and articulatory–acoustic internal models used for sensorimotor control of speech movements. As such, these difficulties may develop during the early childhood period, in which rapid changes in neural and musculoskeletal anatomy and physiology require continuous updating and refining of the internal models. Spontaneous recovery from stuttering during the childhood years may reflect successful acquisition or updating of the required internal models as a result of sensorimotor learning or neurobiological maturation.

14.4.2.2 Genetic factors play a role in the onset and development of stuttering

It has been suggested previously that not stuttering *per se* but a predisposition to develop stuttering may be the hereditary characteristic. It is conceivable that this predisposition may involve a neurologically based sensorimotor limitation that may or may not lead to persistent stuttering, depending on the influence of many other variables. This sensorimotor limitation could consist of difficulties with the learning and updating of stable and correct internal representations of the neural mappings between sensory and motor signals.

14.4.2.3 Stuttering manifests itself as a speech disorder but generalized difficulties may be present

Work by others, as well as from our own laboratory, has demonstrated generalized neuromotor differences between stuttering and nonstuttering individuals. It may be that stuttering individuals' deficiency in acquiring or updating accurate internal models of the neuromotor transformations applies to various effector systems, but that their difficulties are more obvious for speech movements than for nonspeech movements because the former requires representations of additional transformations (articulatory to acoustic). Moreover, speech involves very fast movements, achieved through an intricate coordination of multiple muscle systems. As compared with other motor systems, this may limit the extent to which predictive forward models can be replaced by closed-loop feedback-driven control in the case of incorrect or unstable internal models. In addition, speech is typically performed in the presence of high demands on the available neural resources (i.e. for cognitive–linguistic purposes) and this may limit both the extent to which planned motor commands are evaluated for prediction of the sensory consequences and the extent to which one can rely on online sensory processing for moment-to-moment movement corrections.

14.4.2.4 *DAF, FAF, masking, unison reading, and even visual perception of silent mouth movements have fluency-enhancing effects*

Given that PET studies during speech have indicated a failure to show the normal activation of auditory cortical areas in stuttering subjects, it is possible that the fluency-enhancing effect of delayed auditory feedback (DAF), frequency altered auditory feedback (FAF), masking, and unison reading is not a result of those modifications *per se*, but of their common role in providing an external auditory stimulus that facilitates activation of auditory cortex. This activation may have its fluency-enhancing influence primarily through an improved or even corrected monitoring of efference copies of the motor commands, rather than through altered monitoring of the actual feedback signal (Paus *et al.* 1996). In fact, such a role for the activation of auditory cortex could also explain why masking reduces stuttering and why it does so even when it is present during the *silent* intervals of conversational or read speech (Sutton and Chase 1961). In essence, it is speculated here that stuttering speakers typically fail to activate, or insufficiently activate, auditory cortex, and then adopt motor control strategies that involve longer movement durations to maximally benefit from the use of online proprioceptive feedback, thereby reducing the need to rely on internal models. However, if auditory cortical areas are activated by means of external auditory stimuli, efference copy monitoring may become more efficient and result in the considerable improvements in fluency observed under those conditions.

Interestingly, the above discussion of new insights into cortical activation patterns for speech and nonspeech tasks also made it clear that even visual observation of silent speech movements activates primary and secondary auditory cortex areas. The latter finding could account for a recent report that stuttering individuals show improvements in speech fluency when watching another individual perform silent speech movements (Kalinowski *et al.* 2000).

14.4.2.5 *The adaptation effect: stuttering frequency decreases with repeated practice*

The internal model perspective on stuttering seems highly consistent with the fact that speech production in stuttering individuals typically becomes considerably more fluent with repetitive practice, such as during the repeated readings in a stuttering adaptation paradigm. One could speculate that the repeated performance of the same sequences of articulatory and phonatory movements under unchanged external circumstances would allow more accurate predictions of the sensory consequences of those movements, as well as more accurate selection of motor commands based on the desired sensory consequences. Our previous hypothesis that stuttering adaptation represents a form of motor learning may be rephrased in a more specific way by hypothesizing that this learning comprises the updating and refining of existing internal models. This reasoning is in keeping with the finding that a motorically simplified (i.e. all voiced) speech task does not lead to an immediate decrease in stuttering frequency but to a more rapid learning with repeated practice (Adams and Reis 1974).

14.4.2.6 *Treatment outcome data: overlearning may be a critical component of therapy*

As far as stuttering in children is concerned, more treatment outcome data are available about the Lidcombe program, developed by Onslow and colleagues, than about any other treatment program (Onslow 1997). These clinical data suggest that the Lidcombe program, an operant conditioning approach, is highly effective in improving speech fluency in young children. To date, the reasons for this success are unclear, and research by the developers of the program has failed to show treatment-related changes in temporal measures of speech (Onslow *et al.* 2002). As part of the Lidcombe therapy, parents learn to 'correct' some of their child's moments of stuttering by pointing out in appropriate language that a moment of stuttering occurred and then asking the child to repeat the word in a fluent way. Some fluent productions are then repeated more than once with each production, followed by the necessary praise. It is suggested here that these repetitions of fluent productions may have a therapeutic effect as a result of a form of overlearning that contributes to the development of more stable or more accurate internal models. Indirect evidence in support of this position can be found in data on behavioral improvements in nonhuman primate arm movements that were performed while the animal was wearing prism glasses (Yin and Kitazawa 2001). Findings demonstrated that even when movements were practiced until movement error disappeared, the effects were transient, and that it was only when additional repetitions were performed with approximately zero error that motor memory consolidation occurred.

14.5 Conclusions: toward empirical testing

It is likely that progress in unraveling the mechanisms underlying stuttering would be considerably enhanced if more research programs would include theoretically driven experiments. This requires the availability of theoretical perspectives that have been formulated in a way that is sufficiently general to incorporate various phenomena associated with the disorder, but also sufficiently detailed to derive specific and testable hypotheses. Unfortunately, recent years have witnessed very few attempts of this nature.

In this chapter, I have proposed such a theoretical perspective that is, at this time, largely speculative. That is, although the perspective has its foundation in, and is compatible with, a large body of speech and nonspeech motor control research with both stuttering and nonstuttering individuals, to date there have been no empirical tests of hypotheses specifically derived from this perspective. However, its main value lies in the fact that several such testable hypotheses can be generated and subjected to empirical verification.

Although generating those specific hypotheses is beyond the scope of this chapter, some general suggestions follow readily from a summary of the main components of the proposed perspective. In essence, I have suggested the possibility that the onset of stuttering may be related to difficulties with the formation, consolidation, and/or updating of internal models that correspond to neural mappings between central motor commands and the sensory consequences resulting from those movements. The core characteristics of the disorder (speech dysfluencies) would be considered maladaptive attempts to correct for (correctly or incorrectly) perceived discrepancies between the anticipated sensory consequences that were predicted on the basis of an efference copy of the central motor commands and the actual sensory consequences of the unfolding movements. Therefore, speech and nonspeech experiments could be designed to test whether stuttering children and/or adults have difficulty learning, consolidating, or updating the relationship between motor commands and movement consequences in sensorimotor learning and sensorimotor adaptation paradigms. Furthermore, speech and nonspeech experiments could be designed to test whether stuttering and nonstuttering children and/or adults differ with regard to how much detail about the movement consequences is taken into account during motor planning (for example, the effects of movement kinematic parameters on aerodynamic conditions in the vocal tract). Another line of possible experiments could be related to the modulation of auditory cortex activity that takes place both prior to and during speech production, and that is apparently associated with anticipation of the expected auditory feedback (Houde *et al.* 2002).

In the end, the potential for success of the proposal described herein should be measured not by its accuracy or completeness, as clearly neither of those two ideals has been achieved at this time. Instead, if this perspective will contribute to generating more specific hypotheses that are subsequently subjected to empirical testing, this work will have achieved its goal.

Acknowledgement

Writing of this chapter was supported, in part, by NIH Grant DC 03102.

References

Adams, M.R. and **Reis, R.** (1974). Influence of the onset of phonation on the frequency of stuttering: a replication and reevaluation. *Journal of Speech and Hearing Research,* **17**, 752–4.

Alfonso, P.J. (1991). Implications of the concepts underlying task-dynamic modeling on kinematic studies of stuttering. In H.F.M. Peters, W. Hulstijn and C.W. Starkweather, eds. *Speech motor control and stuttering,* pp. 79–100. Elsevier, Amsterdam.

Balasubramanian, V., Max, L., Van Borsel, J., Rayca, K.O. and **Richardson, D.** (2003). Acquired stuttering following right frontal and bilateral pontine lesion: a case study. *Brain and Cognition,* in press.

Berardelli, A., Hallett, M., Rothwell, J.C., Agostino, R., Manfredi, M., Thompson, P.D. and **Marsden, C.D.** (1996). Single-joint rapid arm movements in normal subjects and in patients with motor disorders. *Brain,* **119**, 661–74.

Bhushan, N. and **Shadmehr, R.** (1999). Computational nature of human adaptive control during learning of reaching movements in force fields. *Biological Cybernetics,* **81**, 39–60.

Binkofski, F., Amunts, K., Stephan, K.M. *et al.* (2000). Broca's region subserves imagery of motion: a combined cytoarchitectonic and fMRI study. *Human Brain Mapping,* **11**, 273–85.

Bishop, J.H., Williams, H.G. and **Cooper, W.A.** (1991). Age and task complexity variables in motor performance of stuttering and nonstuttering children. *Journal of Fluency Disorders,* **16**, 207–17.

Blakemore, S.J., Goodbody, S.J. and **Wolpert, D.M.** (1998*a*). Predicting the consequences of our own actions: the role of sensorimotor context estimation. *Journal of Neuroscience,* **18**, 7511–18.

Blakemore, S.-J., Wolpert, D. and **Frith, C.** (1998*b*). Central cancellation of self-produced tickle sensation. *Nature Neuroscience,* **1**, 635–40.

Blakemore, S.-J., Frith, C.D. and **Wolpert D.M.** (2001). The cerebellum is involved in predicting the sensory consequences of action. *NeuroReport,* **12**, 1879–84.

Bloodstein, O. (1995). *A handbook on stuttering* (5th edn). Singular, San Diego.

Borden, G.J. and **Armson, J.** (1987). Coordination of laryngeal and supralaryngeal behavior in stutterers. In H.F.M. Peters and W. Hulstijn, eds. *Speech motor dynamics in stuttering,* pp. 209–14. Springer-Verlag, Wien.

Borden, G.J., Kim, D.H. and **Spiegler, K.** (1987). Acoustics of stop consonant-vowel relationships during fluent and stuttered utterances. *Journal of Fluency Disorders,* **12**, 175–84.

Boutsen, F. (1995). A comparative study of stress timing of stutterers and nonstutterers. *Journal of Fluency Disorders,* **20**, 145–56.

Brashers-Krug, T., Shadmehr, R. and **Bizzi, E.** (1996). Consolidation in human motor memory. *Nature,* **382**, 252–5.

Braun, A.R., Varga, M., Stager, S. et al. (1997). Altered patterns of cerebral activity during speech and language production in developmental stuttering: An $H_2(^{15})O$ positron emission tomography study. *Brain*, **120**, 761–84.

Buccino, G., Binkofski, F., Fink, G.R. et al. (2001). Action observation activates premotor and parietal areas in a somatotopic manner: an fMRI study. *European Journal of Neuroscience*, **13**, 400–4.

Calvert, G.A., Bullmore, E.T., Brammer, M.J., et al. (1997). Activation of auditory cortex during silent lipreading. *Science*, **276**, 593–6.

Campbell, R., MacSweeney, M., Surguladze, S. et al. (2001). Cortical substrates for the perception of face actions: an fMRI study of the specificity of activation for seen speech and for meaningless lower-face acts (gurning). *Cognitive Brain Research*, **12**, 233–43.

Caruso, A.J., Gracco, V.L. and **Abbs, J.H.** (1987). A speech motor control perspective on stuttering: preliminary observations. In H.F.M. Peters and W. Hulstijn, eds. *Speech motor dynamics in stuttering*, pp. 245–58. Springer-Verlag, Wien.

Caruso, A.J., Abbs, J.H. and **Gracco, V.L.** (1988a). Kinematic analysis of multiple movement coordination during speech in stutterers. *Brain*, **111**, 439–56.

Caruso, A.J., Conture, E.G. and **Colton, R.H.** (1988b). Selected temporal parameters of coordination associated with stuttering in children. *Journal of Fluency Disorders*, **13**, 57–82.

Conture, E.G., Colton, R.H. and **Gleason, J.R.** (1988). Selected temporal aspects of coordination during fluent speech of young stutterers. *Journal of Speech and Hearing Research*, **31**, 640–53.

Curio, G., Neuloh, G., Numminen, J., Jousmäki, V. and **Hari, R.** (2000). Speaking modifies voice-evoked activity in the human auditory cortex. *Human Brain Mapping*, **9**, 183–91.

De Nil, L. (1995). The role of oral sensory feedback in the coordination of articulatory movements in adults who stutter: a hypothesis. In C.W. Starkweather and H.F.M. Peters, eds. *Proceedings of the First World Congress on Fluency Disorders*, pp. 19–22. University of Nijmegen, Nijmegen, The Netherlands.

De Nil, L.F. and **Abbs, J.H.** (1991). Kinaesthetic acuity of stutterers and non-stutterers for oral and non-oral movements. *Brain*, **114**, 2145–58.

De Nil, L.F., Kroll, R.M., Kapur, S. and **Houle, S.** (2000). A positron emission tomography study of silent and oral single word reading in stuttering and nonstuttering adults. *Journal of Speech, Language, and Hearing Research*, **43**, 1038–53.

De Nil, F., Kroll, R. M. and **Houle, S.** (2001). Functional neuroimaging of cerebellar activation during single word reading and verb generation in stuttering and nonstuttering adults. *Neuroscience Letters*, **302**, 77–80.

Fattapposta, F., Pierelli, F., My, F., et al. (2002). L-dopa effects on preprogramming and control activity in a skilled motor act in Parkinson's disease. *Clinical Neurophysiology*, **113**, 243–53.

Flament, D., Ellermann, J.M., Kim, S.G., Ugurbil, K. and **Ebner, T. J.** (1996). Functional magnetic resonance imaging of cerebellar activation during the learning of a visuomotor dissociation task. *Human Brain Mapping,* **4**, 210–26.

Flanagan, J.R. and **Lolley, S.** (2001). The inertial anisotropy of the arm is accurately predicted during movement planning. *Journal of Neuroscience,* **21**, 1361–9.

Forster, D.C. and **Webster, W.G.** (2001). Speech-motor control and interhemispheric relations in recovered and persistent stuttering. *Developmental Neuropsychology,* **19**, 125–45.

Fox, P.T., Ingham, R.J., Ingham, J.C., *et al.* (1996). A PET study of the neural systems of stuttering. *Nature,* **382**, 158–61.

Fox, P.T., Ingham, R.J., Ingham, J.C., Zamarripa, F., Xiong, J.-H. and **Lancaster, J.L.** (2000). Brain correlates of stuttering and syllable production: a PET performance-correlation analysis. *Brain,* **123**, 1985–2004.

Gracco, V.L. (1994). Some organizational characteristics of speech movement control. *Journal of Speech and Hearing Research,* **37**, 4–27.

Grafton, S.T., Woods, R.P. and **Tyszka, M.** (1994). Functional imaging of procedural motor learning: relating cerebral blood flow with individual subject performance. *Human Brain Mapping,* **1**, 221–34.

Grosjean, M., van Galen, G.P., de Jong, P., van Lieshout, P.H.H.M. and **Hulstijn, W.** (1997). Is stuttering caused by failing neuromuscular force control? In W. Hulstijn, H.F.M. Peters and P.H.H.M. van Lieshout, eds. *Speech production: motor control, brain research and fluency disorders,* pp. 197–204. Elsevier, New York.

Hallett, M. and **Khoshbin, S.A.** (1980). A physiological mechanism of bradykinesia. *Brain,* **103**, 301–14.

Hefter, H., Arendt, G., Stremmel, W. and **Freund H.J.** (1993). Motor impairment in Wilson's disease, I: slowness of voluntary limb movements. *Acta Neurologica Scandinavia,* **87**, 133–47.

Hickok, G., Erhard, P., Kassubek, J. *et al.* (2000). A functional magnetic resonance imaging study of the role of left posterior superior temporal gyrus in speech production: implications for the explanation of conduction aphasia. *Neuroscience Letters,* **287**, 156–60.

Houde, J.F. and **Jordan, M.I.** (1998). Sensorimotor adaptation in speech production. *Science,* **279**, 1213–16.

Houde, J.F., Nagarajan, S.S., Sekihara, K. and **Merzenich, M.M.** (2002). Modulation of the auditory cortex during speech: an MEG study. *Journal of Cognitive Neuroscience,* **14**, 1125–38.

Howell, P., Sackin, S. and **Rustin, L.** (1995). Comparison of speech motor development in stutterers and fluent speakers between 7 and 12 years old. *Journal of Fluency Disorders,* **20**, 243–56.

Huda, K., Salunga, T.L. and **Matsunamic, K.** (2001). Dopaminergic inhibition of excitatory inputs onto pyramidal tract neurons in cat motor cortes. *Neuroscience Letters,* **307**, 175–8.

Hutchinson, J.M. and **Watkin, K.L.** (1976). Jaw mechanics during release of the stuttering moment: some initial observations and interpretations. *Journal of Communication Disorders,* **9**, 269–79.

Imamizu, H., Miyauchi, S., Tamada, T., *et al.* (2000). Human cerebellar activity reflecting an acquired internal model of a new tool. *Nature,* **403**, 192–5.

Ingham, R.J. (2001). Brain imaging studies of developmental stuttering. *Journal of Communication Disorders,* **34**, 493–516.

Ingham, R.J., Fox, P.T., Ingham, J.C. and **Zamarripa, F.** (2000). Is overt stuttered speech a prerequisite for the neural activations associated with chronic developmental stuttering? *Brain and Language,* **75**, 163–94.

Jahanshahi, M., Rowe, J. and **Fuller, R.** (2001). Impairment of movement initiation and execution but not preparation in idiopathic dystonia. *Experimental Brain Research,* **140**, 460–8.

Jäncke, L., Bauer, A., Haakert, O. and **Kalveram, K.** (1995*a*). Patterns of interarticulator phasing relations in stutterers and nonstutterers. In C.W. Starkweather and H.F.M. Peters, eds. *Proceedings of the First World Congress on Fluency Disorders,* pp. 23–6. University of Nijmegen, Nijmegen, The Netherlands.

Jäncke, L., Kaiser, P., Bauer, A. and **Kalveram, T.** (1995*b*). Upper lip, lower lip, and jaw peak velocity sequence during bilabial closures: no differences between stutterers and nonstutterers. *Journal of the Acoustical Society of America,* **97**, 3900–3.

Jeannerod, M. (2001). Neural simulation of action: a unifying mechanism for motor cognition. *NeuroImage,* **14**, S103–S109.

Kalinowski, J., Stuart, A., Rastatter, M.P., Snyder, G. and **Dayalu, V.** (2000). Inducement of fluent speech in persons who stutter via visual choral speech. *Neuroscience Letters,* **281**, 198–200.

Kawato, M. and **Wolpert, D.M.** (1998). Internal models for motor control. In M. Glickstein, ed. *Sensory guidance of movement,* pp. 291–307. Wiley, Chichster, UK.

Kent, R.D. and **Vorperian, H.K.** (1995). Development of the craniofacial-oral-laryngeal anatomy: a review. *Journal of Medical Speech-Language Pathology,* **3**, 145–90.

Kleinow, J. and **Smith, A.** (2000). Influences of length and syntactic complexity on the speech motor stability of the fluent speech of adults who stutter. *Journal of Speech, Language, and Hearing Research,* **43**, 548–59.

Lotze, M., Montoya, P., Erb, M., *et al.* (1999). Activation of cortical and cerebellar motor areas during executed and imagined hand movements: an fMRI study. *Journal of Cognitive Neuroscience,* **11**, 491–501.

Loucks, T.M.J. and **De Nil, L.F.** (2001). Oral kinesthetic deficit in stuttering evaluated by movement accuracy and tendon vibration. In B. Maassen, W. Hulstijn, R. Kent, H. F. M. Peters and P. H. H. M. van Lieshout, eds. *Speech motor control in normal and disordered speech,* pp. 307–10. Vantilt, Nijmegen, The Netherlands.

Maguire, G.A., Riley, G.D., Franklin, D.L. and **Gottschalk, L. A.** (2000). Risperidone for the treatment of stuttering. *Journal of Clinical Psychopharmacology,* **20**, 479–82.

Mattay, V.S., Tessitore, A., Callicott, J.H., *et al.* (2002). Dopaminergic modulation of cortical function in patients with Parkinson's disease. *Annals of Neurology,* **51**, 156–64.

Max, L. and **Caruso, A.J.** (1998). Adaptation of stuttering frequency during repeated readings: associated changes in acoustic parameters of perceptually fluent speech. *Journal of Speech, Language, and Hearing Research,* **41**, 1265–81.

Max, L. and **Glass, N.P.** (2001). Relative timing of oral and laryngeal speech movements in individuals who stutter. In H.G. Bosshardt, J.S. Yaruss and H.F.M. Peters, eds. *Proceedings of the Third World Congress on Fluency Disorders,* pp. 78–82. University of Nijmegen, Nijmegen, The Netherlands.

Max, L., and **Gracco, V.L.** (2003). *Coordination of oral and laryngeal movements in the perceptually fluent speech of adults who stutter,* submitted.

Max, L. and **Yudman, E.M.** (2003). Accuracy and variability of isochronous rhythmic movement timing across motor systems in stuttering versus nonstuttering individuals. *Journal of Speech, Language, and Hearing Research,* **46**, 146–63.

Max, L., Caruso, A.J. and **Vandevenne, A.** (1997). Decreased stuttering frequency during repeated readings: a motor learning perspective. *Journal of Fluency Disorders,* **21**, 1–17.

Max, L., Caruso, A.J. and **Gracco, V.L.** (2003*a*). Kinematic analyses of speech, orofacial nonspeech, and finger movements in stuttering and nonstuttering individuals. *Journal of Speech, Language, and Hearing Research,* **46**, 215–32.

Max, L., Gracco, V.L., Guenther, F.H., Ghosh, S.S. and **Wallace, M.E.** (2003*b*). *A sensorimotor model of stuttering: Insights from the neuroscience of motor control,* In A. Packman, A. Meltzer and H.F.M. Peters (Eds.), *Proceedings of the 4th World Congress on Fluency Disorders.* Montreal, Canada.

Max, L., Wallace, M.E. and **Vincent, I.** (2003*c*). Sensorimotor adaptation to auditory perturbations during speech: acoustic and kinematic experiments. In M. J. Solé, D. Recasens and J. Romeno (Eds.), *Proceedings of the 15th International Congress of Phonetic Sciences* (pp. 1053–1056). Barcelona, Spain.

McClean, M.D. (1996). Lip-muscle reflexes during speech movement preparation in stutterers. *Journal of Fluency Disorders,* **21**, 49–60.

McClean, M.D., Kroll, R.M. and **Loftus N.S.** (1990). Kinematic analysis of lip closure in stutterers' fluent speech. *Journal of Speech and Hearing Research,* **33**, 755–60.

Medland, S.E., Geffen, G. and **McFarland, K.** (2002). Lateralization of speech production using verbal/manual dual tasks: meta-analysis of sex differences and practice effects. *Neuropsychologia,* **40**, 1233–9.

Miall, R.C., Weir, D.J., Wolpert, D.M. and **Stein J.F.** (1993). Is the cerebellum a Smith predictor? *Journal of Motor Behavior,* **25**, 203–16.

Mikheev, M., Mohr, C., Afanasiev, S., Landis, T. and **Thut, G.** (2002). Motor control and cerebral hemispheric specialization in highly qualified judo wrestlers. *Neuropsychologia,* **40**, 1209–19.

Mink, J.W. and **Thach, W.T.** (1991). Basal ganglia motor control. III. Pallidal ablation: normal reaction time, muscle cocontraction, and slow movement. *Journal of Neurophysiology*, **65**, 330–51.

Neilson, M.D. and **Neilson, P.D.** (1987). Speech motor control and stuttering: a computational model of adaptive sensory-motor processing. *Speech Communication*, **6**, 325–33.

Neilson, M.D. and **Neilson, P.D.** (1991). Adaptive model theory of speech motor control and stuttering. In H.F.M. Peters, W. Hulstijn and C.W. Starkweather, eds. *Speech motor control and stuttering*, pp. 149–56. Elsevier, Amsterdam, The Netherlands.

Numminen, J., Salmelin, R. and **Hari, R.** (1999). Subject's own speech reduces reactivity of the human auditory cortex. *Neuroscience Letters*, **265**, 119–22.

Onslow, M. (1997). Long-term outcome of early intervention for stuttering. *American Journal of Speech-Language Pathology*, **6**, 51–8.

Onslow, M., Stocker, S., Packman, A. and **McLeod, S.** (2002). Speech timing in children after the Lidcombe Program of early stuttering intervention. *Clinical Linguistics and Phonetics*, **16**, 21–33.

Paus, T., Perry, D.W., Zatorre, R.J., Worsley, K.J. and **Evans, A.C.** (1996). Modulation of cerebral blood flow in the human auditory cortex during speech: role of motor-to-sensory discharges. *European Journal of Neuroscience*, **8**, 2236–46.

Peters, H.F.M. and **Hulstijn W.** (1987). Programming and initiation of speech utterances in stuttering. In H.F.M. Peters and W. Hulstijn, eds. *Speech motor dynamics in stuttering*, pp. 185–96. Springer-Verlag, New York.

Riley, G., Maguire, G. and **Wu, J.C.** (2001). Brain imaging to examine a dopamine hypothesis in stuttering. In B. Maassen, W. Hulstijn, R. Kent, H.F.M. Peters and P.H.H.M. van Lieshout, eds. *Speech motor control in normal and disordered speech*, pp. 156–58. Vantilt, Nijmegen.

Seitz, R.J., Canavan, A.G., Yaguez, L., *et al.* (1994). Successive roles of the cerebellum and premotor cortices in trajectorial learning. *NeuroReport*, **5**, 2541–4.

Shadmehr, R. and **Brashers-Krug, T.** (1997). Functional stages in the formation of human long-term motor memory. *Journal of Neuroscience*, **17**, 409–19.

Shadmehr, R. and **Mussa-Ivaldi, F.A.** (1994). Adaptive representation of dynamics during learning of a motor task. *Journal of Neuroscience*, **14**, 3208–24.

Shaywitz, B.A., Shaywitz, S.E., Pugh, K.R. *et al.* (1995). Sex differences in the functional organization of the brain for language. *Nature*, **373**, 607–9.

Smith, A. and **Kleinow, J.** (2000). Kinematic correlates of speaking rate changes in stuttering and normally fluent adults. *Journal of Speech, Language, and Hearing Research*, **43**, 521–36.

Sutton, S. and **Chase, R.A.** (1961). White noise and stuttering. *Journal of Speech and Hearing Research*, **4**, 72.

Swinnen, S.P., Van Langendonk, L., Verschueren, S., Peeters, G., Dom, R. and **De Weerdt, W.** (1997). Interlimb coordination deficits in patients with Parkinson's disease during the production of two-joint oscillations in the sagittal plane. *Movements Disorders*, **12**, 958–68.

Thompson, P.D., Berardelli, A., Rothwell, J.C., *et al.* (1988). The coexistence of bradykinesia and chorea in Huntington's disease, and its implications for theories of basal ganglia control of movement. *Brain*, **111**, 223–44.

Thoroughman, K.A. and **Shadmehr, R.** (1999). Electromyographic correlates of learning an internal model of reaching movements. *Journal of Neuroscience*, **19**, 8573–88.

van Mier, H., Tempel, L.W., Perlmutter, S.J., Raichle, M.E. and **Petersen, S.E.** (1998). Changes in brain activity during motor learning measured with PET: effects of hand of performance and practice. *Journal of Neurophysiology*, **80**, 2177–99.

Wang T., Dordevic, G.S. and **Shadmehr, R.** (2001). Learning the dynamics of reaching movements results in the modification of arm impedance and long-latency perturbation responses. *Biological Cybernetics*, **85**, 437–48.

Webster, W.G. (1997). Principles of human brain organization related to lateralization of language and speech motor functions in normal speakers and stutterers. In W. Hulstijn, H.F.M. Peters and P.H.H.M. van Lieshout, eds. *Speech production: motor control, brain research and fluency disorders*, pp. 119–39. Elsevier, Amsterdam, The Netherlands.

Webster, W.G. and **Ryan, C.R.L.** (1991). Task complexity and manual reaction times in people who stutter. *Journal of Speech and Hearing Research*, **34**, 708–14.

Wild, B., Klockgether, T. and **Dichgans, J.** (1996). Acceleration deficit in patients with cerebellar lesions: a study of kinematic and EMG-parameters in fast wrist movements. *Brain Research*, **713**, 186–91.

Wing, A.M. and **Kristofferson, A.B.** (1973). Response delays and the timing of discrete motor responses. *Perception and Psychophysics*, **14**, 5–12.

Wolpert, D.M., Miall, R.C. and **Kawato, M.** (1998*a*). Internal models in the cerebellum. *Trends in Cognitive Science*, **2**, 338–47.

Wolpert, D.M., Goodbody, S.J. and **Husain, M.** (1998*b*). Maintaining internal representations: the role of the human superior parietal lobe. *Nature Neuroscience*, **1**, 529–33.

Wu, J.C., Maguire, G., Riley, G., *et al.* (1995). A positron emission tomography [^{18}F]deoxyglucose study of developmental stuttering. *NeuroReport*, **6**, 501–5.

Wu, J.C., Maguire, G., Riley, G., *et al.* (1997). Increased dopamine activity associated with stuttering. *NeuroReport*, **8**, 767–70.

Yin, P.-B. and **Kitazawa, S.** (2001). Long-lasting aftereffects of prism adaptation in the monkey. *Experimental Brain Research*, **141**, 250–3.

Yoshioka, H. and **Löfqvist, A.** (1981). Laryngeal involvement in stuttering: a glottographic observation using a reaction time paradigm. *Folia Phoniatrica*, **33**, 348–57.

Zebrowski, P.M., Conture, E.G. and **Cudahy, E.A.** (1985). Acoustic analysis of young stutterers' fluency: preliminary observations. *Journal of Fluency Disorders*, **10**, 173–92.

Zelaznik, H.N., Smith, A. and **Franz, E.A.** (1994). Motor performance of stutterers and nonstutterers on timing and force control tasks. *Journal of Motor Behavior*, **26**, 340–7.

Zelaznik, H.N., Smith, A., Franz, E. and **Ho., M.** (1997). Differences in bimanual coordination associated with stuttering. *Acta Psychologica*, **96**, 229–43.

Zimmermann, G. (1980). Articulatory dynamics of fluent utterances of stutterers and nonstutterers. *Journal of Speech and Hearing Research*, **23**, 95–107.

CHAPTER 15

THE DIFFERENTIAL DIAGNOSIS OF APRAXIA OF SPEECH

MALCOLM R. MCNEIL, SHEILA R. PRATT, AND TEPANTA R.D. FOSSETT

15.1 Introduction

The study of apraxia of speech (AOS) has received renewed interest in the past 5 or 6 years, as evidenced by several large critical reviews (McNeil *et al.* 1997, 2000; Code 1998; Ballard *et al.* 2000; Miller 2000). This interest was preceded by earlier description (e.g. Itoh *et al.* 1979; Katz 1987; Odell *et al.* 1990, 1991), experimentation (e.g. Monoi *et al.* 1983) and hypotheses about the nature of AOS (e.g. Darley *et al.* 1975; Kelso and Tuller 1981; Wertz *et al.* 1984) and has been expressed in a recent flurry of theoretical formulations (van der Merwe 1997; Dogil and Mayer 1998; Whiteside and Varley 1998; Rogers and Storkel 1999; Miller 2002; Ziegler 2002, 2003*a, b*; Ballard *et al.* 2003). These formulations follow a history, encompassing 30 years and more, of perceptual, acoustic and physiologic descriptions of AOS, and comparisons to other similar populations. In spite of this rich history and the renewed interest in AOS, theoretical developments and experimental research are not likely to advance understanding of this theoretically interesting and clinically challenging entity much beyond what is currently known without a substantive change in the behavioral criteria by which subjects are identified for study. Likewise, while accidents of nature (e.g. strokes, penetrating brain injuries, tumors) rarely produce isolated and one-dimensional categories of speech and language pathology, it is critical for clinical purposes to make differential diagnoses. A change in the clinical criteria by which AOS patients are selected for treatment is required for this to be effective. It is the thesis of this argument that it is not a lack of theory or the inability to select the correct theory from the known alternatives that limits understanding of AOS, although these issues are also challenges. Neither is it the inability to construct critical experiments, nor the inability to select the appropriate level of description or contrast with the appropriate comparison group that limits understanding of AOS. It is, likewise, not the lack of neurologic or anatomic instantiation that limits AOS understanding. The most important impediment to theoretical and clinical advancement in AOS is, however, the lack of a comprehensive and clear definition that leads to an agreed-upon set of criteria for subject selection. Although it has historical legitimacy, the perpetuation of this overriding problem will continue to diminish, confound and block the study of, and clinical advancements in, AOS. In spite of this overriding problem, there is sufficient coherence among the many studies investigating the entity across the psycholinguistic, acoustic, and physiologic (kinematic, aerodynamic, electromyographic) levels of description to characterize both the unique and shared features of the disorder. Importantly, recent models of speech production are consistent with the differential attribution of the core behaviors characterizing AOS to motoric versus linguistic levels of processing. Taken together, these theoretical advances, along with the slow accumulation of data on a few carefully selected and described subjects, and the sifting and winnowing of recurrent attributes from the not-so-carefully defined and selected subject populations, make it possible to propose a set of criteria for the diagnosis of AOS. Additionally, these theoretical advances aid differential diagnosis among AOS and its nearest clinical neighbors. Below we outline the historical antecedents for the current diagnostic dilemma in AOS. We also offer evidence that the current criteria for diagnosis are seriously confounded. This evidence comes from the most popular definition of AOS, criteria currently used for the diagnosis of AOS, experimental data, and lesion location evidence. Finally, criteria for diagnosis will be proposed that are consistent with the differential assignment of speech errors to phonologic and motoric mechanisms, and models of speech production that are based on a summary of evidence derived from recurring experimental findings.

15.2 Brief historical context

Sound-level speech-production deficits following neurological insult had a two-part supraordinate classification for most theorists and clinicians preceding Darley's (1968) observations and seminal paper on apraxia of speech. Although others likely observed patients that challenged the aphasia/dysarthria dichotomy, the critical observation of behaviors and the attempt to connect them to a theoretical mechanism (e.g. impaired motor programming) is correctly attributed to Darley. With this early formulation came a program of studies by Darley and his protégées designed to describe the phenomenon, outline its differences from dysarthria and the conditions under which it was elicited and modified. As noted by McNeil *et al.* (1997), the question for Darley and his colleagues is the question confronted by any clinical pioneer. That is, on what basis is the selection of subjects made when trying to identify and characterize a new clinical entity?

> Without established inclusional and exclusional criteria, derived from
> careful experimentation, usually accumulated over a long period of
> time, and founded on well-established models that specify the levels of

breakdown and the potential mechanisms responsible for the phenomena (neither of which were available during Darley's early formulations
of AOS), it is difficult or impossible to have confidence that the individuals and groups actually represent the subjects of interest.

(McNeil *et al.* 1997, p. 315).

This possibility did not escape the AOS critics, perhaps most notably Martin (1974),
who objected to the application of the term AOS to the subjects selected for study
to that point in time. It is important to recognize that Martin did not object to the
existence of AOS, nor did he believe that AOS was actually aphasia. He recognized
that AOS was, by definition, a disorder of motor programming. As discussed below,
there is in fact indirect evidence that ambiguous behavioral criteria, along with the
lack of models used to guide error elicitation and attribution, led Darley and many
that followed to a set of subject classification criteria that has been at the heart
of much of the controversy surrounding AOS since its recognition and early
characterizations.

Speech-production models that clearly differentiated phonologic from motoric
deficits at the time of Darley's proposal of AOS were, for the most part, non-existent. Those that were available addressed little of relevance to the differential diagnosis of AOS. At that time, aphasia was characterized within the two-stage model
as a disorder at the linguistic level. Within this model, a phonological deficit, as
with deficits at all linguistic levels, was characterized as a competence-based or
language *representation* deficit, suggesting that when language was impaired with
adult-acquired onset, the deficits resulted in a supramodal disorder that crossed all
modalities and levels of language (Schuell *et al.* 1964; Brown 1968). Phonological-
level production disorders would necessarily be accompanied by comparable auditory perceptual disorders. Separate phonological input and output systems were
not entertained in the language models at the time that Darley recognized this
non-aphasic/non-dysarthric entity. The consequence of this inability to identify
selective phonological output disorders that occurred without comparable phonological perceptual and/or comprehension problems was that they were subsumed
within this newly recognized category that was presumed and intended to be *not
aphasia* and *not dysarthria*.

The dysarthrias were generally regarded as a family of disorders that existed at
the *execution* level of the motor system. The execution level of the speech-production model was conceived of as operating from information derived from the
language system that was simply carried out to the muscles for movement. Only
the basic physiology of the nervous system (tone, reflexes, nerve conduction time,
etc.) and the muscles (neuromuscular transmitter, fiber type and size, etc.) and
their biomechanical properties were said to affect the coordinated movements
within and between muscles at this stage of production. The assumption was that
language and other cognitive factors did not have an affect at this stage of speech

production. At this stage of the model, errors across the speech systems (phonation, resonance, articulation, and prosody) were accounted for as errors of timing, range, rate, force, steadiness, and direction of movement, both within and across articulators and speech systems. These movement errors resulted in speech errors of distortion (predominantly), substitution, omission, and addition (rarely). While a third motor programming level existed for the limb system in the form of limb apraxias, it did not exist for the speech-production system. It was only with Darley's proposal of AOS as a unique disorder of motor programming, that the two-level neuropsychological model underpinning speech-production disorders was challenged. This three-level model of sound-level speech-production disorders has survived without serious challenge until recently. In 1997, van der Merwe proposed an explicit division of speech motor *planning* from speech motor *programming*, which, until this time, had routinely been used synonymously and interchangeably. This model, described in greater detail below, provides an important fourth level to account for sound-level speech-production disorders, and makes a clear assignment of the apraxic speech errors to the motor level of impairment.

15.3 Experimental evidence for confounded selection criteria

Without a priori selection criteria, it is difficult or impossible to know if the individuals selected for any particular study of AOS actually represent the population of interest. A study by Halpern *et al.* (1976) is one example of many such studies (e.g. Rochon *et al.* 1991; Dronkers 1997) providing evidence that the generally accepted diagnostic criteria not only include subjects with phonemic paraphasias (PP), but that they perhaps guarantee their admission. Halpern *et al.* (1976) asked whether persons with aphasia actually make phonological production errors, and if they do, if there is a pattern to the errors. They carefully excluded subjects with dysarthria and with AOS so as to test the hypothesis of interest. Subjects were excluded if they 'made articulation errors referable to significant weakness, slowness, incoordination or alteration of tone of the speech muscular' (p. 366) so as to eliminate persons with dysarthria. They also excluded subjects if they 'showed groping, off target, highly inconsistent articulatory errors—primarily substitutions, additions, prolongations and repetitions—in attempting target words in the context of islands of fluent speech, these errors being especially evident on repetition tasks and increasing in incidence with increase in length of word' (p. 366). The results of the study were that 93% of the subjects made *no* phonemic errors. Of the errors that were produced by the two subjects who did make phonemic errors, 75% were attributable to word-level errors. The authors concluded: 'Aphasic behavior is not characterized by significant breakdown of articulatory performance' (p. 371). As there is abundant evidence that phonemic errors are not an infrequently observed error in most persons with aphasia, especially those labeled as *conduction aphasia*, it seems likely that the criteria set for the exclusion of the subjects with AOS eliminated all subjects with phonological-level impairments as well as those with AOS. In addition, many of the behaviors used to exclude persons with AOS are strikingly similar (some identical) to the behaviors that Goodglass (1992) used to describe and classify the speech-production impairments of persons with conduction aphasia (e.g. phoneme and syllable omissions, substitutions, repetition deficits, increased errors with increased word length, unsuccessful repeated attempts at self-correction). Indeed, the definitions of AOS and the error patterns used for its diagnosis support the conclusion that the AOS database is likely greatly confounded. In addition, as discussed above, some error types used to identify AOS are frankly inconsistent with the mechanisms prescribed by the term. Evidence for differential patterns of speech errors across patients or hypothesized populations is necessary to establish a coherent clinical category. Additionally, the validity of the behavioral patterns is fortified when appropriately well-developed and instantiated models provide coherence with error generation and assignment at a specific level of the model. Such models and coherence do exist. These issues will be addressed following a brief discussion of a definition of AOS and the primary speech characteristics that historically have been attributed to the disorder, those that are unique to the disorder as revealed through a careful sifting and winnowing of the literature, and those that are theoretically coherent with the disorder as a motor speech disorder.

15.4 Speech characteristics and definition of AOS

Perhaps the most cited and influential definition of AOS is that of Wertz *et al.* (1984). They defined AOS as 'a neurogenic *phonologic* disorder resulting from sensorimotor impairment of the capacity to select, program and/or *execute* in coordinated and normally timed sequences, the positioning of the speech musculature for the *volitional* production of speech sounds' (p. 4). Assigning the deficit to the *phonologic* level of speech production has caused cognitive dissonance for a number of AOS researchers since the publication of the definition. Likewise, assigning the impairment to the *execution* level of the system has obfuscated the use of this term for the dysarthrias, causing some confusion in differential attribution of behaviors between AOS and several of the dysarthrias. Further, these authors described the speech behaviors of AOS as those dominated by deficits of speech initiation, selection and sequencing difficulties with a predominance of phoneme substitutions, abnormal prosody, and infrequent metathetic errors. These proposed core features and mechanisms have added to the list of behaviors that are now the widely accepted behaviors used for diagnosing AOS. These behaviors, taken from perhaps the most widely used (at least in the United States) assessment tool for AOS, the *Apraxia Battery for Adults-2* (Dabul 2000), are summarized in Table 15.1. Included is a proposed reassignment of these error types to the phonological-level of process-

Table 15.1 Dabul's (2000) inventory of articulation characteristics of apraxia of speech (AOS) and a current proposed assignment of these characteristics to AOS, phonemic paraphasia (PP) or both populations

Dabul's apraxic speech characteristics	AOS	PP	Both
Phonemic *anticipatory* errors (g**r**een glass → g**l**een glass)		X	
Phonemic *perseverative* errors (boo**t** → boo**b**)		X	
Phonemic *transposition* errors (Af**ri**ca → A**rif**ca)		X	
Phonemic *voicing* errors (**p**en → **b**en)			X
Phonemic *vowel* errors (m**a**n → m**oa**n)			X
Visible/audible *searching*			X
Numerous and varied *off-target attempts* at the word			X
Highly *inconsistent* errors			X
Increased errors as phonemic sequence increases (*phoneme length effects*)			X
Fewer errors in *automatic versus volitional* speech			X
Marked *initiation* difficulty			X
Intrusive schwa /ə/ between syllables or within consonant clusters	X		
Abnormal prosodic features	X		X?
Error awareness and *inability to correct*			X
Receptive–expressive gap			X

ing (i.e. PP) to the motor planning/programming level of speech production (i.e. AOS), or to both levels.

Implied in Table 15.1, and of primary relevance to setting the criteria for the identification of AOS, is the differential assignment of several speech sound error types to various levels of the speech-production system/model. *Sound substitutions* were traditionally attributed to the phonological-level of speech production, whereby individual phoneme-sized units are incorrectly selected and produced in place of the intended sounds. However, Itoh *et al.* (1979), and McNeil and Kent (1990), among others, have argued that sound substitutions also can be attributed to motoric as well as phonological selection and sequencing mechanisms. Therefore, sound substitutions, whether consonant or vowel, do not serve as convincing evidence for one level of system impairment, and consequently do not serve as reliable criteria for differentiating AOS from phonemic paraphasia.

Consistent with the leading descriptions of AOS (Wertz *et al.* 1984; Dabul 2000) and the nominal criteria for subject selection based upon these definitions, most researchers use *phonemic anticipatory, perseverative*, and *transposition* errors as part of the criteria for AOS subject selection. As discussed in greater depth below, models of phonemic assembly for speech production are reasonably united in their attribution of these error types to the level of speech processing that precedes motor planning and programming. Likewise, models of motor planning and programming do not appear to be capable of explaining well-formed phoneme-sized units of displaced (errors of sequence) speech sounds at motoric planning or programming levels. Data from well-selected subjects also are consistent with this attribution of these error types to phonological encoding. Indeed, Monoi *et al.* (1983) reported anticipation, perseveration and full exchange errors to occur frequently (44%) in those with conduction aphasia. Odell *et al.* (1990, 1991) found no more serial-order sequencing error types in their subjects with pure AOS than one would anticipate in a normal population.

The majority of the other error types or abnormal behaviors, such as searching, numerous and varied off-target attempts at the correct target, inconsistent errors, length effects, automatic versus volitional speech differences, and initiation difficulties, are not unique to AOS, PP, or to some of the dysarthrias. While these behaviors are frequently seen in persons with AOS, they must be used as identifying features of the disorder with the greatest of caution. Three features that are both consistent with speech-production models and characteristic of persons with *pure* AOS, and that are not seen in PP, are sound distortions, prolonged segment durations, and prolonged intersegment durations (sound/syllable/word segregation). A fourth characteristic involving disturbed prosody is also included in the list of primary and necessary identifying features of the disorder. However, prosody is such a complex and task-dependent/interactive feature of speech production that it has been very difficult to describe the specific prosodic features that are unique to AOS and assign them with confidence to a single level of the speech-production system. Although the speech production of the person with phonemic paraphasia is not typically described as having a disorder of the prosodic aspect of speech, the frequently recognized segmental errors do cause disruptions of flow of speech that might legitimately be characterized as dysprosody. While sound distortions and prolonged segment durations are features shared with some of the dysarthrias, when used in combination with the unique identification of sound, syllable, or word segregation, and with the other shared features, a cluster of AOS behaviors is identifiable. This cluster is unique and can yield a reliable differential diagnosis from its nearest clinical neighbors. Additionally, the required absence of muscle tone and reflex deficits adds to the confidence in the differential diagnosis of AOS from the dysarthrias. AOS, PP, and dysarthria frequently (perhaps nearly always) coexist in some combination. This makes the differential diagnosis difficult, but not impossible to achieve.

Sound distortions have been traditionally argued as evidence for a motoric-level impairment, at least in the phonologically mature speaker. There is little disagreement about this level of assignment, even in those theoretical accounts for AOS that attribute its base mechanisms to the phonological-level of impairment (e.g. Dogil and Mayer 1998; Whiteside and Varley 1998). While early descriptions of AOS did not describe sound-level distortions as an attribute of AOS, several factors may have contributed to this omission. First, Darley and protégé's conceptualization of motor speech disorders reserved distortions for the dysarthrias. The serious consideration of distortions as an attribute of AOS was practically unthinkable for

Darley's generation. Secondly, broad phonetic transcription of speech errors does not account for sound distortions. This fact, along with a tendency for categorical speech perception leads to the categorization of many sound-level distortions as sound substitutions. Thirdly, the likely inclusion of subjects with substantive amounts of phonemic paraphasia may have actually produced samples with predominant sound substitutions. More recent perceptual characterizations of carefully selected subjects with AOS but without concomitant aphasia and dysarthria have used narrow phonetic transcription and have found sound distortion as a predominant error type in AOS and dysarthria but not in persons with phonemic paraphasia (Odell *et al.* 1991). These sound distortions are at least partially a result of deficits in anticipatory coarticulation and extended segment and intersegment durations (sound and syllable segregation).

Extended segment and intersegment durations found with AOS are distinguished by a unique combination of measurable perceptual, acoustical, and physiological features. While slowed speech is generally believed to be a characteristic of many of the dysarthrias, both prolonged consonant and vowel durations (in multisyllabic words) have been found repeatedly to be characteristic of persons identified as having AOS. Abnormally lengthened intersegment durations have also been identified as a characteristic of AOS, and not associated with other sound-level production disorders. Ziegler and von Cramon (1985) first identified the presence and importance of disturbed anticipatory coarticulation in AOS and their results were subsequently replicated (Katz 1987; McNeil *et al.* 1994; Southwood *et al.* 1997). This attribute of AOS, while not unique to the neuropathologies of speech, offers an explanation for many of the identifiable timing errors and one source of the characteristic sound-level distortions of AOS when found in combination with some of the other features.

Prosodic deficits, whether a result of a deficit at a level preceding a motoric level (Dogil and Mayer 1998; Varley and Whiteside 2001), at the mental syllabary (Levelt 1989), at the level of motor planning and programming (van der Merwe 1997; Boutsen and Christman 2003), or at a level yet to be determined (Rogers and Storkel 1998, 1999) are an integral and necessarily observed characteristic for the diagnosis of AOS. The disturbed prosodic component of the apraxic speaker gives the perception of a choppy or syllable-by-syllable, word-by-word, or phrase-by-phrase (depending on the severity of deficit) quality. Additionally, the extended segments can reduce speaking rate (e.g. syllables per minute) and increase the perception of distortion of phonemically correct and identifiable segments (both consonants and vowels). The slowed speech rate does not appear to be one of a primary inability to produce movements within the requirements of the task. McNeil *et al.* (1989) have shown that persons with *pure* AOS can generate a normal average or peak velocity while generating a segment with an overall abnormally long duration. Additionally, the available evidence suggests that apraxic speakers are not able to increase their speech rate while maintaining segmental or prosodic integrity (Kent and McNeil 1987). The primary consistent prosodic feature identifiable with AOS is, however, the tendency to unstress typically stressed syllables, which yields a tendency to perceive an equal stress pattern (Odell *et al.* 1991).

However, error type assignment alone may be insufficient for a diagnosis of AOS. The diagnosis requires a demonstration that the person with suspected AOS has: (1) the intent to move (to communicate); (2) underlying linguistic representations; (3) *fundamental* sensory and motor abilities for movement (speech); and (4) *normal automatic*—but not *volitional*—movements. In general, the same underlying assumptions need to be satisfied for the diagnosis of phonemic paraphasia, and with the exception of (3), for the dysarthrias. Normal automatic and volitional movement in the dysarthrias is a requirement that is certainly open to further discussion and experimentation. Additionally, there are a number of psycholinguistic variables that should not be affected if one is able to confidently assign the specific speech errors to the motor system and consequently make the diagnosis of AOS. Likewise, it may be reasonable to expect impairments at these levels if one is to confidently assign the speech errors to the linguistic system, and hence to the phonemic paraphasia. For example, the so-called *lexicality effect* (the tendency to make a sound-level error that produces a real word instead of a nonword), the *phonological similarity effect* (poorer performance on a task when the items to be recalled are phonologically similar to one another), and the word-length effect (memory span for words decreases as spoken word duration increases) (Baddeley *et al.* 1975, 1984; Dell 1986) should be intact in the person with AOS and impaired in the person with PP. It also should be mentioned that the status of these effects, as unambiguously belonging to the premotor level of processing, might not be as secure as their original formulations would suggest. The challenges of Ziegler (2002), and those implied by articulatory phonology (Browman and Goldstein 1992), suggest that these effects are in need of experimental verification for their role in defining pathological categories. While these psycholinguistic variables may play a role in the differential diagnosis of AOS from PP, their full discussion is beyond the scope of this chapter.

15.4.1 Definition of AOS

From these error patterns and their coherence with models of phonological processing and motor control described below, AOS is best considered a phonetic–motoric (motor planning and programming) disorder of speech production caused by inefficiencies in the translation of a well-formed and filled phonologic frame to previously learned kinematic parameters assembled for carrying out the intended movement (i.e. problems accessing motor plans and programs). These inefficiencies result in temporal and spatial segmental distortions and prosodic distortions evidenced within and across articulators. AOS is characterized by distortions of consonant and vowel segments. These distortions are often perceived as sound substitutions, *mis-assignment* of stress, and other phrasal and sentence-level prosodic abnormalities. Impairments in intersegment transitionalization result in extended durations between sounds, syllables, and words. Errors are relatively consistent in location within the utterance and relatively invariable in type. AOS is not attributable to deficits of muscle tone or reflexes, or to deficits in the processing of auditory, tactile, kinesthetic, proprioceptive, or language information. This is not meant to suggest, however, that kinematic parameters are intact in individuals with AOS. Intra- and inter-articulator kinematics are disturbed, as reflected in variability of peak velocities, measurements of movement durations, dysmetria, and displacement. Moreover, the role of on-line sensory updating of the motor plan/program requires considerable experimentation before these subclinical aspects of the sensorimotor system can be fully exonerated as a mechanism in AOS. In its extremely rare *pure* form, AOS is not accompanied by the above listed deficits of motor physiology, perception, or language (McNeil *et al.* 1997, p. 329).

It should be noted that many of the characteristics of AOS are similar to those used to characterize ataxic dysarthria. However, similarity among the characteristics is not surprising as ataxic dysarthria results from damage to the cerebellum or its rich connections to other sensorimotor control centers. The cerebellum itself is a complex structure, integral to the regulation of movement (Cannito and Marquardt 1997). As indicated above, many of the characteristics associated with AOS involve timing. Errors in timing also occur in many of the dysarthias, but the speech behaviors associated with ataxic dysarthria look more similar to those identified for AOS than those from other types of dysarthria. However, ataxic dysarthria is not identical in character to AOS and clinically differentiable. In addition to the differences in pathophysiology and the diverse etiologies relevant for ataxic dysarthria, but not AOS, the lack of occurrence of behaviors such as the terminal crescendo aspect of dysmetria, and speech characteristics such as phonatory–prosodic insufficiency and excess and equal stress (although equal stress is a frequently occurring sign) in AOS, aid differential diagnosis between the disorders. It is important to remember that differential diagnosis is not based on one speech behavior, but on a constellation of behaviors. Although important, further elaboration of the perceptual and physiological differences between AOS and ataxic dysarthria is beyond the scope of this discussion.

Table 15.2 summarizes the proposed list of inclusional acoustic/physiologic features and their perceptually derived consequences for differentiating AOS from PP. It also includes those features that are frequently occurring in AOS but that are shared with PP.

It is essential to reconcile the observed characteristics with the speech-production models that can account for their differential assignment to various levels/processes of the model. Below is a brief description of the most relevant models of speech production that provide a guide to these differential diagnostic features.

Table 15.2 Proposed necessary and sufficient characteristics for the differential diagnosis of apraxia of speech (AOS) from phonemic paraphasia and normal speech

AOS characteristics	Realized and perceived speech characteristic
Kernel acoustic/physiologic features	Kernel perceptual features
Lengthened segment durations (vowels in multisyllabic words or words in sentences), in consonants and in both phonemically 'on target' and 'off target' syllables, words, phrases and sentences	Overall slowed rate Distorted speech Prosodic abnormalities
Lengthened intersegment durations	Sound, syllable and word segregation Intrusive schwa Prosodic abnormalities → errors on stressed syllables → equal stress Overall slowed rate
Spectrally distorted (in movement transitions) *phonemically on target* (broadly transcribed) *utterances*	Distorted speech (unusual accent, stress and/or dialect)
Distorted sound substitutions, (excluding anticipations, perseverations and exchanges)	Distorted sound substitutions (frequently devoiced phonemes)
	Morphological and derived lexical errors
Frequently co-occurring features – shared with phonemic paraphasia	Frequently co-occurring perceptual features – shared with phonemic paraphasia
Inability to increase speech rate and maintain phonetic and phonemic integrity	Prevailing slowed speech
Islands of 'less impaired' speech	Infrequent, relatively intact productions of nonpropositional, serial, short, phonetically easy or prosodically modified speech
Frequent *unsuccessful self-initiated trials to repair* errors	Trial and error struggle behavior Audible and visible groping and searching Increased effort
Relatively *consistent location of errors* on repeated trials of the same segment	
Relatively *non-variable error types* on repeated trials of the same segment	
Segment *length* and phonetic *difficulty effects*	Increased errors with increased speech demands

15.5 Speech-production models and error assignment

Even the highly influential speech-production models that were developed subsequent to the early studies on AOS, such as those of Dell (1986, 1988), Garrett (1980, 1984), and Levelt (1989, 1992), have largely (perhaps egregiously) underspecified the motor level of speech production. Likewise, the models that have focused on speech motor control and pathology (e.g. van der Merwe 1997; Perkell, *et al.* 2000) have generally underspecified the phonologic, morphologic, and syntactic demands on speech production and interactions among levels and processes. However, taken together, these models offer a plausible and coherent account for a variety of speech sound-level errors. Furthermore, this differentiation is consistent with rarely occurring but isolatable patterns of perceptual, acoustic, kinematic and physiologic impairments found among the pure cases of dysarthrias, AOS and PP.

15.5.1 Phonological encoding processes

An examination of various speech-production models reveals that sound production errors may be generated at various levels of the speech-production system (Shattuck-Hufnagel 1979; Garrett 1980; 1984; Dell 1986; Levelt 1989; Dell *et al.* 1997). Virtually all speech-production models describe the speech/language-production system as being composed of separate levels of representation (conceptual, syntactic, phonologic, etc.), with specific processes or processing demands being assigned to each of these levels. Models differ in the degrees to which the levels interact, whether information is processed in serial or parallel fashion, and whether processing is conceptualized as discrete or cascading in nature. They also differ as to whether they are general or limited to a specific level of processing, to the specificity of the operating mechanism, and on multiple other dimensions. Among those models that consider speech errors as evidence, they typically assign segmental speech errors to the level of phonological planning: the level at which an abstract representation of the target utterance is formed (Wheeldon and Levelt 1995). Additionally, most traditional speech production models (Garrett 1980, 1984; Dell 1986; Levelt 1989) conceive of the phonologic level of representation with an independently retrieved frame or set of slots along with the segments that fill those slots (the phonological lexicon or dictionary).

15.5.2 Garrett and colleagues

Garrett (1980, 1984) proposed a general spoken-language-production model that has provided a conceptual basis for succeeding models. This model does not, however, provide any comprehensive discussion of motor-level processes and thus does not contribute to an understanding of the differences between the sound error characteristics of aphasia and AOS. A brief review of this model is warranted, however, as it does provide the framework within which more recent models have been developed. Garrett's general sentence production model consists of five processing levels. Sound-level (positional level) production errors occur after the intended message to be communicated has been generated (message level) and following the development of the form or syntax for the message and choosing of the necessary lexical items to communicate the intended message (functional level). In this model, sound-level errors occur during the translation from the functional level to the positional level, which is characterized by the retrieval of segmental structures and specification of the parameters for the frame that segments will fill. With a primary focus on sound-exchange errors (errors involving two sound units), Garrett (1980, 1984) proposes that the mechanism for this error type is the disruption of lexical item assignment during phrasal planning processes. Less focus is placed on other phonological error types (e.g. anticipations, perseverations). Other speech-production models provide a more specified description of the mechanism responsible for different types of phonological errors.

15.5.3 Shattuck–Hufnagel

Shattuck–Hufnagel (1979, 1987) developed a speech production model specific to the phonologic encoding level. This model proposes a *scan-copier* mechanism that offers a plausible explanation for serial order segmental errors. In this account, phoneme-sized slots are constructed and ordered along with a copier mechanism and two monitoring devices. The copier scans the target abstract lexical representation in which ordered segments are represented, chooses the appropriate segment, and places it in the ordered slot of the phonological representation for that lexical item. A monitor checks off the selected unit and another monitor checks for errors in the selection. When there is a failure of one of these devices, sound anticipation, perseveration, or exchange errors occur, as well as sound addition and deletion errors. While this model provides a mechanism that can account for the occurrence of specific phonologic error types, it is less able to provide an explanation for the observed distribution patterns of these error types or interactions of phonological processes with other levels of the production system. More comprehensive speech production models have been proposed by Dell (Dell 1986, 1988; Dell *et al.* 1997) and Levelt and colleagues (Levelt 1989; Roelofs 1997; Levelt *et al.* 1999) that provide better prediction of at least some sound segment errors and patterns of errors generated at the level of phonologic encoding.

15.5.4 Dell and colleagues

Dell (1986) proposed a general speech production model that has been extended (Dell *et al.* 1997) and adapted during the course of its development. This psycholinguistic model addresses sentence production from the semantic to phonologic levels of production, with specific focus on phonologic encoding. In this connectionist model, nodes represent linguistic units (i.e. morphemes, phonemes) with links between nodes, some stipulating the relation and the order of the connecting nodes. As with the model of Levelt and colleagues, units are selected by the mechanism of spreading activation where higher-level units activate lower-level units. Spreading activation and decay rates reflect the rate of processing that is assumed to be constant. Spreading activation is bi-directional, thereby allowing feedback among syntactic, morphologic, and phonological levels of representation. Parallel processing occurs among levels, allowing processing at lower levels of representation to begin before units are fully processed at higher levels. While parallel processing occurs among levels of representation, a notable adaptation from the original (Dell 1986) model specifies serial encoding of segments within the phonological level (Dell 1988). Morpheme nodes are connected to syllable nodes and segments and frames are identified for their appropriate positional category (e.g. onset, nucleus, or coda). In this model, unlike that of Levelt and colleagues, syllable structure for a word is assumed to be stored in the mental lexicon. Phoneme units are chosen and assigned based on their positional category in the frame. Category information and spreading activation level determine serial order processing. That is, segments that are activated and that have the highest level of activation are selected and assigned to their specified positions in the frame.

Dell defines phonologic encoding as the spelling out of the sounds of a morpheme. This process includes retrieving, ordering, and organizing phonemes for articulation. According to Dell (1986), speech errors generated at this pre-motoric level occur when there are higher levels of activation for the incorrect unit than for the target unit. Higher levels of activation for incorrect units may result from background activation or during parallel processing of units among production levels. He provides a specific explanation of how serial order (anticipations, perseverations, exchanges) segment errors can be generated by spreading activation levels. According to this theory, anticipation errors occur when an item later in the target production has a higher level of activation than the target unit. Perseveration errors occur when the activation level of a previously selected item remains high and is higher than the correct item at the time of selection. Exchange errors are described as the result of both anticipation and perseveration errors, whereby a later unit in the target production has a higher activation level than the correct item. The incorrect item is selected and thus the correct item remains available to be selected in the position of the initially incorrect selected item. The frequency of occurrence of these errors is related to many factors, including, but not limited to, background activation, parallel processing, environmental similarity, speaking rate (Dell 1986), and practice (Dell *et al.* 1997). The conceptual framework of Dell's (1986) model has been extended and modified to describe the types and proportions of serial-order errors produced by individuals with aphasia and to hypothesize explanations for the effects of brain damage on the production system (Dell *et al.* 1997). This spreading activation model provided an account of how serial order in the language production system operated in the context of activation and time (past, present, and future). Of primary importance for the maintenance of serial order in this model is the production system's ability to deactivate the past, and activate the present and the future. It was hypothesized that persons with aphasia would produce more serial-order errors than normal language users, and importantly, more errors of perseveration than anticipation. Experimental evidence supported the prediction that more error-producing conditions (i.e. brain damage, increased speaking rate), resulted in a higher perseveration to anticipation error ratio. The authors hypothesize that the performance of persons with aphasia may be attributed to either decreased connection weight strengths among nodes or to the slow development of activation in the linguistic network. The authors state that it would be difficult to connect the specific parameters of their model to any specific theoretical explanations for aphasic behavior. However, regardless of the correct physiological explanation, this model and its assumptions further contribute to the conceptualization of the role of serial order in the language production system. This model (Dell 1986; Dell *et al.* 1997), like the model of Levelt and colleagues (Levelt 1989; Roelofs 1997; Levelt *et al.* 1999), assigns phoneme-size serial-order errors to the level of phonological encoding. However, unlike Levelt and colleagues, these serial-order errors are assigned at the level of phono-logical retrieval. A limitation of this model is its restricted account of post-phono-logic encoding processes. In order to fully and accurately account for the array of speech production errors evidenced by both normal and brain-damaged popula-tions, a more complete model will necessarily explicate the bi-directional relation-ship between phonology and motor planning, as well as the translation of the phonological code into the motor domain.

15.5.4 Levelt and colleagues

Levelt (1989) proposed a model similar to Garrett's model (1980, 1984) in that it addresses multiple levels of the speech production system. Levelt and colleagues (Levelt and Wheeldon 1994; Roelofs 1997; Levelt *et al.* 1999) subsequently elaborated this general speech production model. One such elaboration, the WEAVER Model (Roelofs 1997), refined the phonologic encoding level and proposed a perspective on the relationship of phonologic and motor-level processing and how the phonologic code is translated for motor processing. In fact, Roelofs (1997) identifies the lack of integration of the process of phonetic encoding in other speech-production models as one of the motivating factors for the development of the WEAVER model. This model is conceived of as a network of nodes and links that code the information that is used to guide unit selection. Importantly, unlike other models (e.g. Dell 1986), this model incorporates labels that directly state the relationship between morphemes and phoneme segments. As in Dell (1986), spreading activation is assumed to be the mechanism that enables units to be retrieved. Unit selection is based on activation levels and a verification process that determines if the resulting form is licensed (Roelofs 1997). In general, the verification process determines whether a selected unit is truly linked to the immediately preceding level of representation. Occasionally the verification process fails and segment errors result. In this model, similar to others, phonologic encoding follows lemma activation, which provides information about the syntactic properties of the target utterance. Using information from the lemma level of representation (e.g. noun/verb, tense, gender), morphophonological encoding is initiated and made available for phonologic/word form encoding. As with other models, the level of phonologic encoding consists of metrical and segmental spellout, and the eventual assembly of these two processes. Labeled links are used to code the relationship between nodes, and once the morpheme node is derived, it points to its metrical structure and the segments that compose the phonological form of the morpheme. The morpheme node links directly to its segments, with no interceding level of syllable representation. Links between the morpheme and segment nodes identify the serial positions of phonemes within the morpheme. Links between segment and syllable program nodes (i.e. mental syllabary) further constrain the possible syllable positions of the segments. A phoneme is selected if its node is linked to the level above it and if its activation level exceeds threshold. According to Roelofs and Meyer (1998), segment association for syllable position is not stored, but rather guided by the syllabification rules of the language. Syllabification processes sequentially associate the segments to the syllable nodes in the phonological word. A phonological word results from metrical spellout and is a pronounceable metrical pattern that reveals syllabification, codes word stress and may consist of one or more lexical item (Levelt 1992). In this model, syllable position is coded after syllabification occurs and syllabification is an on-line process that occurs after segment and metrical spellout. Because this speech production model does not have a separate syllable level representation following the morphologic representation, and segments are directly linked to the morpheme, segments are not coded for position until syllabification occurs. According to Roelofs (1997) serial-order segment errors (exchanges, anticipations, and perseverations) result from the failure of verification processes. With syllabification, phonological words are constructed and the assumed stored motor programs for phonological syllables are accessed. Thus, phonetic encoding of the phonological word results from accessing the mental syllabary or the 'syllable-based articulatory programs for each of the phonological syllables' (Roelofs 1999, p. 180). These stored motor programs are assumed to contain information about the gestures involved and their temporal relationships. Relative to sound production characteristics, Roelofs suggests that the occurrence of assimilation in speech production may be accounted for by overlapping gestures. While Roelofs and colleagues have not developed this model with the goal of applying it to disordered speech production, the inclusion of such specificity about the translation of phonological code information to motor level information invites this consideration. With considerable specificity at the phonologic level of the model, WEAVER, like the Dell (1986) model, is easily able to account for serial-order errors of phonologic encoding that may occur in normal or pathological productions (specifically not limited to aphasia). The conceptualization of the phonologic to motor-level code translation in WEAVER also promotes hypothesizing about processing to be developed for normal speech production. With continued development, experimentation, and verification, this model has the potential to inform the motor planning processes involved in speech production disorders (i.e. AOS). For example, Roelofs states that in WEAVER there is competition among motor programs and that the speed of choosing a motor program depends on the activity level of other motor programs. If Roelof's assumptions are correct, and if the speed of choosing a motor program is slowed, the resulting effect might be realized as increased intersegment time, extended sound/syllable durations that may include prolonged movement transitions. These behaviors are consistent with some of the previously described characteristics of AOS. However, while a level of phonetic encoding is incorporated in the WEAVER mode, experimental verification has focused primarily on phonologic encoding processes.

15.5.5 Locus of error generation

There is a great deal of agreement across models of phonological encoding that serial-order speech-production errors involving well-articulated phoneme-sized units of information are generated at this level of processing. If this has been convincingly demonstrated, the question then arises as to the generator(s) of other errors that characterize AOS. Rogers and Storkel (1999) proposed a reduced buffer capacity that could accommodate a number of errors, but perhaps most readily the syllable segregation that is typically attributed to the apraxic speaker. However, their model is silent about where in the linguistic/motoric speech production system this reduced buffer might exist. Stated another way, a reduced buffer capacity at any level or stage of the speech production system could account for the errors as conceived in this model. Additionally, Deger and Ziegler (2002) have correctly challenged the validity of the reduced buffer interpretation of the studies by Rogers and Storkel, further minimizing this account as a plausible explanation for error assignment in AOS. Dogil and Mayer (1998) have proposed a phonological overspecification model to account for some of the features of the apraxic speaker. Whiteside and Varley (1998) have proposed a dual route model of phonological access whereby the apraxic speaker has lost access to the direct route and must rely on the indirect route, with the consequence of having to assemble each sequence of phonemes anew, thereby giving rise to the variety of segmental and prosodic features that characterize the disorder. Still other theories or hypotheses have been advanced but none, save the proposal of Dogil and Mayer, makes explicit attribution of the apraxic errors to the phonological-level of speech production.

15.5.6 Motor planning and programming

While neuromotor accounts of AOS have been proposed that assign or hypothesize it as a disorder of motor programming, or specify the site of lesion as being consistent with a motor programming disorder (Mlcoch and Noll 1980), these models generally provide little guidance or prediction about the speech errors generated by disturbances with these processes or lesion sites. Guenther and colleagues (Guenther 1995; Perkell *et al.* 1997, 2000; Guenther *et al.* 1998) have developed a detailed model of motor control that describes how speech sound acquisition occurs, as well as those processes involved in speech motor planning and programming. While this model addresses phenomena that may be relevant in the differential diagnosis of motor speech disorders (i.e. motor equivalence, articulatory variability, coarticulation, and speech rate effects), in its current stage of development it has not been extended to make claims about the relationship between disrupted processing and speech errors in motor speech disorders.

van der Merwe (1997) offered what is perhaps the most detailed, and psychologically and neurologically instantiated, model of motor speech processes, and a model to which specific speech error types can be assigned. She proposed a three-stage or process division of the speech motor system with speech planning, programming, and execution components. A strength of the model is not only its justification, but also the fact that many assumptions at each level of the model are made explicit. At the planning stage, the model assumes that the phoneme is the basic unit of planning. However, in normal speakers, the planned unit is usually several words in size. There are *invariant* spatial and temporal specifications for each sequence of phonemes that are adapted by their context. Sensorimotor memory, in the form of proprioceptive, tactile, and auditory engrams associated with the learned phonemes is accessed during speech production. Motor plans occur sequentially and are articulator-specific, *not muscle-specific*. The movement parameters derived from the specific sequence of phonemes being planned are adapted by the context in which they occur. These contexts include: (1) the sound environment; (2) the co-articulatory requirements of the task; (3) motor equivalence (achieving articulatory/acoustic goals via several different movement patterns); (4) a variety of phonetic influences on segmental duration, such as speaking intensity or changes in speech rate; (5) linguistic influences on segmental duration, such as final segment lengthening and linguistic stress effects; and (6) elocutionary factors, such as the need for *clear* or *formal* speech such as that encountered while making a public address versus that used during casual or conversational speech. van der Merwe's speech *planning* model proposes that adaptations (or perhaps compensations) result in: (1) shortening the *chunks* or units in the plan yielding sound, syllable, and word segregation; (2) slowed speech rate; (3) sound-level distortions resulting from disturbed coarticulation and mis-assigned movement trajectories; (4) a reduced number of phonological targets within a word; and (5) duplicating sounds within a word. Additionally, the model links these speech and movement errors to specific neuroanatomical systems, derived by logical association primarily, though not exclusively, from the literature on limb and other nonspeech structure motor control. Speech *planning* is proposed to occur in the motor association areas, including the premotor (lateral area 6), Broca's area (posterior two-thirds of the third frontal convolution), supplementary motor area (medial area 6), prefrontal and parietal association areas (areas 5 and 7), caudate circuit of the basal ganglia, and Wernicke's area (area 22). The speech-production patterns that characterize AOS are consistent with all of these planning consequences, the speech errors that they generate, and the anatomical areas proposed to house them.

Motor programming is mediated at the middle levels of this three-stage motor hierarchy. This level of the model defines programming as 'a set of muscle commands that are structured before a movement sequence begins which can be delivered without reference to external feedback' (Marsden 1984, p. 228). Importantly, programs specify muscle tone, movement direction, force, range, rate and mechanical stiffness of joints. Also importantly, this model of programming does not assume the strong form of motor programming whereby sensory feedback cannot be used once the movement is initiated, but only that it does not have to be used to initiate or unpack a motor program. While motor plans are analogous to *strategies*, motor programs are analogous to *tactics*. This conception of motor programs may approximate Allen and Tsukahara's (1974) and Gracco and Abbs' (1987) notion of *preprogramming*, Evarts' (1982) *central programs*, and Schmidt's (1982) *generalized motor programs*. Speech *programming* occurs in the motor cortical association areas including the basal ganglia (caudate and putamen), lateral cerebellum, supplementary motor areas, premotor cortex, primary motor cortex, and the frontolimbic system.

What is immediately clear from this definition of motor programming is that the speech errors that would be generated from these processes and from these anatomical structures are consistent with the dysarthrias (previously ascribed to the execution level of the system) and perhaps with some behaviors consistent with AOS. Attempts to sort these difference have been addressed elsewhere (e.g. McNeil *et al.* 2000) and will not be reviewed here. The assumption with this model and with the proposed definition of AOS is that at both the speech planning and programming levels, phonologically intact information has been made available to, or transcoded as input to, the pre-learned routines and subroutines of the sensorimotor system for carrying out precisely timed and coordinated movements within and between articulators and muscles used for speech. Further, a direct relationship exists between the linguistic units and the implementation of the motor system that cannot be replicated without these specific inputs. A primary implication of this assumption is that speech planning and programming is highly specialized for these specific inputs and that clear dissociations between movements of the shared structures used for speech and nonspeech activities should be realized.

The models of phonological encoding discussed here, specifically that of Dell (Dell 1986; Dell, *et al.* 1997), provide a theoretically consistent explanation for the occurrence of anticipation, perseveration, and exchange serial-order phonemic errors. This hierarchically structured model of speech production is consistent with the notion that serial-order phonemic errors cannot be attributed to any level of processing that can be conceived of as controlling motoric processes of speech production (motor planning, programming, and execution). Thus, a disorder of motor control of the articulators and muscles used for speech cannot reasonably account for these types of phoneme-sized serial-order errors. Models derived from the conceptualizations of the sort discussed in this chapter are often referred to as *box and arrows* models. Box and arrow models schematize the proposed operations as levels of representation or computation, which are symbolized as boxes, with the *products* from these computations being fed to subsequent levels of computation/representation via hypothesized *processes*, symbolized as arrows.

It is important to the eventual integrity of the error assignment proposed here that this box and arrows approach readily acknowledges the possible interaction among linguistic and motoric levels. Indeed, the phonological encoding models reviewed are considered connectionist models. However, the levels of representation and/or computation in these distributed processing models are the boxes in the box and arrow models. The fact that dissociations have been demonstrated for these various levels of the models, and clinically *pure* cases do exist that conform to the models, provides instantiation for the models and for the specific differential diagnostic categories and criteria outlined above. Conceptualizing the speech production system as composed of interacting levels does not mean that the effects of disruption at one level of the system must result from processing inefficiencies or impaired computational operations at all levels of the system. This perspective suggests that disorders can be separated. If impairments at one level of the system can be shown to cause impairments at another level of the system, there may be sufficient justification for proposing a new disorder. If disorders or impairments tend to co-occur that can be attributed to two or more separate mechanisms or levels of the system, a syndrome might be proposed. However, an indirect effect of a phonological encoding disorder on motor speech control does not make the motor speech consequences of this interaction, a phonological disorder. Disturbances in speech motor control that may co-occur with a phonological disorder are not part of the phonological disorder but reflect a separate level of disturbance; a disturbance of speech motor control. Conversely, an indirect effect of motor speech impairment on the processing of phonological information does not make this disorder a motor speech disorder.

15.6 Summary

The confusion and ambiguity surrounding the identification, diagnosis, and study of AOS can be traced back to the failure of the defining features first formulated by Darley (1968), and later incorporated into Dabul's (2000) criteria and Wertz *et al.*'s (1984) definition, to clearly separate the speech production levels and processes associated with AOS from those that can be attributable to near clinical neighbors.

This early work not only contributed to confusion regarding the criteria necessary for differential diagnosis and treatment of AOS, but also impeded the understanding and study of the disorder. As a result, much of the past literature on AOS is confounded by erroneous subject selection criteria that produced conflicting results and prevented the formulation of a clear clinical entity. However, increased understanding of the phonological and speech motor systems and how they interact, as well as the development of models of speech production with greater explanatory power, has stimulated renewed interest in the nature of AOS. This growth argues for the development of a set of criteria that can be used to diagnose AOS with more specificity and sensitivity. While the kernel characteristics used for the diagnosis of AOS proposed by McNeil *et al.* (1997) are experimentally justified and theoretically coherent, we recognize that they are likely to be modified as more is learned about normal and disordered speech production.

Current models of speech production (in isolation and in combination) provide an improved framework from which speech characteristics consistent with AOS can be compared to those associated with other disorders. With increased understanding of the workings of the phonological and speech motor systems, speech errors, and the conditions under which they are elicited can be more easily assigned to specific levels and processes. Development and refinement of models, such as that proposed by van der Merwe (1997), has helped to disambiguate AOS from phonemic paraphasia by clearly distinguishing between functions and structure associated with motor planning, programming, and execution. Models focusing on phonological encoding, such as those developed by Dell (1986, 1988), Levelt (1989), and colleagues (Levelt *et al.* 1999) provide a theoretical structure for distinguishing phonemic dysfunctions from those of motor processing, thereby allowing for easier distinction between behaviors attributable to AOS from those characteristic of phonemic paraphasia. Within the context of these explanatory models of speech production, a clear and consistent set of diagnostic criteria should allow our research and understanding of AOS to proceed in a manner more straightforward than has previously been observed.

References

Allen, G.I. and **Tsukahara, N.** (1974). Cerebrocerebellar communication systems. *Physiological Review*, 54, pp. 957–997.

Baddeley, A. D., Thomson, N., and **Buchanan, M.** (1975). Word length and the structure of short-term memory. *Journal of Verbal Learning and Verbal Behavior*, 14, pp. 575–589.

Baddeley, A., Lewis, V., and **Vallar, G.** (1984). Exploring the articulatory loop. *The Quarterly Journal of Experimental Psychology*, 36A, pp. 233–252.

Ballard, K.J., Granier, J.P., and **Robin, D.A.** (2000). Understanding the nature of apraxia of speech: theory, analysis, and treatment. *Aphasiology*, 14, pp. 969–995.

Ballard, K.J., Robin, D.A., and Folkins, J.W. (2003). An integrative model of speech motor control: a response to Ziegler. *Aphasiology*, 17, pp. 37–48.

Boutsen, F. and Christman, S. (2002). Prosody in apraxia of speech. *Seminars in Speech and Language*, 23, 245–256.

Browman, C.P. and Goldstein, L. (1992). Articulatory phonology: an overview. *Phonetica*, 49, pp. 155–180.

Brown, J.R. (1968). *A model for central and peripheral behavior in aphasia.* Paper presented at the Annual Meeting of Academy of Aphasia, Rochester, MN, October, 1968.

Cannito, M.P. and Marquardt, T.P. (1997). Ataxic Dysarthria. In M.R. McNeil, ed. *Clinical management of sensorimotor speech disorders*, pp. 217–247. Thieme, New York, NY.

Code, C. (1998). Models, theories and heuristics in apraxia of speech. *Clinical Linguistics and Phonetics*, 12, pp. 47–65.

Dabul, B. (2000). *Apraxia battery for adults-2*. Pro-Ed, Austin, TX.

Darley, F.L. (1968). Apraxia of speech: 107 years of terminological confusion. Paper presented to the American Speech and Hearing Association Convention, Denver (unpublished).

Darley, F.L., Aronson, A.E. and Brown, J. (1975). *Motor speech disorders*. Saunders, Philadelphia, PA.

Deger, K. and Ziegler, W. (2002). Speech motor programming in apraxia of speech. *Journal of Phonetics*, 30, 321–335.

Dell, G.S. (1986). A spreading-activation theory of retrieval in sentence production. *Psychological Review*, 96, pp. 283–321.

Dell, G.S. (1988). The retrieval of phonological forms in production: tests of prediction from a connectionist model. *Journal of Memory and Language*, 27, pp. 124–142.

Dell, G.S., Burger, L.K., and Svec, W. R. (1997). Language production and serial order: a functional analysis and a model. *Psychological Review*, 104, pp. 123–147.

Dogil, G. and Mayer, J. (1998). Selective phonological impairment: a case of apraxia of speech. *Phonology*, 15, pp. 143–188.

Dronkers, N.F. (1997). A new brain region for coordinating speech coordination. *Nature*, 384, pp. 159–161.

Evarts, E.V. (1982). Analogies between central motor programs for speech and for limb movements. In S. Grillner, B. Lindblom, J. Lubker, and A. Persson, eds. *Speech motor control*, vol. 36. Pergamon Press, Oxford.

Garrett, M.F. (1980). Levels of processing in sentence production. In B. Butterworth, ed. *Language production: Volume 1, Speech and talk*, pp. 177–220. Academic Press, London.

Garrett, M.F. (1984). The organization of processing structure for language production: applications to aphasic speech. In D. Caplan, A.R. Lecours, and A. Smith, eds. *Biological perspectives on language*, pp. 172–193. MIT Press, Cambridge, MA.

Goodglass, H. (1992). Diagnosis of conduction aphasia. In S.E.Kohn, ed. *Conduction aphasia*, pp. 3–50. Lawrence Erlbaum Associates, Hillsdale, NJ.

Gracco, V.L. and **Abbs, J.H.** (1987). Programming and execution processes of speech movement control: potential neural correlates. In E. Keller and M. Gopnik, eds. *Motor and sensory processes of language*. Lawrence Erlbaum Associates, Hillsdale, NJ.

Guenther, F.H. (1995). Speech sound acquisition, coarticulation, and rate effects in a neural network model of speech production. *Psychological Review*, 102, pp. 594–621.

Guenther, F.H., Hampson, M., and **Johnson, D.** (1998). A theoretical investigation of reference frames for the planning of speech movements. *Psychological Review*, 105, pp. 611–633.

Halpern, H., Keith, R., and **Darley, F.L.** (1976). Phonemic behavior of aphasic subjects without dysarthria or apraxia of speech. *Cortex*, 12, pp. 365–372.

Itoh, M., Sasanuma, S., and **Ushijima, T.** (1979). Velar movements during speech in a patient with apraxia of speech. *Brain and Language*, 7, pp. 227–239.

Katz, W.F. (1987). Anticipatory labial and lingual coarticulation in aphasia. In J.H. Ryalls, ed. *Phonetic approaches to speech production in aphasia and related disorders*, pp. 221–242. College-Hill Press, Boston, MA.

Kelso, J.A.S. and **Tuller, B.** (1981). Toward a theory of apractic syndromes. *Brain and Language*, 12, pp. 224–245.

Kent, R.D. and **McNeil, M.R.** (1987). Relative timing of sentence repetition in apraxia of speech and conduction aphasia. In J.H. Ryalls, ed. *Phonetic approaches to speech production in aphasia and related disorders*, pp. 181–220. College-Hill Press, Boston, MA.

Levelt, W.J.M. (1989). *Speaking: from intention to articulation*. MIT Press, Cambridge, MA.

Levelt, W.J.M. (1992). Accessing words in speech production: stages, processes, representation. *Cognition*, 42, pp. 1–22.

Levelt, W.J.M. and **Wheeldon, L.** (1994). Do speakers have access to a mental syllabary? *Cognition*, 50, pp. 239–269.

Levelt, W.J.M., Roelofs, A. and **Meyer, A.S.** (1999). A theory of lexical access in speech production. *Behavioral and Brain Sciences*, 22, pp. 1–75.

Marsden, C.D. (1984). Which motor disorder in Parkinson's disease indicates the true motor function of the basal ganglia? In *Functions of the basal ganglia*, Ciba Foundation Symposium 107. Pitman, London.

Martin, A.D. (1974). Some objections to the term apraxia of speech. *Journal of Speech and Hearing Disorders*, 39, pp. 53–64.

McNeil, M.R. and **Kent, R.D.** (1990). Motoric characteristics of adult aphasic and apraxic speakers. In G.E. Hammond, ed. *Cerebral control of speech and limb movements*, pp. 349–386. Elsevier Science Publishers, North Holland.

McNeil, M.R., Caliguiri, M., and **Rosenbek, J.C.** (1989). A comparison of labio-mandibular kinematic durations, displacements, velocities and dysmetrias in apraxic and normal adults. *Clinical Aphasiology*, 22, pp. 203–218.

McNeil, M.R., Hashi, M., and **Southwood, H.** (1994). Acoustically derived perceptual evidence for coarticulatory errors in apraxic and conduction aphasic speech production. *Clinical Aphasiology*, 22, pp. 203–218.

McNeil, M.R., Robin, D.A., and **Schmidt, R.A.** (1997). Apraxia of speech: definition, differentiation, and treatment. In M.R. McNeil, ed. *Clinical management of sensorimotor speech disorders*, pp. 311–344. Thieme, New York, NY.

McNeil, M.R., Doyle, P.J., and **Wambaugh, J.** (2000). Apraxia of speech: a treatable disorder of motor planning and programming. In S.E. Nadeau, L.J. Gonzalez Rothi and B. Crosson, eds. *Aphasia and language: theory to practice*, pp. 221–266. The Guilford Press, New York, NY.

Miller, N. (2000). Changing ideas in apraxia of speech. In I. Papathanasiou, ed. *Acquired neurogenic communication disorders*, pp. 173–202. Whurr, London.

Miller, N. (2002). The neurological bases of apraxia of speech. *Seminars in Speech and Language*, 23, 223–230.

Mlcoch, A.G. and **Noll, J.D.** (1980). Speech production models as related to the concept of apraxia of speech. In N.J. Lass, ed. *Speech and Language: advances in basic research and practice*, pp. 201–238. Academic Press, New York, NY.

Monoi, H., Fukusako, Y., and **Itoh, M.** (1983). Speech sound errors in patients with Conduction and Broca's aphasia. *Brain and Language*, 20, pp. 175–294.

Odell, K., McNeil, M.R., Rosenbek, J.C., and **Hunter, L.** (1990). Perceptual characteristics of consonant production by apraxic speakers. *Journal of Speech and Hearing Disorders*, 55, pp. 345–359.

Odell, K., McNeil, M.R., Rosenbek, J.C., and **Hunter, L.** (1991). Perceptual characteristics of vowel and prosody production in apraxic, aphasic, and dysarthric speakers. *Journal of Speech and Hearing Research*, 34, pp. 67–80.

Perkell, J., Matthies, M., Lane, H., Guenther, F., Wilhelms-Tricarico, R., Wozniak, J., and **Guiod, P.** (1997). Speech motor control: acoustic goals, saturation effects, auditory feedback and internal models. *Speech Communication*, 22, pp. 227–250.

Perkell, J.S., Guenther, F.H., Lane, H., Matthies, M.L., Perrier, P., Vick, J., Wilhelms-Tricarico, R., and **Zandipour, M.** (2000). A theory of motor control and supporting data from speakers with normal hearing and with profound hearing loss. *Journal of Phonetics*, 28, pp. 233–272.

Rochon, E., Caplan, D., and **Waters, G.S.** (1991). Short-term memory processes in patients with apraxia of speech: implications for the nature and structure of the auditory verbal short-term memory system. *Journal of Neurolinguistics*, 5, pp. 237–264.

Roelofs, A. (1997). The WEAVER model of word-form encoding in speech production. *Cognition*, 64, pp. 249–284.

Roelofs, A. (1999). Phonologic perseveration al segments and features as planning units in speech production. *Language and Cognitive Processes*, 14, pp. 173–200.

Roelofs, A. and **Meyer, A. S.** (1998). Metrical structure in planning the production of spoken words. *Journal of Experimental Psychology: Learning, Memory and Cognition*, 24, pp. 922–939.

Rogers, M.A. and **Storkel, H.** (1998). Reprogramming phonologically similar utterances: the role of phonetic features in pre-motor encoding. *Journal of Speech and Hearing Research*, 41, pp. 258–274.

Rogers, M.A. and **Storkel, H.L.** (1999). Planning speech one syllable at a time: the reduced buffer capacity hypothesis in apraxia of speech. *Aphasiology*, 13, pp. 793–805.

Schmidt, R.A. (1982). *Motor control and learning: A behavioral emphasis*. Human Kinetics Publishers, Champaign.

Schuell, H., Jenkins, J., and **Jimenez-Pabon, E.** (1964). *Aphasia in adults*. Harper, New York, NY.

Shattuck-Hufnagel, S. (1979). Speech errors as evidence for a serial order mechanism in sentence production. In W.E. Cooper and E.C.T Walker, eds. *Sentence processing: psycholinguistic studies presented to Merrill Garrett*, pp. 295–342. Lawrence Erlbaum Associates, Hillsdale, NJ.

Shattuck-Hufnagel, S. (1987). The role of word-onset consonants in speech production planning: new evidence from speech error patterns. In E. Keller and M. Gopnik, eds. *Motor and sensory processes of language*, pp. 17–51. Lawrence Erlbaum Associates, Hillsdale, NJ.

Southwood, H.M., Dagenais, P.A., Sutphin, S.M., and **Mertz Garcia, J.** (1997). Coarticulation in apraxia of speech: a perceptual, acoustic and electropalatographic study. *Clinical Linguistics and Phonetics*, 11, pp. 179–203.

van der Merwe, A. (1997). A Theoretical framework for the characterization of pathological speech sensorimotor control. In M.R. McNeil, ed. *Clinical management of sensorimotor speech disorders*, pp. 1–25. Thieme, New York.

Varley, R. and **Whiteside, S.P.** (2001). What is the underlying impairment in acquired apraxia of speech? *Aphasiology*, 15, pp. 39–84.

Wertz, R.T., LaPointe, L.L., and **Rosenbek, J.C.** (1984). *Apraxia of speech in adults: the disorder and its management*. Grune and Stratton, Orlando, FL.

Wheeldon, L.R. and **Levelt, W.J.M.** (1995). Monitoring the time course of phonological encoding. *Journal of Memory and Language*, 34, pp. 311–334.

Whiteside, S.P. and **Varley R.A.** (1998). A reconceptualisation of apraxia of speech: a synthesis of evidence. *Cortex*, 34, pp. 221–231.

Ziegler, W. (2002). Psycholinguistic and motor theories of AOS. *Seminars in Speech and Language*, 23, 245–256.

Ziegler, W. (2003a). Speech motor control is task-specific: evidence from dysarthria and apraxia of speech. *Aphasiology*, 17, 3–36.

Ziegler, W. (2003b). To speak or not to speak: distinctions between speech and nonspeech motor control. *Aphasiology*, 17, 99–105.

Ziegler, W. and **von Cramon, D.** (1985). Anticipatory coarticulation in a speaker with apraxia of speech. *Brain and Language*, 26, pp. 117–130.

CHAPTER 16

THE ROLE OF THE SYLLABLE IN DISORDERS OF SPOKEN LANGUAGE PRODUCTION

WOLFRAM ZIEGLER AND BEN MAASSEN

16.1 Introduction

The syllable plays an important role in the production and the understanding of spoken language, as well as in language acquisition. Evidence for this comes from different sources: from phonological theory, from phonetics, from theories of language development, and from psycholinguistic studies of speaking and of language comprehension in adults. This chapter gives an overview of data demonstrating that the syllabic organization of speech also influences the way in which spoken language breaks down in conditions of an impaired phonological or speech motor system in children and adults. It reviews results from studies of aphasic patients with phonological encoding problems, from patients with apraxia of speech, or with other motor speech problems, and from children with developmental speech motor disorders, which demonstrate that the error patterns seen in these groups reflect the structural principles of syllabicity.

As an introduction to this, the role of syllabic units in phonology and phonetics and in modern psycholinguistic accounts of spoken language production and language acquisition, will be outlined.

16.2 Phonology

Whereas the traditional phonemic approach and generative phonological theories of the sound pattern of English (SPE) type (Chomsky and Halle 1968) dispensed with syllabic units, modern phonology now recognizes the syllable as a hierarchical unit in phonological representation and as a natural domain of many phonological regularities. Rules such as the final devoicing rule, for instance, can be formulated most parsimoniously when the syllable is postulated as the domain of its application (Wiese 2000). In addition to this, the introduction of the syllable as a separate representational tier was motivated by cross-linguistic observations of asymmetries in the distribution of consonants in syllable-initial versus syllable-

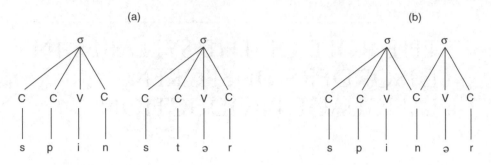

Fig. 16.1 A non-linear representation of syllable structure (as proposed, for instance, by Clements and Keyser 1983). The left panel (a) contains an example with complex onsets, the right panel (b) contains an ambisyllabic consonant.

final position, by phonotactic considerations, and by considerations relating to the assignment of stress and tones to words (Goldsmith 1990).

In non-linear phonological approaches (e.g. Clements and Keyser 1983) the syllable is considered as a superordinate structural unit which dominates the segments belonging to it. Figure 16.1 gives an example of a non-linear model of syllable-based phonological representations.

Such models of the syllable provide a suitable framework for the formulation of phonotactic constraints and the explanation of probabilistic asymmetries (Kessler and Treiman 1997). An important principle here is that the sequencing of a syllable's segments follows a sonority hierarchy: from syllable onset to the nucleus the segments become increasingly sonorous, and sonority decreases again towards the coda. Although there is no generally accepted phonetic criterion which defines sonority, a conventional ordering of segment classes by increasing sonority is: obstruents–nasals–liquids–glides–high vowels–mid/low vowels (e.g. Wiese 2000). The sonority principle regulates, for instance, that the consonants /p/ and /r/ can combine to /#pr/ in the onset (e.g. *prompt*) or to /rp#/ in the coda of a syllable (e.g. *sharp*), whereas /rp/-onsets or /pr/-codas are not well formed. Moreover, it contributes to the assignment of syllable boundaries in multisyllabic words. Most theories assume that a word's syllabification is completely rule-governed and need not be specified in the word's underlying form.

However, problems of syllable boundary assignment exist in words like *spinner* (Fig. 16.1), where a single intervocalic consonant follows a short vowel. Assignment of the consonant to either the first or the second syllable would violate at least one of the syllable assignment rules, which led many phonologists to postulate an ambisyllabic status for such consonants, i.e. its affiliation to both syllables simultaneously (cf. Fig. 16.1).

Based on cross-linguistic observations of distributions of syllable types, theories of syllable markedness posit that syllables with a particularly sharp sonority rise in the onset, and a particularly smooth sonority decline in the coda, are *unmarked* (Vennemann 1988). Thus, markedness theory would classify CV-syllables like /tu:/ (a type which occurs in all languages of the world) as particularly 'good' exemplars, while /tu:θ/, /u:z/, /tru:θ/ or /trʌst/ are increasingly less frequent structure types. Even more, /tu:/ is better than /ju:/ because the sonority distance between onset and nucleus is greater in the former than in the latter.

16.3 Phonetics

Inspired by phonological evidence, phoneticians have made considerable attempts at establishing a phonetic theory of the syllable. As mentioned above, some efforts were made to find a phonetic correlate of the sonority hierarchy, e.g. in terms of perceptual salience or of articulatory ease. Ladefoged (2001), for instance, proposed a sonority-ordering of phonemes based on acoustic measures of loudness, but this approach remained incomplete. Further research was devoted to the problem of finding phonetic markers of the boundaries between adjacent syllables, e.g. on the basis of acoustic or kinematic data, but these investigations also failed to come to a satisfying solution. Neither can the speech signal be dissected into discrete syllabic units nor is there any straightforward evidence of syllable boundaries in the movement trajectories of the articulators. An overview of this research is given by Krakow (1999).

In a different approach, phoneticians attempted to demonstrate that articulatory timing is more stable within syllables than across syllable boundaries (*syllable timing hypothesis*). However, in its general form this hypothesis also remains unproven. Browman and Goldstein (1988), for instance, who looked at articulatory trajectories in neologistic pairs like [pi.splats] versus [pis.plats], found that the onset of the first post-vocalic consonant had a relatively stable time locking with the preceding vowel, regardless of its syllable affiliation. Byrd (1995) who made electro-palatographic measurements on similar pairs of bisyllabic utterances, found a higher stability of consonant onset timing relative to the *following* vowel, with at least some effect of syllabic structure. Schiller *et al.* (1999) used electromagnetic articulography to examine the timing of articulatory movements for intervocalic consonants in Dutch triplets such as

(1)   /ka:.mər/–/kɑm.fər/–/kɑ[m] ən/,

with the hypothesis that the timing between /k/ and /m/ is more stable in /kɑm.fər/ than in /ka:.mər/, because the two consonants belong to the same syllable in the former. Contrary to expectations, however, the timing of consonants within syllables was no more stable than the timing of consonants across syllable boundaries.

A more successful series of investigations focused on examinations of the phonetic properties of syllable-initial versus syllable-final consonants. Krakow (1999) reviews a number of examinations of velar, lingual, labial, and mandibular movements, which consistently demonstrate that syllable onsets and syllable offsets can be distinguished by their articulatory patterns. Generally speaking, onset consonants are characterized by tighter constrictions and a closer between-articulator and between-gesture coupling than coda consonants. Differential behaviour of onset and coda consonants was also demonstrated by De Jong (2001), who used a metronome-controlled repetitive speech production task to show that internal temporal consistency was higher for nucleus-coda relationships than for onset-nucleus relationships. A conclusion from this observation was that the timing of vowel–consonant (VC) combinations is governed by local constraints, whereas consonant–vowel (CV) timing follows more global task constraints. This result conforms to data from quantitative phonology, according to which VC connections are stronger than CV connections (Kessler and Treiman 1997).

On the whole, phonetic evidence for a role of the syllable in speech motor control is focused less on the articulatory coherence of syllabic units or the dissection of neighbouring syllables by clear demarcations, and more on the asymmetric shape of onset and offset movements. Yet, the evidence existing so far is still not entirely convincing, since some investigations have led to contradictory positions (e.g. Tuller and Kelso 1990).

16.4 Psycholinguistics

The syllabic organization of spoken language is discussed in many areas of psycholinguistic theory: First, the syllable is acknowledged as an important primitive in adult speech production. Secondly, the syllable is also considered to be an early building block in models of language acquisition. Thirdly, the segmentation of words into syllables may guide lexical access in spoken language comprehension (Pitt *et al.* 1998) and may even play a role in visual word recognition. In the following, only production-related evidence will be reviewed.

16.4.1 Speech production in normal adults

To begin with, evidence for a syllable-based organization of speech production can be inferred from statistical considerations. In a statistical analysis of a Dutch text corpus, Schiller *et al.* (1996) demonstrated that a relatively small inventory of 500 syllables suffices to cover 85% of the Dutch lexicon. Similar results can be obtained from word counts in German and English corpora (cf. Schiller 1998). It is tempting to conclude from this that speech production is based on a 'library of articulatory routines' of syllabic size, i.e. a 'mental syllabary', an idea that is among the core elements of the word-production model formulated by W. J. M. Levelt *et al.* (1999).

More influential evidence for the syllable as a representational unit in speech production came from analyses of segmental speech errors in normal speakers. A frequently occurring class of errors, so-called movement errors, is considered sensitive to syllable structure, i.e. onsets tend to interact with onsets (2a), codas with codas (2b), and nuclei with nuclei (2c) (all examples of slips are from a personal corpus of the first author).

(2a) /pɔst.kʊtʃə/ (mail-coach) → [kɔst.pʊtʃə]

(2b) /aʊf.aʊs.lɛndɐ/ (on foreigners) → [aʊs.aʊf.lɛndɐ]

(2c) /tir.ʃʏtsɐ/ (animal protector) → [tyr.ʃɪtsɐ].

The observation that segmental slips obey a 'syllable position constraint' had a major influence on the emergence of 'slot-and-filler-models' of speech production. These models postulate that speech production involves the generation of syllabic frames consisting of slots for syllable onsets, nuclei, and codas, which are then filled with the appropriate segments (for a comprehensive review see Meyer, 1992). Dell's interactive model of speech production, too, acknowledges the specific role of syllable constituents by assigning them a separate representational layer and by specifying segments for syllable positions (Dell 1986). Several criticisms have been expressed against these theories. First, a principal objection was raised against the formulation of language-production models on the basis of speech errors alone. Some of the devices and functions postulated in speech-error-based models have been introduced solely to account for the occurrence of slips, with no useful function otherwise. This is an apparent paradox in the modelling of normal processes of spoken language production. Secondly, many of the data relating to syllable onsets were observed in word-initial position. A considerable proportion of the evidence for a syllable position constraint can therefore be explained by postulating a distinguished position for word- rather than syllable onsets, and a further part of the data can be accounted for by simply assuming that vowels and consonants occupy different slots on a linear string of segment-sized slots (cf. Meyer 1992).

A third source of evidence for the psychological reality of syllabic units in spoken language production comes from metalinguistic syllabification tasks. A variety of 'word-game' tasks have been developed which require subjects to produce polysyllabic words in a scanning manner, to dissect them by inserting pauses, or to reverse or reduplicate the parts of a bisyllabic word (Treiman 1983). Schiller *et al.* (1997), who reported on six word-game experiments, demonstrated that adult native speakers of Dutch largely conform to phonological syllable structure constraints in reversal tasks, reversing words like /ka:.mər/ into /mər.ka:/ and /ka[m]ər/ into /mər.kam/. Yet, in a noticeable number of cases the branching rhyme constraint (which rules out that open syllables end in a short vowel) was violated in their experiments, e.g. when /kI[k]ər/ was reversed to /kər.kI/ instead of /kər.kIk/. Schiller *et al.* (1997) concluded from their results that syllabification regularities reflect *preferences* rather than *strict rules*, which weakens the evidence coming from studies of this kind.

Content *et al.* (2001) chose a different approach to investigate the explicit status of syllable representations. They abandoned the search for clear syllable boundaries, adopting the view that the syllables of a word may overlap, i.e. that the offset of a syllable may not coincide with the onset of the following syllable. The results of their experiments corroborated this view, showing that syllable-onset decisions in word games are more stable than syllable-offset decisions. Multiple factors determine how subjects locate syllable offsets in metalinguistic tasks, e.g. the length and quality of the vowel, the sonority of the intervocalic consonant, lexical stress, orthography, and the nature of the task, while onset decision remains invariant under these factors (Content *et al.* 2001). The result that onset determination prevails over offset determination is consistent with the phonetic findings mentioned earlier, according to which syllable initial consonants have more distinct phonetic properties than coda consonants. It also fits a view which considers onsets more freely movable than coda consonants (Kessler and Treiman 1997).

All studies based on *explicit* manipulations of syllables have in common that these tasks are performed *offline* and may therefore rely on strategies that play no role in spoken language production. The results of such investigations can be influenced by experimental artefacts such as working memory constraints, response-dependency constraints (avoidance of geminates or of phoneme repetitions), or orthographic rules (for a discussion, see Schiller *et al.* 1997). To circumvent these shortcomings, effects of syllabic structure were investigated by *priming* paradigms. Ferrand *et al.* (1996) required subjects to name written or pictured words preceded by masked orthographic primes. These primes either shared the first syllable with the target, e.g. the prime PAR in the (French) word PAR.TI.SAN, or they crossed a syllable boundary, e.g. the same prime in the word PA.RA.SITE. In other cases, a prime matched the first syllable of the target (PA in PA.RA.SITE) or only part of it (PA in PAR.TI.SAN). The authors found that naming was facilitated by matching relative to non-matching syllable primes. They concluded that the syllable represents a functional unit of output phonology in French. These results were also extended to English (Ferrand *et al.* 1997), with the additional result that syllabic targets ending with an ambisyllabic consonant (CV[C]) were equally facilitated by their corresponding CV or CVC primes, respectively. However, in a further series of experiments based on the masked priming technique, Schiller (1998) failed to replicate the syllabic priming effect in Dutch speakers. A conclusion from this may be that the role of syllabic units, at least at the particular processing stage addressed by the masked syllable priming paradigm, is not homogeneous across languages.

However, a more recent study by Brand *et al.* (2002) even failed to replicate the syllable priming effect in French.

Despite the fact that the evidence provided by these and other studies is not unequivocal, the syllable plays a crucial role as a processing unit in the speech production model proposed by W. J. M. Levelt *et al.* (1999). The phonological encoding component of this model focuses on the problem of how a speaker transforms discrete word representations into strings of fluently pronounceable syllables. A basic assumption is that we speak *in syllables*. When the word forms stored in our long-term memory are retrieved serially, discontinuities of syllabicity may arise at the boundaries between morphemes, e.g. when the German plural form "pilots" would surface as * /pilot–ən/. To guarantee fluency of articulation, the segment sequences retrieved from the lexicon must be restructured, and much of this restructuring occurs across morpheme or word boundaries, e.g. turning <pilot> + <en> into /pi.lo.tən/. Thus, the phonological encoding component is viewed as an interface mechanism that maps the segmental constituents of lexical representations serially on to a metrical frame. As in most of the theories described above (except for Dell's theory) syllabification is achieved by a deterministic algorithm, i.e. syllables are not specified at the level of the lexicon but are generated 'on the fly' during word form encoding.

W. J. M. Levelt *et al.* (1999) postulate that syllables—at least those occurring frequently in a language—constitute articulatory primitives in the sense that their learned motor programmes are stored in a mental syllabary. In an influential series of reaction-time experiments Levelt and Wheeldon (1994) had found that words with a given word frequency were named faster when they consisted of frequently occurring syllables than when they were composed of low-frequency syllables. This finding, which still waits to be replicated, provided the basis for the assumption that the gestural scores (see Browman and Goldstein, 1989) for frequent syllables are retrieved from a mental syllable lexicon, while those of infrequent syllables must be assembled from smaller units. The direct access to ready-made motor programmes of syllabic size allows a considerable reduction of the computational load of the motor programming routines in speaking.

16.4.2 Theories of spoken language acquisition

Studies of the relation between babbling and early speech in normal development show that there is a continuous developmental progression from oral motor behaviour during the first year of life to early speech in the second year (Kent 1981; Koopmans-van Beinum *et al.* 1986; Mitchell and Kent 1990). Vocal development during the first year of life seems to be robust with respect to conditions of rearing, in particular socio-economic status and bilingual or monolingual environment (Oller *et al.* 1997), but other factors than ambient language affect infant speech development. Thus, severe hearing impairment, or mild and variable hearing loss due to episodes of otitis media, have been shown to affect babbling (Shriberg *et al.* 2000). This supports the view that the first year of speech development is dominated by perceptual–motor learning principles, which remain important during the years to follow, but in normal development are gradually dominated by phonological aspects: expanding the repertoire of speech sounds, and particularly speech sound combinations.

Thus, babbling and infant speech can be considered to consist of articulomotor patterns. The typical motoric pattern comprises a closing and opening gesture, perceived by adults as syllables. Oller *et al.* (1997, 1999) demonstrated a developmental transition at the age of about 10 months towards 'canonical' babbling, which is defined in the articulatory domain by a full (consonant-like) closure followed by a full (vowel-like) opening, and in the acoustic domain by a typical durational pattern, and typical fundamental frequency and formant trajectories. C. C. Levelt *et al.* (1999) showed that at the earliest stage of speech development the child produces a restricted set of syllable-sized articulatory forms. During this stage, place of articulation is not varied phoneme-by-phoneme but syllable-by-syllable, with the result that back consonants are combined with back vowels (in syllables such as [go]), front consonants with front vowels ([di]), and labial consonants with low-central vowels ([ba]). In a multi-session study on the babbling of six infants aged between 6.5 and 8 months of age, MacNeilage and Davis (2001*a*) not only corroborated these findings with respect to the front–back dimension, but in addition demonstrated that consonantal contexts that involve lingual occlusion at the roof of the mouth—coronal and dorsal—tend to favour high vowels. In contrast, in the labial context, in which the tongue is not required for the consonant, there is a complementary preference for the tongue to remain in a relatively low position. The authors interpreted these observations as strong evidence for 'lingual inertia' during this babbling stage.

Consonant–vowel productions at two distinct stages of language development were studied in a single female child by Sussman *et al.* (1996). Also in this study, an association was found between frequency of occurrence between consonant and vowel, in that at 12 months of age the velar consonant /g/ tended to be followed by a back or mid-central vowel, as compared to high-front and mid-low front vowels after bilabial /b/ and alveolar /d/. At 21 months of age, this tendency had disappeared. Assimilation of place between consonant and vowel was expressed in the frequency of co-occurrence of consonant and vowel with similar place, but not in acoustic overlap between segments. That is, only slight lingual anticipatory coarticulation in canonical babbling at 12 months of age and first words at 21 months of age was found during labial occlusion in, for instance, [bV] syllables. Similarly, a relatively constant alveolar locus was maintained across vowel contexts in [dV] syllables. Only [gV] syllables showed adult-like locus equation functions at 12 and 21 months. Thus, for some consonantal contexts this infant produced *weaker* coarticulation than adults, which at first sight seems at odds with the 'lingual inertia' hypothesis cited above. However, MacNeilage and Davis (2001*a*) based their conclusion on relative frequencies of productions, whereas the locus equations in the study of Sussman *et al.* are derived from all productions, frequent and rare. The solution to this apparent paradox might be that the tendency of 'lingual inertia' only applies to speech patterns that are produced frequently and can therefore be considered automatic. The relatively novel speech patterns occurring in a more diverse set of utterances, are produced in a more protracted manner, leading to the weaker coarticulation found by Sussman *et al.* (1996). We suggest that a second factor determining coarticulation is whether the speech pattern is homorganic or heterorganic. In the *homorganic* utterance /gV/, the tongue body is the main articulator involved in both the velar occlusion and the vowel. In contrast, for the production of *heterorganic* /bV/ and /dV/, apart from tongue body, a different main articulator is involved, namely lips for /b/ and tongue tip for /d/. Due to kinematic restrictions, the production of strong coarticulation in homorganic speech patterns requires less fine-tuned coordination than the production of weak coarticulation. For instance, to produce /gy/ with the same place of velar plosive constriction as /gu/ would require a rapid, well-coordinated tongue-body movement, whereas a more coarticulated pattern with slight fronting of velar constriction requires only a tongue body dropping gesture. In contrast, to produce strong coarticulation in heterorganic contexts requires fine-tuning of both articulators involved, in particular well-timed anticipation of the upcoming tongue body gesture during labial (/bV/) or alveolar (/dV/) occlusion. We will return to the issue of homorganic versus heterorganic in the discussion of speech disorders.

Further details of the acquisition process at a slightly later developmental stage have been studied by Nittrouer and collaborators (Nittrouer *et al.* 1989, 1996; Nittrouer, 1993), who provided evidence that the unit in children's speech develops from the syllable to the phoneme. The evidence comes from acoustic analyses of coarticulation in speech production and coarticulatory effects in perception. As an example of production studies, Nittrouer (1993) requested 10 adults and 30 children, ranging in age from 3 to 7 years, to produce an utterance such as: 'It's a CV Bob', in which C stand for one of the consonants /s, ʃ, t, d, k/ and V for one of the vowels /a, i, u/. Acoustical analyses were conducted on the fragment: [ə]-CV. It was shown that, for instance, in the word set: 'she' (/ʃi/), 'shoe' (/ʃu/), 'see' (/si/), and 'Sue' (/su/) children produced more coarticulation between vowel and consonant than adults, and less distinction in spectral characteristics of the fricative. Nittrouer *et al.* (1996) drew a parallel with motor development in newborns, in that global movements of the infant are refined into more precise and more differentiated coordinative structures, and that, at the same time, these increasingly differentiated movements are assembled into large functional units. Following our suggestion above, the developmental pattern seems to be one of increasing coarticulation during automation, followed by decreasing coarticulation during differentiation.

W. J. M. Levelt *et al.* (1999) suggested that the earliest meaningful speech production emerges from coupling lexical concepts to a repository of speech motor

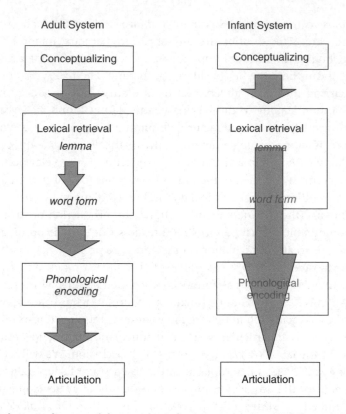

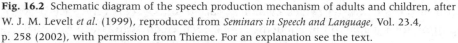

Fig. 16.2 Schematic diagram of the speech production mechanism of adults and children, after W. J. M. Levelt *et al.* (1999), reproduced from *Seminars in Speech and Language*, Vol. 23.4, p. 258 (2002), with permission from Thieme. For an explanation see the text.

patterns, called a 'protosyllabary'. Until then, lexical concepts and speech motor patterns coexisted as two independent systems. Thus, as the models in Fig. 16.2 show, the young child's production system can be characterized by a simplified model, consisting of a direct route between lexical concepts and articulatory forms, without the intermediate stages of the full-fletched adult system: word form retrieval and phonological encoding (see also Maassen 2002). Only at a later stage of development, under the communicative pressure of the growing vocabulary, the combinatorial possibilities of speech sounds expand, first of all by variation within the syllable of the feature place of articulation, later by other complicating processes such as the production of consonant clusters. From this expansion, which yields a tremendous increase in the productive power of the speech mechanism, a word-form lexicon and a phonological encoding system emerge.

Maturation and development of articulo-motor control plays a persisting role in the progress to adult speech. A first observation is that, at the stage at which children produce intelligible speech, the maturation of speech motor control continues. Clear indices of continuing maturation have been demonstrated until the age of 7 years, possibly continuing up to the age of 12 years (Kent 1997). Smith and Goffmann (Chapter 10, this volume) present evidence showing maturation up to 16 years of age. During this developmental period, (certain aspects of) the variability in speech production decreases, resulting in stabilization of speech patterns increasingly similar to the adult patterns.

Also, at the phonological level, syllabic effects can be demonstrated. Above, we saw that in non-linear phonology, in which the syllable is considered as a superordinate structural unit, asymmetries in the distribution of consonants across syllable-initial and syllable-final position occur. In the phonological development of children such asymmetries are clearly reflected. Based on data from a group of 12 children aged between 1 and 2 years of age, C. C. Levelt *et al.* (1999) found a consistent order of acquisition of syllabic structures across children (CV–CVC–V–VC) followed by either CVCC–VCC–CCV–CCVC or CCV–CCVC–CVCC–VCC. Thus, consonants and consonant clusters are not acquired at the same moment in syllable-initial and syllable-final position. These data allowed for the construction of a developmental grammar for syllable structure in the production of child language, and the concept of syllable complexity.

Taking a different approach, so-called 'syllable structure processes' during phonological development in early childhood further demonstrate syllabic constraints. Thus, all children go through a stage during which they produce many adult target forms without the consonant in syllable-final position (normal process 'final consonant deletion'), but not without the consonant in syllable-initial position (abnormal process 'initial consonant deletion'). Reduplication of syllable structures and omission of weak syllables are further examples of syllable structure processes during normal phonological development (Beers 1995). In the developmental trajectory the role of phonetic and phonological influences remain to be disentangled.

16.5 The role of syllables in acquired disorders of speech and language production

Turning now to the role of the syllable in aphasic speech, several lines of evidence can be followed. The discussion here is organized by two major symptoms of aphasic spoken output disorders, i.e. phonemic paraphasia and neologistic jargon on the one hand, and speech automatisms on the other.

16.5.1 Syllable structure constraints in phonemic paraphasia

First, one may ask whether phonemic paraphasic errors, similar to normal slips, are sensitive to syllable structure. An important observation here is that ill-formed syllable structures rarely, if ever, occur in paraphasic speech. In phonemic substitutions, consonants are regularly substituted by consonants and vowels by vowels, and phonemic errors usually respect phonotactic constraints. Further, as in normal slips, phonemes involved in cross-syllable transposition errors most often retain their syllable constituency, i.e. onset and coda consonants move to syllable onsets and codas, respectively (see examples (2a)–(2c) above). Movement errors within syllables may occur as well, e.g. when /ʃa:f/ (German for *sheep*) is pronounced as /ʃa:ʃ/.

There are several possible explanations for the preservation of phonotactic constraints in phonemic paraphasia:

1. An error-creating mechanism may respect syllable structure because it operates on the constituents of fully syllabified representations. Within the framework of Dell's spreading activation model, for instance, phonemes or consonant clusters involved in a phonemic error will be inserted into appropriate syllable slots because they are marked for syllable constituency (Dell 1986). Explanations relating to the copying and check-off mechanism of the classical slot-and-filler model follow a similar logic (Buckingham 1993).
2. Errors occurring at a stage where phonological representations are not yet syllabified, e.g. in the output lexicon, may create phoneme strings that cannot be parsed by the normal syllabification algorithm. In such a case, later occurring repair processes must be postulated which lead to a graceful restitution of pronounceability. As an example, vowel epenthesis may occur when the normal syllabification mechanism fails (Béland 1990).
3. Within the framework of the Nijmegen model of speech production, phonemic errors are ascribed to an *indexing failure*, i.e. a problem at the point where the syllabary is accessed for the selection of a target syllable (Roelofs 2000). Thus, a phonemic error of the kind

    (3)   /to.ma.tə/ (tomato's) → /mo.ta.tə/

    would be explained by erroneous selection of the syllable /mo/ for /to/ and of /ta/ for /ma/. Here, syllable structure constraints are preserved by virtue of the fact that the system operates on a 'lexicon' of overlearned, syllable-sized motor programmes. This framework does not predict, however, that syllable structure is still preserved if encoding errors occur in low-frequent syllables, i.e. when the syllabary is circumvented and syllables must be assembled phoneme by phoneme.

16.5.2 Syllable structure constraints in neologistic jargon

Patients with severe fluent aphasia may produce 'abstruse' neologisms with very little or no similarity to target word forms. If a patient's speech output is dominated by such extremely aberrant forms, the syndrome is termed *neologistic jargon*. A

THE ROLE OF THE SYLLABLE

striking feature of abstruse neologisms is that they conform to syllable structure regularities as well. The fact that neologisms are phonotactically well formed has even become a part of their definition (Ryalls *et al.* 1988).

The creation of neologistic jargon is tentatively explained by two major theories. One theory postulates that the occurrence of neologistic forms is associated with the condition of anomia. In cases where lexical access fails entirely, a 'random generator' steps in and generates new strings of phonemes (Butterworth 1979). In its original form, this device was conceived as a segment-based generator, and an additional mechanism was assumed which aligns the segments in a phonotactically regular manner in a buffer (Butterworth 1979). To avoid the strong assumption of a separate machinery generating phonotactic well-formedness, Buckingham (1987) proposed that the random generator produces entire syllables. Borrowing from the Levelt model, one might say that the deadlocked situation of impaired lexical access triggers some default production mechanism to randomly select syllables from the syllabary. A second theory of neologistic jargon assumes that neologisms result from a disinhibition mechanism. In this model, the fact that the unintended utterances conform to phonotactic constraints is ascribed to an intact sound-sequencing mechanism which is governed by syllable structure principles (cf. Butterworth 1979).

16.5.3 Markedness effects in phonemic paraphasia

A large part of the literature concerned with syllable structure in paraphasic speech refers to the concept of syllabic *markedness*. Blumstein (1973), who examined phonemic errors in Broca's, Wernicke's, and conduction aphasia, found that patients from all syndrome groups had a tendency to decrease the markedness of syllable structures. According to these data, aphasic patients not only avoid illegal syllable structures, but they also avoid rare structures, such as VC or CVCC, and preferentially create unmarked syllables of the CV type. Since Blumstein's work, syllable markedness effects in paraphasic speech were replicated in patients from different syndrome groups, such as conduction aphasia (Béland *et al.* 1990), 'fluent aphasia' (Christman 1992), or Broca's aphasia (Romani and Calabrese 1998). Only Favreau *et al.* (1990) found that *fluent* aphasics may often *increase* syllable markedness by adding consonants in onset or coda positions.

It should be mentioned that cluster reduction alone (e.g. CCV → CV or CVCC → CVC) does not necessarily require a syllable-based explanation, since it is also consistent with a simplification mechanism operating on linear phonemic structures. Convincing evidence for a role of the syllable in phonemic paraphasia can only be inferred from observations demonstrating that aphasic patients avoid deleting or inserting segments to create more marked syllable structures. The conduction aphasic described by Béland *et al.* (1990), for instance, produced a noticeable number of vowel omissions, but he avoided omissions of the type

(4a) /palɛ/ (French for *palace*) → * [plɛ],

where an increase in syllable complexity would result. At the same time, this patient occasionally added vowels to create less complex structures, as in

(4b) /stʀi/ (French for *scratch*) → [sœ.tʀi].

   Similar to (4b), aphasic speakers of German or English may frequently reduce clusters by schwa insertion between clustering consonants.

   Syllable structure effects can also be postulated when phonemic paraphasias lead to a systematic increase of the sonority gradient at syllable onset and a sonority decrease at syllable offset. A frequent observation is, for instance, that consonant deletions in obstruent–liquid onset clusters preferentially concern the liquid and not the obstruent, i.e.

(5a) /plчi/ (French for *rain)* → [pчi]

but not

(5b) /plчi/ → * [lчi]

(see Béland *et al*. 1990; Romani and Calabrese 1998).

   The tendency of certain aphasic patients to reduce syllabic markedness is considered to characterize the mechanism of error creation as basically a reduction of phonological complexity. Blumstein (1973), on the basis of her data, speculated that phonemic errors in all aphasic syndromes can be accounted for by a single *simplification* mechanism operating on syllabic structure. Béland *et al*. (1990) claimed that the conduction aphasic patient described in their report avoided marked syllable structures because he had a problem of applying the difficult syllabification rules associated with complex syllable structures. In their view, markedness reduction occurs at a rather abstract representational level. In contrast, Favreau *et al*. (1990), who failed to observe markedness reduction in patients with fluent aphasia, speculated that markedness reduction only occurs in patients with *lower-level* encoding problems and that it reflects a major problem of these patients with articulatory complexity. Romani and Calabrese (1998), too, pledged for an articulatory–motor interpretation of markedness effects and claimed that patients with Broca's aphasia may simplify complex syllabic structures in anticipation of their motor problems of realizing these structures. Their assumption is that a deficit at the level of articulatory planning leads to a simplification of higher-level representations. It should be mentioned that this explanation implies a bottom-up flow of information across the boundary between phonological encoding and articulation, which is not allowed for by conventional models of spoken language production (Ziegler 2002).

16.5.4 Syllable structure constraints and markedness in speech automatisms

Syllable structure preservation is also observable in a most severe form of spoken output disturbance in aphasia, i.e. in speech automatisms. Speech automatisms, or *recurring utterances*, are stereotypical and repetitive, lexical or neologistic, utterances, which mostly predominate a patient's speech output or even constitute her or his only verbal means (Blanken *et al.* 1990). In their lexical form, speech automatisms consist of regularly formed real words or of short phrases (e.g. *macht nix*; German for *doesn't matter*), while non-lexical recurring utterances consist of concatenations of nonsense syllables (e.g. [da da]) (both examples of automatisms are from Blanken and Marini 1997). In their meta-analysis of speech automatisms and recurring utterances in global aphasia, Code *et al.* (1994) reported that phonotactic constraints are rigidly adhered to, even in non-lexical forms. A further important result of their analysis was that unmarked forms occur more frequently in these utterances than more marked forms. In particular, the CV structure clearly predominates, which may mean that the production of speech automatisms is entertained by some kind of *proto-syllabary* (cf. Section 16.4.2). According to a theory proposed by Blanken (1991), severe damage to neural structures supporting the articulatory buffer may prevent the assembly of new articulatory programmes and thereby lead to a stereotyped reiteration of default material stuck in the buffer. In a review of syllable-related mechanisms in speech and language disorders, Code (2002) evaluates more comprehensively the findings and theories about this aphasic symptom.

16.5.5 Apraxia of speech

The syndrome of apraxia of speech (AOS) has traditionally been related to a stage where speech motor programmes are constructed or pre-existing articulatory routines are accessed. Some of the symptoms of AOS have an obvious surface-relation to syllabic units: apraxic speakers often dissect the flow of speech into segregated syllables, with a reduced coarticulation across syllable boundaries (Ziegler and von Cramon 1985) or even with short intersyllabic pauses (Kent and Rosenbek 1982, 1983) .

The observation of a syllable-by-syllable mode of articulation has stimulated hypotheses postulating a restricted programming window in AOS speakers. Rogers and Storkel (1999) explicitly formulated a *reduced buffer capacity hypothesis*, saying that AOS patients have a restricted articulatory buffer and are therefore required to plan and programme utterances on a syllable-by-syllable basis. In their experiment, patients had to produce, as quickly as possible, two monosyllabic words appearing on a computer screen. Apraxic speakers demonstrated a phonological similarity effect in their response delays, which was interpreted as an inhibitory effect occurring after the first word had been programmed. The inhibitory mechanism, in their theory, prevented AOS patients from loading a new programme sharing one or more features with a programme already residing in the buffer.

The assumption that AOS patients plan speech 'one syllable at a time' is inconsistent with the results of a simple reaction experiment published recently (Deger and Ziegler 2002). In this experiment, preparation for speech was examined in two types of motor responses: in pseudowords consisting of alternating syllables (e.g. /daba/) and in reiterations of a single syllable (/dada/). A group of apraxic speakers had increased simple reaction times to the heterogeneous sequences, indicating that they had a problem of 'chunking' two different syllables into a complex integrated motor programme. They appeared to require extra time for the 'unpacking' of a programme component regulating the transition between two subsequent syllables. This finding suggests that intersyllabic programming routines may play a role in phonetic planning, and that these routines (in addition to syllabic or segmental routines) are affected in AOS.

According to a theory formulated by Varley and Whiteside (2000), the problem patients with AOS are faced with is one of accessing the programme routines for linguistic units of the size of a word. This hypothesis borrows from Levelt's account of a mental syllabary (W. J. M. Levelt et al., 1999), but is not confined to the level of syllables. In the view of Varley and Whiteside (2000), AOS patients have lost the ability to use stored 'movement gestalts' for frequently occurring words and are instead required to assemble, via an 'indirect route', each utterance from smaller units. This was inferred from the results of a preliminary study (Whiteside and Varley 1998), in which AOS patients failed to demonstrate a frequency effect similar to the one described by Levelt and Wheeldon (1994), but on word, not syllable frequency. Others have been opposed to Varley and Whiteside's position, saying that destruction of a 'direct' encoding route in apraxic speakers might perhaps explain some dysfluency in their articulation, but it cannot explain their extremely laborious, effortful, groping, and distorted speech (Miller 2001; Ziegler 2001).

Aichert and Ziegler (2003) examined syllable frequency effects on speech errors in 10 patients with AOS. On a word list controlled for phonological structure and word frequency, apraxic patients made significantly more errors on syllables with low frequency as compared to highly frequent syllables. At the same time, syllable structure effects were found in the segmental errors of apraxic speakers. For instance, patients with AOS made significantly more errors on syllable-initial consonant clusters than on consonant clusters crossing a syllable boundary, and syllable boundary clusters were more error prone than coda clusters. This finding is not consistent with a model postulating that AOS patients are confined to a phoneme-by-phoneme assembly route. Instead, it suggests that syllabic representations are accessed during phonetic encoding, but that these representations may contain incomplete or distorted gestural information and force patients to reconstruct parts of the syllabic motor programme from smaller units.

16.5.6 Repetitive speech disorders

In rare cases, after acquired brain lesions, patients present with a pattern of speech impairment that is predominated by the occurrence of repetitive elements. Although there is no general agreement on how these disorders should be classified, several clinical patterns can be distinguished (cf. Wallesch 1990). One of the criteria used in differential diagnosis refers to the *size* of the reiterated element. Since repetitive syndromes may originate at different levels of the speech production system, the implication of syllabic units in repetitive behaviour may shed light on the locus of the impairment.

16.5.6.1 Repetitive speech disorders following supplementary motor area lesions

Speech impairments subsequent to lesions of the supplementary motor area (SMA) have inconsistently been associated with aphasia ('transcortical motor aphasia'), dysfluency ('stuttering'), or disordered movement initiation. A variety of different symptoms can be observed in patients with left SMA lesions, including mutism, hypophonia, reduced speech production, and iterative and dysfluent articulation (cf. Laplane *et al.* 1977; Gelmers 1983; Goldberg 1985). An relevant observation here is that patients with lesions to mesio-frontal cortical areas of the left hemisphere may, during the course of their disorder, develop dysfluent, iterative, or even stuttering-like speech (e.g. Ackermann *et al.* 1996).

Ziegler *et al.* (1997) described a patient with a haemorrhagic lesion undercutting the left SMA, who was not aphasic, but who had a reduced language output and was dysfluent. She had intersyllabic and interword pauses of increased frequency and length, false starts, and repetitions of syllables and whole words. Her articulation was otherwise undisturbed. Repetition of words was largely normal, while repetition of non-words longer than three syllables was severely compromised. In a series of simple reaction tasks including syllable sequences of different lengths (/dada/ versus /dadada/) or different segmental content (/dada/ versus /daba/), the SMA patient demonstrated a clear length effect on reaction time (*syllable latency effect*), but no effect of segmental complexity. This finding, which contrasted with the pattern found in apraxic speakers (Deger and Ziegler 2002), was attributed to a deficit at the level of the articulatory buffer, in particular to the unpacking of a fully specified sequence of syllable-sized motor programmes (Ziegler *et al.* 1997). It was concluded that the SMA plays a role in the preparation of sequential articulations for multisyllabic strings. Together with the observation that intra-operative electrical stimulation of the SMA may elicit rhythmic repetitions of CV syllables, this case report provides evidence for a frame-content dualism, with a major role of mesio-frontal cortical and striatal structures in the generation of syllabic frames (MacNeilage and Davis 2001*b*).

16.5.6.2 Palilalia

A rare but very remarkable variant of repetitive speech is *palilalia*, i.e. the compulsive repetition of words or phrases. Unlike the automatisms of aphasic patients, palilalic iterations are not stereotyped, but based on contextually adequate speech. An Italian patient reported by Gorno *et al.* (1997), for instance, who was asked to repeat the sentence 'oggi è una bella giornata' (it's a nice day today), produced:

(6a) oggi oggi gi oggi è una bella è una bella è una bella bella giornata giornata oggi è una bella giornata oggi è una bella giornata;

or a Japanese patient who, on a question about his well-being, produced the utterance

(6b) guai guai guai guai ima ima ima ima toku toku toku tokuni ii-desu

instead of the answer 'guai ima tokuni ii-desu' (Yasuda *et al.* 1990). Often, such sequences are produced with a gradually increasing speech rate and a decreasing voice volume, although other variants are discussed as well (Benke and Butterworth 2001). Palilalia has been described in postencephalitic parkinsonism, progressive supranuclear palsy, thalamic and midbrain infarcts, and in degenerative disorders, and as a side-effect of pharmacologic agents (for a review, see Wallesch 1990). Most authors assume that bilateral striatal ventral-thalamic circuits are implicated in the genesis of palilalic speech (Yasuda *et al.* 1990). The frequent co-occurrence with dysexecutive symptoms might suggest that palilalia results from a loss of frontal inhibitory control on spoken language production.

The unit of palilalic iteration is usually larger than the syllable. In most examples documented in the literature, palilalic repetitions encompass syllables, multisyllabic words or word parts, or even whole phrases (cf. the examples (6a) and (6b) above or the speech samples presented by Benke and Butterworth 2001). Articulation is well formed and the iterative cycle rarely cuts through a syllable. If we assume that syllables constitute the predominant unit of speech motor programming, the finding of preserved syllable integrity is consistent with the view that the iteration mechanism operates on strings of fully encoded speech and does not interrupt the articulatory implementation of pre-programmed units. Garratt *et al.* (1999) assume that palilalic reiteration originates at the level of the articulatory buffer and is due to a disinhibition of the downloading process. Benke and Butterworth (2001) discuss a failure of central executive functions implicated in the monitoring or, more specifically, the termination of articulation-based processes. The case described by Ackermann *et al.* (1989), who presented with palilalia as a symptom of pharmacologically induced hyperkinesia, suggests an explanation based on striatal mechanisms of motor inhibition. More systematic investigations of the 'loop size' of repetition cycles are required to examine these hypotheses.

16.5.6.3 Acquired stuttering

While stuttering is a very frequent transient condition during language acquisition (which sometimes even persists during adulthood), it is an extremely rare consequence of lesions to the adult brain. Acquired neurogenic stuttering may occur after left or right hemisphere infarction, head injury, or in basal ganglia disorders, e.g. parkinsonism (Helm *et al.* 1978; Koller 1983; Fleet and Heilman 1985; Hertrich *et al.*, 1993), but it is not clear whether the reported cases pertain to a unitary syndrome. Several pathomechanisms were named to account for acquired stuttering-like behaviours, e.g. damage to callosal pathways coordinating the activity of the two hemispheres (Soroker *et al.* 1990), a dyskinetic condition caused by dysfunctions at the mesothalamic or striatal level (Andy and Bhatnagar 1992), or an interruption of thalamic projections to the supplementary motor area (Abe *et al.* 1993).

The speech pattern of acquired neurogenic stuttering is often dominated by iterations, although the occurrence of tonic blocks has also been reported. In most case descriptions, the size of the reiterated units is specified as phonemic or syllabic: In a patient with a right-hemisphere stroke, Ardila and Lopez (1986) reported percentages of 31 and 34 for phoneme and syllable iterations, respectively, and considerably smaller percentages for part-word, word, and phrase repetitions. A patient with Parkinson's disease reported by Hertrich *et al.* (1993) had more than 95% CV repetitions, and the patient described by Fleet and Heilman (1985) 'almost always' stuttered on initial phonemes or syllables. Similar observations were made in other case studies, and the low incidence or the absence of iterations of word or phrase size was often regarded as an operational criterion for the exclusion of palilalia. Therefore, it appears safe to say that the repetitive disorder classified as acquired neurogenic stuttering differs from other syndromes by the relative amount of syllabic and sub-syllabic units involved in the iterations. Moreover, not all iterations classified as 'syllabic' are iterations of the full target syllable, e.g. when /lam.pə/ (*lamp*) is stuttered as [lə lə lə lampə], where the unit of repetition is the phoneme /l/ rather than the syllable /lam/. If syllables are the building blocks of speech motor programming, the frequent occurrence of subsyllabic repetitions suggests that the oscillator involved in acquired stuttering must operate on units of motor execution rather than on full motor programmes. The implication of a striato-thalamo-cortical loop postulated by some authors would suggest that the pathomechanism underlying acquired neurogenic stuttering is similar to the pathomechanism underlying palilalia, but the former presumably operates on a lower motor level than the latter. From this point of view, the dysfluent speaking seen in patients with lesions to the SMA (see above) might be considered as another variation of the same theme.

16.5.7 Dysarthria

Dysarthria results from an impairment of the motor processes involved in the *execution* (as opposed to the programming) of speech movements. The major pathomechanisms underlying the dysarthrias are paresis, rigidity and akinesia, dyskinesia, tremor, and ataxia. From the viewpoint of the Nijmegen model of speech production discussed above, these pathophysiological conditions must be considered to influence the speech mechanisms at the level of the *articulator*. Given that the input to the articulator is comprised of sequences of syllable-sized motor programmes, the function of this component is to transform the pre-programmed information into action. Unfortunately, it is not known what precisely must be prescribed in the phonetic plan of an utterance and how much is left to the function of the skilful articulatory motor system (for a discussion, see Levelt 1989). Regarding the role of syllabic units, W. J. M. Levelt *et al.* (1999) speculated that between-syllable coarticulation processes are not included in the phonetic encoding process but are left over to the functioning of the articulators. However, this part of Levelt's theory is not substantiated by experimental data. Results from reaction time experiments reported by Deger and Ziegler (2002) rather suggest that between-syllable adjustments are part of the phonetic plan rather than being regulated by motor execution processes, since patients with apraxia of speech required considerable extra time for the concatenation of consecutive syllables in initiating heterogeneous syllable sequences (e.g. /daba/ as opposed to /dada/). It should be mentioned here that these issues arise only through the assumption of a prescriptive relation between motor planning and motor execution. In task-dynamic models of speech motor control, such regularities are explained as emergent properties of a self-organizing system (see Chapter 3, this volume).

Data from dysarthric speakers are equivocal at this point. Patients with ataxic dysarthria may often demonstrate *scanning speech*, i.e. a syllable-by-syllable mode of speaking with an equal pacing of stressed and unstressed syllables (Kent and Rosenbek 1982). Perceptually, the syllables of an utterance are not smoothly integrated into a continuous stream, but are clearly separated from each other, and sometimes short intersyllabic pauses are perceptible. This might indicate a specific failure of between-syllable coarticulatory adjustments. Yet, a different interpretation would ascribe the segregation of syllables in ataxic dysarthria to a compensation for ataxic symptoms like tremor or dysmetria. It is a rather common clinical observation that patients with severe dysarthrias of almost all aetiologies take care to maintain the syllabicity of their spoken output. For instance, patients whose articulatory capacity of realizing consonantal occlusions is almost completely wiped out may often tend to vocalize each syllable separately, and patients with severe respiratory disorders most often take their breaths between, not within, syllables (Ziegler *et al.* 1990). This behaviour may express a patient's attempt to optimize intelligibility and maintain some speech-like quality in his or her severely distorted output, rather than a problem of specifying the motor adjustments for the concatenation of consecutive syllables. A pattern that is seen in Parkinson's disease demonstrates that not all patients dispose of such compensatory resources. The speech of many patients with Parkinson's disease is characterized by an increase in syllabic rate, often to the extent that consecutive syllables virtually merge (Ackermann and Ziegler 1992). This pattern indicates an extremely high degree of between-syllable motor integration and a loss of control over the sequential ordering of syllabic movement cycles. It is only by the use of assistive devices, e.g. external pacemakers or delayed auditory feedback, that these patients can temporarily regain control over the rhythmic pace of their spoken output.

16.6 The role of syllables in disorders of speech development

Normal speech and language development comprises the acquisition of increasingly complex patterns, in which newly acquired skills build upon the then available repertoire. In this paragraph we discuss phonological and speech motor control aspects of developmental speech disorders, and the issue of differential diagnosis between a phonological disorder as a consequence of specific language impairment (SLI) and children with the speech motor disorder, developmental apraxia of speech (DAS), with special emphasis on the role of the syllable.

The motor speech disorder which has undoubtedly been the most disputed in the past two decades, since the provocative publication by Guyette and Diedrich (1981), is developmental apraxia of speech. Guyette and Diedrich argued that all the symptoms of DAS referred to in the literature, were not exclusive for DAS, but also occurred in other speech disorders in children. This lack of 'pathognomonic' symptoms led them to conclude that the evidence for a diagnostic category, DAS, is insufficient. Since then many studies have been conducted with the aim of establishing the symptomatology of DAS, and discussion has concentrated on whether DAS is a syndrome or a specific function disorder.

From a developmental perspective, it is reasonable to assume that the origin of this diagnostic confusion—which may well apply to other developmental speech disorders—is the changing symptomatology that can be expected even under the supposition of a stable underlying impairment. Above, we saw that, in normal speech motor development, differentiation and dissociation of articulatory gestures is a process that extends over years (approximately from age 1;6 to 7 or even 12 years of age). Now suppose that the inability to make progress in this important speech motor acquisition process is the core feature of DAS. The immediate first implicational hypothesis is that all children, normally developing as well as speech delayed, go through a stage of development in which they show speech characteristics that are similar to those seen in DAS. If a severity index or progression index could be found reflecting this aspect of speech motor acquisition, then an early diagnostic characteristic would be available. However, the supposition that both children with DAS and normally speaking children show similar characteristics at that particular acquisition stage, makes one realize that differential diagnosis is particularly complicated, or even impossible.

16.6.1 Segments

What is the role of the syllable in this discussion? To date, no longitudinal studies are available in which children with DAS are followed from babbling to early speech. The problem, of course, is that DAS is only diagnosed at a later age, typically not younger than 4 years. The most extensive overview of speech–language characteristics of children with DAS, or, more cautiously, 'suspected DAS', by Shriberg *et al.* (1997*a*), showed no characteristics at the segmental level differentiating speech by children with suspected DAS from speech by children with speech delay (SD). Thus, the speech profiles for both groups were similar, both with respect to frequency of intended consonants in spontaneous speech, as with respect to the intended syllable and word forms. Some differences in error pattern were found between DAS and SD, such as a lower percentage of vowels correct in DAS, but effects of syllabic structure, if any, were identical. Thus, some processes were insensitive to syllable structure in both groups, such as palatal fronting and liquid simplification, which occurred equally frequently in syllable-initial and syllable-final position. Other processes showed a preference for a particular syllabic position, examples are cluster reduction and stopping, which occurred predominantly in syllable-initial position. However, the crucial finding was that these symmetries and asymmetries were identical for DAS and SD.

Similar results were obtained by Thoonen *et al.* (1994) and Maassen *et al.* (1997) in an analysis of articulation test data from 23 children with DAS (age 4;11–6;10 years) as compared to 23 children with SD (age 4;06–7;0) and 25 normally speaking (NS) children (age 4;09–6;10). There were substantial differences between groups with respect to rates of consonant substitutions and omissions, cluster errors and error types, but all contextual analyses yielded negative results. Thus, similar relative frequencies of syllable initial (many) as compared to syllable final (few) consonant substitutions, and syllable initial (few) as compared to syllable final (many) consonant omissions were found for all three groups. Likewise, similar relative frequencies of syntagmatic consonant substitution (around 2/3, dominated by syllable initial anticipations and perseverations) as compared to paradigmatic (1/3) substitution rates were found for both DAS and NS. Thus, there is no indication that the syllable plays a differential role in the segmental spellout processes (Levelt 1989) of children with DAS as compared to other speech disorders, or as compared to (younger) normally speaking children.

16.6.2 Prosody

However, at the prosodic level, a recent study by Shriberg *et al.* (1997*b*) indicates a possible role of the syllable in DAS, based on the stress patterns of utterances from children with suspected DAS, yielding the following categories: inappropriate multisyllabic word stress; reduced–equal stress; excessive–equal–misplaced stress; combinations of these. Excessive–equal–misplaced stress was the predominant behaviour coded as inappropriate. In a cross-validation study (Shriberg *et al.* 1997*c*), approximately 50% of the children referred to the clinic with the diagnosis 'suspected DAS' showed this typical profile, comprising inappropriate stress in combination with adequate phrasing, adequate rate, and adequate voice characteristics. Stress assignment is assumed to be part of the syllabification process in Levelt's model (W. J. M. Levelt *et al.* 1999). Now the question is whether these symptoms are primary or secondary. In earlier publications on clinical characteristics of DAS, the question was raised whether inappropriate stress is a compensatory behaviour, and thus secondary to some primary deficit. Shriberg *et al.* (1997*c*) provide two findings they consider as counter-evidence for the 'compensatory strategy' explanation of inappropriate stress. First, if excessive–equal stress is a learned behaviour to enhance intelligibility or to compensate for some segmental production deficit, one would expect older children to exhibit most evidence of long-term adoption of this type of compensatory pattern. However, inappropriate stress was unrelated to age. A second finding viewed as inconsistent with the compensatory behaviour explanation is that inappropriate stress was observed not only in long and complex utterances, but also in brief and simple utterances.

Velleman and Shriberg (1999) compared the speech of children with DAS and speech delay, using analytic procedures from metrical phonology. The lexical stress errors of both groups of children were found to conform to patterns identified in metrical studies of younger normally developing children, confirming the applicability of this approach to children with disorders. Lexical metrical patterns did not differentiate the groups from each other. However, syllable omissions persisted at much later ages in the children with DAS, especially those children previously identified as having inappropriate phrasal stress.

Results further corroborating a prosodic involvement in DAS were obtained in a study by Nijland et al. (2003). Children with DAS, 5 years of age, produced brief utterances in which the syllabic structure was systematically varied. The crucial elements were the consonants /s/ and /x/, which were produced either as a syllable–initial consonant cluster (utterances of the form: $/zV_1/$ # $/sxV_2t/$, in which # is the syllable boundary, example: /zə/ # /sxit/, meaning: 'she shoots'), or as abutting consonants in different syllables ($/zV_1s/$ # $/xV_2t/$, example: /zʉs/ # /xit/, meaning: 'sister pours'). Below we will discuss coarticulation effects within and between syllables, but at this point two results are relevant. First, it was observed that of the six children with DAS, three were not able to produce /sx/ as a cluster, but did produce /sx/ as abutting consonants without any pauses or other acoustically measurable differences. The typical cluster error was cluster reduction, which can be considered a normal phonological process. Thus, these data can be interpreted to show that syllabic structure does play a role in the generation of speech by children with DAS, in a manner similar to that of younger, normally speaking children, cluster reduction being a normal developmental process. Secondly, for the total group of children with DAS, it was found that they do not distinguish between iambic (unstressed /zə/ followed by stressed /sxit/) and spondaic (equal stress on /zʉs/ and /xit/) utterances. NS children systematically and significantly made durational differences between these two patterns.

16.6.3 Coarticulation

From a motor perspective, the phonemic segment is not the unit of articulation. Rather, successive articulatory gestures are highly dependent on the phonemic context and extend across phonemes, which results in articulatory overlap or coarticulation (Browman and Goldstein 1997). In this view, problems in planning and programming of speech movements leave their traces in the coarticulatory cohesion of the utterances. Hertrich and Ackermann (1995), for example, found that, in normal speech, slowed speech rate resulted in a decrease of perseveratory coarticulation and, against their expectations, unaltered or even increased anticipatory coarticulation. Above we cited studies demonstrating that the amount of coarticulatory overlap changes during the developmental process from babbling, to infant speech, and to fully mature speech. Thus, coarticulation phenomena can tell us something about speech motor control and speech motor development.

Although only a few studies have been conducted on coarticulation patterns in children with DAS (e.g. Sussman *et al.* 2000), studies on coarticulation in AOS in adults are mentioned frequently. These studies have reported divergent results. Whereas some researchers found a lack of coarticulatory cohesion in apraxic patients (Ziegler and Von Cramon 1985, 1986; Dogil *et al.* 1996; Whiteside and Varley 1998), others did not (Katz and Baum 1987; Katz 1988). The data of Southwood *et al.* (1996) showed that speaking rate and articulators involved might be one of the sources of the different coarticulation patterns in apraxic speech. Furthermore, divergent problems underlying AOS were suggested, varying from inappropriately phasing speech gestures (Ziegler and Von Cramon 1985, 1986) and lack of automation (Whiteside and Varley 1998), to phonological overspecification (Dogil *et al.* 1996).

Recently, Nijland *et al.* (2002*a*) conducted a series of experiments to study coarticulation within and across syllables in children with DAS. Considering the divergent results on AOS, either *weaker* or *stronger* coarticulation in children with DAS as compared to normally speaking children was expected. Weaker coarticulation in DAS would correspond to the frequently reported clinical impression of slow and protracted speech, due to a protracted segment-to-segment motor planning or programming. Stronger coarticulation effects could be predicted under the hypothesis that motor control in children with DAS is not fully developed, corresponding to a more global planning of the utterances similar to the speech of younger, normally speaking children. By using formant frequency measurements, Nijland *et al.* (2002*a*) found that normally speaking

(NS) children and adult women displayed highly similar patterns of F2 ratios. In contrast to the NS children and adults, the children with DAS produced idiosyncratic coarticulation patterns, suggesting that gestural control in children with DAS is not only delayed, but also deviant. This result was confirmed in a second study in which utterances produced with and without a bite-block were compared (Nijland *et al.* 2002*b*). As demonstrated by a significant change in F2, NS children compensated to a lesser extent than adult women, who were able to fully compensate for the bite-block, but both groups showed similar coarticulation patterns. However, the children with DAS also produced aberrant coarticulation patterns, as well as higher variability caused by the bite-block, suggesting specific deficits in speech motor control. A third study was designed specifically to demonstrate syllabic effects, by measuring coarticulation in utterances of the form /zV₁/ # /sxV₂t/ as compared to /zV₁s/ # /xV₂t/ (for examples see above). Based on the syllabic organization of gestures, stronger coarticulation within syllables than between syllables was predicted; in this case, stronger anticipatory coarticulation from /V₂/ on /s/ in /zV₁/ # /sxV₂t/, where these segments belong to the same syllable, than in /zV₁s/ # /xV₂t/, where /V₂/ and /s/ belong to different syllables. Although systematic coarticulation effects were found, no such syllabic difference could be demonstrated, neither in the children with DAS nor in the NS children and adult women. Quite unexpectedly, however, syllabic structure did show an effect on anticipatory coarticulation from /V₂/ on /V₁/, which was stronger in iambic unstressed /zə/ followed by stressed /sxV₂t/ than in spondaic equal stressed /zʉs/ and /xV₂t/ utterances. In explaining this effect, the quality of V₁ seems to be important. Although the average second formant values of V₁ in the open syllable context (/zə/) were equal to the values in the closed syllable (/zʉs/), there seem to be other differences. The syllables differ in phonological specification of V₁ and in a prosodic sense. First, the phonologically more specified vowel /ʉ/ possibly allows for less coarticulation than the neutral vowel /ə/. This finding corresponds to the principle of underspecification (Keating 1988), which suggests that phonologically unmarked features remain unspecified in phonetic realizations. The underspecified /ə/ is more easily influenced by context (the following/preceding consonant and vowel) than specified /ʉ/.

Secondly, the syllables differ in prosodic sense. Vowels in a prosodically stronger position are expected to exhibit less coarticulation than those in weaker positions (de Jong *et al.* 1993; Cho 1999). Above, we saw that the closed syllable (/zʉs/) was stressed, whereas the open syllables /zə/ did not have stress in these utterances. Both interpretations, phonological underspecification as well as difference in prosodic processing, might account for the effect of our experimental manipulation of syllable structure on the coarticulation in V₁.

To conclude, children with speech disorders demonstrate syllabic effects at the segmental level, the prosodic level, and at the level of phonetic planning and motor programming. To some extent, effects originating from each of these processing levels can be distinguished, forming the methodological basis for delineating the underlying deficits in DAS. Only recently, attempts to explore the developmental trajectory have been undertaken, addressing questions related to, for instance, determination of segmental and syllable-structure deviations by speech motor factors.

16.7 Concluding remarks

This chapter was an introduction into current discussion of the role of the sylla-ble as an organizing structure in spoken language production and its disorders. Since, in many types of normal linguistic performance, syllables apparently play a prominent role, modern phonological theory, phonetic experimentation, and psycholinguistic modelling have focused strongly on syllabic representations. It was shown here that the patterns of breakdown of language production in chil-dren and adults with brain lesions, as well as developmental patterns during infancy and early speech in both normal and disordered speech acquisition, provide additional evidence for the assumption that speaking is based heavily on the rhythmical structure of syllabified language. 'Protosyllables' of maximal simplicity form the basis of early language development, and may constitute the last remnants in the communicative inventory of persons with global aphasia. Syllabic well-formedness survives in severe phonological impairment and remains a characteristic feature of spoken language, even in patients who produce completely unintelligible neologistic jargon. This may mean that, in the on-line speech-production process, syllabicity constitutes itself at a rather late stage of output planning, i.e. at a stage where learned speech motor programmes are accessed. Modern accounts of apraxia of speech are consistent with this view. Not much attention was paid to the role of the syllable in fluency disorders. Investigations into the various types of developmental and acquired fluency disorders may help to determine more precisely the conditions under which the integrity of syllabic units can be broken up.

References

Abe, K., Yokoyama, R., and **Yorifuji, S.** (1993). Repetitive speech disorder resulting from infarcts in the paramedian thalami and midbrain. *Journal of Neurology, Neurosurgery, and Psychiatry, 56,* 1024–1026.

Ackermann, H. and **Ziegler, W.** (1992). Articulatory deficits in Parkinsonian dysarthria: an acoustic analysis. *Journal of Neurology, Neurosurgery, and Psychiatry, 54,* 1093–1098.

Ackermann, H., Ziegler, W., and **Oertel, W. H.** (1989). Palilalia as a symptom of levodopa induced hyperkinesia in Parkinson's disease. *Journal of Neurology, Neurosurgery, and Psychiatry, 52,* 805–807.

Ackermann, H., Hertrich, I., Ziegler, W., Bitzer, M., and Bien, S. (1996). Acquired dysfluencies following infarction of the left mesiofrontal cortex. *Aphasiology, 10,* 409–417.

Aichert, I. and Ziegler, W. (2003). Syllable frequency and syllable structure in apraxia of speech. *Brain and Language* (in press).

Andy, O. J. and Bhatnagar, S. C. (1992). Stuttering acquired from subcortical pathologies and its alleviation from thalamic perturbation. *Brain and Language, 42,* 385–401.

Ardila, A. and Lopez, M. V. (1986). Severe stuttering associated with right-hemisphere lesion. *Brain and Language, 27,* 239–246.

Beers, M. (1995). *The phonology of normally developing and language-impaired children.* Amsterdam: IFOTT.

Béland, R. (1990). Vowel epenthesis in aphasia. In J.-L. Nespoulous and P. Villiard (Eds.), *Morphology, phonology, and aphasia.* (pp. 235). New York: Springer.

Béland, R., Caplan, D., and Nespoulous, J.-L. (1990). The role of abstract phonological representations in word production: evidence from phonemic paraphasias. *Journal of Neurolinguistics, 5*(2/3), 125–164.

Benke, T. and Butterworth, B. (2001). Palilalia and repetitive speech: two case studies. *Brain and Language, 78*(1), 62–81.

Blanken, G. (1991). The functional basis of speech automatisms (recurring utterances). *Aphasiology, 5,* 103–127.

Blanken, G. and Marini, V. (1997). Where do lexical speech automatisms come from. *Journal of Neurolinguistics, 10*(1), 19–31.

Blanken, G., Wallesch, C. W., and Papagno, C. (1990). Dissociations of language functions in aphasics with speech automatisms (recurring utterances). *Cortex, 26,* 41–63.

Blumstein, S. E. (1973). *A phonological investigation of aphasic speech.* The Hague: Mouton.

Brand, M., Rey, A., and Peereman, R. (2002). Where is the syllable priming effect in visual word recognition? *Journal of Memory and Language, 48,* 435–443.

Browman, C. P. and Goldstein, L. (1988). Some notes on syllable structure in articulatory phonology. *Phonetica, 45,* 140–155.

Browman, C. P. and Goldstein, L. (1989). Articulatory gestures as phonological units. *Phonology, 6,* 201–251.

Browman, C. P. and Goldstein, L. (1997). The gestural phonology model. In W. Hulstijn, H. F. M. Peters, and P. H. H. M. van Lieshout (Eds.), *Speech production: motor control, brain research and fluency disorders* (pp. 57–71). Amsterdam: Elsevier Science BV.

Buckingham, H. W. Jr (1987). Phonemic paraphasias and psycholinguistic production models for neologistic jargon. *Aphasiology, 1,* 381–400.

Buckingham, H. W. Jr (1993). Disorders of word-form processing in aphasia. In G. Blanken, J. Dittmann, H. Grimm, J. C. Marshall, and C.-W. Wallesch (Eds.), *Linguistic disorders and pathologies. An international handbook.* (pp. 187–196). Berlin: W. de Gruyter.

Butterworth, B. (1979). Hesitation and the production of verbal paraphasias and neologisms in jargon aphasia. *Brain and Language, 8,* 133–161.

Byrd, D. (1995). C-centers revisited. *Phonetica, 52,* 285–306.

Cho, T. (1999). Effects of prosody on vowel-to-vowel coarticulation in English. In Anonymous, *Proceedings of the International Congress of Phonetic Sciences.* (pp. 459–462). San Francisco: University of California.

Chomsky, N. and **Halle, M.** (1968). *The Sound Pattern of English.* New York: Harper & Row.

Christman, S. S. (1992). Uncovering phonological regularity in neologisms: contributions of sonority theory. *Clinical Linguistics and Phonetics, 6*(3), 219–247.

Clements, G. N. and **Keyser, S. J.** (1983). *From CV phonology: a generative theory of the syllable.* Cambridge, MA: MIT Press.

Code, C. (2002). Syllables in the brain: evidence from brain damage. In R. J. Hartsuiker, R. Bastiaanse, A. Postma, and F. N. K. Wijnen (Eds.), *Phonological encoding and monitoring in normal and pathological speech.* Hove: Psychology Press.

Code, C. and **Ball, M. J.** (1994). Syllabification in aphasic recurring utterances: contributions of sonority theory. *Journal of Neurolinguistics, 8,* 257–265.

Content, A., Kearns, R. K., and **Frauenfelder, U. H.** (2001). Boundaries versus onsets in syllabic segmentation. *Journal of Memory and Language, 45,* 177–199.

De Jong, K., Beckman, M. E., and **Edwards, J.** (1993). The interplay between prosodic structure and coarticulation. *Language and Speech, 36*(2,3), 197–212.

Deger, K. and **Ziegler, W.** (2002). Speech motor programming in apraxia of speech. *Journal of Phonetics, 30,* 321–335.

Dell, G. S. (1986). A spreading-activation theory of retrieval in sentence production. *Psychological Review, 93,* 283–321.

Dogil, G., Mayer, J., and **Vollmer, K.** (1996). A representative account for apraxia of speech. In T. W. Powell (Ed.), *Pathologies of speech and language: contributions of clinical phonetics and linguistics* (pp. 95–99). New Orleans: LA, ICPLA.

Favreau, Y., Nespoulous, J.-L., and **Lecours, A.** (1990). Syllable structure and lexical frequency effects in the phonemic errors of four aphasics. *Journal of Neurolinguistics, 5,* 165–187.

Ferrand, L., Segui, J., and **Grainger, J.** (1996). Masked priming of word and picture naming: the role of syllabic units. *Journal of Memory and Language, 35,* 708–723.

Ferrand, L., Segui, J., and **Humphreys, G. W.** (1997). The syllable's role in word naming. *Memory and Cognition, 25,* 458–470.

Fleet, W. S. and **Heilman, K. M.** (1985). Acquired stuttering from a right hemisphere lesion in a right-hander. *Neurology, 35,* 1343–1346.

Garratt, H., Bryan, K., and **Maxim, J.** (1999). Palilalia in progressive supranuclear palsy: failure of the articulatory buffer and subcortical inhibitory systems. In B. Maassen and P. Groenen (Eds.), *Pathologies of Speech and Language. Advances in Clinical Phonetics and Linguistics.* (pp. 245–252). London: Whurr.

Gelmers, H. J. (1983). Non-paralytic motor disturbances and speech disorders: the role of the supplementary motor area. *Journal of Neurology, Neurosurgery, and Psychiatry, 46,* 1052–1054.

Goldberg, G. (1985). Supplementary motor area structure and function: review and hypotheses. *The Behavioral and Brain Sciences, 8,* 567–616.

Goldsmith, J. A. (1990). *Autosegmental and metrical phonology.* Oxford: Basil Blackwell.

Gorno, M. L., Miozzo, A., Mattioli, F., and **Cappa, S. F.** (1997). Isolated palilalia: a case report. *European Journal of Neurology, 4,* 94–96.

Guyette, Th. and **Diedrich, W. M.** (1981). A critical review of developmental apraxia of speech. In N. J. Lass (Ed.), *Speech and Language. Advances in basic research and practice.* (pp. 1–49). New York: Academic Press.

Helm, N. A., Butler, R. B., and **Benson, D. F.** (1978). Acquired stuttering. *Neurology, 28,* 1159–1165.

Hertrich, I., Ackermann, H., Ziegler, W., and **Kaschel, R.** (1993). Speech iterations in Parkinsonism: a case study. *Aphasiology, 7,* 395–406.

Hertrich, I. and **Ackermann, H.** (1995). Coarticulation in slow speech: durational and spectral analysis. *Language and Speech, 38,* 159–187.

Katz, W. F. (1988). Anticipating coarticulation in aphasia: Acoustic and perceptual data. *Brain and Language, 35,* 340–368.

Katz, W. F., and **Baum, S. R.** (1987). Compensatory articulation in Broca's aphasia: the facts aren't in yet. A reply to Sussman *et al. Brain and Language, 30,* 367–373.

Keating, P. A. (1988). Underspecification in phonetics. *Phonology, 5,* 275–292.

Kent, R. D. (1981). Articulatory–acoustic perspectives on speech development. In R. E. Stark (Ed.), *Language behavior in infancy and early childhood.* (pp. 105–126). New York: Elsevier North-Holland.

Kent, R. D. and **Rosenbek, J. C.** (1982). Prosodic disturbance and neurologic lesion. *Brain and Language, 15,* 259–291.

Kent, R. D. and **Rosenbek, J. C.** (1983). Acoustic patterns of apraxia of speech. *Journal of Speech and Hearing Research, 26,* 231–249.

Kent, R. D. (1997). Speech motor models and developments in neurophysiological science: new perspectives. In W. Hulstijn, H. F. M. Peters, and P. H. H. M. van Lieshout (Eds.), *Speech production: motor control, brain research and fluency disorders* (pp. 13–36). Amsterdam: Elsevier.

Kessler, B. and **Treiman, R. (1997).** Syllable structure and the distribution of phonemes in English syllables. *Journal of Memory and Language, 37,* 295–311.

Koller, W. C. (1983). Dysfluency (stuttering) in extrapyramidal disease. *Archives of Neurology, 40,* 175–177.

Koopmans-van Beinum, F. J., Jansonius-Schultheiss, K., and **van der Stelt, J. M.** (1986). Early stages of speech movements. In B. Lindblom and R. Zetterstrom (Eds.), *Precursors of early speech.* (pp. 37–50). Basingstoke: MacMillan Press.

Krakow, R. A. (1999). Physiological organization of syllables: a review. *Journal of Phonetics, 27,* 23–54.

Ladefoged, P. (2001). *A course in phonetics.* (4th edn). Orlando, FL: Harcourt College Publishers.

Laplane, D., Talairach, J., Meininger, V., Bancaud, J., and **Orgogozo, J. M.** (1977). Clinical consequences of corticectomies involving the supplementary motor area in man. *Journal of the Neurological Sciences, 34,* 301–314.

Levelt, C. C., Schiller, N. O., and **Levelt, W. J. M.** (1999). A developmental grammar for syllable structure in the production of child language. *Brain and Language, 68,* 291–299.

Levelt, W. J. M. (1989). *Speaking. From intention to articulation.* Cambridge, MA: MIT Press.

Levelt, W. J. M. and **Wheeldon, L. R.** (1994). Do speakers have access to a mental syllabary? *Cognition, 50,* 239–269.

Levelt, W. J. M., Roelofs, A., and **Meyer, A. S.** (1999). A theory of lexical access in speech production. *Behavioral and Brain Sciences, 22,* 1–38.

Maassen, B. (2002). Issues contrasting adult acquired versus developmental apraxia of speech. In M. R. McNeil (Ed.), *Apraxia of speech: from concept to clinic (Seminars in Speech and Language).* (pp. 257–266). New York: Thieme.

Maassen, B., Thoonen, G., and **Boers, I.** (1997). Quantitative assessment of dysarthria and developmental apraxia of speech. In W. Hulstijn, H. F. M. Peters, and P. H. H. M. van Lieshout (Eds.), *Speech production: motor control, brain research and fluency disorders.* (pp. 611–619). Amsterdam: Elsevier Science BV.

MacNeilage, P. F. and **Davis, B. L.** (2001*a*). Relations between consonants and vowels in babbling: the vowel height dimension. In B. Maassen, W. Hulstijn, R. D. Kent, H. F. M. Peters, and P. H. H. M. van Lieshout (Eds.), *Speech Motor Control in Normal and Disordered Speech. Proceedings of the 4th International Speech Motor conference, Nijmegen, June 13–16, 2001.* (pp. 49–51). Nijmegen: Uitgeverij Vantilt.

MacNeilage, P. F. and **Davis, B. L.** (2001*b*). Motor mechanisms in speech ontogeny: phylogenetic, neurobiological and linguistic implications. *Current Opinion in Neurobiology, 11,* 696–700.

Meyer, A. S. (1992). Investigation of phonological encoding through speech error analyses: achievements, limitations, and alternatives. *Cognition, 42,* 181–211.

Miller, N. (2001). Dual or duel route? *Aphasiology, 15*(1), 62–68.

Mitchell, P. R. and **Kent, R. D.** (1990). Phonetic variation in multisyllabic babbling. *Journal of Child Language, 17,* 247–265.

Nijland, L., Maassen, B., van der Meulen, Sj., Gabreëls, F., Kraaimaat, F. W., and **Schreuder, R.** (2002*a*). Coarticulation patterns in children with developmental apraxia of speech. *Clinical Linguistics and Phonetics, 16,* 461–483.

Nijland, L., Maassen, B., and **van der Meulen, Sj.** (2002*b*). Speech motor subprocesses in DAS studied with a bite-block. In F. Windsor, L. Kelly, and N. Hewlett (Eds.), *Investigations in clinical phonetics and linguistics.* (pp. 257–266). Mahwah, New Jersey: Lawrence Erlbaum.

Nijland, L., Maassen, B., van der Meulen, Sj., Gabreëls, F., Kraaimaat, F. W., and **Schreuder, R.** (2003). Planning of syllables in children with developmental apraxia of speech. *Clinical Linguistics and Phonetics, 17,* 1–24.

Nittrouer, S. (1993). The emergence of mature gestural patterns is not uniform: evidence from an acoustic study. *Journal of Speech and Hearing Research, 36,* 959–972.

Nittrouer, S., Studdert-Kennedy, M., and **McGowan, R. S.** (1989). The emergence of phonetic segments—evidence from the spectral structure of fricative-vowel syllables spoken by children and adults. *Journal of Speech and Hearing Research, 32,* 120–132.

Nittrouer, S., Studdert-Kennedy, M., and **Neely, S. T.** (1996). How children learn to organize their speech gestures: further evidence from fricative-vowel syllables. *Journal of Speech and Hearing Research, 39*(2), 379–389.

Oller, D. K., Eilers, R. E., Urbano, R., and **Cobo-Lewis, A. B.** (1997). Development of precursors to speech in infants exposed to two languages. *Journal of Child Language, 24*(2), 407–425.

Oller, D. K., Eilers, R. E., Neal, A. R., and **Schwartz, H. K.** (1999). Precursors to speech in infancy: the prediction of speech and language disorders. *Journal of Communication Disorders, 32,* 223–245.

Pitt, M. A., Smith, K. L., and **Klein, J. M.** (1998). Syllabic effects in word-processing: evidence from the structural induction paradigm . *Journal of Experimental Psychology-Human Perception and Performance, 24*(6), 1596–1611.

Roelofs, A. (2000). WEAVER++ and other computational models of lemma retrieval and word-form encoding. In L. Wheeldon (Ed.), *Aspects of language production.* (pp. 71–114). Hove: Psychology Press.

Rogers, M. A. and **Storkel, H. L.** (1999). Planning speech one syllable at a time: the reduced buffer capacity hypothesis in apraxia of speech. *Aphasiology, 13*(9–11), 793–805.

Romani, C. and **Calabrese, A.** (1998). Syllabic constraints in the phonological errors of an aphasic patient. *Brain and Language, 64*(1), 83–121.

Ryalls, J., Valdois, S., and **Lecours, A. R.** (1988). Paraphasia and jargon. In F. Boller and R. Grafman (Eds.), *Handbook of Neuropsychology, Volume 1.* (pp. 367–375). Amsterdam: Elsevier.

Schiller, N. O. (1998). The effect of visually masked syllable primes on the naming latencies of words and pictures. *Journal of Memory and Language, 39*(3), 484–507.

Schiller, N. O., Meyer, A. S., Baayen, R. H., and **Levelt, W. J. M.** (1996). A comparison of lexeme and speech syllables in dutch. *Journal of Quantitative Linguistics, 3*(1), 8–28.

Schiller, N. O., Meyer, A. S., and **Levelt, W. J. M.** (1997). The syllabic structure of spoken words: Evidence from the syllabification of intervocalic consonants. *Language and Speech, 40,* 103–140.

Schiller, N. O., van Lieshout, P. H. H. M., Meyer, A. S., and **Levelt, W. J. M.** (1999). Does the syllable affiliation of intervocalic consonants have an articulatory basis? Evidence from electromagnetic midsagittal articulography. In B. Maassen and P. Groenen (Eds.), *Pathologies of speech and language. advances in clinical phonetics and linguistics.* (pp. 342–350). London: Whurr.

Shriberg, L. D., Aram, D. M., and **Kwiatkowski, J.** (1997*a*). Developmental apraxia of speech: I. Descriptive and theoretical perspectives. *Journal of Speech, Language, and Hearing Research, 40*(2), 273–285.

Shriberg, L. D., Aram, D. M., and Kwiatkowski, J. (1997*b*). Developmental apraxia of speech: II. Toward a diagnostic marker. *Journal of Speech, Language, and Hearing Research, 40*(2), 286–312.

Shriberg, L. D., Aram, D. M., and Kwiatkowski, J. (1997*c*). Developmental apraxia of speech: III. A subtype marked by inappropriate stress. *Journal of Speech, Language, and Hearing Research, 40* (2), 313–337.

Shriberg, L. D., Friel-Patti, S., Flipsen, P., and Brown, R. L. (2000). Otitis media, fluctuant hearing loss, and speech-language outcomes: A preliminary structural equation model. *Journal of Speech, Language, and Hearing Research, 43*(1), 121–128.

Soroker, N., Bar-Israel, Y., Schechter, I., and Solzi, P. (1990). Stuttering as a manifestation of right-hemispheric subcortical stroke. *European Neurology, 30,* 268–270.

Southwood, M. H., Dagenais, P. A., Garcia, J. M., and Sutphin, S. M. (1996). Coarticulation in apraxia of speech: an electro-palatographic and perceptual study. In T. W. Powell (Ed.), *Pathologies of speech and language: contributions of clinical phonetics and linguistics* (pp. 247–254). New Orleans: LA: ICPLA.

Sussman, H. M., Minifie, F. D., Buder, E. H., Stoel-Gammon, C., and Smith, J. (1996). Consonant–vowel interdependencies in babbling and early words: preliminary examination of a locus equation approach. *Journal of Speech and Hearing Research, 39,* 424–433.

Sussman, H. M., Marquardt, T. P., and Doyle, J. (2000). An acoustic analysis of phonemic integrity and contrastiveness in developmental apraxia of speech. *Journal of Medical Speech-Language Pathology, 8,* 301–313.

Thoonen, G., Maassen, B., Gabreëls, F., and Schreuder, R. (1994). Feature analysis of singleton consonant errors in developmental verbal dyspraxia (DVD). *Journal of Speech and Hearing Research, 37,* 1424–1440.

Treiman, R. (1983). The structure of spoken syllables: evidence from novel word games. *Cognition, 15,* 49–74.

Tuller, B. and Kelso, J. A. S. (1990). Phase transitions in speech production and their perceptual consequences. In M. Jeannerod (Ed.), *Attention and performance XIII* (pp. 429–452). Hillsdale, NJ: Erlbaum.

Varley, R. A. and Whiteside, S. P. (2000). What is the underlying impairment in acquired apraxia of speech? *Aphasiology, 15,* 39–49.

Velleman, S. L. and Shriberg, L. D. (1999). Metrical analysis of the speech of children with suspected developmental apraxia of speech. *Journal of Speech, Language, and Hearing Research, 42,* 1444–1460.

Vennemann, T. (1988). *Preference laws for syllable structure and the explanation of sound change.* Berlin: Mouton.

Wallesch, C. W. (1990). Repetitive verbal behaviour: functional and neurological considerations. *Aphasiology, 4,* 133–154.

Whiteside, S. P. and Varley, R. A. (1998). A reconceptualization of apraxia of speech: a synthesis of evidence. *Cortex, 34*(2), 221–231.

Wiese, R. (2000). *The phonology of German.* Oxford: Oxford University Press.

Yasuda, Y., Akiguchi, I., Ino, M., Nabatabe, H., and **Kameyama, M.** (1990). Paramedian thalamic and midbrain infarcts associated with palilalia. *Journal of Neurology, Neurosurgery, and Psychiatry, 53,* 797–799.

Ziegler, W. and **von Cramon, D. Y.** (1985). Anticipatory coarticulation in a patient with apraxia of speech. *Brain and Language, 26,* 117–130.

Ziegler, W. and **Cramon, D. Y. V.** (1986). Disturbed coarticulation in apraxia of speech: acoustic evidence. *Brain and Language, 29,* 34–47.

Ziegler, W., Hartmann, E., Hoole, P., and **von Cramon, D.** (1990). *Entwicklung von diagnostischen Standards und von Therapieleitlinien für zentrale Stimm- und Sprechstörungen (Dysarthrophonien).* München: GSF.

Ziegler, W., Kilian, B., and **Deger, K.** (1997). The role of the left mesial frontal cortex in fluent speech: evidence from a case of left supplementary motor area hemorrhage. *Neuropsychologia, 35*(9), 1197–1208.

Ziegler, W. (2001). Apraxia of speech is not a lexical disorder. *Aphasiology, 15*(1), 74–77.

Ziegler, W. (2002). Psycholinguistic and motor theories of apraxia of speech. *Seminars in Speech and Language, 23*(4), 231–243.

INDEX